D0201293

PUBLIC HEALTH LAW AND POLICY IN CANADA

SECOND EDITION

Tracey M. Bailey
Timothy Caulfield
Nola M. Ries

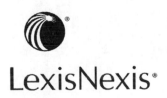

LexisNexis®

Public Health Law and Policy in Canada, Second Edition
© LexisNexis Canada Inc. 2008
December 2008

All rights reserved. No part of this publication may be reproduced, stored in any material form (including photocopying or storing it in any medium by electronic means and whether or not transiently or incidentally to some other use of this publication) without the written permission of the copyright holder except in accordance with the provisions of the Copyright Act. Applications for the copyright holder's written permission to reproduce any part of this publication should be addressed to the publisher.

Warning: The doing of an unauthorized act in relation to a copyrighted work may result in both a civil claim for damages and criminal prosecution.

Members of the LexisNexis Group worldwide

Canada	LexisNexis Canada Inc, 123 Commerce Valley Dr. E. Suite 700, MARKHAM, Ontario
Australia	Butterworths, a Division of Reed International Books Australia Pry Ltd, CHATSWOOD, New South Wales
Austria	ARD Betriebsdienst and Verlag Orac, VIENNA
Czech Republic	Orac, sro, PRAGUE
France	Éditions du Juris-Classeur SA, PARIS
Hong Kong	Butterworths Asia (Hong Kong), HONG KONG
Hungary	Hvg Orac, BUDAPEST
India	Butterworths India, NEW DELHI
Ireland	Butterworths (Ireland) Ltd, DUBLIN
Italy	Giuffré, MILAN
Malaysia	Malayan Law Journal Sdn Bhd, KUALA LUMPUR
New Zealand	Butterworths of New Zealand, WELLINGTON
Poland	Wydawnictwa Prawnicze PWN, WARSAW
Singapore	Butterworths Asia, SINGAPORE
South Africa	Butterworth Publishers (Pty) Ltd, DURBAN
Switzerland	Stämpfli Verlag AG, BERNE
United Kingdom	Butterworths Tolley, a Division of Reed Elsevier (UK), LONDON, WC2A
USA	LexisNexis, DAYTON, Ohio

Library and Archives Canada Cataloguing in Publication

Public health law and policy in Canada / [edited by] Tracey M. Bailey, Timothy Caulfield, Nola M. Ries — 2nd ed.

Includes index.
ISBN 978-0-433-45817-3

1. Public health laws — Canada. 2. Public health — Government policy — Canada. I. Bailey, Tracey M. II. Caulfield, Timothy A., 1963- III. Ries, Nola M. (Nola Maria), 1972-

KE3575.P82 2005   344.7104   C2005-904461-6
KF3775.ZA2P82 2005

Printed and bound in Canada.

ABOUT THE GENERAL EDITORS

Nola M. Ries, B.A. (Hons.), LL.B., M.P.A., LL.M. is Research Associate with the Health Law Institute, University of Alberta and Adjunct Assistant Professor, University of Victoria, where she teaches health law in the Faculty of Law and School of Health Information Science. Her research focuses on public health law; health system reform; privacy of health information; and legal issues in genetics and biotechnology.

Timothy Caulfield, B.Sc., LL.B., LL.M., FRSC is Canada Research Chair in Health Law and Policy; Professor, Faculty of Law and School of Public Health, University of Alberta; Research Director of the Health Law Institute, University of Alberta; and Senior Health Scholar, Alberta Heritage Foundation for Medical Research. Professor Caulfield's research has focused on two general areas: genetics, ethics and the law; and the legal implications of health care reform in Canada.

Tracey M. Bailey, B.A., LL.B. is Executive Director of the Health Law Institute at the University of Alberta. Ms. Bailey is also Adjunct Assistant Professor with the Faculty of Medicine & Dentistry, as well as the John Dossetor Health Ethics Centre, and a Sessional Lecturer with the Faculty of Law. She is a former Chair of the Canadian Bar Association's National Health Law Section.

CONTRIBUTORS

Solomon R. Benatar, MB.ChB. DSc (Med), FFA (SA), FRCP, FRS SAfr is Emeritus Professor of Medicine and Director of the Bioethics Centre, University of Cape Town and Professor, Dalla Lana School of Public Health, University of Toronto. He was President of the International Association of Bioethics from 2001 to 2003. He is also a member of the University of Toronto Joint Centre for Bioethics.

Jamie Benidickson, B.A. (Trent), LL.B. (Toronto), LL.M. (Harvard) is Professor, Faculty of Law, University of Ottawa and author of *Environmental Law* (Irwin Law, 2008).

Mary Anne Bobinski, B.A., J.D., LL.M. is Dean and Professor at the Faculty of Law at the University of British Columbia. She is a co-author of *Health Care Law & Ethics* (Aspen Publishers, 2007). She previously served as John and Rebecca Moores Professor of Law and Director of the Health Law & Policy Institute at the University of Houston Law Center.

Abdallah S. Daar, FRS(C), D.Phil. (Oxon), F.R.C.P. (Lon), F.R.C.S., F.R.C.S.C. is Professor of Public Health Sciences and of Surgery at the University of Toronto. He is co-director of the Program on Life Sciences, Ethics and Policy at the McLaughlin-Rotman Centre for Global Health, University Health Network, and Director of Ethics and Policy, McLaughlin Centre for Molecular Medicine, University of Toronto. He is also a member of the University of Toronto Joint Centre for Bioethics.

Ronald L. Doering, B.A., LL.B, M.A., LL.D. is a partner in the Ottawa office of Gowling Lafleur Henderson where he practises with the Government Relations and Regulatory Affairs Group. Dr. Doering is the former President of the Canadian Food Inspection Agency.

Louis Hugo Francescutti, M.D., Ph.D., M.P.H., F.R.C.P.C., F.A.C.P.M. is Professor, University of Alberta, Founder of the Coalition for Cellphone Free Driving, Founder of injuryearth.com and an emergency medicine and preventive medicine physician at the Royal Alexandra Hospital in Edmonton.

Elaine Gibson, LL.B., LL.M. is Associate Director of the Dalhousie Health Law Institute and Associate Professor of Law, with a cross-appointment to the Faculty of Health Professions, Dalhousie University. She is co-editor (with Jocelyn Downie) of *Health Law at the Supreme Court of Canada* (Irwin Law, 2007).

Constance MacIntosh, B.A., M.A., LL.B. is Associate Professor of Law at Dalhousie University, and a Faculty Associate with Dalhousie's Health Law Institute. Professor MacIntosh was formerly an associate lawyer with Mandell Pinder, a boutique firm specializing in Aboriginal law, and her graduate work was in the area of medical anthropology.

Stephanie Nixon, B.H.Sc. (P.T.), M.Sc., Ph.D. is an Assistant Professor in the Department of Physical Therapy at the University of Toronto, and a Research Associate at the Health Economics and HIV/AIDS Research Division (HEARD) at the University of KwaZulu-Natal in South Africa. She is also a member of the University of Toronto Joint Centre for Bioethics.

Patricia Peppin, B.A. (Hons.), M.A., LL.B. is Professor in the Faculty of Law at Queen's University, with a cross-appointment to the Department of Family Medicine. In the School of Medicine, she is director of the Law program in the undergraduate curriculum. Her research focuses on pharmaceutical law and women's health.

Wayne N. Renke, B.A. (Hons.), M.A., LL.B., LL.M. is Professor and Vice-Dean, Faculty of Law, University of Alberta. Professor Renke's teaching and research is in the areas of Criminal Law, Evidence and Counter-Terrorism. Professor Renke was a member of Alberta's 2007 Crime Reduction and Safe Communities Task Force.

Ann Robertson, M.Sc., DrPH is Professor at the Dalla Lana School of Public Health at the University of Toronto and a member of the University of Toronto Joint Centre for Bioethics.

Trevor L. Strome, M.Sc. (Medical Sciences — Public Health Sciences) is Informatics and Process Improvement Lead with the Winnipeg Regional Health Authority Emergency Program. He holds an appointment as Lecturer in the Department of Emergency Medicine, Faculty of Medicine, University of Manitoba, and is a member of the University of Manitoba Emergency Medicine Research Committee.

Alison K. Thompson, Ph.D. is an Assistant Professor in the Leslie Dan Faculty of Pharmacy at the University of Toronto, cross-appointed to the Dalla Lana School of Public Health and a member of the University of Toronto Joint Centre for Bioethics.

Barbara von Tigerstrom, B.A., M.A., LL.B., Ph.D. is Assistant Professor at the University of Saskatchewan College of Law and School of Public Health, where she teaches health law and international law.

Ross Upshur, B.A. (Hons.), M.A., M.D., M.Sc., C.C.F.P., F.R.C.P.C. is the Canada Research Chair in Primary Care Research, Director of the University of Toronto Joint Centre for Bioethics, Director, Primary Care Research Unit, Sunnybrook Health Sciences Centre and Associate

Professor, Departments of Family and Community Medicine and Public Health Sciences at the University of Toronto.

Kumanan Wilson, M.D., M.Sc., F.R.C.P.(C) is a specialist in internal medicine at the Ottawa Hospital and Associate Professor in the Department of Medicine at the University of Ottawa. He holds the Canada Research Chair in Public Health Policy.

THE CORE VALUES OF PUBLIC HEALTH LAW AND ETHICS

Lawrence O. Gostin

Population health, and the law that nourishes (or starves) that enterprise, is experiencing a renaissance. One can sense the changes from within nation states and the international community. National public health law reform efforts are emerging in North America, Europe, the Commonwealth, and Asia.[1] The World Health Organization is implementing the new International Health Regulations. The WHO is embarking on a major law reform project: "Reaching the Millennium Development Goals (MDGs) Through Public Health Law — A WHO Model Public Health Act to Advance the MDGs." Private foundations are also supporting a new "Global Exchange on Population Health Law."

Much of the stimulus for public health law reform comes from the salience of infectious diseases — both intentionally inflicted and naturally occurring. Although the probability of bioterrorism is comparatively low, the consequences of a successful attack are high. Even low-level events, such as the anthrax attacks in the United States, engender fear and foster instability. Politicians have rushed to increase preparedness, including the adoption of emergency health powers. This kind of legislation has

---

[*] Associate Dean (Research and Academic Programs) and the Linda D. and Timothy J. O'Neill Professor of Global Health Law, Georgetown University Law Center; Professor, The Johns Hopkins Bloomberg School of Public Health; Director, Center for Law & the Public's Health; Visiting Professor, Oxford University.

[1] See, *e.g.*, Stephen Monaghan, Dyfed Huws & Marie Navarro, *The Case for a New UK Health of the People Act* (London: The Nuffield Trust, 2003); Lawrence O. Gostin, *et al.*, "The Model State Emergency Health Powers Act: Planning and Response to Bioterrorism and Naturally Occurring Infectious Diseases" (2002) 288 Journal of the American Medical Association 622.

instigated contentious debates about the powers of the state and the liberties of individuals in liberal democracies.[2]

Even if the risk of bioterrorism is uncertain, new or re-emerging naturally occurring infectious diseases are inevitable. Ancient, constant, and abiding fatal diseases still represent a deep burden, particularly in developing countries (*e.g.*, malaria, tuberculosis, and HIV/AIDS). Endemic diseases have re-emerged in more virulent, multi-drug resistant forms. Diseases once endemic only in the Third World have arrived in the First World (*e.g.*, West Nile virus and monkeypox). Emerging infections have been newly identified in humans (*e.g.*, hemorrhagic fevers and SARS), animals (*e.g.*, bovine spongiform encephalopathy), and across species (*e.g.*, avian influenza), some with devastating consequences for world health, international trade, and tourism. The legislative and regulatory changes in Canada and elsewhere resulting from the SARS outbreaks illustrate the striking potential of epidemics to influence social policy.[3]

A further important stimulus for public health law reform is the increase in chronic diseases, many of which are partially caused by behaviour and exacerbated by transformations in culture and advertising. Tobacco, sedentary lifestyle, and high fat/high caloric foods have all contributed to the rise in non-communicable diseases such as cancers, cardiovascular disease, and diabetes. Societies are debating the appropriate legal responses, and raising profound issues of efficacy, cost, and justice. Should the law be used to make it easier for people to choose a more active lifestyles and better nutrition, while also restricting smoking and alcohol consumption? Central to these debates are arguments about personal responsibility, which leads to disturbing social fault lines based on politics and ideology. Are individuals responsible for their own behaviour or are they influenced by social and cultural factors that can, and should, be changed?

Much of this debate is about the role of law as a tool for change. Elsewhere, I have offered a taxonomy of legal powers to protect and promote the public's health:[4]

---

[2]   Lawrence O. Gostin, "Public Health Law in an Age of Terrorism: Rethinking Individual Rights and Common Goods" (2002) 21 Health Affairs 79.

[3]   Report of the National Advisory Committee on SARS and Public Health, *Learning from SARS – Renewal of Public Health in Canada* (Ottawa: Health Canada, October 2003); Lawrence O. Gostin, *et al.*, "Ethical and Legal Challenges Posed by Severe Acute Respiratory Syndrome: Implications for the Control of Severe Infectious Disease Threats" (2003) 290 Journal of American Medical Association 3229.

[4]   Lawrence O. Gostin, "Law and Ethics in Population Health" (2004) 28 Aust. & N.Z. J. Pub. Health 7.

- tax and spend — *e.g.*, tobacco taxes and health care spending
- alter the informational environment — *e.g.*, restrictions on advertising
- alter the built environment — *e.g.*, zoning, occupational safety, and housing codes
- alter the socioeconomic environment — decrease disparities
- direct regulation — *e.g.*, quarantine, licenses, and inspections
- indirect regulation through the tort system — *e.g.*, tobacco and firearm litigation
- deregulation — *e.g.*, legalise distribution and possession of drug injection equipment.

Here, it may be helpful to offer a brief account of the core values in the field of public health law and policy. This account may help frame the rich analysis and set of arguments presented by the authors in *PUBLIC HEALTH LAW & POLICY IN CANADA, SECOND EDITION*. The core values of the field include: the collective responsibility for health and well-being, the population focus, community involvement, the prevention orientation, and social justice.

COLLECTIVE RESPONSIBILITY FOR HEALTH AND WELL-BEING

The Institute of Medicine ("IOM"), in its seminal report *THE FUTURE OF PUBLIC HEALTH*, proposed one of the most influential contemporary definitions of public health: "Public health is what we, as a society, do collectively to assure the conditions for people to be healthy."[5] The IOM's definition can be appreciated both by observing its emphasis on co-operative and mutually-shared obligation ("we, as a society"), and by focusing on the collective responsibility for healthy populations (*e.g.*, governments and communities). The definition also makes clear that even the most organized and socially conscious society cannot guarantee complete physical and mental well-being. The role of public health, therefore, is to "assure the conditions for people to be healthy". These conditions include a variety of educational, economic, social, and environmental factors that are necessary for good health.

[5]   Institute of Medicine, *The Future of the Public's Health in the 21st Century* (Washington, D.C.: National Academy Press, 2003).

THE POPULATION FOCUS

Perhaps the single most important feature of public health is that it strives to improve the functioning and longevity of populations. The field's purpose is to monitor and evaluate the health status of populations as well as to devise strategies and interventions designed to ease the burden of injury, disease, and disability and, more generally, to promote the public's health and safety. Public health interventions reduce mortality and morbidity, thus saving lives and preventing disease on a population level. These reductions save real lives and prevent real disease, but the benefits often cannot be linked to specific persons.

Public health differs from medicine, which has the individual patient as its primary focus. The physician diagnoses disease and offers medical treatment to ease symptoms and, where possible, to cure disease. Public health, on the other hand, seeks to understand the conditions and causes of ill-health (and good health) in the populace as a whole. It seeks to assure a favourable environment in which people can maintain their health.

COMMUNITY INVOLVEMENT AND CIVIC RESPONSIBILITY

Public health is interested in how communities function to protect and promote (or, as is too often the case, endanger) the health of their members. A community has a life in common which stems from such things as a shared history, language, and values. Public health officials want to understand what health risks exist among varying populations, and, of equal importance, why differences in health risks exist: who engages in risk behaviour, and who suffers from high rates of disease? Public health professionals often observe differences in risk behaviour and disease based on race, sex, or socioeconomic status. Understanding the mechanisms and pathways of risk is vital to developing interventions to improve health within communities.

Beyond understanding the variance of risk within groups, public health encourages individual attachment to the community. Individuals who feel they belong to a community are more likely to strive for health and security for all members. Viewing health risks as common to the group, rather than to individuals, helps foster a sense of collective responsibility for the mutual well-being of *all* individuals. Finding solutions to common problems can forge more cohesive and meaningful community associations.

THE PREVENTION ORIENTATION

The field of public health is often understood to emphasize the prevention of injury and disease, as opposed to their amelioration or cure. Public health historians often tell a classic story of the power of prevention. In September 1854, John Snow wrote, "the most terrible outbreak of cholera which ever occurred in this Kingdom, is probably that which took place in Broad Street, Golden Square [Soho, London], and the adjoining streets, a few weeks ago".[6] Snow, a celebrated epidemiologist, linked the cholera outbreak to a single source of polluted water, the Broad Street pump. He convinced the Board of Guardians of St. James's Parish, in whose parish the pump fell, to remove the pump handle as an experiment. Within a week, the outbreak was all but over, with the death toll standing at 616 Sohoites.

Public health prevention may be defined as interventions designed to avert the occurrence of injury or disease. Many of public health's most potent activities are oriented toward prevention: vaccination against infectious diseases, health education to reduce risk behaviour, fluoridation to avert dental caries, and seat belts or motor cycle helmets to avoid injuries.

The public health sciences — epidemiology and biostatistics — are emblematic of the field's mission, functions, and services. These are the sciences that are concerned with the distribution and determinants of health in populations, and drawing inferences when only a subset of the population is observed. The public health sciences, then, enable the field to better understand the causes of, and response to, risk in society. These sciences dovetail nicely with each of the major attributes of the field of public health law and ethics — collective responsibility for health and well-being, the population focus, community involvement, and the prevention orientation.

SOCIAL JUSTICE

Social justice has been viewed as so central to the mission of public health that it has been described as the field's core value: "The historic dream of public health ...is a dream of social justice."[7] The idea of "justice" is complex and multifaceted, but it remains at the heart of public health's mission. Justice is fair, equitable, and appropriate treatment in

---

[6]   Judith Summers, *Soho: A History of London's Most Colourful Neighborhood* (London: Bloomsbury Pub. Ltd., 1989) at 113-17.

[7]   D.E. Beauchamp, "Public health as social justice", in D.E. Beauchamp and B. Steinbock, eds., *New Ethics for the Public's Health* (New York and Oxford: Oxford University Press, 1999) at 105.

light of what is due or owed to individuals and groups. Justice does not require universally equal treatment, but does require that similarly situated people be treated equally. Justice, in other words, requires that equals are treated the same and unequals are treated differently.

Justice, which is the fair and proper administration of laws, has three important attributes of special relevance to public health. Perhaps the most important aspect of justice is *non-discrimination* — treating people equitably based on their individual characteristics rather than membership in a socially distinct group such as race, ethnicity, sex, religion, or disability. It cautions against public health judgments based on prejudice, irrational fear, or stereotype such as singling out persons living with HIV/AIDS for adverse treatment.

A second important aspect of justice is *natural justice* — affording individuals procedural fairness when imposing a burden or withholding a benefit (due process). The conduct of legal proceedings according to established rules and principles for the protection and enforcement of individual rights lies at the heart of due process. The elements of due process include notice, trial rights including an attorney, and a fair hearing. Natural justice requires public health officials to afford individuals procedural safeguards in conjunction with the exercise of compulsory powers, such as isolation or quarantine.

The final aspect of justice is *distributive justice* — fair disbursement of common advantages and sharing of common burdens (fair allocation of risks, burdens, and benefits). This form of justice requires that officials act to limit the extent to which the burden of disease falls unfairly upon the least advantaged, and ensure that the burden of interventions themselves are distributed equitably. Coercive public health powers, therefore, should not be targeted against vulnerable groups such as injection drug users, prostitutes, or gays without good cause based on careful risk assessments. Distributive justice also requires the fair distribution of public health benefits such as vaccines and medical treatment. This principle might apply, for example, to the fair allocation of vaccines or antiviral medications during a major influenza outbreak. Public health actions, moreover, must be seen to be fair. For example, the U.S. government's decision during the anthrax outbreak to aggressively screen and treat congressional staffers, but not poor postal workers in Washington, D.C., was perceived to be discriminatory.

These are the quintessential values of public health law — collective responsibility for health, populations, communities, prevention, and social justice.

AN ENDURING CONTRIBUTION TO THE FIELD OF PUBLIC HEALTH LAW AND POLICY

In this second edition of their text, Tracey M. Bailey, Timothy Caulfield and Nola M. Ries continue to make a fundamentally important contribution to the advancement of knowledge and innovation in public health law. It is one of only a handful of books to cover the field in the English-speaking world, and the first to offer a systematic account from a Canadian perspective.[8] To be sure, books on law, medicine, and ethics abound. But this text is remarkable for its authentic understanding of the health of populations. The authors present a vision of a healthy and secure public, with government and its partners serving the common good. The book carefully demonstrates the power of law to achieve that vision, and the ethical values that must guide that vision — indeed, an extraordinarily important achievement that should be read and savoured by scholars, practitioners, public officials, and the public.

---

[8]   See, *e.g.*, Lawrence O. Gostin, *Public Health Law: Power, Duty, Restraint* (Berkeley: University of California Press, 2nd ed. 2008); Christopher Reynolds, *Public Health Law and Regulation* (Sydney, Australia: The Federation Press, 2004).

ACKNOWLEDGMENTS

We express immense gratitude to the authors who contributed their knowledge and time to the second edition of this book. After working tirelessly on the first edition, they all responded positively to our invitation to participate in this edition and the depth of analysis and insight in each revised and updated chapter in this text is due to their expertise. Many authors rely enormously on the tireless work of research assistants and students — thanks to all those affiliated with our institutes, faculties and firms for their contributions.

Special thanks to Nina Hawkins, who keeps everything running smoothly at the University of Alberta Health Law Institute. It was a pleasure to work again with Danann Hawes, our liaison with the publisher, and we thank him for his encouragement and patience as we worked to complete this edition. We acknowledge generous financial support of the Alberta Law Foundation and the Alberta Heritage Foundation for Medical Research which facilitate everything our Health Law Institute tackles. In addition, the Canadian Institutes of Health Research contributed to this project and we are extremely grateful. Finally, we express our gratitude to our families for their tolerance and support.

TABLE OF CONTENTS

TABLE OF CASES

INTRODUCTION TO THE
SECOND EDITION

Nola M. Ries, Timothy Caulfield and Tracey M. Bailey
Co-Editors

The first edition of this book was published in the wake of the 2003 SARS outbreak, an event that put Canadian and international public health systems under intense scrutiny. The various reports that investigated the response to SARS in Canada and our local, provincial and national capacity to deal with novel disease outbreaks emphasized the need for greater attention to laws that impact public health activities.[1] After all, "[l]aw is an essential tool for public health. Law sets the structure within which public health officials, regulators and private citizens act to protect

---

[1] National Advisory Committee on SARS and Public Health, *Learning from SARS: Renewal of Public Health in Canada* (Ottawa: Health Canada, 2003) (Chair: Dr. D. Naylor); Honourable Mr. Justice Archie Campbell, Commissioner, "The SARS Commission Interim Report: SARS and Public Health in Ontario" (2004) online: Ministry of Health and Long-Term Care < http://www.health.gov.on.ca/english/public/pub/ministry_reports/campbell04/campbell04.pdf>; Honourable Mr. Justice Archie Campbell, Commissioner, "The SARS Commission Second Interim Report: SARS and Public Health Legislation" (2005) online: Ministry of Health and Long-Term Care < http://www.health.gov.on.ca/english/public/pub/ministry_reports/campbell05/campbell05.pdf >; Honourable Mr. Justice Archie Campbell, Commissioner, "The SARS Commission Final Report: Spring of Fear" (2006) online: Ministry of Health and Long-Term Care < http://www.health.gov.on.ca/english/public/pub/ministry_reports/campbell06/online_rep/V1Cover.html>; Ontario Expert Panel on SARS and Infectious Disease Control, *For the Public's Health: A Plan of Action* (Toronto: Ministry of Health and Long-Term Care, 2004).

the population's health. Law can impede that process ...or it can enhance it ...".[2]

Despite the critical functions law plays in creating and maintaining conditions that promote health, public health law has been an under-analyzed area of law in Canada. With publication of the first edition of this text, we aimed to help fill this gap and provide a resource for scholars, practitioners, students and others. This second edition will provide readers with analyses of important developments in legislation, case law and policy in a wide range of topics relevant to public health. Since the first edition of this text, legislators across the country have developed new laws and regulations that change and modernize various public health programs and policies. Courts have ruled on important disputes that clarify — or, in some cases, raise new questions — about the role and authority of governments in assuring conditions for health, about individual rights and liberties in public health contexts, and duties and liabilities of those whose activities can create health risks.

The first three chapters are intended to be overview chapters that set the stage for the topical chapters that follow. Chapter 1 presents the legal foundations of public health in Canada, focusing on issues such as constitutional division of powers, rights guaranteed under the *Canadian Charter of Rights and Freedoms*, emergency powers and liability of government authorities for public health failures. As public health actions involve intertwining issues of law and ethics, we felt it was important to include a discussion of ethical issues in public health. Chapter 2 distinguishes public health ethics from clinical ethics, identifies philosophical roots and theories for public health ethics, and analyzes frameworks for public health ethics. Because much of public health is concerned with issues of risk perception, analysis and management, we include a chapter that addresses this complex topic. Chapter 3 uses public health case studies to present evidence-based decision-making in risk management, discuss the precautionary principle as an alternative paradigm, and identify limitations of both approaches.

The rest of the text is devoted to topical chapters that address issues of critical public health importance. With the proliferation of privacy laws across the country, many express concerns about the ability of public health officials to collect, use and share personal information for surveillance and other public health purposes. Chapter 4 discusses legal principles relevant to protection of personal information and grapples with major issues related to privacy and confidentiality in the public

---

[2]   Gene W. Matthews *et al.*, "Legal Preparedness in Bioterrorism" (2002) 30:3 J.L. Med. & Ethics 52 at 53.

health context, including mandatory reporting, contact notification, and surveillance and epidemiologic research activities.

Chapter 5 addresses legal issues associated with vaccination, including controversy over mandatory vaccine and vaccine-related harms. Noting criticism about the lack of coordinated vaccine policy across the country, structural changes to achieve greater harmonization are discussed.

The emergence of HIV/AIDS was one of the largest public health concerns in the last two decades of the 20th century and controlling the spread of this disease remains a significant public health priority. Chapter 6 analyzes major legal issues related to HIV/AIDS, including challenges associated with testing, confidentiality, contact tracing and the role of law in strategies to reduce transmission of the disease.

Thousands of Canadians suffer harm associated with tobacco use and exposure. Chapter 7 explores legal aspects of reducing demand for and supply of tobacco products, protection against "second hand" smoke, and litigation against tobacco companies.

Each year, numerous Canadians are injured in their homes, workplaces, automobiles and other settings. Preventable injuries are a major public health concern and Chapter 8 addresses the role of law in injury prevention and control, with reference to issues such as mandatory seatbelt legislation, occupational health and safety codes, and consumer product safety laws.

Rising rates of obesity among Canadians, especially children and youth, are a major public health concern. Obesity is a risk factor for serious medical conditions including diabetes, cardiovascular disease and some cancers, and numerous public health initiatives encourage healthier eating and physical activity. Chapter 9, a new chapter in this edition, explores the role of legal tools to influence food environments and eating behaviour, including food product and menu-labelling laws, restrictions on food advertising, and price and access controls on foods. It also briefly discusses the use of litigation to assign responsibility for obesity.

The health status of Canada's Aboriginal peoples has been described as a public health disgrace. The urgency of this problem merits special attention and Chapter 10 addresses the role of law and legal mechanisms in influencing conditions that affect the health status of Canada's Aboriginal peoples. It discusses relevant legislation and treaties and the role of Aboriginal self-governance in improving health status.

As individuals can only be as healthy as their environment, Chapter 11's analysis of environmental law and public health is critical. As do many chapters in the text, this chapter uses case studies, including mercury pollution, pesticide exposure, drinking water contamination and poor air quality, to demonstrate the complex interrelationship between law, the environment and health. Just as environmental exposures may harm human health, so may the food we ingest. Drawing attention to the shocking incidence of food-borne illness, Chapter 12 explains the food safety regulation system in Canada and analyzes a number of current issues, including investigation, traceability and recalls of food, and international trade issues.

Many areas of law are relevant in the public health context and Chapter 13 focuses specifically on the use of criminal law as a measure to deter and punish human behaviour in order to achieve public health goals. This chapter compares and contrasts elements of the public health system and the criminal justice system, and explores a range of issues including the incorporation of public health approaches in criminal justice procedures and the criminal justice system as a source of public health risks.

Turning an eye to the impact of emerging genetic advances on public health, Chapter 14 analyzes complex legal issues that arise in population genetic research and comments on contemporary concerns regarding eugenics, race and public health genetics.

As disparate as these topics may appear at first glance, they raise common themes. Many public health activities involve a fundamental tension between individual interests in freedom and liberty and the community interest in protecting and promoting health. Public health emphasizes the health of populations and because of its population focus, public health must often confront a dilemma — both from a legal and ethical perspective — of when it is legitimate to infringe on the rights of one person or a few in the interests of protecting or promoting the broader health of a community. It is often said that the interests of the few must give way to safeguard the interests of the many and nowhere is this axiom more apparent than in public health.

Public health activities are, indeed, of undeniable importance: "[a]n effective public health system is essential to preserve and enhance the health status of Canadians, to reduce health disparities, and to reduce the costs of curative health services".[3] Yet the capacity to protect and promote health is only as strong as the resources available, including appropriate legislation, trained workers, up-to-date infrastructure, and finances.

---

[3] National Advisory Committee on SARS and Public Health, *Learning from SARS: Renewal of Public Health in Canada* (Ottawa: Health Canada, 2003) (Chair: Dr. D. Naylor) at 163.

The first edition of this book was published after the 2003 SARS outbreak; now, as the second edition goes to press in winter 2008, Canadian food safety regulators and the processed meat industry are dealing with a listeriosis outbreak that has affected consumers across the country, causing illness and at least 20 confirmed deaths. A massive recall of potentially contaminated products has occurred, but critics charge this outbreak reveals flaws in food inspection systems and constraints on the autonomy of the Public Health Agency of Canada.[4] The Prime Minister and federal Agriculture Minister have promised a full investigation into the outbreak and emphasize the need to maintain public confidence in the safety of our food supply. So, much as there have been changes in public health law and policy since the first edition, some things remain constant: threats to public health persist and can arise from acts as simple and routine as eating a bologna sandwich at a summer picnic, drinking a glass of water, travelling by airplane, driving a car, having sex and breathing air. Law, in many forms and contexts, plays a critical role in protecting the public from known and emerging threats and promoting conditions for health.

---

[4]   See *e.g.*, Kumanan Wilson & Jennifer Keelan, "Learning from *Listeria*: the Autonomy of the Public Health Agency of Canada" (2008) C.M.A.J. (released online 17 September 2008).

1

LEGAL FOUNDATIONS OF PUBLIC HEALTH IN CANADA

Nola M. Ries[*]

I. INTRODUCTION

Law plays a critical role in public health but often operates in the background, receiving little attention until a new health threat emerges and prompts scrutiny of the adequacy of existing public health tools — including law — to protect and promote health of the population. Canada's experience with the 2003 outbreak of severe acute respiratory syndrome ("SARS") focused attention on the need for public health renewal, including public health legal renewal.[1] Since then, various federal, provincial and territorial governments have undertaken initiatives to modernize outdated public health statutes, develop new programs to address contemporary public health issues, and establish collaborative arrangements with other levels of government to put policies and procedures in place to facilitate more effective, coordinated responses to threats to the health of Canadians.

Law and legal instruments at all levels — from international agreements to local government by-laws — play a key role in public

---

[*] Research Associate with the Health Law Institute, University of Alberta; Adjunct Assistant Professor, University of Victoria.

[1] Joe Sornberger, "SARS silver lining: a renewal of public health" (2004) 171 Canadian Medical Association Journal 1160. The report of the National Advisory Committee on SARS and Public Health pointed out that "the legal issues raised by SARS speak to the need for a thorough review of the broader constitutional and statutory framework governing infectious disease management in Canada": see National Advisory Committee on SARS and Public Health, *Learning from SARS: Renewal of Public Health in Canada* (Ottawa: Health Canada, 2003) (Chair: Dr. D. Naylor) at 163.

health. At the international level, Canada is a member state of the World Health Organization ("WHO") and a signatory to various international instruments and agreements that aim to address global health concerns. As discussed in more detail in subsequent chapters, the WHO is active in coordinating measures to address infectious disease threats and working with countries to develop global strategies directed at contemporary health problems associated with tobacco use, improper nutrition and inadequate physical activity. Many lofty global goals are realized at the local level, where trends such as no-smoking by-laws have stretched across Canada and factors such as urban planning enhance or impede opportunities for healthier lifestyles. As this chapter focuses primarily on federal and provincial/territorial legal issues, analysis of international law and local public health activities are outside the scope of this chapter, though other chapters comment on those areas in specific public health contexts.

At the national level, Canada's Constitution divides powers between the federal and provincial governments. As health is not a topic specifically enumerated in the *Constitution Act, 1867*,[2] both levels of government exercise legal authority in regard to public health concerns. The lack of clear authority can lead to federal-provincial disputes and impede a timely response to public health concerns, particularly during outbreak situations. Many public health organizations and commentators in Canada have called for improved harmonization or interoperability of public health legislation, policies and programs across the country.[3]

This chapter begins by canvassing the constitutional dimensions of public health law in Canada, focusing on the division of powers between federal and provincial governments. The chapter then summarizes common features of federal and provincial public health laws and also discusses emergency powers legislation. An Appendix to this chapter lists relevant federal, provincial and territorial public health and emergency statutes.

The chapter next discusses the application of the *Canadian Charter of Rights and Freedoms*[4] in the public health context. The *Charter*, part of Canada's Constitution, guarantees specific individual rights against government infringement. Aside from the extreme example of abrogating individual rights and liberties during a time of emergency — caused either by the outbreak and spread of virulent disease or an act of bioterrorism —

---

2   *Constitution Act, 1867* (U.K.), 30 & 31 Vict., c. 3, reprinted in R.S.C. 1985, App. II, No. 5.

3   See *e.g.*, Canadian Coalition for Public Health in the 21st Century, *Consultation on Strengthening the Pan-Canadian Public Health System and Meeting with the Minister of State (Public Health)* (10 March 2004), Special Insert in (2004) 95 Canadian Journal of Public Health.

4   Part I of the *Constitution Act, 1982*, being Schedule B to the *Canada Act 1982* (U.K.), 1982, c. 11 [*Charter*].

public health actions often impinge on freedoms we value. However, just as we value certain liberties, we also value public health activities that protect and promote conditions for health. Consequently, assertions that public health officials have infringed on individual rights must be weighed against the motivations behind their action and its expected benefits.

The last substantive section of this chapter examines the issue of potential legal liability of public health actors for failing to protect individuals from public health threats. In particular, this section considers tort claims that assert the government owes a private law duty of care to protect individuals from public health risks. The chapter closes with some observations on intergovernmental relations in the public health context.

II. CONSTITUTIONAL DIMENSIONS OF PUBLIC HEALTH LAW

Canada's Constitution divides authority between the federal and provincial governments,[5] but "health" is not an enumerated topic specifically assigned to one level of government. Consequently, both levels of government may legislate in regard to public health matters,[6] though the provinces have been recognized as having primary authority over medical care and services by virtue of their powers in regard to hospitals, property and civil rights in the province and matters of a local nature. The Supreme Court of Canada has noted, however, that "[h]ealth is not a matter which is subject to specific constitutional assignment but instead is an amorphous topic which can be addressed by valid federal or provincial legislation, depending in the circumstances of each case on the nature and scope of the health problem in question".[7]

The influential 1974 Lalonde Report[8] on the health of Canadians emphasized the importance of understanding the legal framework for public health in Canada. The report notes that "[a]ny comprehensive review of health activities and policies must, of course, take into full

---

5   *Constitution Act, 1867* (U.K.), 30 & 31 Vict., c. 3, ss. 91 and 92, reprinted in R.S.C. 1985, App. II, No. 5.

6   For further analysis of the constitutional division of powers in regard to health, see *e.g.*, Martha Jackman, "Constitutional Jurisdiction Over Health in Canada" (2000) 8 Health L.J. 95 and Commission on the Future of Health Care in Canada, *Health and the Distribution of Powers in Canada, Discussion Paper No. 2* by André Braën (Saskatoon: Commission on the Future of Health Care in Canada, 2002).

7   *Schneider v. British Columbia*, [1982] S.C.J. No. 64, [1982] 2 S.C.R. 112 at 142 (S.C.C.). See also *RJR-MacDonald Inc. v. Canada (Attorney General)*, [1995] S.C.J. No. 68, [1995] 3 S.C.R. 199 (S.C.C.).

8   Marc Lalonde, *A New Perspective on the Health of Canadians* (Ottawa: Department of National Health and Welfare, 1974), online: Health Canada <http://www.hc-sc.gc.ca/hcs-sss/alt_formats/hpb-dgps/pdf/pubs/1974-lalonde/lalonde-eng.pdf>.

account the division of powers under the Canadian constitution". Lalonde further observed that:

> Since the role of the State was so modest, the subject of health could not be expected to claim an important place in the discussions leading up to Confederation ... because the Fathers of Confederation could not have foreseen the pervasive growth and range of health care needs of a large industrialized urban society, the advances of medical sciences, nor the public expenditures required to maintain high quality health care.[9]

While this statement comments primarily on the complexities of a modern system of physician and hospital care, it is equally relevant to contemporary public health systems. Infectious diseases were an inescapable fact of life when the Constitution was drafted in 1867 (indeed, much more so than they were for the latter half of the 20th century), but the mechanisms of disease transmission and prevention were poorly understood. Today, we contend with new and emerging infectious diseases,[10] omnipresent threat of a worldwide influenza pandemic, the rise of multi-drug resistant bacteria,[11] as well as the existence of a global HIV/AIDS pandemic. As well, chronic diseases — cancer, cardiovascular disease, diabetes, obesity — constitute a continuing and growing health threat. Preventable accidents and injuries are also a leading cause of morbidity and mortality.

The National Advisory Committee on SARS and Public Health observed that "[j]urisdictional ambiguities and tensions have long bedevilled public health activities and programs. ... However, attempts at unilateral centralization of authority in a fragile federation with a complex division of powers and responsibilities are generally a prescription for conflict, not progress. Measures to create collegiality, consensus, and commonality of purpose can lead to collaborative work that overcomes jurisdictional tensions".[12]

---

[9]   *Ibid.*, at 43.
[10]   Not just matters of academic interest, these issues garner increasing attention through the popular press: see *e.g.*, Laurie Garrett, *The Coming Plague: Newly Emerging Diseases in a World Out of Balance* (New York: Farrar, Straus & Giroux, 1994) and Elinor Levy & Mark Fischetti, *The New Killer Diseases: How the Alarming Evolution of Mutant Germs Threatens Us All* (New York: Crown Publishers, 2003).
[11]   Again, this issue is addressed in popular science writing. See *e.g.*, Michael Shnayerson & Mark J. Plotkin, *The Killers Within: The Deadly Rise of Drug-Resistant Bacteria* (Boston: Little, Brown & Company, 2002).
[12]   National Advisory Committee on SARS and Public Health, *Learning from SARS: Renewal of Public Health in Canada* (Ottawa: Health Canada, 2003) (Chair: Dr. D. Naylor) at 79.

(a) Constitutional Authority

Under the *Constitution Act*, the federal government has jurisdiction over various areas relevant to public health. These include authority to legislate in regard to "Quarantine and the Establishment and Maintenance of Marine Hospitals",[13] criminal law,[14] "the Peace, Order and good Government of Canada",[15] "Indians, and Lands reserved for the Indians",[16] and all matters not exclusively assigned to provincial authority.[17] As well, federal spending power confers authority to act in the health domain.[18] Under authority of these various heads of power, the federal government has enacted numerous laws that seek to protect and promote public health. These include the *Public Health Agency of Canada Act*,[19] the *Department of Health Act*,[20] the *Quarantine Act*,[21] the *Food and Drugs Act*,[22] the *Tobacco Act*,[23] the *Hazardous Products Act*,[24] the *Pest Control Products Act*,[25] the *Canadian Environmental Protection Act, 1999*,[26] the *Health of Animals Act*[27] and the *Canadian Food Inspection Agency Act*.[28]

The provinces, in turn, have authority over "the Establishment, Maintenance and Management of Hospitals, Asylums, Charities and Eleemosynary Institutions in and for the Province, other than Marine Hospitals",[29] "Property and Civil Rights in the Province",[30] "Municipal Institutions in the Province",[31] and "Generally all Matters of a merely local or private Nature in the Province".[32] In accordance with these powers, provinces have enacted statutes dealing with communicable

---

[13] *Constitution Act, 1867* (U.K.), 30 & 31 Vict., c. 3, s. 91(11), reprinted in R.S.C. 1985, App. II, No. 5.

[14] *Ibid.*, s. 91(27). Issues related to the intersection of criminal law and public health are analyzed in detail in a subsequent chapter, so will not be discussed here.

[15] *Ibid.*, s. 91, preamble.

[16] *Ibid.*, s. 91(24).

[17] *Ibid.*

[18] Spending power is derived from ss. 91(1A) [power related to public debt and property], 91(3) [taxation powers] and 106 [Parliamentary appropriations for public services], *ibid.*

[19] S.C. 2006, c. 5.

[20] S.C. 1996, c. 8.

[21] S.C. 2005, c. 20.

[22] R.S.C. 1985, c. F 27.

[23] S.C. 1997, c. 13.

[24] R.S.C. 1985, c. H-3.

[25] S.C. 2002, c. 28.

[26] S.C. 1999, c. 33.

[27] S.C. 1990, c. 21.

[28] S.C. 1997, c. 6.

[29] *Constitution Act, 1867* (U.K.), 30 & 31 Vict., c. 3, s. 92(7), reprinted in R.S.C. 1985, App. II, No. 5.

[30] *Ibid.*, s. 92(13).

[31] *Ibid.*, s. 92(8).

[32] *Ibid.*, s. 92(16).

disease control, drinking water safety, emergency planning and response, environmental protection, food safety, and many other public health concerns. Provincial legislation also confers authority on municipal governments to enact by-laws with a local purpose to protect and promote health and safety of persons and property.[33]

The following sections provide an overview of federal and provincial laws that establish public health institutions, officials and programs. Legislation dealing with emergency planning and response is also discussed here. Subsequent chapters provide detailed discussion of legislation relevant to topics such as communicable diseases, environmental protection, food safety, tobacco control, vaccination and many other important public health issues.

(b) Federal Public Health Legislation

Before 2004, Canada did not have a national public health agency. In contrast, the United States Centers for Disease Control and Prevention ("CDC") has existed since 1946. The establishment of the Public Health Agency of Canada was a significant development following the 2003 SARS outbreak. The National Advisory Committee on SARS and Public Health emphatically recommended the need for a national agency: "The Government of Canada should move promptly to establish a Canadian Agency for Public Health, a legislated service agency, and give it the appropriate and consolidated authorities necessary to provide leadership and action on public health matters...".[34] The Public Health Agency of Canada was established by Order-in-Council in September 2004, though legislation formalizing its powers did not come into force until December 2006.

The preamble to the *Public Health Agency of Canada Act* describes the federal government's desire to collaborate with provincial/territorial governments, foreign governments, and international organizations in public health activities. The Act creates the national public health agency and appoints a Chief Public Health Officer to "contribute to federal efforts to identify and reduce public health risk factors and to support national readiness for public health threats".[35] The Public Health Agency of Canada has programs that address infectious and chronic diseases, emergency preparedness and health promotion.

---

[33]   See *e.g.*, Alberta *Municipal Government Act*, R.S.A. 2000, c. M-26, s. 7, which provides that "[a] council may pass bylaws for municipal purposes respecting the following matters: (a) the safety, health and welfare of people and the protection of people and property...".

[34]   National Advisory Committee on SARS and Public Health, *Learning from SARS: Renewal of Public Health in Canada* (Ottawa: Health Canada, 2003) (Chair: Dr. D. Naylor) at 214.

[35]   *Public Health Agency of Canada Act*, S.C. 2006, c. 5, preamble.

In his first report to Canadians in June 2008, Chief Public Health Officer David Butler-Jones focused on the persistent problem of health inequities in Canada. He noted that "the majority of Canadians enjoy good to excellent physical and mental health" but says "[t]he bad news is that not all health trends are improving, and not all Canadians are benefiting to the same degree...".[36] Butler-Jones emphasized that inequalities in income, education, employment, social supports, food security and access to health care are all important influences on health.

Federal jurisdiction over public health matters is also governed by the *Department of Health Act*. This statute establishes a broad federal mandate to protect against the spread of disease, to engage in health surveillance activities, to conduct public health research, and to promote the physical, mental and social well-being of Canadians.[37]

The capacity to respond promptly and effectively to disease outbreaks is a critical responsibility of public health systems, and the SARS outbreak exposed deficiencies at all levels of government in Canada. Modernized, federal quarantine legislation was enacted in the wake of SARS.[38] The quarantine law was first enacted in 1872 and authorized federal officials to establish quarantine stations at entry points to Canada and inspect conveyances (ships, trains, and later aircraft and motor vehicles) and decontaminate them in cases of infestation. Individuals entering the country could also be screened and detained in cases of suspected infectious disease.

In introducing new quarantine legislation in the Canadian Parliament in 2004, Carolyn Bennett (the then Minister of State for Public Health) remarked that the *Quarantine Act* was first drafted at

> ... a time when automobiles and jetliners were the stuff of science fiction. Needless to say, times have changed. We live in an age when people move from continent to continent in hours and days rather than weeks or months, often in airplanes and ships whose confined spaces provide a perfect breeding ground for highly communicable diseases to spread. Infectious diseases move like wildfire across the planet today. Diseases

---

[36]   *The Chief Public Health Officer's Report on the State of Public Health in Canada 2008*, online: Public Health Agency of Canada <http://www.phac-aspc.gc.ca/publicat/2008/cpho-aspc/pdf/cpho-report-eng.pdf> at i-ii.

[37]   These general functions are set out in s. 4 of the *Department of Health Act*, S.C. 1996, c. 8. In regard to health research, the *Canadian Institutes of Health Research Act*, S.C. 2000, c. 6 created the Canadian Institutes of Health Research, a major federal health funding body that supports Canadian research in a vast range of health fields. In particular, the CIHR have an Institute devoted to population and public health, the mandate of which is to support research into the range of interactions and factors that influence individual and population heath. See <http://www.cihr-irsc.gc.ca/e/13777.html>.

[38]   *Quarantine Act*, S.C. 2005, c. 20.

do not respect borders, so we know that we will face repeated threats to public health in the future. Among the hard lessons learned from the experience of SARS is the need to strengthen our quarantine legislation to help prevent the introduction and spread of both emerging and re-emerging communicable diseases.[39]

The updated federal *Quarantine Act* places more attention on air travel as the major mode of global disease transmission, applies to a broader number of infectious diseases, permits establishment of quarantine facilities anywhere in the country, and allows further limits on entry into Canada of persons or goods where necessary to control the spread of disease.[40]

(c)   Provincial Public Health Laws

Each province and territory has public health legislation that establishes public health officials and institutions to carry out various functions to protect and promote health. For example, the objectives of Ontario's *Health Protection and Promotion Act* are stated as follows: "The purpose of this Act is to provide for the organization and delivery of public health programs and services, the prevention of the spread of disease and the promotion and protection of the health of the people of Ontario".[41]

Public health statutes grant various powers to health officials and also impose obligations on them and others. Each statute establishes the Office of a Chief Provincial Health Officer, whose duties generally include monitoring the health of residents, providing independent advice to the government on public health issues in the province, and superintending health officers and inspectors who carry out key functions related to communicable disease control and health hazard mitigation.

In regard to disease control, health officers may enter premises to inspect for and control health hazards. In regard to persons who pose a health threat to others because of communicable disease, health officers may order individuals to undergo medical testing and treatment, and to be isolated or quarantined to prevent spread of disease.[42] The circumstances when such powers are authorized vary from jurisdiction to jurisdiction.

---

[39]   House of Commons Debates, *Hansard*, No. 055 (14 May 2004) at 1250 (Hon. Carolyn Bennett), online: <http://www.parl.gc.ca/37/3/parlbus/chambus/house/debates/055_2004-05-14/han055_1250-E.htm>.

[40]   See Public Health Agency of Canada, News Release, "Questions & Answers — The *Quarantine Act*" (2006), online: <http://www.phac-aspc.gc.ca/media/nr-rp/2006/2006_10bk1-cng.php>.

[41]   R.S.O. 1990, c. H.7, s. 2.

[42]   The term "isolation" refers to the segregation of a person who is known to be infected with a communicable disease, and the term "quarantine" refers to the segregation of a person who is suspected of having been exposed to a communicable disease.

For example, in Québec, the power to compel a person to undergo medical treatment without a court order is available only for tuberculosis.[43] In Newfoundland and Labrador, quarantine orders may only be issued in "a case of actual or apprehended emergency".[44] Individuals who suspect they may be infected with a communicable disease often have a statutory duty to seek and submit to appropriate medical care.[45]

Public health laws impose reporting obligations on health care providers and others to notify health officials of individuals who are infected with, or suspected to be infected with, a communicable disease.[46] Health officials may also have a statutory duty to notify third parties who have been in contact with an infected person. In Saskatchewan, for example, persons who are diagnosed with certain communicable diseases must communicate that information to their contacts, or must request a physician or nurse to do so.[47] The physician or nurse must communicate with the contacts or provide a list of contacts to a public health officer for follow-up.[48]

Under public health statutes, an order made by a health officer may be enforceable in court. Individuals who breach orders may face penalties ranging from fines to terms of imprisonment. Public health officials themselves are generally protected from legal liability for their actions, unless they act in bad faith.

Individuals who are subject to public health orders, such as isolation or quarantine orders, typically have appeal rights guaranteed by statute. In some cases, the individual may appeal the order to the provincial superior court or to an administrative tribunal.[49] In some circumstances, the appeal right is illusory as the subject individual may have to comply with the order while awaiting her or his appeal hearing. By the time the appeal is

---

[43]   See *Public Health Act*, R.S.Q. c. S-2.2, Chapter IX ("Compulsory Treatment and Prophylactic Measures for Certain Contagious Diseases or Infections") and *Minister's Regulation under the Public Health Act*, M.O. 2003-011, s. 9.

[44]   See *Communicable Diseases Act*, R.S.N.L. 1990, c. C-26, s. 30.

[45]   See *e.g.*, Saskatchewan *Public Health Act, 1994*, S.S. 1994, c. P-37.1, s. 33 and Yukon *For the Control of Communicable Diseases, Regulations*, Y.C.O. 1961/048, s. 3, made under authority of the *Public Health and Safety Act*, R.S.Y. 2002, c. 176.

[46]   Individuals with this obligation include health care providers, heads of medical laboratories, school principals and teachers, heads of institutions (such as a correctional centre) and householders. See *e.g.*, Alberta *Public Health Act*, R.S.A. 2000, c. P-37, s. 22 and Ontario *Health Protection and Promotion Act*, R.S.O. 1990, c. H.7, ss. 25, 27-29.

[47]   See *Public Health Act, 1994*, S.S. 1994, c. P-37.1, s. 33(4)(c).

[48]   *Ibid.*, s. 34.

[49]   See *e.g.*, Ontario *Health Protection and Promotion Act*, R.S.O. 1990, c. H.7, s. 44, which grants a right of appeal to the Health Services Review and Appeal Board (established under the *Ministry of Health Appeal and Review Boards Act*, S.O. 1998, c. 18), provided the appeal request is filed within 15 days of the order being served.

heard, the issue may be moot if, for example, the person has already served a required quarantine period.

In addition to empowering health officials to take action to control health hazards and disease threats, public health statutes may also authorize the establishment of health registries, including cancer registries, to collect population data on certain health conditions for research and statistical purposes.[50] These registries provide critical epidemiological information to assist health officials in tracking disease patterns in the population and identifying emerging health concerns.

Finally, public health laws confer broad authority on government to make regulations on a vast range of topics relevant to controlling disease.[51] Regulations may establish various categories of communicable diseases, prescribe time periods for isolation and quarantine, specify details regarding appropriate sanitary conditions for various premises such as restaurants, and stipulate qualifications of public health workers.

III. EMERGENCY POWERS

Emergency legislation is relevant in the public health context, particularly when officials decide that a public health threat warrants the declaration of an emergency. Use of emergency powers is frequently contentious, particularly when coercive measures restrict individual liberties. Emergency situations may also raise federal-provincial jurisdictional disputes in Canada, particularly when an event like an infectious disease outbreak within a province threatens to spread beyond provincial borders. As will be discussed below, some commentators argue that collaborative arrangements are inadequate to address public health emergencies and the federal government should be more aggressive in taking charge to control health threats.

(a)   Federal Emergency Powers

Federal statutes for emergency planning and response are the *Emergency Management Act*[52] ("*EMA*") and the *Emergencies Act*[53] ("*EA*"). The *EMA* deals with preparation of emergency management

---

[50]   See *e.g.*, Québec *Public Health Act*, R.S.Q. c. S-2.2, Chapter V ("Collection of Information and Registries"). Some jurisdictions have enacted separate registry legislation for cancer, communicable diseases or other conditions: see *e.g.*, Alberta *Cancer Programs Act*, R.S.A. 2000, c. C-2, Northwest Territories *Disease Registries Act*, R.S.N.W.T. 1988, c. 7 (Supp.).

[51]   Regulations are a form of subordinate legislation that may be enacted and amended much more quickly than statutes.

[52]   *Emergency Management Act*, S.C. 2007, c. 15.

[53]   *Emergencies Act*, R.S.C. 1985, c. 22 (4th Supp.), s. 2.

plans, coordination of intergovernmental activities during emergencies, and information-sharing among levels of government to enhance emergency response. This statute defines a provincial emergency as "an emergency occurring in a province if the province or a local authority in the province has the primary responsibility for dealing with the emergency"[54] and stipulates that federal institutions "may not respond to a provincial emergency unless the government of the province requests assistance or there is an agreement with the province that requires or permits the assistance".[55] On provincial request, the federal government may provide financial assistance if the provincial emergency is declared under the *EMA* to be "of interest" to the federal government;[56] otherwise, non-financial assistance may be provided.[57]

The *EA*, which replaced the *War Measures Act* in 1988, authorizes federal actions to respond to a national emergency, which is defined as

> ... an urgent and critical situation of a temporary nature that
>
> (a) seriously endangers the lives, health or safety of Canadians and is of such proportions or nature as to exceed the capacity or authority of a province to deal with it, or
>
> (b) seriously threatens the ability of the Government of Canada to preserve the sovereignty, security and territorial integrity of Canada
>
> and that cannot be effectively dealt with under any other law of Canada.[58]

The Governor in Council may declare a public welfare emergency, which includes a real or imminent emergency caused by disease "that results or may result in a danger to life or property, social disruption or a breakdown in the flow of essential goods, services or resources, so serious as to be a national emergency".[59] The Governor in Council must have reasonable grounds to believe that such an emergency exists and the declaration must specify the nature of the emergency, the measures necessary to deal with it, and the area of Canada affected by the

---

[54]   *Emergency Management Act*, S.C. 2007, c. 15, s. 2.

[55]   *Ibid.*, s. 6(3).

[56]   *Ibid.*, s. 4(1)(j).

[57]   *Ibid.*, s. 4(1)(i).

[58]   *Emergencies Act*, R.S.C. 1985, c. 22 (4th Supp.), s. 3.

[59]   *Ibid.*, s. 5. Other categories of emergencies under the *EA* are a public order emergency (defined in s. 16 as "an emergency that arises from threats to the security of Canada and that is so serious as to be a national emergency"), an international emergency (defined in s. 27 as "an emergency involving Canada and one or more other countries that arises from acts of intimidation or coercion or the real or imminent use of serious force or violence and that is so serious as to be a national emergency), and a war emergency (defined in s. 37 as "war or other armed conflict, real or imminent, involving Canada or any of its allies that is so serious as to be a national emergency").

emergency. Before declaring the emergency, the Governor in Council must consult with the affected provinces and an emergency cannot be declared where "the direct effects of the emergency are confined to, or occur principally in, one province"[60] unless the province advises the federal government that it does not have capacity to respond. During an emergency period, the Governor in Council may, *inter alia*, regulate or prohibit travel, establish emergency hospitals, direct persons to provide essential services, and make emergency payments.[61]

The *EA* has never been used in Canada, which is not surprising considering the high threshold that must be met. Following the 2003 SARS outbreak, some commentators proposed the federal government should enact public health emergency legislation that would involve "graded increases in federal responsibility and jurisdiction as the scope and scale of an emergency spreads".[62] The National Advisory Committee on SARS and Public Health cautioned that Ottawa's "effectiveness in coordinating health emergencies on a national basis is arguably compromised by the lack of specific legislation"[63] and recommended the federal government consider enacting such statutory power.

Some scholars in Canada have argued that the federal government should assert a more active role, particularly in regard to public health emergencies and surveillance activities.[64] It has been contended that restricting federal authority to a national emergency precludes action "to tackle a disease outbreak while it remains small, manageable, and confined to one province".[65] By analogy to medical practice, it is argued that "this is rather similar to a surgeon declining to operate on a patient's cancer when it is small and confined to a single diseased organ, preferring to wait until tumours have grown and the cancer has metastasized throughout the body. A surgeon applying that logic could be considered unethical, if not medically negligent, and so similar logic cannot ethically be accepted in law for public health emergencies".[66] This argument may, however, be unconvincing to a judge who must apply the plain text of ss.

---

[60]   *Ibid.*, s. 14(2).

[61]   *Ibid.*, s. 8(1). Those who contravene an order may face fines from $500 to $5,000 and/or imprisonment from six months to five years.

[62]   National Advisory Committee on SARS and Public Health, *Learning from SARS: Renewal of Public Health in Canada* (Ottawa: Health Canada, 2003) (Chair: Dr. D. Naylor) at 177, summarizing the Canadian Medical Association's proposal for federal public health emergency legislation.

[63]   *Ibid.*

[64]   See *e.g.*, Sina A. Muscati, "POGG as a Basis for Federal Jurisdiction over Public Health Surveillance" (2007) 16 Const. Forum 41.

[65]   Amir Attaran & Kumanan Wilson, "A Legal and Epidemiological Justification for Federal Authority in Public Health Emergencies" (2007) 52 McGill L.J. 381 at 385.

[66]   *Ibid.*

91 and 92 of the *Constitution Act* in reviewing any challenge to federal actions taken in response to disease outbreaks or other public health emergencies.

Regardless of one's view of how far Ottawa should push the constitutional envelope, it is clear that federal capacity to respond to public health emergencies remains constrained in some respects. For example, a 2008 Auditor General of Canada report investigated the surveillance capacities of the Public Health Agency of Canada.[67] The report noted that the Agency depends on provincial and territorial "goodwill" in sharing of public health surveillance data. Deficiencies persist in readiness to share information during public health emergencies:

> ... critical arrangements — such as procedures for notifying other parties, and protocols affecting the collection, use, and disclosure of personal information — still need to be sorted out. The 2003 SARS crisis demonstrated why such arrangements were needed. Until these arrangements are in place, it may be more difficult for the Agency to obtain the information needed to prevent and respond to a disease outbreak.[68]

In regard to emergency preparedness, the federal government also has an important role in establishing relationships with international jurisdictions to coordinate emergency activities in the event of a disease outbreak or other public health emergency that is not contained within domestic boundaries. In November 2007, the Canadian, American and Mexican governments signed a Memorandum of Understanding ("MOU"), the Mutual Aid Declaration, to enhance cross-border coordination and cooperation for infectious disease surveillance, prevention and control. Pursuant to the MOU, the three countries agree to improve public health emergency preparedness (*e.g.*, through joint emergency training exercises) and to strengthen information sharing procedures (*e.g.*, sharing of infectious disease testing methods and laboratory results).[69] Further, the three countries must establish protocols to share resources during an emergency, including health professional personnel, medical supplies and laboratory specimens.

---

[67]   Auditor General of Canada, *Report of the Auditor General of Canada to the House of Commons, Chapter 5: Surveillance of Infectious Diseases — Public Health Agency of Canada* (May 2008), online: <http://www.oag-bvg.gc.ca/internet/docs/aud_ch_oag_200805_05_e.pdf>.

[68]   *Ibid.*, at 2.

[69]   United States Department of Health and Human Services, News Release, "United States, Canada and Mexico Agree to Mutual Assistance" (1 November 2007), online: <http://www.hhs.gov/news/press/2007pres/11/pr20071101a.html>.

(b) Provincial Emergency Powers

Provinces and territories throughout Canada also have legislation that requires the development of emergency plans and authorizes the use of emergency powers.[70] An emergency is typically defined as an accidental or intentional state of affairs that requires immediate attention to protect the health, safety or welfare of people and/or to minimize property damage. Such legislation generally authorizes the responsible Minister of government to require that provincial departments and agencies, municipalities, and other organizations take steps to address the emergency.

Depending on the jurisdiction, the Minister, the Premier, or the Lieutenant Governor in Council may declare a state of emergency within part or all of the province. Once a state of emergency is declared, response measures that are considered necessary may be implemented, including restrictions on travel, destruction of property, and orders to provide needed services, such as medical assistance. Government authorities may require that prices for essential goods, such as medical supplies, remain fixed to ensure that those who need them do not face inflated prices by those who wish to profit from high demand fuelled by emergency.

Declarations of states of emergency are typically for a time-limited period (ranging from 15, 30 to 90 days depending on the jurisdiction) and may either be renewed if conditions persist or cancelled if the situation giving rise to the emergency dissipates.

Public health statutes in various jurisdictions contain provisions specific to public health emergencies. For example, public health statutes in Alberta and Nova Scotia allow the Lieutenant Governor in Council and Minister of Health, respectively, on the advice of the Chief Medical Officer, to declare a provincial public health emergency.[71] When a public health emergency is in effect, powers like those listed above may be exercised — including conscripting persons to render assistance and to distribute necessary medical and other supplies.

At present, emergency powers legislation across the country varies from jurisdiction to jurisdiction and events like the SARS outbreak have underscored the need for greater coordination. Public health experts in the United States have developed model state legislation specific to emergency health powers that may be required in the face of a serious

---

[70]   See Appendix to this chapter.

[71]   Alberta *Public Health Act*, R.S.A. 2000, c. P-37, ss. 52.1-52.91; Nova Scotia *Health Protection Act*, S.N.S. 2004, c. 4, s. 53.

infectious disease outbreak or a bioterrorism event.[72] The stated goal of the model statute is "to facilitate the detection, management, and containment of public health emergencies while appropriately safeguarding personal and proprietary interests".[73]

The authors of the model statute emphasize that it

> ... is designed to be triggered by an extreme public health emergency comparable with the sudden, devastating epidemics of the 19th century. Emergency health powers by definition are a concession to the fact that normal systems of civil governance may break down under the pressure of widespread sudden death or illness, even as the outbreak demands a decisive response.[74]

The authors acknowledge the need to respect individual rights and to guard against "the serious threats to individual freedoms posed by the exercise of governmental power in a perceived emergency".[75] Numerous states have adopted all or part of the model legislation into law.[76]

IV. LIMITS ON THE EXERCISE OF PUBLIC HEALTH AUTHORITY

The law imposes various limits on the exercise of state authority, notably through constitutional and administrative law principles. The *Canadian Charter of Rights and Freedoms*, adopted as part of Canada's Constitution in 1982, entrenches numerous individual rights in relation to governmental authority.[77] As discussed below, numerous *Charter* rights

---

[72]   See Lawrence O. Gostin *et al.*, "The Model State Emergency Health Powers Act" (2002) 288 Journal of the American Medical Association 622. For critique of the model statute, see *e.g.*, George Annas, "Bioterrorism, public health, and civil liberties" (2002) 346 New Eng. J. Med. 1337.

[73]   *Ibid.*, at 625.

[74]   *Ibid.*, at 626.

[75]   *Ibid.*

[76]   For details of state legislative activity regarding the *Model State Emergency Health Powers Act*, see the following information published by The Centers for Law & the Public's Health at Georgetown and Johns Hopkins Universities, online: <http://www.publichealthlaw.net/ModelLaws/MSEHPA.php>.

[77]   It is important to note that the *Charter* applies only to governmental action. Section 32(1) specifies:

> 32(1) This Charter applies
> > (*a*) to the Parliament and the government of Canada in respect of all matters within the authority of Parliament...; and
> > (*b*) to the legislature and government of each province in respect of all matters within the authority of the legislature of each province.

For a brief discussion of what constitutes "government" for *Charter* purposes, see *e.g.*, Robert J. Sharpe, Katherine E. Swinton & Kent Roach, *The Charter of Rights and Freedoms*, 2d ed. (Toronto: Irwin Law, 2002) at 85-96.

may be implicated by the exercise of public health authority. Administrative law principles are also relevant in superintending the exercise of statutory authority.[78] This chapter will focus on *Charter* limits on the exercise of public health authority.

Various *Charter* rights may come into play when public health rules and interventions constrain or compel action. These include: freedom of expression, assembly and association (s. 2); mobility rights (s. 6); rights to liberty and personal security (s. 7); security against unreasonable search or seizure (s. 8); freedom from arbitrary detention (s. 9); freedom from cruel and unusual treatment (s. 12); and equality rights (s. 15).

Other chapters in this volume explore *Charter* issues in specific public health contexts, such as tobacco control initiatives, surveillance and other activities involving collection, use and disclosure of personal information, and the intersection between public health and criminal law. Before turning to a brief discussion of several case examples, it is important to keep in mind that *Charter* rights are not absolute and may be justified under s. 1 of the *Charter*, which states:

> The *Canadian Charter of Rights and Freedoms* guarantees the rights and freedoms set out in it subject only to such reasonable limits prescribed by law as can be demonstrably justified in a free and democratic society.[79]

Under s. 1, a governmental entity may justify infringing a *Charter*-protected right if it meets the criteria set out by the Supreme Court of Canada in *R. v. Oakes*.[80] First, the impugned governmental action must be directed at a pressing and substantial concern; second, its goal must be rationally connected to the limitation imposed on an individual's rights; third, the limitation must impair the individual's right in a minimal fashion; and, fourth, there must be proportionality between the benefits of the limitation and its harmful impact.

In evaluating whether a limit on a *Charter* right is justified, a court will assess the individual right or freedom at issue against a competing societal interest as it is expressed through government action. The Supreme Court of Canada has stated that the government need not provide

---

[78]   For further discussion, see *e.g.*, Nola M. Ries, "Legal Issues in Disease Outbreaks: Judicial Review of Public Health Powers" (2007) 16:1 Health Law Review 11. Administrative law has been defined as addressing "the legal limitations on the actions of governmental officials, and on the remedies which are available to anyone affected by a transgression of these limits. The subject invariably involves the question of the lawful authority of an official to do a particular act which, in the absence of such authority, might well be illegal (or *ultra vires*) and give rise to an actionable wrong": David Phillip Jones & Anne S. de Villars, *Principles of Administrative Law*, 4th ed. (Scarborough, Ont.: Carswell, 1999) at 3.

[79]   Part I of the *Constitution Act, 1982*, being Schedule B to the *Canada Act 1982* (U.K.), 1982, c. 11.

[80]   [1986] S.C.J. No. 7, [1986] 1 S.C.R. 103 (S.C.C.) [*Oakes*].

"scientific demonstration" to justify its infringement of a *Charter* right; instead, it can defend its actions "by the application of common sense to what is known, even though what is known may be deficient from a scientific point of view".[81] Clearly, in responding to novel public health threats, authorities will often lack scientific facts and must make judgment calls about restricting individual liberties for the sake of protecting the population as a whole. As Chief Justice Laskin observed in *Oakes*: "It may become necessary to limit rights and freedoms in circumstances where their exercise would be inimical to the realization of collective goals of fundamental importance".[82] Some public health statutes explicitly recognize the need to balance individual liberties. For example, Nova Scotia's *Health Protection Act* instructs: "Restrictions on private rights and freedoms arising as a result of the exercise of any power under this Act shall be no greater than are reasonably required, considering all of the circumstances, to respond to a health hazard, notifiable disease or condition, communicable disease or public health emergency".[83]

In the United States, courts have also addressed the need to balance competing interests in the public health context. As a general rule, a judge reviewing the action of health officials "must defer to public health authorities on their choice of public health strategies. Public health orders get the most permissive judicial review ... because they are based on objective criteria, are usually of limited duration, and are necessary to prevent imminent harm".[84] As highlighted below, such factors could warrant a more lenient application of the *Oakes* criteria in *Charter* challenges to public health actions that infringe individual liberties.

(a) Case Examples

Charter challenges have arisen in various public health contexts in Canada. The following section summarizes several pertinent cases and additional examples are discussed in subsequent chapters.

The most common basis for a constitutional challenge to public health interventions is likely s. 7 of the *Charter*, which states: "Everyone has the right to life, liberty and security of the person and the right not to be deprived thereof except in accordance with principles of fundamental

---

[81]   *RJR-MacDonald Inc. v. Canada (Attorney General)*, [1995] S.C.J. No. 68 at para. 137 (S.C.C.).

[82]   [1986] S.C.J. No. 7, [1986] 1 S.C.R. 103 at 136 S.C.R. (S.C.C.).

[83]   S.N.S. 2004, c. 4, s. 2.

[84]   Edward P. Richards & Katharine C. Rathbun, "Making State Public Health Laws Work for SARS Outbreaks" (2004) 10 Emerging Infectious Diseases 356 at 356, online: United States Centers for Disease Control and Prevention <http://www.cdc.gov/ncidod/EID/vol10no2/03-0836.htm>.

justice". Section 7 protects against unreasonable, state-imposed restraints on liberty as well as government action that imposes severe psychological stress.[85]

In two cases where courts have balanced claims of individual *Charter* rights against a broader public health interest, the latter has prevailed. The 1995 Ontario court decision in *Canadian AIDS Society v. Ontario*[86] involved HIV testing of stored blood that had been donated some 11 years previously. When the blood was collected from the donors between 1984 and 1985, they were not advised the blood would be tested for HIV as no such testing capacity existed at that time. When testing became available, the Canadian Red Cross Society tested the stored samples to trace any recipients of contaminated blood. Twenty-two HIV-positive donors were identified; nine of whom had previously been identified, leaving 13 remaining donors. The issue that arose in this case was whether the Red Cross should notify the donors and report them to the Province of Ontario in accordance with the *Health Protection and Promotion Act*. The Canadian AIDS Society objected to donor notification and reporting on the basis that the donors had not consented to testing their blood for HIV and notification and reporting would violate the donors' privacy rights.

The Court accepted that s. 7 of the *Charter* may be interpreted to recognize a blood donor's privacy interest in regard to personal information revealed through testing their blood samples. However, the Court went on to rule that the public interest in mandatory reporting of HIV cases to public health authorities outweighed the individual donors' privacy interests. The Court noted that "although due consideration will be given to the privacy rights of individuals, the state objective of promoting public health for the safety of all will be given great weight".[87]

In 2002, a court in Ontario applied similar logic in adjudicating a *Charter* challenge by a tuberculosis patient who was under detention for treatment.[88] The patient, who had consented to a four-month detention and treatment order by the medical health officer, challenged a four-month extension to the order that health professionals believed was necessary to control his tuberculosis. The patient, who had been physically restrained during several violent outbursts, and was routinely restrained during "smoke breaks" to prevent escape (which he had done once to buy beer),

---

[85] See *e.g.*, *New Brunswick (Minister of Health and Community Services) v. G. (J.)*, [1999] S.C.J. No. 47, [1999] 3 S.C.R. 46 (S.C.C.) and *Blencoe v. British Columbia (Human Rights Commission)*, [2000] S.C.J. No. 43, [2000] 2 S.C.R. 307 (S.C.C.).
[86] [1995] O.J. No. 2361, 25 O.R. (3d) 388 (Ont. Gen. Div.), aff'd [1996] O.J. No. 4184 (Ont. C.A.).
[87] *Ibid.*, at para. 133.
[88] *Toronto (City, Medical Officer of Health) v. Deakin*, [2002] O.J. No. 2777 (Ont. C.J.).

argued the restraints and continued detention violated his constitutional liberty rights. In a brief judgment, the Court accepted his rights were violated, but concluded the infringement was justified under s. 1 of the *Charter*. The Court stated:

> What was done to [the patient] was carried out for the protection of public health and the prevention of the spread of tuberculosis, a disease that [a medical specialist] described as extremely contagious. [The patient] is in the early stages of the disease, it is eminently treatable now, but will become less responsive and more virulent if not treated.[89]

In addition to s. 7, other *Charter* provisions may be raised to challenge public health actions. For example, in 2003, the Ontario Restaurant Hotel & Motel Association ("ORHMA") argued that a City of Toronto by-law requiring public disclosure of health inspections of food premises violated, *inter alia*, the *Charter*'s free expression provisions.[90] Under the by-law, restaurants must display the inspection result in a publicly prominent location. The results are conveyed through a coloured notice (green, yellow and red for a pass, conditional pass and fail, respectively) that details any food safety infractions. Specifically, the ORHMA asserted that the by-law "constitutes forced expression in that a restaurant owner is compelled to convey the city's message, a message which in the case of the yellow and red notices, the owner would not have chosen to convey".[91]

This claim was dismissed at first instance and on appeal. The Divisional Court dismissed the ORMHA's s. 2 argument, explaining that forced expression occurs when the government's intent is to put unwanted words into the mouth of another. In this case, the City's intent was to protect the public from potential health dangers, to provide information to allow the public to make an informed dining decision, and to encourage restaurateurs to maintain appropriate food safety standards. Further, the by-law does not prohibit a restaurant from posting a reply to the inspection notice. Considering all these factors, the Court ruled the by-law

---

[89]   *Ibid.*, at para. 26.

[90]   *Ontario Restaurant Hotel & Motel Assn. v. Toronto (City)*, [2004] O.J. No. 190 (Ont. Div. Ct.), aff'd [2005] O.J. No. 4268, 258 D.L.R. (4th) 447 (Ont. C.A.), application for leave to appeal dismissed [2006] S.C.C.A. No. 45, 223 O.A.C. 399n (S.C.C.). The ORHMA also argued, on administrative law grounds, that the City lacked jurisdiction to enact the by-law and the by-law was unreasonable. In regard to the *Charter*, it also argued the by-law violated s. 7 because it was allegedly vague and overbroad. However, this latter ground of attack was bound to fail as the Supreme Court of Canada has ruled that a corporation is not entitled to the rights protected under s. 7: *Irwin Toy Ltd. v. Québec (Attorney General)*, [1989] S.C.J. No. 36, [1989] 1 S.C.R. 927 (S.C.C.). The ORHMA did not pursue the s. 7 claim in argument before the Ontario Court of Appeal.

[91]   *Ontario Restaurant Hotel & Motel Assn. v. Toronto (City)*, [2004] O.J. No. 190 at para. 37 (Ont. Div. Ct.).

did not violate s. 2 of the *Charter* and, even if it did, the violation would be saved under s. 1.[92]

In the context of *Charter* challenges to public health action, it appears courts will recognize the need to balance competing interests and will likely give deference to health officials who must act to safeguard the public's health, sometimes during difficult times of uncertainty and possible emergency. Only in situations involving arbitrary or unreasonable exercise of public health powers are courts likely to find a breach of rights protected under the *Canadian Charter of Rights and Freedoms*.

V. GOVERNMENT TORT LIABILITY FOR PUBLIC HEALTH FAILURES

Where public health systems are perceived to have failed, individual citizens may pursue legal action against governmental bodies and individuals who are allegedly responsible for the failure. Typically, such challenges proceed as tort law claims in which individuals argue public health officials owed them a duty of care and failed to discharge that duty in accordance with an appropriate standard. Class action lawsuits are used with increasing frequency to pursue such claims.

Establishing tort liability against a governmental authority is not a straightforward legal task:

> Tort claims against governments have spawned special problems. While many have urged that governments should be liable in tort the same way as anyone else, others have contended that government business is different from ordinary business and therefore must, in many cases, be judged differently. ... as usual, a compromise has been reached: some types of activities, policy functions, have been rendered immune from negligence law whereas others, operational functions, have been subjected to it.[93]

The Supreme Court of Canada has explained the rationale for distinguishing between policy and operational decisions by observing that "the Crown is not a person and must be free to govern and make true policy decisions without becoming subject to tort liability as a result of

---

[92]   In reaching this opinion, the court considered evidence that "there are 2.2 million cases of food poisoning annually with an economic cost of $1 billion approximately. Evidence filed establishes that restaurants are the cause of the highest incidence of food poisoning outbreaks". *Ibid.*, at para. 53.

[93]   Allen M. Linden *et al.*, *Canadian Tort Law: Cases, Notes & Materials*, 12th ed. (Markham, Ont.: Butterworths, 2004) at 491.

those decisions".[94] A policy decision is typically one that involves the exercise of discretion regarding matters such as budgetary allocations. In contrast, operational decisions relate to putting government policy into practice. For example, a government decision to allocate resources to road maintenance is a policy decision; decisions about how to carry out the maintenance activities, such as selection of staff and equipment to carry out needed work, are generally operational matters.

Litigation regarding the Ontario government's response to West Nile virus highlights the challenges of tort litigation in the public health context. Persons affected by the WNV outbreak in Ontario during summer 2002 launched approximately 40 lawsuits alleging the provincial government was negligent in implementing a plan to combat the disease. The province sought a court order dismissing the cases on the basis that they did not disclose a legal cause of action.[95] The government argued its response to the virus constituted a policy decision that is immune from judicial review. In adjudicating the dismissal motion, Justice Speigel observed that "[t]here is no dispute that a private law duty of care may only arise when a government is carrying out its policy decisions at the operational level. As with many principles of law, however, it is easier to state the principle than to actually draw the line between policy and operations".[96] As a court will only dismiss a claim prior to trial if it is plain and obvious it will not succeed,[97] Speigel J. was unwilling to dismiss the actions, ruling that the government may have owed a duty of care to the plaintiffs in relation to its plan to address the WNV threat.

While Speigel J.'s ruling marked "the first time that a court in Canada has found that a public authority can be held liable in tort for failing to prevent the spread of disease",[98] the Ontario Court of Appeal ultimately ruled the claim raised no private law duty of care and, moreover, policy considerations militated against recognizing private law obligations in these circumstances. Writing for the Court, Sharpe J.A. stated:

> ... no doubt there is a general public law duty that requires the Minister to endeavour to promote, safeguard, and protect the health of Ontario

---

[94]   *Just v. British Columbia*, [1989] S.C.J. No. 121, [1989] 2 S.C.R. 1228 at para. 16 (S.C.C.), *per* Cory J.

[95]   *Eliopoulos v. Ontario (Minister of Health and Long Term Care)*, [2004] O.J. No. 3035 (Ont. S.C.J.).

[96]   *Ibid.*, at para. 40.

[97]   *Hunt v. Carey Canada Inc.*, [1990] S.C.J. No. 93, [1990] 2 S.C.R. 959 (S.C.C.). The Supreme Court of Canada has also noted that even a "germ" or a "scintilla" of a cause of action is sufficient to proceed with a claim. See *Operation Dismantle Inc. v. Canada*, [1985] S.C.J. No. 22, [1985] 1 S.C.R. 441 (S.C.C.).

[98]   *Eliopoulos Estate v. Ontario (Minister of Health and Long Term Care)*, [2004] O.J. No. 4396 at para. 3 (Ont. Div. Ct.).

residents and prevent the spread of infectious diseases. However, a general public law duty of that nature does not give rise to a private law duty sufficient to ground an action in negligence. I fail to see how it could be possible to convert any of the Minister's public law discretionary powers, to be exercised in the general public interest, into private law duties owed to specific individuals.[99]

In regard to policy considerations, Sharpe J.A. cautioned that, in regard to policy choices, "[p]ublic health authorities should be left to decide where to focus their attention and resources without the fear or threat of lawsuits".[100]

Litigation arising from the SARS outbreak also advanced claims in negligence. Approximately 200 individuals who were infected with SARS or otherwise affected by the outbreak filed a class action lawsuit against the City of Toronto and the federal and Ontario governments. This claim, seeking $6 million in compensation, alleged that the various levels of government breached their legal duties by not sustaining adequate measures to control the disease. In a press release, counsel for the plaintiffs declared:

> While front line doctors and nurses were heroically battling this infection and trying to save people's lives, the defendants too quickly jumped to the conclusion that SARS was under control. Our public health officials flipped from SARS panic to SARS denial within a few days. The protection of public health took a back seat to political considerations such as the rehabilitation of Toronto's image.[101]

In a preliminary ruling, the Ontario Superior Court of Justice dismissed the claims against the City of Toronto and federal government, but permitted the claim against Ontario to proceed.[102]

In related litigation, over 50 nurses who were employed at hospitals in Ontario during the SARS outbreak alleged the provincial government was negligent and breached the nurses' s. 7 *Charter* rights by failing to take sufficient steps to protect their health and safety.[103] The government issued directives under the provincial *Emergency Management Act*

[99] *Eliopoulos v. Ontario (Minister of Health and Long Term Care)*, [2006] O.J. No. 4400, 82 O.R. (3d) 321 at para. 17 (Ont. C.A.), leave to appeal to S.C.C. dismissed [2006] S.C.C.A. No. 514 (S.C.C.).

[100] *Eliopoulos v. Ontario (Minister of Health and Long Term Care)*, [2006] O.J. No. 4400, 82 O.R. (3d) 321 at para. 33 (Ont. C.A.).

[101] Roy Elliott Kim O'Connor LLP, Press Release, "Toronto area resident starts $600 million dollar SARS 2 class action law suit" (23 February 2004), online: <http://www.reko.ca/html/sars_pr_feb21_2004.pdf>, quoting lawyer Douglas Elliott.

[102] *Williams v. Canada (Attorney General)*, [2005] O.J. No. 3508, 76 O.R. (3d) 763 (Ont. S.C.J.).

[103] *Abarquez v. Ontario*, [2005] O.J. No. 3504, 257 D.L.R. (4th) 745 (Ont. S.C.J.).

regarding hospital activities during the outbreak. The plaintiffs argued these directives were deficient and amounted to negligence in operational activities that resulted in reasonably foreseeable harm to them. The court rejected Ontario's preliminary dismissal application.

While the courts ultimately rejected negligence claims regarding WNV, the outcomes of the SARS litigation may be significant in clarifying when governmental bodies owe (or do not owe) a private law duty of care to protect individuals from public health threats.

VI. INTERGOVERNMENTAL RELATIONS IN PUBLIC HEALTH

Although this chapter focuses on legal dimensions of public health in Canada, law, in and of itself, leaves many ambiguities and cannot provide a complete framework for intergovernmental relations in the public health context. In others words, while the Constitution divides authority over health matters, public health concerns demand an approach that moves beyond assertions of legal turf. Consequently, this chapter will conclude with a few observations regarding intergovernmental relations in public health.

It has been argued that "effective intergovernmental cooperation is one of the most significant challenges facing public health today".[104] Legal ambiguities and resulting interjurisdictional and interorganizational tensions were highlighted in the various reports arising from the SARS outbreak.[105] In regard to the Canadian public health system, the National Advisory Committee on SARS and Public Health observed:

> What exist now are separate systems within each of the provinces and territories, as well as a federal system that operates primarily at Canada's international borders. These systems are connected by a limited number of intergovernmental agreements, rather than through a systemic set of intergovernmental agreements oriented around an agreed strategic plan or

---

[104]   Kumanan Wilson, "The Complexities of Multi-level Governance in Public Health" (2004) 95 Canadian Journal of Public Health 409.

[105]   For example, in 2004, the Ontario SARS Commission, chaired by the Honourable Mr. Justice Archie Campbell, identified the following questions as critical to learning lessons from SARS: "Who legally was in charge of the outbreak? Who had the ultimate responsibility for the classification of a case: the local jurisdiction or the province? What was the legal authority for issuing directives to hospitals? What were the consequences of not following those directives? What specific information had to be transmitted, by whom, when and to whom?" See Ontario SARS Commission, *SARS and Public Health in Ontario* (Ontario Ministry of Health, 15 April 2004) at 126, online: <www.health.gov.on.ca/english/public/pub/ministry_reports/campbell04/campbell04.pdf>.

through formal legal instruments that enable the systems to operate collectively and detect and address common challenges.[106]

In developing systems or programs to address public health issues in Canada, at least four governance models are available,[107] each with advantages and disadvantages. On the first model, governments work independently from one another within their areas of constitutional jurisdiction. This approach may avoid legal disputes over jurisdiction, but may perpetuate or exacerbate fragmentation and lack of coordination. The second model is based on a clear hierarchy where the federal government has a strong leadership role and the authority to require provincial participation in federal initiatives. This model may generate legal disputes if federal authority is challenged, but could promote greater national consistency in those areas of public health where the federal government decides to act. The third model envisages collaboration across all levels of government to develop and implement public health programs. This model has a clear benefit of averting legal jurisdictional disputes, but requires political will to collaborate and establish agreements among governments. Finally, a confederated model involves interprovincial collaboration on public health issues, but minimal or no involvement of the federal government. This approach may promote consistency across provinces, but may overlook important areas of federal responsibility and capacity.

In light of constitutional ambiguities in public health, the focus of federal and provincial relationships has largely been collaborative,[108] an approach emphasized by the Public Health Agency of Canada. For example, a September 2004 federal news release states that "the creation of the Public Health Agency of Canada marks the beginning of a new approach to federal leadership and collaboration with provinces and territories on public health", "public health strategies will be supported by a new level of coordination and collaboration", and, finally, the Agency will respond to recommendations for "improved collaboration within and between jurisdictions".[109] The federal *Department of Health Act* also emphasizes "cooperation with provincial authorities with a view to the

---

[106]   See National Advisory Committee on SARS and Public Health, *Learning from SARS: Renewal of Public Health in Canada* (Ottawa: Health Canada, 2003) (Chair: Dr. D. Naylor) at 163-64.

[107]   These four models are identified by Kumanan Wilson: see "A Canadian Agency for Public Health: Could it Work?" (2004) 170 Canadian Medical Association Journal 222.

[108]   For further discussion, see *e.g.*, Kumanan Wilson, "The Complexities of Multi-level Governance in Public Health" (2004) 95 Canadian Journal of Public Health 409.

[109]   Public Health Agency of Canada, News Release, "The Public Health Agency of Canada — Information September 2004 Backgrounder", online: <http://www.phac-aspc.gc.ca/media/nr-rp/2004/phac-eng.php>.

coordination of efforts made or proposed for preserving and improving public health".[110]

However, establishing effective collaboration is more easily said than done. Indeed, in March 2005, two years after the SARS outbreak, David Naylor, Chair of the National Advisory Committee on SARS and Public Health, criticized the federal public health agency for moving too slowly in developing regional operations across the country.[111] Regional centres were intended "to have federal officials working side-by-side with provincial counterparts in a bid to eliminate jurisdictional tensions that had been a serious impediment to information flow during SARS".[112] Yet, Dr. Naylor reportedly commented that "the longer we wait, the more the chance there will be a certain degree of cynicism about whether the notion of regional hubs and a truly co-ordinated federal-provincial public health response is going to happen".[113] The 2008 report of the Auditor General of Canada also criticized slowness in establishing public health information sharing agreements with the provinces.[114] It appears that a collaborative approach to public health reform is likely to continue in Canada, albeit too slowly for many.

VII.   CLOSING COMMENTS

This chapter has provided an overview of legal foundations of public health in Canada, with particular emphasis on the role of law both in empowering and constraining public health activities. While legal issues in public health have typically attracted little analysis, that situation is now changing; unfortunately, we needed the dramatic emergence of new disease threats to prompt that attention. As federal, provincial/territorial

---

[110]   S.C. 1996, c. 8, s. 4(*i*).

[111]   "Health agency architect says progress too slow" *Canadian Press* (13 March 2005).

[112]   *Ibid.*

[113]   *Ibid.*

[114]   Auditor General of Canada, *Report of the Auditor General of Canada to the House of Commons, Chapter 5: Surveillance of Infectious Diseases — Public Health Agency of Canada* (May 2008), online: Office of the Auditor General of Canada <http://www.oag-bvg.gc.ca/internet/docs/aud_ch_oag_200805_05_e.pdf>.

and local levels of government work to improve public health systems and capacity in this country, legal issues will continue to arise. It is worth reflecting on the legal rules and provisions that gird the system — from constitutional law, including the *Charter*, to public health and emergency statutes, and also private law duties — to permit more informed response to public health legal problems that will inevitably require solutions.

APPENDIX

PUBLIC HEALTH LEGISLATION IN CANADA

Jurisdiction	Public Health Statutes General	Emergency Statutes	Other Public Health Statutes
Alberta	**Public Health Act**, R.S.A. 2000, c. P-37	**Emergency Management Act**, R.S.A. 2000, c. E-6.8	
British Columbia	Health Act, R.S.B.C. 1996, c. 179 New legislation pending: **Public Health Act**, S.B.C. 2008, c. 28 (Bill 23; received Royal Assent May 2008)	**Emergency Program Act**, R.S.B.C. 1996, c. 111	**Venereal Disease Act**, R.S.B.C. 1996, c. 475 (to be repealed by new **Public Health Act**)
Manitoba	**Public Health Act**, C.C.S.M. c. P210 New legislation pending: **Public Health Act**, S.M. 2006, c. 14	**Emergency Measures Act**, C.C.S.M. c. E80 **Public Health Act**, S.M. 2006, c. 14, Part 6 (not yet in force) deals with public health emergencies	

Jurisdiction	Public Health Statutes General	Emergency Statutes	Other Public Health Statutes
New Brunswick	Health Act, R.S.N.B. 1973, c. H-2 Public Health Act, S.N.B. 1998, c. P-22.4	Emergency Measures Act, S.N.B. 1978, c. E-7.1	Venereal Disease Act, R.S.N.B. 1973, c. V-2
Newfoundland and Labrador	Health and Community Services Act, S.N.L. 1995, c. P-37.1 Communicable Diseases Act, R.S.N.L. 1990, c. C-26	Emergency Measures Act, R.S.N.L. 1990, c. E-8	Venereal Disease Prevention Act, R.S.N.L. 1990, c. V-2
Northwest Territories	Public Health Act, R.S.N.W.T. 1988, c. P-12 A new Public Health Act received assent in August 2007 and will come into force on order of the Commissioner of the Northwest Territories	Civil Emergency Measures Act, R.S.N.W.T. 1988, c. C-9	Disease Registries Act, R.S.N.W.T. 1988, c. 7 (Supp.)

Jurisdiction	Public Health Statutes General	Emergency Statutes	Other Public Health Statutes
Nova Scotia	**Health Protection Act**, S.N.S. 2004, c. 4	**Emergency Management Act**, S.N.S. 1990, c. 8	
Nunavut	**Public Health Act**, R.S.N.W.T. 1988, c. P-12, as duplicated for Nunavut by s. 29 of the **Nunavut Act**, S.C. 1993, c. 28	**Civil Emergency Measures Act**, R.S.N.W.T. 1988, c. C-9, as duplicated for Nunavut by s. 29 of the **Nunavut Act**, S.C. 1993, c. 28	**Disease Registries Act**, R.S.N.W.T. 1988, c. 7 (Supp.), as duplicated for Nunavut by s. 29 of the **Nunavut Act**, S.C. 1993, c. 28
Ontario	**Health Protection and Promotion Act**, R.S.O. 1990, c. H.7	**Emergency Management and Civil Protection Act**, R.S.O. 1990, c. E.9	
Prince Edward Island	**Public Health Act**, R.S.P.E.I. 1988, c. P-30	**Emergency Measures Act**, R.S.P.E.I. 1988, c. E-6.01	

Jurisdiction	Public Health Statutes General	Emergency Statutes	Other Public Health Statutes
Québec	An Act respecting health services and social services, R.S.Q. c. S-4.2 Public Health Act, R.S.Q. c. S-22 An Act respecting Institut national de santé publique du Québec, R.S.Q. c. I-13.1.1	Civil Protection Act, R.S.Q. c. S-2.3	
Saskatchewan	Public Health Act, 1994, S.S. 1994, c. P-37.1	Emergency Planning Act, S.S. 1989-90, c. E-8.1	
Yukon	Public Health and Safety Act, R.S.Y. 2002, c. 176	Civil Emergency Measures Act, R.S.Y. 2002, c. 34	
Federal	Public Health Agency of Canada Act, S.C. 2006, c. 5 Department of Health Act, S.C. 1996, c. 8	Emergencies Act, R.S.C. 1985, c. 22 (4th Supp.) Emergency Management Act, S.C. 2007, c. 15	Quarantine Act, S.C. 2005, c. 20

2

PUBLIC HEALTH ETHICS

Stephanie Nixon, Ross Upshur, Ann Robertson, Solomon R. Benatar, Alison K. Thompson and Abdallah S. Daar[*]

I. INTRODUCTION

In 2003, Canada and the world were suddenly awakened by the emergence of a highly infectious disease called SARS. It moved around the globe at an incredible pace and seemed to have a high fatality rate. Toronto was hit hard. Little was known about the causative agent or the epidemiology in the early days of the outbreak. Yet public health authorities had to make critical decisions on how to contain the spread of the disease and protect the public. It was not easy.

Questions included: To what extent should individual freedoms be limited for the collective good? In the absence of good diagnostic testing, effective treatment and only vague insight into this new disease, is it

[*] All authors are affiliated with the Joint Centre for Bioethics at the University of Toronto. Stephanie Nixon is an Assistant Professor in the Department of Physical Therapy at the University of Toronto and a researcher with the Health Economics and HIV/AIDS Research Division ("HEARD") at the University of KwaZulu-Natal. Ross Upshur is Director of the Joint Centre for Bioethics and is supported by a Canada Research Chair in Primary Care Research. Ann Robertson is a Professor in the Dalla Lana School of Public Health at the University of Toronto. Solomon R. Benatar is Emeritus Professor of Medicine at the University of Cape Town and a Professor in the Dalla Lana School of Public Health at the University of Toronto. Alison K. Thompson is an Assistant Professor in the Faculty of Pharmacy at the University of Toronto. Abdallah S. Daar is co-director of the Program on Life Sciences, Ethics and Policy ("PLEP") of the McLaughlin-Rotman Centre for Global Health, University Health Network and University of Toronto. PLEP receives most of its funding from Genome Canada through the Ontario Genomics Institute, the Ontario Research Fund, and the Bill and Melinda Gates Foundation. A full list of funders is available online at <http://www.mrcglobal.org/about/funding>. Dr. Daar is also supported by the McLaughlin Centre for Molecular Medicine at the University of Toronto. The authors would like to thank Shari Gruman and Carly Bolshin for their expert help in preparing the manuscript.

justified to quarantine all people exposed to the virus and keep them away not only from the public but also from family and friends? If so, what is owed, if anything, to those individuals to compensate them for the burden they shoulder on society's behalf? To what extent should health care providers be forced to care for people with SARS when the little evidence available indicated a very high risk of acquiring the disease, transmitting it to family and contacts, and perhaps even dying from it? How should information relating to such an outbreak be communicated to a nervous public? How should the Province of Ontario relate to the Canadian federal government when it was the latter that had to deal with the World Health Organization, which had passed a controversial advisory against travel to Toronto?

In the aftermath of the outbreak, what should have been the responsibility of the municipal, provincial or federal governments to financially assist businesses that experienced massive economic losses as a result of real or perceived threats of contagion? Furthermore, if, rather than an anomaly, the emergence of a highly infectious agent like SARS foreshadows a future trend on the planet, what should we be learning about the links between globalization and health security? What can we learn from reflecting on the magnitude of response that was mounted against this global infectious disease that predominantly affected the rich world and killed a relatively small number of people, compared to the kind of response that is being mounted against infectious diseases like HIV, TB and malaria that predominantly affect the developing world but kill many thousands of people every day? These are some of the ethical questions that arise within the sphere of public health, ranging from questions about how we should treat individuals to new ways of thinking about the health impacts of today's globalizing world.

This chapter examines this relatively unexplored terrain by first describing public health ethics in contrast to clinical bioethics. Next, we examine the historical roots of public health ethics, followed by contemporary perspectives on "what public health ethics is". We then discuss the philosophical underpinnings of the field and some of the frameworks that have been developed to inform public health ethics analysis. We finish with a discussion of the importance of moving the discourse in public health ethics to the global level and of some of the morally relevant factors that need to be taken into consideration when examining global public health issues.

II.   FROM BIOETHICS TO PUBLIC HEALTH ETHICS

Public health ethics, as envisaged here, is a recent field of scholarly interest, unlike the more established field of bioethics. Since its inception in the middle of the last century, the field of bioethics has focused upon ethical issues pertaining to the practice of clinical medicine (*e.g.*, physician-patient relationships) and to medical research (*e.g.*, protection of human research subjects). Consequently, bioethics as a discipline has focused almost exclusively upon individualistic concerns, primarily the notion of autonomy, which has become a leading concern in the West. While this focus is understandable, given the impetus promoting modern bioethics since the Nuremberg Trials, the Tuskegee Syphilis study and patient rights movements in the 1960s, Onora O'Neill has argued that bioethics has been "damagingly preoccupied" with not only the autonomy of individual patients but also with the requirements for justice within, but not between, states.[1]

Until relatively recently, the development of a broader public health ethics discourse has been largely ignored. However, this is beginning to change. Since the mid-1990s, there has been growing engagement with public health ethics as a field. The increasing recognition that the approaches that underpin clinical bioethics cannot simply be transposed to public health ethics has led to a number of publications that have begun to articulate and develop the theoretical, conceptual and substantive parameters of the field.[2] At the same time, there have been several efforts to develop specific curricula in public health ethics for graduate education at schools and departments of public health.[3] Other initiatives include: increased instruction on public health ethics amongst public health practitioners;[4] development of a draft Public Health Code of

---

[1] Onora O'Neill, "Public Health or Clinical Ethics: Thinking Beyond Borders" (2002) 16 Ethics & International Affairs 35.

[2] Solomon R. Benatar, "Prospects for Global Health: Lessons from Tuberculosis" (1995) 50 Thorax 487; Solomon R. Benatar, "Global Disparities in Health and Human Rights: A Critical Commentary" (1998) 88 American Journal of Public Health 295; Lawrence O. Gostin, "Public Health, Ethics, and Human Rights: A Tribute to the Late Jonathan Mann" (2001) 29 J.L. Med. & Ethics 121; Nancy E. Kass, "An Ethics Framework for Public Health" (2001) 91 American Journal of Public Health 1776; Daniel Callahan & Bruce Jennings, "Ethics and Public Health: Forging a Strong Relationship" (2002) 92 American Journal of Public Health 169; James F. Childress *et al.*, "Public Health Ethics: Mapping the Terrain" (2002) 30 J.L. Med. & Ethics 170; R.E.G. Upshur, "Principles for the Justification of Public Health Intervention" (2002) 93 Canadian Journal of Public Health 101; D. Wikler & R. Cash, "Ethical Issues in Global Public Health" (2003) in Robert Beaglehole, ed., *Global Public Health: A New Era* (Oxford: Oxford University Press, 2003) at 226; Angus Dawson & M Verweij, *Ethics, Prevention and Public Health* (New York: Oxford University Press, 2007); Nuffield Council on Bioethics, *Public Health: Ethical Issues* (London: Nuffield Council on Bioethics, 2007), online: Nuffield Council on Bioethics <http://www.nuffieldbioethics.org/fileLibrary/pdf/Public_health_-_ethical_issues.pdf>.

[3] Association of Schools of Public Health, *Ethics and Public Health: Model Curriculum* (2003), online: <http://www.asph.org/document.cfm?page=782>. At the University of Toronto Department of Public Health Sciences, a course on public health ethics began in 2003.

[4] Steven S. Coughlin *et al.*, *Case Studies in Public Health Ethics* (Washington, D.C.: American Public Health Association, 1997); Steven S. Coughlin *et al.*, "Ethics Instruction at Schools of Public Health in the United States. Association of Schools of Public Health

Ethics;[5] and the emergence of research and policy symposia on public health ethics, such as the international meeting, *Public Health Ethics: Towards a Research Agenda,* held at the University of Toronto in May 2002[6] as well as the first national roundtable on public health ethics held in Montreal in November 2007.   The Nuffield Council on Bioethics recently released a report focusing on public health ethics issues in which they have developed: (a) a "stewardship model" that sets out guiding principles for making decisions about public health policies; and (b) an "intervention ladder" that provides a way of thinking about the acceptability of different public health measures.[7]

There are a number of reasons for the increasing interest in the field of public health ethics. In Canada in particular, there have been a number of recent public health "crises" that have indicated a need for an articulated public health ethics. The tainted blood scandal and the subsequent Krever Commission report were harbingers of future public health crises.[8] In May 2000, in the town of Walkerton, Ontario, a waterborne *E. coli* outbreak resulting from inadequate health protection measures was responsible for seven deaths and the infection of almost half the town's population.[9] As noted, the recent SARS outbreak in Canada not only highlighted the lack of preparation of public health authorities for major infectious disease threats, but also raised fundamental ethical issues about the appropriate scope and limitation of individual liberty and autonomy by public health authorities for the control of disease and public health protection. As a result, in 2003, a major commission made recommendations for sweeping changes to the governance, legal structure, and training and practice of public health in Canada.[10]

Education Committee" (1999) 89 American Journal of Public Health 768; Anthony S. Kessel, "Public Health Ethics: Teaching Survey and Critical Review" (2003) 56 Social Science & Medicine 1439.

[5]   Public Health Leadership Society, *Principles of the Ethical Practice of Public Health* (New Orleans, LA: Public Health Leadership Society, 2002), online: American Public Health Association <http://www.apha.org/NR/rdonlyres/1CED3CEA-287E-4185-9CBD-BD405FC60856/0/ethicsbrochure.pdf>.

[6]   A. Thompson *et al.*, "Public Health Ethics: Towards a Research Agenda" (2003) 9 Acta Bioethica 157.

[7]   Nuffield Council on Bioethics, *Public Health: Ethical Issues* (London: Nuffield Council on Bioethics, 2007), online: Nuffield Council on Bioethics <http://www.nuffieldbioethics.org/fileLibrary/pdf/Public_health_-_ethical_issues.pdf>.

[8]   Horace Krever, *Final Report: Commission of Inquiry on the Blood System in Canada* (Ottawa, 1997).

[9]   Canadian Broadcasting Corporation, "Inside Walkerton: Canada's Worst Ever *E. Coli* Contaminiation" (20 December 2004), online: <http://www.cbc.ca/news/background/walkerton>.

[10]   National Advisory Committee on SARS and Public Health, *Learning from SARS: Renewal of Public Health in Canada (A Report of the National Advisory Committee on SARS and Public*

At a more global level, the variable means by which public health exercised its authority in response to SARS has underscored the need for a sustained international dialogue on the ethical aspects of disease control and its relation not only to diverse and culturally based ethical norms, but also to universal human rights standards. In addition, the emerging field of genomics raises profound ethical issues for public health, both nationally and internationally, related to potential population-based genetic screening programs and genetic data banks. There are also public health concerns, such as the emergence of infectious disease pandemics (*e.g.*, multi-drug and extensive drug resistant TB), the neglected epidemic of chronic diseases, the potential threat of bioterrorism that needs to be balanced by the legitimate need of developing countries to benefit from modern biotechnology,[11] and the alarming increase in global health inequities, all of which call for a broad normative discourse. It is clear from these and other instances that the existing frameworks and tools developed by bioethicists are not easily adapted to deal with ethical issues in public health, nor is it appropriate to attempt to do so, given the individualistic focus of much of clinical bioethics.

III. THE HISTORICAL ROOTS OF PUBLIC HEALTH ETHICS

Although the scholarly field of public health ethics has only recently begun to emerge, ethics issues in public health and their management are far from novel concerns. In order to provide a foundation for the discussion that follows, this section will trace the historical underpinnings of public health ethics.

The historical roots of public health ethics lie in the varied origins of public health itself. While a fuller discussion of the history of contemporary public health is beyond the scope of this chapter,[12] there are three general streams within public health that are of particular relevance to public health ethics. The first is an early historical stream that underscores the more authoritarian, even coercive, aspects of public health. According to one version, the origins of public health lie, in part, in the creation of a new kind of public official that emerged in the 17th

---

Health, October 2003) (Ottawa: Health Canada, 2003) (Chair: Dr. D. Naylort), online: Public Health Agency of Canada <http://www.phac-aspc.gc.ca/publicat/sars-sras/naylor/index.html>.

[11]   Calestous Juma & Ismail Serageldin, *Freedom To Innovate: Biotechnology in Africa's Development. Report of the High-Level African Panel on Modern Biotechnology* (Addis Ababa, Ethiopia: African Union and Pretoria, South Africa: New Partnership for Africa's Development, 2007).

[12]   See *e.g.*, George Rosen, *A History of Public Health* (Baltimore: Johns Hopkins University Press, 1993).

century known as "police",[13] whose duties included enforcing public health measures such as quarantine. Indeed, other than the police (in its modern form), the military and child protection agencies, public health is one of the few contemporary public institutions that holds a delegated legal authority to enforce certain kinds of actions or behaviours (*e.g.*, restaurant closures, individual quarantine, treatment in certain cases). Of course, the exercise of this authority can — and does — have negative consequences, a point which will be discussed more fully below.

A second historical stream in public health is aligned with more progressive social reform movements. This was the case during the last half of the 19th century when public health officials, particularly in Great Britain, directed their attention and actions to tackling the worst consequences of industrial capitalism that had created a large population of urban poor. This was a period of great "sanitary reform" (the "hygienist movement"), often referred to as the "Golden Age" of public health, during which much of what we associate with contemporary public health had its origins: public water and sewage systems (commonly referred to as "mains and drains"), housing regulations and inspections, improvements in working conditions, and maternal and child health services (including "lady health visitors").[14] This tradition in public health is not without its own more questionable consequences in terms of the "management", however well-intended, of large sectors of society, predominantly the working class and the poor.[15] Nevertheless, the point remains that public health has had a long association with social reform, social action, and social justice. Indeed, it has been argued that public health *is* social justice.[16]

A third, more recent stream is the somewhat subversive shift away from the holistic, universal and implied horizontal approach to improving global health that was initially supported by the World Health Organization and articulated in the Alma Ata Declaration in 1978, in favour of increasingly selective, vertical and privatized health programs. The latter were promoted through the increasing influence of the World Bank, International Monetary Fund and the United States Treasury (through a policy doctrine often called the "Washington Consensus"), as

---

[13]   Michel Foucault, "The Politics of Health in the Eighteenth Century" in Paul Rabinow, ed., *The Foucault Reader* (New York: Pantheon Books, 1984) at 273.

[14]   Simon Szreter, "The Importance of Social Intervention in Britain's Mortality Decline, C. 1850-1914. A Reinterpretation of the Role of Public Health" (1988) 1 Social History of Medicine 1.

[15]   David Armstrong, *The Political Anatomy of the Body* (Cambridge: Cambridge University Press, 1983).

[16]   Dan E. Beauchamp, "Public Health as Social Justice" (1976) 13 Inquiry 3.

well as powerful philanthropy, which have been able to wield more power than the World Health Organization.[17]

Given the multiple and interwoven historical roots of public health, it should not be surprising that public health ethics emerges as extremely complex and full of uncertainties, ambiguities, paradoxes and even contradictions. To begin to explore this nascent field more fully, it may be useful to start with the mandate of public health. Through its focus on societal rather than individual actions, public health seeks to improve the well-being of communities and populations through activities such as immunization and ensuring a safe water supply. Information to guide public health is obtained largely through epidemiological research exploring the physical, psychological, environmental and social conditions that underlie and give rise to health and disease.[18] These ideas are captured succinctly in the Institute of Medicine's definition of public health: "... what we, as a society, do collectively to assure the conditions for people to be healthy".[19]

Given this definition of public health, it could be argued that public health ethics is most closely related to the ethical tradition of utilitarianism. For example, Edwin Chadwick, who was the architect of the *Poor Law Amendment Act* and one of the founders of the hygienic movement in Great Britain in the 1830s and 1840s, was profoundly influenced by the thinking of Jeremy Bentham, the founder of utilitarianism.[20] Although controversial in his time, Chadwick's recognition that acute infectious diseases were fatal to many, and that the death of working men left their families disadvantaged, led to the Report of the Health of Towns Committee in 1840, followed by the Sanitary Report in 1842. These reports, along with a series of Public Health Acts, were instrumental in the development of the hygienic movement in Great Britain and the justification for state involvement in public health with the goal of improving the health of the population.[21] It also established a tradition of public health paternalism and state intervention in health, a legacy that continues to the present. The control of communicable diseases entailed the use of state functions for promoting and protecting

---

[17]   Italian Global Health Watch, "From Alma Ata to the Global Fund: The History of International Health Policy" (2008) 3 Social Medicine 36.

[18]   Nancy E. Kass, "An Ethics Framework for Public Health" (2001) 91 American Journal of Public Health 1776.

[19]   Institute of Medicine, *The Future of Public Health* (Washington, D.C.: National Academy Press, 1988) at 19.

[20]   Iqbal Sram & John Ashton, "Millennium Report to Sir Edwin Chadwick" (1998) 317 British Medical Journal 592.

[21]   Simon Szreter, "The Importance of Social Intervention in Britain's Mortality Decline" (1988) 1 Society for Social History of Medicine 1.

health, which included the curtailment of civil liberties for the aim of disease control.

Sheila Rothman has documented this in her illustration of the history of tuberculosis control in the early 20th century. She notes that public health authorities aggressively pursued restrictive interventions and government intrusion as a means of disease control. She quotes Hermann Biggs, of the New York City Department of Health:

> The cry has been raised again and again ... that for humanity's sake pulmonary consumption must not be pronounced a communicable disease, and the friends of patients often declare that they prefer to expose themselves to the chance of infection rather than have their dear ones banished, or treated as if they were plague-stricken; but this is all the sheerest nonsense. ... The government of the United States is democratic ... but the sanitary measures adopted are sometimes autocratic, and the functions performed by sanitary authorities paternal in character. We are prepared, when necessary, to introduce and enforce, and the people are ready to accept, measures which might seem radical and arbitrary, if they were not plainly designed for the public good, and evidently beneficent in their effects.[22]

Throughout the latter half of the 20th century, as communicable diseases were seemingly controlled, there was a diminishing use of extraordinary public health measures such as detention and seizure of property and forcible removal of humans that characterized the control of typhoid, tuberculosis and cholera in earlier times. The profile of public health actions and their ethical dimensions were not revisited until the HIV/AIDS pandemic in the 1980s and 1990s. At first, the pandemic disproportionately affected homosexual men and there was tremendous debate about the use of state powers to control the epidemic, such as the closure of bathhouses. It was often thought during this phase that a double discrimination existed and that the activism of affected communities led to a policy of "AIDS exceptionalism" that altered the way that public health has managed that pandemic.[23]

However, in the two decades subsequent to the emergence of HIV/AIDS, the optimism concerning the control of communicable diseases has given way to the recognition that emerging and re-emerging infectious diseases will continuously be with us. In particular, the 2002–2003 global outbreak of SARS and the more recent emergence of extensive drug resistant tuberculosis (XDR-TB) have driven this lesson home. In addition, other global chronic disease pandemics, such as those

---

[22]   Sheila M. Rothman, "Seek and Hide: Public Health Departments and Persons with Tuberculosis, 1890-1940" (1993) 21 J.L. Med. & Ethics 289 at 291.

[23]   Ronald Bayer, "Clinical Progress and the Future of HIV Exceptionalism" (1999) 159 Archives of Internal Medicine 1042.

associated with tobacco and obesity, require us to reflect on the legitimacy of certain kinds of interventions aimed at improving public health.

Global pandemics, however, are not simply the result of diseases that have spread evenly around the world. Rather, in many cases they are the result of global inequities in wealth and power that have created the conditions in which poverty and disease can flourish. Thus, it is relevant to consider not only the kinds of public health issues that affect developed societies, but also the burden of illness and death that disproportionately affects the poorest parts of the world, and important moral questions about how it came to be this way. This issue will be addressed in detail later in the chapter. First, however, we will turn to a discussion of the field of public health ethics as it is evolving today.

IV. WHAT IS "PUBLIC HEALTH ETHICS"?

As discussed earlier, traditional ethical concerns in health arose from issues raised by the care and/or research of individuals. Clinical ethics, and the sets of ethical frameworks created for reflection upon related issues, have focused on problems such as end of life care, micro level resource allocation and problems inherent in the provider-patient relationship, to name but a few. Attempting to use the frameworks of clinical ethics to deal with public health results in an imperfect fit. Public health practice and clinical practice are different in terms of context, mandate and range of activities. For instance, clinical ethics are rooted in the fiduciary responsibility of the clinician in his or her therapeutic contract with the patient that is legitimized by the informed consent of the patient. Conversely, public health practice assumes a population focus whereby the contract is with society as a whole and is legitimized by the policies and law of government. The approaches also differ in their patterns of practice. In clinical practice, the patient seeks out the clinician for a service and may accept or reject advice given. In public health, the patient is sought by the public health practitioner and may not be able to refuse the treatment being delivered.[24]

As such, different kinds of ethical issues may arise in public health. As Gostin notes, "[t]o defend the common welfare, political communities assert their collective power to tax, inspect, license, regulate, and coerce".[25] These concepts underscore one of the primary ethical debates in public health: the tension from the predominant orientation in clinical

---

[24]   Richard Schabas, "Is Public Health Ethical?" (2002) 93 Canadian Journal of Public Health 98.

[25]   Lawrence O. Gostin, "Public Health Law in a New Century: Part 1: Law as a Tool to Advance the Community's Health" (2000) 283 Journal of the American Medical Association 2837 at 2840.

bioethics in favour of civil liberties and individual autonomy versus the utilitarian, paternalistic and communitarian orientations that mark the field of public health.[26]

Public health ethics may be approached by examining the range of topics that fall within this field. In an early effort to map the field, the Kennedy Institute of Ethics generated a list of public health ethics concerns under the following categories: general literature, epidemiology, health promotion and education, public health administration, philosophical and ethics issues, socio-economic and legal perspectives, individual versus societal rights, risk, the media and personal choice, and genetics and public health.[27] This kind of approach offers no coherent theoretical foundation underlying the subject, and may even be misleading with respect to the meaning of the categories, but it does offer a point of departure for thinking about the kinds of issues encountered in the field.

Recently, there have been several attempts to articulate more general constitutive features of public health ethics. For example, Gostin has advanced thinking about the field by distinguishing between what he terms ethics *in* public health, ethics *of* public health and ethics *for* public health.[28] He describes ethics *in* public health as concerns involving the public health enterprise, including tradeoffs between collective goods and individual interests. This is distinct from the ethics *of* public health, which is concerned with the ethical dimensions of professionalism and moral trust that society invests in professionals to act for the common good. Ethics *for* public health takes into account the value of healthy communities and the interests of populations, with particular emphasis on the oppressed. We allude to this later notion in the section on global considerations.

Callahan and Jennings offer four broad categories for describing the field: health promotion and disease prevention; risk reduction; epidemiology and other public health research; and structural and socio-economic disparities.[29] They use this foundation to illustrate four types of analyses required to respond to concerns within these diverse areas. First, they describe *professional ethics* as based on professional character and virtues and involving ethical principles regarding trust and legitimacy in the profession. Second, *applied ethics* involves reasoning from general

---

[26] Daniel Callaghan & Bruce Jennings, "Ethics and Public Health: Forging a Strong Relationship" (2002) 92 American Journal of Public Health 169.

[27] Martina Darragh & Pat Milmoe McCarrick, "Public Health Ethics: Health by the Numbers" (1998) 8 Kennedy Institute of Ethics Journal 339.

[28] Lawrence O. Gostin, "Public Health, Ethics and Human Rights: A Tribute to the Late Jonathan Mann" (2001) 29 J.L. Med. & Ethics 121.

[29] Daniel Callaghan & Bruce Jennings "Ethics and Public Health: Forging a Strong Relationship" (2002) 92 American Journal of Public Health 169.

ethical theories to inform the profession. *Advocacy ethics* is less theoretical but arguably the most pervasive in public health. This type of analysis has a strong orientation towards equality and social justice. Finally, *critical ethics* describes an approach that attempts to combine the strengths of each of the above. It is practically oriented toward real-life problems, but brings larger social values and historical trends to bear. Critical ethics understands dilemmas not only as the result of behaviours of disease organisms and individuals, but also from institutional arrangements and prevailing structures of cultural attitudes and social power.[30, 31] These attempts to characterize public health ethics can be complemented by an appreciation of the philosophical issues that underpin the field.

V.   PHILOSOPHICAL ISSUES

It has been noted that public health decisions often involve conflicting and contrary ethical principles. One of the most difficult issues is the need to balance what is best for the population with protection for the individual. Roberts and Reich have noted that ethical arguments in public health can be grouped into three main categories, each representing a major theme in contemporary public health discourse: utilitarianism, liberalism and communitarianism.[32]

As indicated earlier, public health has strong utilitarian roots. This is manifested in techniques such as cost benefit analysis, quality adjusted life years or disability adjusted life years as a means of ranking programs and adjudicating decisions. There are concerns about the ability of these metrics to adequately reflect more than merely prevailing prejudgments. As well, there are concerns about how such evidence and data are collected in the first place, and the normative values that go into such ranking decisions.[33] There are also concerns expressed from deontological perspectives about the rights of minorities and how best to protect interests within a theory that has an overarching concern with a maximizing strategy. Although concerns may be expressed about the primacy or absoluteness of a utilitarian perspective, it is clear that in a

[30]   *Ibid.*
[31]   Italian Global Health Watch, "From Alma Ata to the Global Fund: The History of International Health Policy" (2008) 3 Social Medicine 36.
[32]   Marc J. Roberts & Michael R. Reich, "Ethical Analysis in Public Health" (2002) 359 Lancet 1055.
[33]   J. La Puma & E. Lawlor, "Quality-Adjusted Life-Years: Ethical Implications for Physicians and Policymakers" (1990) 263 Journal of the American Medical Association 2917. An example of this on a large scale would be the Oregon project. See *e.g.*, R. Steinbrook & B. Lo, "The Oregon Medicaid Demonstration Project — Will It Provide Adequate Medical Care?" (1992) 326 New Eng. J. Med. 340.

discipline like public health with a strong commitment to the quantitative analysis of health events, utilitarianism will continue to be an influential theory.

Liberalism also underlies some of the major philosophical trends in public health thinking. Liberalism is a 19th century political doctrine that is strongly influenced by Kantian thinking and is concerned, *inter alia*, with issues of liberty and rights. The notion of rights underlies many theories of justice, such as egalitarianism and libertarianism. The work of philosopher John Rawls has been of tremendous influence in this regard, particularly his concept of justice as fairness.[34] These ideas have been extended into health care by commentators such as Amy Gutmann[35] and into priority setting in health care by Norman Daniels.[36] More recent interpretations of justice, such as those described by Amartya Sen, look towards maximizing justice by maximizing capabilities available to individuals, and are likely to prove to be an influential paradigm in the future.[37]

Communitarian perspectives also have a long tradition. The focus in communitarian ethics is on creating a good society in which individuals within that society exemplify virtues appropriate to that society. There are two distinct trends within communitarianism: one more relativistic that sees morality as inherently contextual to the community itself, and the other more universalist that argues there are ideal norms for every society that can be approximated.

More recent analyses have explored the relationship between social justice and public health. Powers and Faden have argued that a theory of social justice provides the moral foundation for public health ethics.[38] They are critical of accounts of justice in public health that focus exclusively on outcomes alone derived from considerations of utility. They argue instead that a social justice perspective addresses the twin moral impulses that animate public health:

> ... to improve human well being by improving health and to do so in particular by focusing on the needs of those who are the most disadvantaged. A commitment to social justice ... attaches a special moral

---

[34]   John Rawls, *A Theory of Justice* (Cambridge, MA: Belknap Press of Harvard University Press, 1999).

[35]   A. Gutmann & D. Thompson, "Just Deliberation About Health Care" in Marion Danis, Carolyn M. Clancy & Larry R. Churchill, eds., *Ethical Dimensions of Health Policy* (New York: Oxford University Press, 2002) at 77.

[36]   Norman Daniels, "Accountability for Reasonableness" (2000) 321 British Medical Journal 1300.

[37]   Amartya Sen, *Development as Freedom* (New York: Knopf, 1999).

[38]   M. Powers & R. Faden, *Social Justice, The Moral Foundations of Public Health and Public Health Policy* (New York: Oxford University Press, 2006).

urgency to remediating the conditions of those whose life prospects are poor across multiple dimensions of well being. Placing a priority on those so situated is a hallmark of social justice.[39]

Central to Powers and Faden's theory is recognition of the interdependence of empirical and conceptual approaches to public health ethics. That is, neither philosophical theories of justice nor measurement of health states is sufficient on its own to build a satisfactory account of public health ethics.

Dawson and Verweij, in a collected set of essays on public health ethics, have expanded and deepened the philosophical discourse to more fully parse out the meaning of public in public health.[40] They have also sought to distinguish between two main senses in which the term has been employed, namely public health as the health of the public and as a set of public or collective interventions aimed at improving health.[41]

It is important to note that often in public health ethics debates, discussions and analyses cross these various philosophical domains with utilitarianism predominating in some analyses, and rights-based approaches or community-based approaches predominating in others. It has been argued that what is most important is explicit discussion of the moral philosophical issues and the will to move towards a coherent position. However, as Roberts and Reich conclude:

> Yet public-health professionals have minimal training in ethical analysis. If health professionals are to develop coherent positions on these issues, and contribute to democratic deliberation about public policies, then they need enhanced skills in applied philosophy. Understanding alternative ethical arguments has become as important as knowing the advantages and disadvantages of different epidemiological techniques.[42]

VI. FRAMEWORKS AND APPLICATIONS

A range of operational frameworks and principles have been proposed for the analysis of ethical issues in public health practice. Nancy Kass has articulated one such ethics framework that provides six primary

---

[39]   *Ibid.*, at 82.

[40]   A. Dawson & M. Verweij, *Ethics, Prevention and Public Health* (New York: Oxford University Press, 2007).

[41]   The collection includes an essay by Bruce Jennings on civic republicanism where he outlines the way in which a civic republican perspective grafts on to philosophical conceptions of public health ethics, and shows how this is an advance on contractarian and liberal perspectives.

[42]   Marc J. Roberts & Michael R. Reich, "Ethical Analysis in Public Health" (2002) 359 Lancet 1055.

questions to be addressed in relation to the ethical dimensions of any proposed public health program:

• What are the public health goals of the proposed program?

• How effective is the program in achieving its stated goals?

• What are the known or potential burdens of the program?

• Can burdens be minimized? Are there alternative approaches?

• Is the program implemented fairly?

• How can the benefits and burdens of the program be fairly balanced?[43]

A second framework articulated by Childress *et al.* enumerates five considerations to be weighed when analyzing the ethical dimensions of public health action: effectiveness, proportionality, necessity, least infringement and public justification.[44] Upshur proposed the following four principles to guide the justification of public health intervention: the harm principle; the principle of least restrictive or coercive means; the reciprocity principle; and the transparency principle.[45] These ideas have not yet been debated regarding their strengths and limitations. However, if the history of debate over principlism in clinical ethics is a guide, one may expect that these principles may be valued for advancing the ethics discourse among public health practitioners in both practice and training settings, but challenged in terms of their relationship to broader moral theory.[46]

Recent events have prompted the development of new applications for ethical analysis of public health issues. For example, Peter Singer (of the University of Toronto) and his colleagues have analyzed ethical dimensions of the SARS epidemic.[47] The point of departure in their analysis was the lack of available evidence when initial decisions and policies were required. There was a need for decision-makers to weigh individual freedoms against the common good, and personal safety against the duty to treat the sick. There was also a concern with risking economic loss to control the spread of a potentially serious epidemic. At the time

---

[43] Nancy E. Kass, "An Ethics Framework for Public Health" (2001) 91 American Journal of Public Health 1776.

[44] James F. Childress *et al.*, "Public Health Ethics: Mapping the Terrain" (2002) 30 J.L. Med. & Ethics 170.

[45] R.E.G. Upshur, "Principles for the Justification of Public Health Intervention" (2002) 93 Canadian Journal of Public Health 101.

[46] T.L. Beauchamp, "Principlism and Its Alleged Competitors" (1995) 5 Kennedy Institute of Ethics Journal 181; K.D. Clouser & B. Gert, "A Critique of Principlism" (1990) 15 Journal of Medicine & Philosophy 219.

[47] Peter A. Singer *et al.*, "Ethics and SARS: Lessons from Toronto" (2003) 327 British Medical Journal 1342.

that decisions had to be made, there were no diagnostic tests or therapeutic agents available and the causative agent was still unclear. Many key epidemiological features of SARS were unknown, including its duration of shedding, communicability and how long immunity was conferred. As a result, it was clear that decision-makers could not rely simply on science in their deliberations. Although public health decision-making always requires value analyses, the scientific uncertainty during SARS and the moral distress suffered by decision-makers, healthcare workers, patients and the public in the wake SARS, brought this aspect of decision-making to the fore.

Singer *et al.*'s ethical analysis of the SARS epidemic drew on elements of the above frameworks. The goal of the analysis was to use normative discourse to illuminate lessons learned, highlight areas where improvements could be made and indicate areas where further research was required. In the lessons learned, five key areas and ten ethical values were identified. The analysis assessed:

(1) the balance between public health interests and civil liberties with respect to quarantine decisions;

(2) the limits of privacy in personal information;

(3) the duty of health care workers to provide care, and the duty of institutions to support them;

(4) collateral damage, such as the restriction of care of others during the SARS outbreak; and

(5) global implications.

The ten key ethical values identified were: individual liberty; privacy; protection of the public from harm; protection of communities from undue stigmatization; proportionality; duty to provide care; reciprocity; equity; transparency; and solidarity.

Building on this work and drawing from the literature on battlefield triage ethics, Upshur *et al.* developed a framework to guide decision-making for pandemic influenza planning.[48] In addition to further articulating both procedural and substantive values identified by Singer *et al.*, it identifies four key ethical issues facing public health, governments and other pandemic planners:

(1) health workers' duty to provide care during a communicable disease outbreak;

---

[48]   Ross E.G. Upshur *et al.*, *Stand on Guard for Thee: Ethical Considerations in Preparedness Planning for Pandemic Influenza. A Report of the University of Toronto Joint Centre for Bioethics Pandemic Influenza Working Group* (Toronto: University of Toronto, 2005).

(2) restricting liberty in the interest of public health by measures such as quarantine;

(3) priority setting, including the allocation of scarce resources such as medicines; and

(4) global governance implications, such governments' responsibilities to their citizenry vs. their international obligations during infectious disease outbreaks of international significance.

Emmanuel and Wertheimer have attempted to provide a framework for deciding who should get an influenza vaccine first, based on what they call the life-cycle principle.[49] This principle is based on the idea that each person should have an opportunity to live through all the stages of life, and thus vaccines should be allocated in such a way as to maximize this principle.

These two examples of frameworks drawn from the ethics of pandemic influenza planning illustrate the different ways in which frameworks can be conceptualized. The framework presented by Upshur *et al.* does not argue for a particular stance; rather, it provides principles to procedurally and substantively guide deliberations by various moral communities. The Emmanuel and Wertheimer framework takes a prescriptive stance on the issue of vaccine allocation. Thus, frameworks can confer moral legitimacy on decisions based on their use in different ways. The Upshur *et al.* framework confers legitimacy to decisions based on a process of moral discernment and deliberation by its community of users; that is, a decision is morally justified to the extent that its authors have engaged with the elements of the framework and used them to inform their deliberations. This is called discursive legitimacy.[50, 51] The Emmanuel and Wertheimer framework depends on the credibility of the authors as moral authorities in the field, and claims to appeal to most people's moral intuitions. Whether or not this claim is true, it is apparent that the system of moral justification is different from that used by Upshur *et al.*

The use of frameworks in public health ethics is an important tool for both policy-makers and practitioners. Frameworks can be evaluative, facilitative or prescriptive, and the ways that they can impart moral legitimacy to decisions can vary. As such, further investigation into how

---

[49]   E.J. Emanuel & A. Wertheimer, "Public Health: Who Should Get Influenza Vaccine When Not All Can?" (2006) 312 Science 854.

[50]   J. Habermas, *Legitimation Crisis* (Boston: Beacon Press, 1975).

[51]   S. Benhabib, "Toward a Deliberative Model of Democratic Legitimacy" in S. Benhabib, ed., *Democracy and Difference* (Princeton: Princeton University Press, 1996).

frameworks can impart legitimacy or morally justify decisions in public health is warranted.

A different kind of framework has been developed by Benatar *et al.* that considers the ethical dimensions of public health at the international and global levels. In attempting to address the moral challenges posed by global health considerations, they have identified several values that need to be widely promoted: respect for all life and universal ethical principles; human rights, responsibilities and needs; equity; freedom; democracy; environmental ethics; and solidarity.[52] They have also suggested a way forward through five transformational approaches: developing a global state of mind; promoting long-term self-interest; striking a balance between optimism and pessimism about globalization and solidarity; strengthening capacity; and enhancing production of global public goods for health.

They propose that such progress could be initiated by expanding the discourse on ethics from interpersonal relationships to the ethics of relationships between institutions, and even to the ethics of relationships between nations. This will require promotion of a deeper understanding of citizenship in an interdependent world, commitment to an extended range of human rights, and new ways of thinking about ourselves, our relationship to others and to the ecological system. In addition, human rights should be linked to a broader moral agenda embracing the duty to meet essential human needs and to achieve greater social justice within and between nations. It is from this springboard that we move to an expanded discussion of public health ethics and its implications at the international and global levels.

VII.   CONSIDERATIONS AT A GLOBAL LEVEL

An account of current issues in public health ethics would be incomplete if it did not recognize the increasingly global nature of health and public health obligations. As both the HIV and SARS pandemics illustrate, there is an intimate and irrevocable sense that the health of humanity is linked. Reciprocal understanding, and solidarity and collaboration in action, are crucial. In recent years there has been an outpouring of generous philanthropic donations directed at improving the health of the poor — with the Bill and Melinda Gates Foundation setting a leading example with donations in the region of $450 million (all figures in this section are in US dollars). However, consideration of the global dimensions of public health, with attendant concern for issues in justice,

---

[52]   Solomon R. Benatar, Abdallah S. Daar & Peter A. Singer, "Global Health Ethics: The Rationale for Mutual Caring" (2003) International Affairs 107 at 109.

equity and the distribution of wealth is incomplete without an analysis of the forces that determine the shape and form of the contemporary global economic landscape.

Despite a more than six-fold increase in the global economy over the past 55 years, the gap between the richest 20 per cent and the poorest 20 per cent of the world's population has widened continuously from nine times at the beginning of the 20th century to over 70 times by 1997, and even more since then. Per capita global wealth increased from $77,000 in 1990 to $96,000 in 2000 (in 2000 constant $), and the number of billionaires in the world increased from 423 in 1996 to 946 in 2006.[53] In 2005, approximately 2.7 billion people lived on less than $2 per day — a rise of 10 per cent since 1987.[54] Many of these people live under conditions of absolute poverty, in circumstances so limited by malnutrition, lack of access to safe water and basic health care, illiteracy, disease, squalid surroundings, high infant mortality and low life expectancy as to be beneath any reasonable definition of decent human living conditions.

Health and poverty are intimately related. Poverty impairs health and poor health sustains poverty. Growing inequalities in the burden of disease and in premature deaths are associated with these growing economic disparities.[55] About one-third of all human deaths each year are related to poverty. Moreover, disparities in wealth are no longer distributed along a "North-South" axis, but now apply within most countries, including the so-called highly developed.

Disparities in wealth and health are accompanied by distorted expenditure on health and medical research. Global expenditure on health amounted to over $2.2 trillion per year in the early 2000s (and has continue to increase since then) with 87 per cent of this expenditure on a mere 16 per cent of the world's population who bear about 7 per cent of the global burden of disease expressed in disability adjusted life years. Annual per capita expenditure on health care around the world ranges from less than $15 to over $5,000. Of more than $80 billion spent annually on medical research, about 90 per cent is devoted to those diseases that account for 10 per cent of the global burden of disease. Of 1,393 new drugs marketed from 1975 to 1999, only 16 were for tropical diseases or tuberculosis. These statistics suggest that medicine and health care as universal moral endeavours are "off the rails".

---

[53]   J.H. Dobryznski, "International philanthropy" (2007) Carnegie Reporter Fall 34.

[54]   Global Health Watch, *Global Health Watch 2005-2006*, online: <http://www.ghwatch.org/2005_report.php>.

[55]   Solomon R. Benatar, "Global Disparities in Health and Human Rights: A Critical Commentary" (1998) 88 American Journal of Public Health 295.

During the second half of the 20th century, the evolution towards a globalized economy has perpetuated and aggravated centuries of exploitative processes that have facilitated the enrichment of some people at the expense of others, both within and between nations. Such exploitation is made possible by processes that devalue and dehumanize the "other" and relegates them to lower standards of life. Over the past 50 years, covert erosion of the economies of many poor countries under the impact of neo-liberal economic policies driving globalization has further obstructed real development and has prevented achievement of widespread access to even basic health care for billions of people.[56] Average national per capita GNP has risen to above $25,000 in some countries while remaining static or dropping to less than $200 in others, and similar disparities can be observed *within* many societies.

The debt owed to rich countries by poor countries amounted to $2.2 trillion in 1997. However, this debt was largely developed and perpetuated through arms trading and ill-conceived "development projects" that did more harm than good and usually benefited developed nations more than those they were allegedly developing. Such debt can never be repaid and perpetuates economic slavery and human misery in more covert guises.[57] Welch describes the links between debt and health as follows:

> The overwhelming debt burdens of poor countries is a major contributor to the crisis that grips the economies of most developing countries today. For the 41 most heavily indebted poor countries, total external debt rose from $55 billion in 1980 to $215 billion by 1995. Debt has continued to climb in most countries. African governments alone now have $350 billion of foreign debt and they have to spend two-fifths of their revenues to service it. As a result, governments have been forced to divert scarce resources away from spending on health, education, environmental protection and other vital social services and instead dedicate them to pay what are essentially unpayable debts. Because of this process, Jubilee 2000 says 13 children die every minute in the 40 poorest nations.[58]

Foreign development aid has also been falling over recent years and is increasingly directed towards humanitarian aid rather than towards sustainable development.[59] Development aid to Africa in 2000 amounted

---

[56]   Richard Falk, *Predatory Globalization: A Critique* (Malden, MA: Polity Press, 1999).

[57]   Ronald Labonte *et al.*, *Fatal Indifference: The G8, Africa and Global Health* (Ottawa: Juta Academic, 2004); Ann Pettifor, *Debt, the Most Potent Form of Slavery: A Discussion of the Role of Western Lending Policies in Supporting the Economies of Poor Countries* (London: Christian Aid Society, Debt Crisis Network, 1996).

[58]   Carol Welch, "A World In Chains: Developing Countries and Debt" (2000), online: The Ecologist <http://findarticles.com/p/articles/mi_m2465/is_6_30/ai_65653648>.

[59]   Carol Lancaster, *Transforming Foreign Aid: United States Assistance in the 21st Century* (Washington, D.C.: Institute for International Economics, 2000).

to $21.2 billion, while sub-Saharan African debt in 2002 was $275.6 billion.

It is against this background that many people in wealthy countries (and many emerging middle-class people elsewhere) are increasingly suffering from diseases of affluence (*e.g.*, obesity, diabetes and cardiovascular diseases),[60] while new infectious diseases with the potential to spread throughout the whole world have been emerging over the past 30 years. These signs of change in the global system result from complex processes that include population growth, rapid urbanization, inequitable economic growth with widening disparities in wealth and health, over- and under-consumption of food and energy, and war and ethnic conflict with resulting migration and displacement of millions of people. Additional forces include profound poverty traps, altered relationships with animals, ecological degradation and a growing informal economy in which drugs, people and sex are traded across the world.[61] Sub-Saharan Africa has been most adversely affected.[62] In a sub-continent where there are 13 million displaced people, 14 million AIDS orphans, 475 million living on less than $2 per day and hunger affecting 40 million, this situation can be viewed as a modern version of the exploitation that characterized the era of slavery.

As Pogge has argued, because wealthy nations and their citizens are implicated in the generation and maintenance of social injustice and poverty, they need to face their responsibilities to alleviate the lives of those most adversely affected.[63] These are crucial challenges for public health ethics. To understand the magnitude of the challenge, we need to understand the dominant values that have shaped our world.

In order to make progress, it is necessary to be able to reflect deeply on the upstream forces that shape human health and well-being, and to attempt to develop constructive solutions. Some illustrative work includes recent publications on the impact on health of international trade rules and the arms trade, and the way in which patterns of wealth and poverty are being locked into place through the "Washington Consensus".[64, 65]

---

[60]   Abdallah S. Daar *et al.*, "Grand Challenges in Chronic Non-Communicable Diseases" (2007) 450 Nature 494.

[61]   Solomon R. Benatar, "The Coming Catastrophe in International Health: An Analogy with Lung Cancer" (2002) LVI Journal of the Canadian Institution of International Affairs 595.

[62]   Peter Schwab, *Africa: A Continent Self-Destructs* (New York: Palgrave, 2001).

[63]   Thomas W. Pogge, "Responsibilities for Poverty-Related Ill Health" (2002) 16 Ethics & International Affairs 71.

[64]   G. Sreenivasan & S.R. Benatar, eds., "Challenges for Global Health in the 21st Century: Some Upstream Considerations" (2006) 27 Theoretical Medicine and Bioethics 3 (Special Issue).

[65]   Italian Global Health Watch, "From Alma Ata to the Global Fund: The History of International Health Policy" (2008) 3 Social Medicine 36.

Jonathan Glover's description of repeated genocide across the world during the 20th century reminds us of the inhumanity of humans to fellow humans, and of how difficult it will be to change dominant ways of thinking. He concludes that it is only our moral imagination — our ability to imagine ourselves in the shoes of others — that could enable us to significantly alter our outlook and actions.[66]

Peter Singer (of Princeton University), in an extension of his previous work on poverty alleviation, asks what a global ethic means in an interdependent world, in which all are linked through exposure to the same atmosphere, global economy, international law, human rights and global community. He does so through a critical and provocative examination of climate change, the World Trade Organization's role, the concept of human rights, the place for humanitarian interventions and shortcomings in foreign aid. He develops the thesis that:

> ... how well we will come through the era of globalization (perhaps whether we come through it at all) will depend on how we respond ethically to the idea that we live in one world. For the rich nations not to take a global ethical viewpoint has long been seriously morally wrong. But now it is also, in the long term, a danger to their security.[67]

Booth, Dunne and Cox[68] remind us that "choice lies at the heart of ethics", that human choices are neither always free nor always determined. History, power, context and biology shape our choices, as do our powers of imagination and our capacity to choose rationally. Every choice also has a price. Politics and ethics are inseparable, like politics and power, and foreign policy should be understood as ethics in action — the challenge being to build a better world.

Crocker poses several questions about development ethics and globalization. What should be meant by development? In what direction and by what means should a society "develop"? Who is morally responsible for beneficial change? What are the obligations, if any, of rich societies to poor societies? How should globalization's impact and potential be assessed ethically?[69] Addressing these questions through the lens of public health ethics could shape new ways of looking at the world. It could also promote deeper understanding of what it means to be a citizen in an increasingly interdependent world and could promote the

---

[66]   Jonathan Glover, *Humanity: A Moral History of the Twentieth Century* (New Haven, CT: Yale University Press, 2000).

[67]   Peter Singer, *One World: The Ethics of Globalization* (New Haven, CT: Yale University Press, 2002).

[68]   Ken Booth, Tim Dunne & Michael Cox, eds., *How Might We Live? Global Ethics in the New Century* (New York: Cambridge University Press, 2001).

[69]   David A. Crocker, "Development Ethics and Globalisation" (2002) 22 Philosophy & Public Policy Quarterly 13.

embrace of renewed concepts of solidarity and concern for others, even those very distant from our own daily lives. New paradigms of thinking could both promote deeper insight into how complex systems function and facilitate novel approaches to international economic arrangements.

An ethical examination of the issues around global and local health disparities raises questions around equity, solidarity and social justice more broadly. Discourse in this domain can be guided by the use of public health ethics frameworks, yet to date the frameworks discussed in this chapter remain "untested" in the global context. The development of public health ethics frameworks that are robust enough to guide our thinking in the moral terrain of global public health have yet to be developed. While it may well be true that some of the values that have emerged from analyses of public health crises such as SARS have moral traction in this context, there is a need to be sensitive to the fact that different cultures and societies may place more moral weight on some values, and less on others. The only way to know this is to encourage a global dialogue on ethical issues in public health with a strong focus on what *public health as social justice* means in this era of globalization and pandemics.

VIII.   CONCLUSIONS

There is always a set of potential conflicts in public health and, hence, the need for balance between such things as collective and personal good, coercion and duty to care, and scientific uncertainty and necessity for action. Future scholarship and research is required to further the conceptual and theoretical basis of public health ethics. Empirical case studies are needed to evaluate the diversity of issues and practices specific to public health ethics. These should illuminate dimensions of public health deliberation at local, national and global levels. For instance, the debate about how best to roll-out anti-retroviral therapy in resource-poor settings to achieve the best public health effects while protecting human rights is illustrative of how the principles of public health ethics can be applied to such dilemmas.[70]

For public health ethics to mature as a discipline requires capacity building with specific attention to curriculum development and funding for research and development. Currently, public health ethics has been poorly represented on the course curricula of schools of public health, but this is rapidly changing. Finally, the use of moral imagination and

---

[70]   Solomon R. Benatar, "Facing Ethical Challenges in Rolling Out Antiretroviral Treatment in Resource-Poor Countries" (2006) 15 Cambridge Quarterly of Healthcare Ethics 322. Also see related articles in the same issue.

demonstration of political courage in an inequitable global economic landscape is required to transform public health ethics beyond a merely academic exercise.

3

RISK, CAUSATION AND PRECAUTION: UNDERSTANDING POLICY-MAKING REGARDING PUBLIC HEALTH RISKS

Kumanan Wilson*

I.   INTRODUCTION

In recent years, Canadian policy-makers have been forced to tackle various challenges related to public health risk, including the emergence of bovine spongiform encephalopathy ("BSE" or "mad cow disease"), West Nile virus and severe acute respiratory syndrome ("SARS"), as well as issues related to genetically modified foods and novel technologies with potential human health impacts. One of the fundamental challenges to establishing effective public health policies to address these problems is determining whether a risk does or does not exist. Often there are high levels of uncertainty surrounding the knowledge of the existence and magnitude of public health risks. In some instances, the presence of a risk is known, but the size of the risk is not. In other instances, the existence of a risk is purely theoretical. In most cases, taking action to protect against the risk does not come without substantial economic and, potentially, health costs.

How then do policy-makers go about making decisions regarding risk? Traditionally, policy-makers have been governed by the evidence-based paradigm to policy-making. According to this paradigm, establishing risk is essentially a question of establishing causation; in other words, determining whether exposure to a risk factor produces an adverse outcome.

Specialist in internal medicine and Associate Professor in the Departments of Medicine and Health Policy Management and Evaluation at the University of Toronto.

Establishing causation is a multi-step process and requires the following three questions to be answered: (1) Is there an association between treatment/exposure and effect? (2) Can this association be due to error (either bias or chance)? and (3) Is there other evidence to support a cause-effect relationship?

This evidence-based approach is fundamentally conservative and errs on the side of omitting the assertion of a potential causal interaction in exchange for reducing the possibility of assuming an erroneous causal relationship (in other words, an error of omission is better than an error of commission). Such a tradeoff, however, may not be appropriate in public health where causal interactions need to be identified early, often in the absence of complete evidence, to prevent large-scale, population-wide exposures to a harmful agent. The precautionary principle has emerged as an alternative decision-making paradigm, reflecting the need to be more aggressive in attributing causation even in the absence of complete evidence.

This chapter discusses these two approaches to decision-making, using case studies to illustrate their application. It begins by describing how a traditional, evidence-based approach would establish whether a causal relationship exists between an exposure and a health hazard. This section presents a case study of a link between a weight loss drug, fenfluramine, and a fatal form of lung disease. The limitations of the evidence-based approach are then discussed, as well as the value of using the precautionary principle to attribute potential causality based on more limited evidence. Potential pitfalls of the precautionary approach are also described. Finally, the chapter concludes with a reconciliation of the evidence-based and precautionary approaches.

II.   CHALLENGES IN DEVELOPING PUBLIC HEALTH POLICY

To understand the challenges in developing public health policy, it is important to first distinguish between public health and health care. One of the key differences is that public health is directed at improving the health of the population as a whole, while health care focuses on the individual patient. Emerging out of its patient-centred focus, formulation of health care policy must respect its fundamental ethical principles, which include autonomy, non-maleficence, beneficence and justice. In particular, the ethical principles of non-maleficence, or "first do no harm", and beneficence are consistent with the adoption of evidence-based approaches for health care delivery.[1] Evidence-based medicine is defined as "the conscientious, explicit, and judicious use of current best evidence in making decisions about the care of individual patients".[2] The paradigm evolved as an alternative to the traditional model of clinical decision-making, which was primarily experience or opinion based. Increasingly, there has been a call for the formulation of evidence-based health policy. Such an approach would require the formulation of clear health policy questions, the identification of all literature concerning the policy problem, an appraisal of the literature and utilization of the evidence to formulate "best policy". In public health, the benefits of adopting a strict, evidence-based approach are not as clear. This is primarily a consequence of the negative impact of delaying measures to protect against a risk, even if those measures may have harm and the existence and magnitude of the risk are uncertain. As a result, public health officials often face the formidable challenge of decision-making in the presence of considerable scientific uncertainty.

The challenge of decision-making concerning risk in public health is well illustrated by describing the response to several recent public health challenges. In the 1980s, public health officials in the United Kingdom identified a BSE outbreak, resulting from an infectious agent known as a prion. The condition was believed to have been transmitted from sheep to cows or from cow to cows through the practice of using sheep and cow remains (offal) in feed. In theory, ingestion of food products from affected cows could potentially infect humans, since the condition was already suspected to have crossed the species barrier once. The policy option to address the risk primarily consisted of introducing a feed ban to prevent transmission of the condition from cow to cow, and a cull of cattle with appropriate compensation for farmers. Despite the lack of definitive evidence of risk, a preliminary decision was made to proceed with the cull and compensation option. However, implementation of this approach was delayed, partly because the risk was theoretical and the cost of the measure was real. Eventually, evidence emerged that BSE could be transmitted to humans in the form of variant Creutzfeldt-Jakob disease (vCJD), a fatal neurodegenerative condition. The delay in implementing the large-scale cull was viewed as a failure of the policy response to the emerging threat. The delay is particularly important because, given the condition's potentially long latency period, it was uncertain as to what

---

[1]   R. Gillon, "Medical ethics: four principles plus attention to scope" (1994) 309 British Medical Journal 184.

[2]   David L Sackett *et al.*, "Evidence Based Medicine: what it is and what it isn't" (1996) 312 British Medical Journal 71.

percentage of the population may have been exposed and would subsequently develop vCJD.[3]

Also in the 1980s, several countries were confronted with the potential threat of new blood-borne infectious conditions, in particular hepatitis C and human immunodeficiency virus ("HIV"). In deciding how to manage these risks, the policy options available included deferring donations from individuals at high risk for the conditions and introducing blood testing of all donors. The latter option had important costs associated with it, and particularly in the case of hepatitis C, the testing would result in discarding many good donations due to the high false positive rate. Some policy-making processes determined that the uncertainty about possible HIV and hepatitis C transfusion transmission, combined with the potential loss of donations from less than perfect tests, indicated these tests should not be adopted. Unfortunately, in some instances where blood testing was delayed until clear evidence was available, thousands of individuals had already been infected.[4]

While the outcomes of these public health responses are known, the implications of more recent public health decisions are less certain. In managing the potential threat associated with genetically modified foods, policy-makers have had to balance the potential benefits of this new technology against theoretical harms that may result from it.[5] New infectious threats have also challenged decision-making. The progressive migration of West Nile virus across the Atlantic Ocean has forced countries to consider the use of potentially toxic pesticides to protect the population.[6] The threat of bioterrorism, as illustrated by the anthrax attacks following the September 2001 terrorist attack in the United States, forced that country to consider the use of smallpox vaccination. In doing so, policy-makers were again balancing a theoretical risk — bioterrorism — against the possible harm associated with small pox vaccination as a policy response.[7] Perhaps the most high profile public health challenge in

---

[3]   The Inquiry into BSE and variant CJD in the United Kingdom, *The BSE Inquiry Report* (London: Stationary Press, 2000), online: The BSE Inquiry Report: Home <http://www.bseinquiry.gov.uk> (Chair: Lord Phillips of Worth Matravers).

[4]   Commission of Inquiry on the Blood System in Canada, *Final Report. Commission of Inquiry on the Blood System in Canada: Towards a New Blood System*, Volume 3, Part VI (Ottawa: Canadian Government Publishing, 1997) (Justice Horace Krever).

[5]   The Royal Society of Canada, *Elements of Precaution: Recommendations for the Regulation of Food Biotechnology in Canada* (Ottawa: The Royal Society of Canada, 2001), online: The Royal Society of Canada: Expert Panel on the Future of Food Biotechnology <http://www.rsc.ca/index.php?lang_id=1&page_id=119>.

[6]   Barbara Sibbald, "Larvicide Debate Marks Start of Another West Nile Virus Summer" (2003) 168 (11) Canadian Medical Association Journal 1455.

[7]   Anthony S. Fauci, "Smallpox Vaccination Policy — The Need for Dialogue" (2002) 346 New Eng. J. Med. 1319.

recent years has been the emergence of SARS, which represented a new infectious condition about which little was known but which appeared initially to be both highly infectious and pathogenic. Decision-making to manage SARS had to consider the use of such coercive measures as quarantine and travel advisories; measures which had clear non-physical harms such as isolation and economic impact.[8]

All these policy responses demonstrate the need to formulate policy in advance of clear evidence about risk. They put forth the question as to what exactly is the appropriate role of evidence in the policy process? When should policy-makers consider the evidence of causation substantial enough to act on it? Under what circumstances would it be premature to address a potential risk? The remainder of this chapter will examine the two dominant paradigms governing decision-making on public health risks: evidence-based models and the precautionary principle. To explain these models, some discussion of statistical concepts and epidemiological research models is required, which may be unfamiliar to some readers. To assist in explaining these concepts, both text and charts are provided.

III. ESTABLISHING CAUSATION — THE EVIDENCE-BASED APPROACH

Evidence-based approaches are often used to establish causation, a central issue in public health policy-making concerning risk. These approaches rely on a hierarchy of evidence, with higher levels of evidence considered to be less susceptible to bias. To illustrate how a strict evidence-based approach would be applied to public health, the case study of a link between a weight loss agent, fenfluramine, and pulmonary hypertension is examined.

Primary pulmonary hypertension is a disease of the blood vessels in the lungs that produces an increase in the blood pressure of these vessels. The condition characteristically occurs in women in their 30s and 40s. Progressive elevation of pulmonary blood pressure in affected persons eventually results in impairment of the right side of the heart (which pumps blood to the pulmonary vessels). Individuals with severe pulmonary hypertension who develop right-sided heart failure have a life expectancy of less than one year. There is no clearly effective, long-term treatment for the condition other than removing potential causes of the

---

[8]   National Advisory Committee on SARS and Public Health, *Learning from SARS: Renewal of Public Health in Canada* (Ottawa: Health Canada, 2003) (Chair: Dr. D. Naylor), online: <http://www.phac-aspc.gc.ca/publicat/sars-sras/pdf/sars-e.pdf>.

elevated pulmonary pressure or considering the patient for a lung transplant.[9]

In the 1960s, policy-makers became concerned that drugs used to help patients lose weight could cause pulmonary hypertension. During this time, the European introduction of a weight-loss agent known as aminorex was associated with a ten-fold increase in pulmonary hypertension. In the 1990s, particular attention was focused on the dietary agent fenfluramine as a potential cause of pulmonary hypertension.[10] Various reports linking the drug with the disease emerged; for example, two people taking a dietary supplement containing fenfluramine were diagnosed with pulmonary hypertension and a study reported that 15 of 73 individuals with pulmonary hypertension had taken fenfluramine. In the face of this information, policy-makers were confronted with two questions: (1) What level of evidence is sufficient to establish a causal relationship between ingestion of fenfluramine and the development of pulmonary hypertension?; and (2) At what point should measures be instituted to protect the public against this risk?

The following sections provide a detailed description of how causality is established. Readers who do not require this level of detail may proceed to the section entitled "Summary: Does Fenfluramine Cause Pulmonary Hypertension?".

(a) Determining if an Association Exists

The first step to determine if a causal relationship exists between two factors is to find evidence of an association. This requires a close examination of information that suggests the possibility of an association. One way to answer this question is to summarize information in a table to allow for a visual assessment of whether or not an association between an exposure and outcome has been demonstrated in the study.

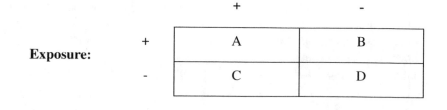

Outcome:

		+	-
Exposure:	+	A	B
	-	C	D

[9]   Lewis J. Rubin, "Primary Pulmonary Hypertension" (1997) 336 New Eng. J. Med. 111.
[10]   Alfred P. Fishman, "Aminorex to Fen/Phen: An Epidemic Foretold" (1999) 99 Circulation 156.

Using this table, it becomes apparent that many decisions are based on evidence summarized either by Block A (individuals exposed who develop an outcome), Block A and B alone (individuals exposed who develop an outcome versus exposed individuals who do not develop the outcome) or Blocks A and C alone (individuals with an outcome who are exposed to the agent of interest compared to individuals with an outcome who are not exposed to the agent of interest). An example of decision-making based solely on Block A would be relying on the report of two individuals who had taken fenfluramine subsequently developed pulmonary hypertension. An example of decision-making based on only Blocks A and C would be basing a decision on the report of 73 patients with pulmonary hypertension, 15 of whom had taken fenfluramine.

However, to determine if an association exists between exposure to fenfluramine and development of pulmonary hypertension, information from all four boxes is needed. Specifically, the following information is needed: of all those exposed to fenfluramine, how many individuals have developed pulmonary hypertension and how many have not (Blocks A and B), and of all those *not* exposed to fenfluramine, how many individuals have developed pulmonary hypertension and how many have not (Blocks C and D)?

Given that the information from the two reports lacks a control population, additional research is needed to establish more clearly whether an association exists between fenfluramine and pulmonary hypertension. A study by Abenhaim and colleagues presents the results of a case-control study that examined 95 patients with pulmonary hypertension and 355 healthy controls matched for sex, age and general practice.[11] The investigators determined what proportion of individuals in each group had taken weight loss agents in the previous year. The results of the study can be summarized in the following table:

---

[11]   Lucien Abenhaim *et al.*, "Appetite-Suppressant Drugs and the Risk of Primary Pulmonary Hypertension" (1996) 335 New Eng. J. Med. 609.

Outcome:

Development of Pulmonary Hypertension

		+	-	**Total**
Exposure: Anorectic Agents	+	30	26	235
	-	65	329	210
Total		95	355	

According to the results of this case-control study, the odds that an individual with pulmonary hypertension had taken a weight loss agent are 30:65 (0.46). The odds for a person without the disease are 26:329 (0.079). Therefore, individuals who have pulmonary hypertension have nearly a six-fold higher chance (technically an increased odds) of having taken a weight loss agent compared to those without the disease. Based on this study, it appears that an association exists between pulmonary hypertension and weight loss drugs.

(b)   Determining the Nature of the Association

The next step to assessing causality is to determine the nature of the association observed in the study. Four distinct possibilities exist to explain the observed association: (1) the observed association is a consequence of chance; (2) the observed association is a consequence of bias; (3) fenfluramine causes pulmonary hypertension; and (4) pulmonary hypertension predisposes towards the use of fenfluramine.

To sort through these four possibilities, the study must first be examined for sources of error, then additional supporting evidence of a causal relationship must be identified. In general, studies are susceptible to two forms of error: systematic and unsystematic. Systematic error, also known as bias, refers to the existence of a variable that consistently distorts the relationship between the two factors of interest towards one direction. Unsystematic error refers to the likelihood that the results of the study occurred by chance.

(i)   Systematic Error or Bias

Bias can occur at two points in the conduct of a study: the selection of subjects and the measurement of study results. Selection bias occurs when subjects in one group (either the exposed group or the control) are systematically different from those in the other group. This systematic difference introduces the potential for confounding — the presence of a third variable related to both the exposure and the result that alters the association between the two. For instance, epidemiological studies have determined an association between cigarette smoking and liver cirrhosis.[12] However, liver disease is probably not a direct effect of smoking but rather occurs because smokers are more likely to consume larger quantities of alcohol. Thus, alcohol is an important confounding variable.

In the fenfluramine study, it is possible that patients who take fenfluramine are obese and obesity is a risk factor for pulmonary hypertension. As a consequence, obesity is a potential confounding variable that could increase the likelihood of observing an association where one does not exist.

Measurement bias occurs when the observations of outcomes in one group are systematically different from observations in the other group. For example, patients who have taken fenfluramine may be more likely to be diagnosed with pulmonary hypertension because they have sought medical assessment after hearing media reports about potential adverse effects of the drugs. The diagnosis may have been less likely to have been suspected in individuals not taking the medication.

Systematic error is controlled primarily through study design. Several different study designs are used to determine if an association exists between two variables. The strongest study design for identifying a causal association is a randomized, controlled trial. This form of study reduces selection bias by randomly allocating subjects to either exposure or control groups. Randomization maximizes the likelihood that known and unknown confounders will be equally distributed between the two groups.

Randomized, controlled trials often cannot be conducted due to cost, logistical or ethical concerns; therefore, public health officials must then rely on observational studies. The observational study with the highest level of validity is a well-designed controlled prospective cohort study in which two groups of individuals are followed for a period of time. Of these two groups, one will be exposed to the agent of interest and the other will not. Outcomes in both groups can then be compared. When the

---

[12]   N.J. Wald & A.K. Hackshaw, "Cigarette Smoking: An Epidemiological Overview" (1996) 52 British Medical Bulletin 3.

outcome of interest is rare or the latency period between exposure and outcome is long, a case-control design is often utilized. In this form of study, investigators begin with individuals who have the condition of interest and healthy controls and then identify what proportion of each group has received the exposure. As efficiency is improved with each of these study designs, the potential for bias also increases.

In the fenfluramine case-control study, the investigators first ensured that the individuals with pulmonary hypertension and the healthy controls were similar with respect to age and sex. They also attempted to adjust for the impact of potential confounding variables. These variables included the following: systemic hypertension, use of cocaine or intravenous drugs, smoking status, high body-mass index, weight-loss behaviour, use of thyroid extracts and possible exposure to other anorectic drugs.[13]

(ii)   Unsystematic Error or Chance

Unsystematic error is an inaccurate association due to chance.[14] Researchers and policy-makers typically must tolerate some degree of uncertainty in examining associations between risks and adverse health outcomes. Factors that influence tolerable levels of uncertainty include: the level of exposure of the risk factor; the potential harm caused by the exposure; the potential for treating the harm caused by the exposure; and the cost, both in economic and health terms, of removing the exposure. Thus, for widespread exposures where the exposure causes a serious adverse effect that is not treatable and the cost of removing the exposure is minimal, a much greater level of uncertainty is acceptable for policy-makers to take action to protect against the risk. This will become an important point in discussing the role of the precautionary principle in influencing decision-making.

For the case of fenfluramine and pulmonary hypertension, the exposure is limited, the impact is severe, the condition is not treatable and the economic cost to society of removing the exposure would be minimal. There is a health consequence of removing the exposure because severe obesity is an important health risk in and of itself. However, evidence indicates that fenfluramine only produces a small weight loss and there are other strategies for losing weight. Given the harms of the exposure, the

---

[13]   It is possible that other unmeasured or unknown confounding variables could still distort the relationship between fenfluramine and pulmonary hypertension.

[14]   The likelihood of this type of error occurring in a study can be identified through statistical tests and is often provided as a "p-value". Traditionally, a p-value is considered significant if it is less than 0.05. This refers to the fact that the likelihood of the results occurring by chance is less than 5 per cent. Of course, there is nothing magical about 5 per cent as a cut-off for significance.

level of certainty provided by the study results would be adequate for demonstrating the existence of an association between fenfluramine and pulmonary hypertension.

(c) Identifying Supporting Evidence of a Causal Relationship

In order to be comfortable about the presence and nature of an association, several supporting pieces of evidence are also required. These are, in approximate order of importance: (1) Did the cause precede the effect? (2) How strong was the association observed? (3) Is increasing exposure more likely to lead to disease? (4) Is there evidence from several different studies (of differing design and study populations) showing the same association? (5) Does withdrawal of the cause result in loss of the effect? (6) Does exposure to the cause result only in the one effect? and (7) Is there a biological model that can explain the causal relationship?

One study alone cannot examine all these questions; rather, evidence is required from several studies. Ideally, this information would be found in a systematic review, "the consolidation of research that incorporates a critical assessment and evaluation of research that attempts to address a focused clinical question using methods designed to reduce the likelihood of bias".[15] In the absence of such a study, policy-makers must identify the information themselves using systematic techniques that will reduce bias in the selection of studies, assess the quality of the studies and evaluate the results

(i) Did the Cause Precede the Effect?

For obvious reasons, for a true causal association to exist, the purported causal exposure must occur before the effect. In the case of fenfluramine and pulmonary hypertension, this would require establishing that individuals with pulmonary hypertension had ingested fenfluramine before the onset of the lung condition. While this may appear to be easy to establish, often conditions exist in pre-clinical stages prior to their clinical diagnosis.

Generally speaking, cohort studies are better than case-control studies at examining this question. However, because pulmonary hypertension is a rare disease, most studies investigating an association have been case-control studies. In these studies, it is possible that

---

[15] Gordon Guyatt & Drummond Rennie, eds., *Users' Guides to the Medical Literature: A Manual for Evidence-Based Clinical Practice* (Chicago: American Medical Association Press, 2002) at 691.

individuals with pulmonary hypertension may have had the condition before ingesting fenfluramine. This would be particularly true in severely obese individuals who are at higher risk for pulmonary hypertension.

(ii)   How Strong was the Association?

In general, the stronger the magnitude of the association, the more likely it is that the association represents a cause and effect relationship. The higher the quality of the study design, the lower the magnitude of effect necessary to be comfortable that a causal relationship exists. In observational studies, to be sufficiently confident that the association is true and not due to bias, the magnitude of effect needs to be in the order of two to four times greater in the group receiving the intervention than in the control group. By this criterion, the odds ratio of 6.3 in the fenfluramine study is sufficiently strong, suggesting the existence of a causal association.

(iii)   Is Increasing Exposure more Likely to Lead to Disease?

Support for a causal association is strengthened if studies demonstrate that increasing exposure is more likely to produce the effect observed. An example of this would be the evidence of increased asbestos exposure and increased likelihood of developing fibrotic lung disease.[16] In the fenfluramine case study, the use of anorectic drugs for less than three months was associated with an odds ratio of 1.8, and the use of the drugs for longer than three months was associated with an odds ratio of 23.1, suggesting a strong association with duration of exposure.

(iv)   Is there Evidence from Other Studies Supporting the Association?

If the association between an intervention and an outcome is found in several studies in different populations, the likelihood that the association represents a causal relationship is increased. There have been few epidemiological studies examining an association between fenfluramine and pulmonary hypertension. However, several case reports exist, demonstrating an apparent temporal association between ingestion of the drug and development of the disease.[17]

---

[16]   Gregory R. Wagner, "Asbestosis and Silicosis" (1997) 349 Lancet 1311.

[17]   H.M. Pouwels et al., "Pulmonary Hypertension and Fenfluramine" (1990) 3 European Respiratory Journal 606; Douglas G. Munor et al., "Pulmonary Hypertension and Fenfluramine" (1981) 283 British Medical Journal 881; F. Brenot et al., "Primary Pulmonary Hypertension and Fenfluramine Use" (1993) 70 British Heart Journal 537; M. Fahlen et al., "Phenformin and Pulmonary Hypertension" (1973) 35 British Heart Journal 824.

(v)   Does Withdrawal of the Cause Result in Loss of the Effect?

If removal of the potential causative agent results in a loss of the effect, the likelihood of causal association is increased. For example, the fact that smoking cessation reduces the risk of cardiovascular disease points to a causal link between smoking and cardiovascular disease.[18] Similarly, case reports have found that pulmonary hypertension improves upon cessation of anorectic drugs and one report found that the condition recurred with re-exposure to these agents.[19] This is strong evidence in favour of causality.

(vi)   Does Exposure to the Cause Result Only in the One Effect?

Generally, the causal argument is strengthened if the exposure only results in one effect, although this is a weaker level of evidence to establish causation. In addition to pulmonary hypertension, fenfluramine is also associated with the development of cardiac valvular lesions,[20] which are likely caused by the same pathophysiological process that produces pulmonary hypertension. However, even if the cause results in several different effects, the possibility of a causal relationship cannot be ruled out. Cigarette smoking is again a good example, as it is associated with several different health conditions (including cancer, lung disease and cardiovascular disease) and is believed to be causally linked to each of them.[21]

(vii)   Is There a Credible Biological Hypothesis That Can Explain the Causal Relationship?

Ideally, the cause and effect relationship makes biological "sense". This, however, is considered by some to be a weak level of evidence to support a causal hypothesis, primarily because we often change our biological hypotheses to support the associations we observe. There are several biological models that could explain the development of pulmonary hypertension with ingestion of fenfluramine. One is that

---

[18]   U.S. Surgeon General, U.S. Department of Health and Human Services, *The Health Consequences of Smoking: Cardiovascular Disease: A Report of the Surgeon General* (Rockville, MD: Public Health Service, Office of the Surgeon General, Department of Health and Human Services, 1983) (DHHS Publication No. (PHS) 84-50204).

[19]   Douglas G. Munor *et al.*, "Pulmonary Hypertension and Fenfluramine" (1981) 283 British Medical Journal 881.

[20]   Heidi M. Connolly *et al.*, "Valvular Heart Disease Associated with Fenfluramine-Phentermine" (1997) 337 New Eng. J. Med. 581 (correction published (1997) 337 (24) New Eng. J. Med. 1783).

[21]   R. Doll *et al.*, "Mortality in Relation to Smoking: 40 Years' Observations on Male British Doctors" (1994) 309 British Medical Journal 901.

fenfluramine acts by elevating serotonin levels and serotonin can cause the blood vessels in the lung to constrict. This, in turn, could trigger a process that obliterates the capillaries, leading to pulmonary hypertension. Furthermore, there is evidence that other anorectic drugs can produce pulmonary hypertension, suggesting the condition may be common to the entire class of drugs.

(d) Summary: Does Fenfluramine Cause Pulmonary Hypertension?

Overall, epidemiological evidence supports the assertion that fenfluramine causes pulmonary hypertension. Specifically, the study identified an association between the exposure and the disease. Potential for bias existed in the conduct of the study, but investigators made efforts to control some of these sources of bias. The magnitude of association in the study was sufficiently large and there was a high level of certainty regarding the existence of an association. Other case reports and case series also suggested a link between the exposure and the development of pulmonary hypertension and demonstrated evidence of reversibility upon removal of the exposure. The study also provided strong evidence of a dose response relationship.

While a causal relationship appears likely, the absolute magnitude of the impact still needs to be determined. Both relative risk and odds ratios are relative measures of association. The actual, absolute, impact in terms of number of individuals affected will depend on the prevalence of the condition. Assuming that the relative risk of people developing pulmonary hypertension is approximately equivalent to the odds ratio, a reasonable assumption in cases of rare diseases, then the impact of the exposure on the overall burden of disease is equivalent to this value multiplied by the prevalence of the condition in the study. In the study, the baseline incidence of the condition was one in 500,000 and the odds ratio was approximately six. Therefore, those taking fenfluramine would have an expected risk of approximately six in 500,000 and the absolute increase in risk would be five in 500,000. This increase in risk would have to be weighed against the potential benefits of the drug.

Using this rationale and despite the evidence of causality, the U.S. Food and Drug Administration approved the use of fenfluramine as a weight loss agent. A few years later, a New England Journal of Medicine study reported that individuals taking these medications were developing heart valve lesions. In September 1997, the FDA withdrew the use of these drugs.[22] In Canada, when evidence of fenfluramine cardiac toxicity became apparent, policy-makers issued a warning against the use of the agent.[23] Prior to this warning, the drug had been approved for short-term treatment of obesity (less than three months).

As an interesting footnote, the issue of the New England Journal of Medicine in which the fenfluramine study was published contained an editorial arguing that while the relative risk of pulmonary hypertension was substantially increased, the absolute increase in risk was small. As such, removing the use of an agent, which could address the major health problem of obesity, was not recommended.[24] A later issue of the New England Journal of Medicine revealed the authors of this editorial had undisclosed financial links to manufacturers of dietary supplements and stated the editorial would not have been published if this had been known.[25]

IV. PROBLEMS WITH EVIDENCE-BASED DECISION-MAKING UNDER CONDITIONS OF SCIENTIFIC UNCERTAINTY

The fenfluramine case demonstrates the classic evidence-based decision-making model for formulating policy on issues of risk. This model, however, has some important limitations in the public health context. In particular, the question arises as to whether, in a widespread exposure with a potentially serious adverse outcome, policy-makers should act on preliminary data suggesting a potential association. For example, in the case of fenfluramine and pulmonary hypertension, were the original case studies adequate to trigger action to restrict the use of fenfluramine, particularly given the evidence of pulmonary hypertension associated with the use of other weight loss agents? Was the well-designed, case-control study adequate to imply a causal relationship? Once a causal association is established or not established, what are the appropriate policies to address the potential risk? Answering these

---

[22]   U.S. Food and Drug Administration, News Release, F97-32 "FDA Announces Withdrawal of Fenfluramine and Dexfenfluramine" (15 September 1997), online: <http://www.fda.gov/bbs/topics/NEWS/NEW00591.html>.

[23]   Health Canada, News Release/Warning, 1997-52 "Warning not to use products containing fenfluramine (PONDERAL, PONDERAL) or dexfenfluramine (REDUX)" (15 September 1997). For access to this document, see online: <http://www.hc-sc.gc.ca/ahc-asc/media/advisories-avis/1997-eng.php>.

[24]   JoAnn E. Manson & Gerald A. Faich, "Pharmacotherapy for Obesity — Do the Benefits Outweigh the Risks?" (1996) 335 New Eng. J. Med. 659.

[25]   Marcia Angell & Jerome P. Kassirer, "Editorials and Conflicts of Interest" (1996) 335 New Eng. J. Med. 1055.

questions requires us to examine the paradigms that influence our use of scientific information.

(a) Challenges in the Use of Scientific Information to Establish Risk

One of the primary limitations to the evidence-based paradigm for establishing risk is that there is often an absence of high quality data on risk. According to evidence-based principles, the "gold standard" study design for establishing causality is the randomized controlled trial ("RCT"). This chapter has already described some of the limitations to relying on RCT evidence to establish risk. Primarily, it is neither ethical nor moral to conduct this form of study to establish risk because it would require knowingly exposing individuals to a potentially harmful agent. Therefore, policy-makers must rely on other, non-experimental evidence to establish causation in questions of risk. Observational studies such as cohort studies and case-control studies have been employed in the past to demonstrate the harms associated with cigarette smoking and other exposures. Of these, the well-designed controlled cohort study is the form of study design least susceptible to bias. However, these studies are logistically challenging to conduct for rare conditions with long latency periods between exposure and onset of disease. In these instances, case-control studies may be more useful. Weaker study designs that have been employed to establish causation include ecological designs (for example, time series) and case series.[26] However, as this chapter has described, these study designs are susceptible to bias and are most useful for generating hypotheses. When no epidemiological evidence exists, individuals may turn to evidence suggested by case reports, from animal

---

[26]   There are a variety of "levels of evidence" rating scales for determining the quality of evidence suggesting causal associations. Randomized controlled trials are considered the highest level of evidence. In this experimental study design, individuals are unpredictably assigned to either a study group or a control group. The use of randomization maximizes the likelihood that other variables (confounders) that could affect the association between intervention and outcome are equally allocated between the intervention and the control group. Among non-experimental study designs, the prospective controlled cohort is considered the highest quality of evidence. In this study, individuals who are exposed and unexposed controls are followed prospectively and the rates of outcomes in each group are then compared. When duration between exposure and outcome is long or the outcome is rare, researchers often rely on case-control studies. In this study design, investigators begin with individuals who have the outcome of interest and unaffected controls. They then retrospectively compare the odds of those with the outcome of interest having been exposed to the odds of those without the outcome of interest having been exposed. Just below these observational study designs are ecological studies. In these forms of studies, investigators look at aggregate exposures, either in a time period (time-series analysis) or in a region (cross-sectional analyses) to determine if there is an association between incidence/prevalence of exposure and incidence/prevalence of outcome.

evidence or biological models. However, there are substantial dangers in relying on these forms of evidence as more than hypothesis generating.

Despite these evidence guides, policy-makers can still face difficulties in determining when a risk moves from being theoretical to real. Often biological models or animal models may suggest potential risk, but there is no higher-level epidemiological evidence supporting the existence of the risk. In some instances, this could simply be because the studies have not yet been conducted. This is often the case with new technologies and new exposures in which harm may take many years to manifest. For example, when BSE was discovered in the United Kingdom, concern arose that the condition may have been transmittable to humans. This concern was based primarily on biological hypotheses, as there were no documented cases of bovine to human transmission.[27] Several years later, this theoretical risk was believed to have become a real risk when the Lancet published a case series of ten individuals with a variant form of Creutzfeldt-Jakob disease.[28] The infectious agent in these individuals was subsequently identified as being the same infectious agent as in BSE.[29]

Policy-makers may also be confronted with a scenario in which lower levels of epidemiological evidence suggest a risk even though higher levels of available evidence do not suggest an association. The current controversy surrounding the measles, mumps and rubella vaccine ("MMR") provides an example. A 1998 Lancet study presented a case series, which was highly criticized for its methodology, of several children who developed a variant form of autism soon after receiving the MMR vaccine.[30] The study hypothesized that a variant form of autism may be associated with the MMR vaccine, which prompted many parents in the U.K. not to have their children vaccinated with the combined vaccine, thereby contributing to the emergence of measles outbreaks.[31] Vaccine refusal has continued despite the fact that several "higher level" epidemiological studies have revealed no evidence of an association.[32]

---

[27] The Inquiry into BSE and variant CJD in the United Kingdom, *The BSE Inquiry Report*, Volumes 3-5 (London: Stationary Press, 2000), online: The BSE Inquiry Report: Home <http://www.bseinquiry.gov.uk> (Chair: Lord Phillips of Worth Matravers).

[28] R.G. Will *et al.*, "A New Variant of Creutzfeldt-Jakob Disease in the UK" (1996) 347 Lancet 921.

[29] Moira E. Bruce *et al.*, "Transmissions to Mice Indicate that 'New Variant' CJD is Caused by the BSE Agent" (1997) 389 Nature 498.

[30] Wakefield A.J. *et al.*, "Ileal-Lymphoid-Nodular Hyperplasia, Non-Specific Colitis, and Pervasive Developmental Disorder in Children" (1998) 351 Lancet 637.

[31] Zosia Kmietowicz, "Government Launches Intensive Media Campaign on MMR" (2002) 324 British Medical Journal 383 (News).

[32] Kumanan Wilson *et al.*, "Association of Autistic Spectrum Disorder and the Measles, Mumps, and Rubella Vaccine: A Systematic Review of Current Epidemiological Evidence" (2003) 157 Archives of Pediatrics & Adolescent Medicine 628.

There are many reasons why the debate continues, including lack of trust of public health authorities and the public's aversion to a potentially catastrophic risk exposure.

On a purely scientific level, ruling out rare effects with epidemiological studies can pose significant challenges due to issues of statistical power.[33] This is also a particularly challenging issue in the context of genetic susceptibility. For example, on a population-wide level no link may be found between an exposure and an outcome. However, a small minority may be genetically predisposed to react adversely to an exposure and, if a study were conducted on this population, an association would be identified.[34] Scientists have argued that individuals who developed pulmonary hypertension from weight loss drugs were genetically susceptible to the exposure. At present, there are substantial limitations in our ability to identify genetically susceptible populations. These are primarily related to the ability of scientists to recognize which genes, combinations of genes or gene/environment interactions combine to produce susceptibility.

(b) Levels of Uncertainty

One of the problems in using evidence-based approaches to establish risk is the fact that an exposure often has both potential risks and potential benefits and there may be scientific uncertainty concerning these risks and benefits. As a result, policy-makers can face one of four levels of uncertainty regarding association of risk and benefit:

---

[33]   The power of a study reflects its ability to identify an effect when one truly exists. For example, a study with 80 per cent power to identify a two-fold relative risk increase in death will identify the existence of that level of risk increase 80 per cent of the time, if it truly exists. Generally, the power of a study increases the larger the sample size and the larger the effect being investigated. Studies inquiring into small relative increase risks require very large sample sizes to be adequately powered.

[34]   M.J. Khoury, R. Davis, M. Gwinn, M.L. Lindegren, P. Yoon, "Do We Need Genomic Research for the Prevention of Common Diseases with Environmental Causes?" (1 May 2005) 161 (9) Am. J. Epidemol 799-805.

Certainty of Risk

		High	Low
Certainty of Benefit	**High**	(1) Fenfluramine	(2) Genetic modification of foods
	Low	(3) Smallpox vaccination	(4) Xeno-transplantation

In scenario one above, high-quality information about both the risk of an exposure/intervention and its benefits may be available. The fenfluramine case provides an example. Research data demonstrates the potential benefit of fenfluramine as a weight loss agent. However, as has been described, well-conducted observational studies have demonstrated a potential serious risk with the exposure.

In the second scenario, the benefits of an intervention may be known but the risks are not or are considered theoretical. For example, genetic modification of food offers a known benefit — enhancing current food production — versus what many would consider the theoretical risk of downstream health and agricultural harm. In the third scenario, policy-makers may be confronted with the challenge of a known risk and an unknown benefit. For example, in deciding whether to embark on mass smallpox immunization to protect against a potential bioterrorist attack, the small but real risk of the vaccine must be balanced against the benefit, which is entirely dependent on the theoretical threat of a bioterrorist attack.

In the final scenario, both the benefits and the potential harms associated with the intervention may be considered uncertain or theoretical. For example, xenotransplantation provides the theoretical benefit of extending the lives of individuals who require organ or tissue transplants by using non-human donors, such as pigs. However, there is considerable concern over the theoretical harm of introducing new animal pathogens to human systems (known as xenozoonoses).

It is important to recognize that no risk falls clearly into any scenario as there is often disagreement over whether a risk or benefit is known or unknown. It is also important to understand that for each scenario, the risk and benefit may occur at different levels. For example, in the case of mass immunization programs, the individual benefits from the immunization directly, but he or she also incurs a potential health risk to benefit others, since immunization programs reduce the incidence of disease in a population, even among non-immunized members of the community.[35]

(c) Alternative Paradigms to Evidence-Based Decision-Making

If there is scientific uncertainty about the risks and benefits of an exposure, evidence-based decision-making models have important limits for assisting decision-makers in balancing these risks and benefits. In scenarios in which both risks and benefits are known, decision-makers can apply risk-benefit analyses. However, if either the risk or benefit is unknown, it becomes difficult to apply this approach. Arguably, if risks are theoretical and based on case series, animal or biological models, while benefits are demonstrated in higher-level epidemiological studies, evidence-based models of decision-making would argue against introducing measures to protect against the risk.

However, past experiences in public health have demonstrated some of the dangers of waiting for definitive evidence of risk before taking measures to protect against the risk. Perhaps the highest profile recent example is the transfusion transmission of hepatitis C and HIV through the blood system in many nations which clearly illustrated the danger of waiting for definitive epidemiological evidence in conditions with long latency periods.[36] In these situations, by the time the association becomes evident, numerous individuals may already have been exposed.

(d) The Precautionary Principle

In an attempt to prevent these problems from manifesting themselves in the future, some members of the public health community have advocated adopting a new paradigm for decision-making based on the "precautionary principle".[37] The precautionary principle is a concept that emerged out of environmental law, has gained widespread acceptance in the environmental movement and is increasingly being used in public health.

---

[35] This phenomenon is often referred to as herd immunity or herd effect: see *e.g.*, T. Jacob John & Reuben Samuel, "Herd Immunity and Herd Effect: New Insights and Definitions" (2000) 16 European Journal of Epidemiology 601.

[36] Peter D. Weinberg *et al.*, "Legal, Financial, and Public Health Consequences of HIV Contamination of Blood and Blood Products in the 1980s and 1990s" (2002) 136 Annals of Internal Medicine 312.

[37] David Kriebel & Joel Tickner, "The Precautionary Principle and Public Health: Reenergizing Public Health through Precaution" (2001) 91 American Journal of Public Health 1351.

As examples of current influence, the principle has been incorporated into the 1992 Rio Declaration on Environment and Development, the Maastricht Treaty establishing the European Community and has been endorsed by the American Public Health Association.

The precautionary principle emerged from concerns about the ability of science to understand complex systems related to risk and from the limitations of evidence in establishing risk. It emphasizes the importance of acting proactively to manage risk, and essentially states that complete evidence of harm does not have to exist before governments should take actions to protect the public from these risks. The Rio Declaration more specifically defined the principle as follows: "Where there are threats of serious or irreversible damage, lack of full scientific certainty shall not be used as a reason for postponing cost-effective measures to prevent environmental degradation."[38]

An alternative but parallel definition provided in the Wingspread Statement defines the precautionary principle as follows:

> Where an activity raises threats of harm to the environment or human health, precautionary measures should be taken even if some cause and effect relationships are not fully established scientifically.
>
> .....
>
> In this context the proponent of an activity, rather than the public bears the burden of proof.[39]

While the precautionary principle has had considerable influence on policy formulation concerning risk, this has not come without controversy. A particular concern with respect to the application of the precautionary principle is the variability in its interpretation. International treaties and declarations vary in the degree to which the burden is transferred from regulators (who generally must demonstrate harm) to proponents of potentially harmful measures who must demonstrate safety.[40] Stronger interpretations of the precautionary principle place the entire burden of responsibility on proponents of potentially harmful measures to demonstrate that these measures are safe. Weaker interpretations of the principle place more of the burden of proof on those

---

[38] UN, Report of the United Nations Conference on Environment and Development, *Rio Declaration on Environment and Development*, UN Doc. A/CONF. 151/26 (Vol. I) (Annex I) (1992), online: <http://www.un.org/documents/ga/conf151/aconf15126-1annex1.htm>.

[39] Nicholas Ashford *et al.*, "Wingspread Statement on the Precautionary Principle" (Statement of the participants in the Wingspread Conference, Wingspread Conference Center, Racine, Wisconsin January 23-25, 1998), online: Global Development Research Center <http://www.gdrc.org/u-gov/precaution-3.html>.

[40] D. VanderZwaag, "The Precautionary Principle in Environmental Law and Policy. Elusive Rhetoric and First Embraces" (1998) 8 J. Envtl. L. & Prac. 355.

arguing for the possibility of harm and open the door to cost-benefit analyses. This variability means policy-makers have had difficulty in agreeing on how much or how little evidence is required to trigger a precautionary action and on the role of the scientific process when the principle is used.[41]

The variability in the interpretation of the principle has also led to accusations that the principle has been used as a mechanism to introduce trade protectionism.[42] Addressing the issue of interpretive variation, the Wingspread Statement states that four core concepts should inform the application of the precautionary principle. These include: advocating anticipatory action to prevent harm; shifting some of the burden of proof to the proponents of new technologies to demonstrate safety; advocating a consideration of all alternatives to a new technology including doing nothing; and incorporation of all affected parties in the decision-making process of adopting a new technology.[43]

In addition, and partially as a consequence of the variable interpretations of the principle, the precautionary principle has been accused of producing over-regulation, denying the public the benefits of new technologies, arousing unnecessary fear in the public about theoretical risks and making the scientific process irrelevant.[44] In particular, there is concern that use of the precautionary principle can deny a population the benefits of a technology and may actually produce harm, a scenario that has emerged in public health.

A high profile current example is in the ongoing debate over the safety of genetically modified organisms ("GMOs"). The European Union, citing the experimental nature of GMOs and having recently experienced the BSE epidemic, had placed a moratorium on the importation of these substances.[45] This attitude has spread to developing

---

[41]   Merle Jacob & Tomas Hellstrom, "Policy Understanding of Science, Public Trust and the BSE-CJD Crisis" (2000) 78 Journal of Hazardous Materials 303 and B.D. Goldstein, "The Precautionary Principle and Scientific Research are not Antithetical" (1999) 107 Environmental Health Perspectives A594.

[42]   For a detailed description of some of the criticisms of the precautionary principle see *e.g.*, Julian Morris, ed., *Rethinking Risk and the Precautionary Principle* (Oxford: Butterworth-Heinemann, 2000).

[43]   Joel Tickner, Carolyn Raffensperger & Nancy Myers, eds., *The Precautionary Principle in Action: A Handbook*, 1st ed. (Ames, IA: Science and Environmental Health Network, 1998).

[44]   See *e.g.*, Julian Morris, ed., *Rethinking Risk and the Precautionary Principle* (Oxford: Butterworth-Heinemann, 2000).

[45]   EC, *Council Directive 90/220/EEC of 23 April 1990 on the deliberate release into the environment of genetically modified organisms* (Article 16) O.J. L. 117/15. This moratorium was effectively terminated by the European Commission decision to license genetically modified corn (Bt11) by the Swiss company Syngenta. See EC, *Commission Decision*

countries, highlighted by the agricultural minister of Zambia refusing a large donation of GM grains intended to feed millions of starving Zambians.[46] Other examples of adverse effects related to precautionary decisions are malaria deaths that resulted from a DDT ban in South Africa and a cholera epidemic that followed the removal of chlorine from water in Peru.[47] Precautionary measures may also harm individual liberty. This issue became apparent in the worldwide response to SARS and, in particular, the use of quarantine as a policy option to halt spread of the disease.[48] Such policies severely restricted the freedom of individuals, induced psychological harm and caused economic harm due to loss of income.[49]

In an attempt to assist policy-makers in overcoming some of these potential pitfalls, the European Community has provided guidelines for applying the precautionary principle. The guidelines incorporate the following key concepts:

Proportionality means tailoring measures to the chosen level of protection. Risk can rarely be reduced to zero, but incomplete risk assessments may greatly reduce the range of options open to risk managers. A total ban may not be a proportional response to a potential risk in all cases. However, in certain cases, it is the sole possible response to a given risk.

Non-discrimination means that comparable situations should not be treated differently, and that different situations should not be treated in the same way, unless there are objective grounds for doing so.

Consistency means that measures should be of comparable scope and nature to those already taken in equivalent areas in which all scientific data are available.

Examining *costs and benefits* entails comparing the overall cost ... of action and lack of action, in both the short and long term. This is not simply an economic cost-benefit analysis: its scope is much broader, and

2004/657/EC of 19 May 2004 authorizing the placing on the market of sweet corn from genetically modified maize line Bt11 as a novel food or novel food ingredient under Regulation (EC) No 258/97 of the European Parliament and of the Council (notified under document number C(2004) 1865), O.J. L. 300/48.

[46] "Famine-hit Zambia rejects GM food aid" BBC News (29 October 2002), online: <http://news.bbc.co.uk/1/hi/world/africa/2371675.stm>.

[47] Amir Attaran & Rajendra Maharaj, "Doctoring Malaria Badly: The Global Campaign to Ban DDT" (2000) 321 British Medical Journal 1403; Henry I. Miller & Gregory Conko, "Precaution Without Principle" (2001) 19 Nature Biotechnology 302.

[48] Lawrence O. Gostin et al., "Ethical and Legal Challenges Posed by Severe Acute Respiratory Syndrome: Implications for the Control of Severe Infectious Disease Threats" (2003) 290 Journal of the American Medical Association 3229.

[49] Laura Hawryluck et al., "SARS Control and Psychological Effects of Quarantine, Toronto, Canada" (2004) 10 Emerging Infectious Diseases 1206.

includes non-economic considerations, such as the efficacy of possible options and their acceptability to the public. ...

Subject to review in the light of new scientific data, means measures based on the precautionary principle should be maintained so long as scientific information is incomplete or inconclusive, and the risk is still considered too high to be imposed on society, in view of chosen level of protection. Measures should be periodically reviewed in the light of scientific progress, and amended as necessary.

Assigning responsibility for producing scientific evidence is already a common consequence of these measures. ... [50]

Of particular importance among these guidelines are the issues of proportionality and the need for policies to be subject to review. Highly aggressive approaches to theoretical risks, as this chapter describes, can result in serious adverse consequences. Thus, it is important for policy-makers to have leeway to introduce a measure that protects partially against the risk and reduces the negative consequences of the protective measure. Similarly, when confronted with a series of equivalent, reasonable policy responses, policy-makers should select the response that is the least restrictive alternative, to protect the liberty and well-being of individuals who may be directly adversely affected by the risk management measure. Alternatively, policy-makers may choose to permit the risk to continue until mechanisms are available to protect against the consequences of removing the risk, an approach being taken with respect to the use of DDT in the developing world.

Once measures are introduced to protect against theoretical risks, governments must also be prepared to revoke these measures if new evidence arises to demonstrate the absence of risk. There can be substantial disincentives for policy-makers to do so as the public may perceive the government is allowing "unsafe" practices to occur. Nevertheless, in the absence of this approach, countries may find themselves facing the economic consequences of mounting regulations that protect against risks, without ever having the option of removing these regulations. Such a perception may actually deter the introduction of protective policies in the first place.

---

[50] EC Commission, Communication on the Precautionary Principle COM (2000) 1 (Brussels: 2 February 2000), online: Europa Gateway to the EU <http://europa.eu.int/comm/dgs/ health_consumer/library/pub/pub07_en.pdf>.

V. RECONCILING EVIDENCE-BASED DECISION-MAKING AND PRECAUTION

The precautionary principle reflects an aggressive approach to risk management and prevents exposures to potential risks. Current applications of evidence-based decision-making, and its reliance on hierarchies of evidence, reflect a more conservative approach to managing potential risks. To develop effective policies in public health concerning risk, a middle ground must be found between strict precaution and strict evidence-based approaches. An example of a middle ground approach is the use of risk modelling techniques. These techniques attempt to manage uncertainty by decomposing a policy problem into a limited number of policy alternatives and the key factors that will influence the choice of alternatives. The expected value of each policy alternative can then be calculated for a given range of values for each factor. However, these models include many assumptions and there is considerable uncertainty in the values of the key factors. Also there is the possibility of "unknown unknowns", important factors that have not been included in the model but have the potential to considerably alter the results of the simulation.

(a) Case Study: Potential Blood Transfusion Transmission of vCJD

Approaches that combine components of risk modelling, precaution and evidence-based decision-making are required to adequately address public health challenges pertaining to risk. Such a combined approach has been utilized by several nations in managing the theoretical risk of variant CJD ("vCJD") to their blood supply. CJD produces progressive neurological deterioration in affected individuals, inevitably resulting in death. While there is no epidemiological evidence that the classical (non-variant) form of CJD could be transmitted through blood transfusions, the risk of blood transmission of vCJD has been believed to be higher because the prion protein infects lymphatic tissue, which is linked with the body's blood supply.

Concern about potential transfusion transmission of the condition prompted the United Kingdom, in 1997, to conduct three blood withdrawals of products linked to vCJD donors.[51] This was followed, in February 1998, by a U.K. decision to import all their plasma requirements. This decision was based on the possibility that an unknown

---

[51]   U.K. Department of Health, Press Release (98/076), "Further Precautionary Measures On Blood Products Announced" (26 February 1998), online: News Distribution Service for Government and Public Sector <http://nds.coi.gov.uk/content/detail.asp?ReleaseID=31884&NewsAreaID=2&NavigatedFromSearch=True>.

portion of the British population could be harbouring vCJD and the potential costs associated with withdrawals of blood derived from donors who were subsequently diagnosed with vCJD.[52] As an additional safety measure, the U.K. also introduced a policy to leukodeplete (remove white blood cells from) blood donations, based on the understanding that the infectious prion was primarily located in white blood cells.[53]

Other nations followed suit and also introduced precautionary measures to protect their blood supplies from vCJD, primarily by restricting donations from individuals who had travelled to the U.K. Both Canada and the United States introduced policies to defer blood donations from individuals who had lived in the U.K. for six months between 1980 to 1996, the peak period of the BSE outbreak.[54] A variety of factors influenced the Canadian decision, including scientific information suggesting a theoretical risk as well as the need to balance blood safety against the impact of donor restrictions on the blood supply. Surveys of Canadian donors suggested the six-month deferral policies could reduce the donor pool by 3 per cent, which policy-makers believed was sustainable.[55] The Canadian vCJD policies have since been made more stringent and now exclude donors who resided in Western Europe as new evidence accumulated on the potential transfusion transmission of vCJD and as the adequacy of the blood supply to sustain reductions in donors was identified.

At the time many of these policies were introduced, the risk of transfusion transmission of vCJD was only theoretical and was primarily based on the discovery of the prion protein in peripheral lymph tissue of persons with vCJD.[56] Increasingly, evidence has accumulated to support the potential transfusion transmission of vCJD. Animal models of

---

[52] U.K. Department of Health, Press Release (98/182), "Committee on Safety and Medicines Completes Review of Blood Products" (13 May 1998).

[53] U.K. Department of Health, Press Release (98/295), "Government Accepts Advice on Leucodepletion from Spongiform Encephalopathy Advisory Committee" (17 July 1998), online: News Distribution Service for Government and Public Sector <http://nds.coi.gov.uk/content/detail.asp?ReleaseID=4583&NewsAreaID=2&NavigatedFromSearch=True>.

[54] Health Canada, Directive D99-02 "Donor Exclusion to Address Theoretical Risk of Transmission of Variant CJD through the Use of Commercial Blood Products" (17 August 1999); U.S. Department of Health and Human Services (Center for Biologics Evaluation and Research), "Guidance for Industry: Revised Preventive Measures to Reduce the Possible Risk of Transmission of Creutzfeldt-Jakob Disease (CJD) and Variant Creutzfeldt-Jakob Disease (vCJD) by Blood and Blood Products" (January 2002), online: <http://www.fda.gov/cber/gdlns/cjdvcjd.pdf>.

[55] Kumanan Wilson et al., "A Policy Analysis of Major Decisions Related to Creutzfeldt-Jakob Disease and the Blood Supply" (2001) 165 Canadian Medical Association Journal 59.

[56] Andrew F. Hill et al., "Diagnosis of New Variant Creutzfeldt-Jakob Disease by Tonsil Biopsy" (1997) 349 Lancet 99.

transmissible spongiform encephalopathies have suggested that these conditions may be transmissible through transfusion. In particular, the transfusion transmission of BSE from both clinically ill and preclinically ill sheep to healthy sheep has been demonstrated.[57] Furthermore, a recent primate study suggests that transfusion exposure to the BSE prion may be at least as efficient as exposure via the oral route, although it is not certain whether an infective dose of BSE exists in human blood.[58] Most recently, four case reports have supported this evidence by indicating that the recipients of blood products from individuals with vCJD have subsequently developed evidence of infection.[59,60,61] Based on the new evidence, the risk of transfusion transmission of vCJD would have to be considered to have moved from theoretical to probable, and transfusion transmission is likely an efficient mechanism by which the infection could be spread. Partly in response to these concerns, and the potential perpetuation of transfusion-derived vCJD, the U.K. is now deferring donations from individuals who have received a previous blood transfusion.[62]

(b) Evaluation of the Precautionary Measures

In retrospect, it appears that countries appropriately introduced precautionary policies to manage the risk of vCJD to the blood supply. Arguably, using an evidence-based model, the decisions would not have been justifiable. Animal and biological models, the primary scientific information that influenced decision-making, would be viewed as too susceptible to bias to be the primary determinants of a policy that had the potential to have negative consequences — these include the costs associated with implementing the policies, reducing the availability of blood products and potentially dissuading future donors. Despite these drawbacks and the limitations of the existing evidence, policies introduced to protect the blood supply would have to be viewed as a success. In

---

[57] F. Houston *et al.*, "Transmission of BSE by Blood Transfusion in Sheep" (2000) 356 Lancet 999; Nora Hunter *et al.*, "Transmission of Prion Diseases by Blood Transfusion" (2002) 83 Journal of General Virology 2897.

[58] C. Herzog *et al.*, "Tissue Distribution of Bovine Spongiform Encephalopathy Agent in Primates after Intravenous or Oral Infection" (2004) 363 Lancet 422.

[59] C.A. Llewelyn *et al.*, "Possible Transmission of Variant Creutzfeldt-Jakob Disease by Blood Transfusion" (2004) 363 Lancet 417.

[60] K. Wilson & M. Ricketts, "A Third Episode of Transfusion-Derived vCJD" (2006) 368 Lancet 2037.

[61] Health Protection Agency, Press Release, "Fourth Case of Variant CJD Infection Associated with Blood Transfusion" (18 January 2007), online: <http://www.hpa.org.uk/webw/HPAweb&HPAwebStandard/HPAweb_C/1195733711457?p=1171991026241>.

[62] C.A. Ludlam & M.L. Turner, "Managing the Risk of Transmission of Variant Creutzfeldt Jakob Disease by Blood Products" (2006) 132 British Journal of Haematology 13.

particular, they have limited the impact of blood recalls that result from donors who later are found to have developed the condition. These occurrences have a particularly significant impact on fractionated products that involve pooling blood from hundreds to thousands of donors. Blood recalls are expensive, can cause short-term shortages in blood products and can introduce complicated ethical issues surrounding the notification of recipients.[63] The second major benefit of the vCJD policies is to maintain the trust of the public by demonstrating that the blood system in acting proactively. This is an essential task due to the legacy of the transfusion transmission of hepatitis C and HIV. Perhaps most importantly, given the current evidence of the probable efficiency of transfusion transmission of the prion, introducing a precautionary policy has helped prevent the perpetuation of vCJD among humans even after bovine to human transmission had ceased.

(c) How Should Precaution be Applied?

The management of the potential threat of transfusion transmission of vCJD provides some guidance on how to appropriately apply precaution and how to reconcile precautionary based policies with evidence-based decision-making. When deciding on the mechanism by which to apply precaution, two questions need to be answered: (1) When should precaution be applied and how should it be applied? (2) In determining when the principle should be applied, the characteristics of the problem being addressed need to be examined.

As stated earlier, when discussing evidence-based decision-making, it is appropriate to act on higher levels of *uncertainty*, measured as increased systematic or unsystematic error, if the following apply: (1) the exposure is widespread; (2) harm caused by the exposure is serious; (3) harm caused by the exposure is not treatable; (4) economic costs of removing the exposure are minimal; and (5) health costs of removing the exposure are minimal.

These conditions, with the possible exception of (4), applied to the threat of vCJD to the blood supply. By introducing partial deferral policies, Canada and the United States protected against shortages, thus ensuring health costs were minimal. Given that the threat of vCJD possessed these characteristics, it was appropriate for decision-makers to act on high levels of uncertainty. In contrast, in the decision to ban DDT from South Africa, the health costs of removing the exposure were

---

[63]   Shelia M. Bird, "Recipients of Blood or Blood Products 'at vCJD risk'" (2004) 328 British Medical Journal 118.

substantial. In this scenario, a higher level of *certainty* of cause and effect needs to exist before taking precautionary actions.

As important as identifying the appropriate time to introduce precautionary measures is determining the mechanism by which the principle should be applied. The E.U. guidelines cited earlier in this chapter provide some direction with respect to this issue and the Canadian vCJD policy followed many of these guidelines. In particular, the policies were proportional and were gradually introduced as more information became available on risk of transfusion transmission and the adequacy of the donor pool. The policies also clearly examined costs and benefits and employed a detailed risk modelling/risk management analysis. To be truly successful, policy-makers will have to be prepared to reduce or remove the policies if evidence accumulates suggesting transfusion transmission of vCJD is not possible.

VI. CONCLUSION

This chapter has highlighted the challenges of public health policy-making concerning risk. It has described the traditional evidence-based approach, limitations with this approach and the use of precaution as an alternative paradigm. It is important to emphasize that, despite its limitations, the evidence-based approach should not be entirely rejected. Identifying and evaluating the best available evidence on a public health risk is still an essential component of any public health decision-making process. However, the precautionary principle can be useful in guiding the formulation of evidence-based public health policy.

In summary, an appropriate combination of precaution and evidence-based models would consider the following points when developing policy. The nature of the risk should determine what level of systematic or unsystematic error decision-makers are willing to accept. Decisions made in response to scientific uncertainty should be proportional to the risk they are managing and take into consideration potential harms associated with the risk. When possible, the least restrictive option should be considered, all other things being equal. Finally, the policy process should be closely linked to the scientific process and scientists should address gaps in knowledge that impair policy development. Similarly, policy-makers must be prepared to respond to new science that emerges on a topic, even if it contradicts previous policy decisions. By following this approach, an effective new policy-making paradigm that incorporates evidence-based decision-making and precaution can be developed.

4

PUBLIC HEALTH INFORMATION PRIVACY AND CONFIDENTIALITY

Elaine Gibson[*]

I.   INTRODUCTION

A complex web of legislation, common law and constitutional issues exists with regard to public health information in Canada. One area of uniformity can be found in the calls for drastic improvement in the infrastructure of reporting of communicable diseases.[1] On the other hand, we have witnessed in recent years a plethora of legislation that is aimed at improving privacy protections for personal health information, accompanied by an increasing concern on the part of Canadians as to whether our highly sensitive health information is receiving adequate protection. These two areas — demand for increased reporting in the area of public health, and greater concern for privacy protections — have not been reconciled. This makes analysis of the sort undertaken in this chapter

[*]   Associate Director of the Health Law Institute, Dalhousie University, and Associate Professor of Law with cross-appointment to the Faculty of Health Professions, Dalhousie University. Thanks to Keri Gammon and Jeff Haylock for their excellent research assistance.
[1]   Canada, Auditor General of Canada, *2008 May Report*, Chapter 5, "Surveillance of Infectious Diseases — Public Health Agency of Canada", online: <http://www.oag-bvg.gc.ca/internet/ English/parl_oag_200805_05_e_30701.html>; National Advisory Committee on SARS and Public Health, *Learning from SARS: Renewal of Public Health in Canada* (Ottawa: Health Canada, 2003) (Chair: Dr. D. Naylor) at 91-112; Honourable Mr. Justice Archie Campbell, Commissioner, "The SARS Commission Interim Report: SARS and Public Health in Ontario" (2004) at 100-30, online: Ministry of Health and Long-Term Care <http://www.health.gov.on.ca/ english/public/pub/ministry_reports/campbell04/campbell04.pdf>; Ontario Expert Panel on SARS and Infectious Disease Control, *For the Public's Health: A Plan of Action* (Toronto: Ministry of Health and Long-Term Care, 2004) esp. at 240 and 251-57.

a major challenge. Thus, the discussion here is by no means exhaustive; this area is worthy of further examination in future.

The early portions of this chapter provide an overview of legal protections for health information in general. The first section explains differences between privacy and confidentiality — concepts that are often blurred. Next I outline major pieces of legislation relevant to health information, including an examination of jurisdictional issues and why there exists at times overlapping federal and provincial legislation pertaining to information. This is followed by a discussion of duties of confidentiality that have developed historically at common law, and a series of exceptions that have been carved out from the duty of confidentiality, both through specific provisions in legislation and through changes in common law. The final section in this portion of the chapter discusses the *Canadian Charter of Rights and Freedoms* and its implications for both the protection of confidentiality and the need for public health information.

The latter portions of the chapter cover specifics of public health legislation pertaining to proper and improper uses of personal health information, and highlight differences between the provinces in their approaches to this topic. First is a discussion of duties on individuals to self-report if they believe they have or may have a communicable disease. Next I cover mandatory reporting by third parties, such as physicians, nurses and directors of laboratories, of the likely presence of a communicable disease. The duty of confidentiality of medical officers of health is reviewed, followed by a discussion of contact notification in the case of communicable disease. Also, I outline statutory provisions for notification of the public by such means as placarding and media releases. Finally, I discuss uses of health information for surveillance, epidemiology and research. The chapter concludes with a review of measures that may be taken *vis-à-vis* uses of information in case of a public health emergency.

II. GENERAL (NON PUBLIC HEALTH SPECIFIC)

(a) Privacy and Confidentiality Distinguished

The terms "privacy" and "confidentiality" are often used in conjunction or interchangeably without an appreciation of their distinct and separate meanings. For purposes of clarity, when I refer in this chapter to privacy, the concept is that the individual or group is entitled (or not) to keep aspects of themselves from being revealed to others if they so choose. Privacy may involve interests that are territorial/spatial, personal or informational.[2] As the focus of this chapter is on public health information, the discussion will centre on informational privacy. This concept was encapsulated by the Supreme Court of Canada in *R. v. Duarte*[3] as being "... the right of the individual to determine for himself when, how and to what extent he will release personal information about himself".[4]

Confidentiality, on the other hand, is the duty owed by another to guard as private information that has been conveyed to that person or organization in circumstances where it is likely that the conveyor of information is not providing such information for public consumption. The quintessential model in health care is that of physician and patient, but a duty of confidentiality may arise not only in the context of any professional/client relationship but also in relationships of other types, such as those between friends. In the medical context, this duty has been described as follows:

> Members of the medical profession have a duty of confidentiality with respect to their patients. They are under restraint not to volunteer information respecting the condition of their patients or any professional services performed by them without their patient's consent. In the absence of such consent, members of the medical profession breach their duty if they disclose such information unless required to do so by due process of law.[5]

Much of this chapter will be concerned with duties of confidentiality, as the discussion primarily centres on information in the hands of others. However, a privacy interest is antecedent to the duty of confidentiality, and in fact such a duty depends on the existence of a perceived privacy interest. Therefore, both privacy and confidentiality are relevant and must be considered in the balance when it comes to personal information and its uses for public health purposes.

---

[2]   *R. v. Dyment*, [1988] S.C.J. No. 82, [1988] 2 S.C.R. 417 at 427, 55 D.L.R. (4th) 503 (S.C.C.), *per* La Forest J.

[3]   [1990] S.C.J. No. 2, [1990] 1 S.C.R. 30, 65 D.L.R. (4th) 240 (S.C.C.) ["*Duarte*" cited to S.C.R.].

[4]   *Ibid.*, at para. 25.

[5]   *Re Inquiry into Confidentiality of Health Records in Ontario*, [1979] O.J. No. 4219, 24 O.R. (2d) 545 at 555 (Ont. C.A.), rev'd on other grounds [1981] S.C.J. No. 95, [1981] 2 S.C.R. 494, 128 D.L.R. (3d) 193 (S.C.C.).

(b) Statutes Aimed at Protection of Information

(i) Jurisdiction

Both informational privacy and public health are areas of mixed jurisdiction between the federal and provincial governments. Information is primarily within provincial jurisdiction by virtue of the mandate provided to the provinces by the *Constitution Act, 1867*[6] to regulate property and civil rights as well as matters of a local or private nature.[7] Thus, a majority of statutes regulating information has been enacted by the provinces/ territories. There are, however, two areas of particular significance where the federal government has asserted jurisdiction *vis-à-vis* information: first, under the federal power over census and statistics,[8] manifested in the *Statistics Act*;[9] and second, under the trade and commerce power.[10] The latter is relied on to support federal legislation, the *Personal Information Protection and Electronic Documents Act ("PIPEDA")*,[11] which regulates information collected, used or disclosed in the course of commercial activity. Note its restriction to commercial activity, as otherwise it would be difficult or impossible to justify as falling legitimately within trade and commerce.[12]

The area of public health, similar to health information, is primarily under provincial jurisdiction. The *Constitution Act, 1867* assigned "quarantine and the establishment and maintenance of marine hospitals"[13] to the federal government. The provinces were assigned power over "the establishment, maintenance, and management of hospitals, asylums, charities and eleemosynary[14] institutions in and for the province, other than marine hospitals".[15] Thus, jurisdiction over health is viewed as falling primarily within provincial jurisdiction due to a combination of the power to regulate hospitals, property and civil rights, and matters of a local or

---

[6]   (U.K.), 30 & 31 Vict., c. 3, reprinted in R.S.C. 1985, App. II, No. 5.

[7]   *Ibid.*, s. 92(13), (16).

[8]   *Ibid.*, s. 91(6).

[9]   R.S.C. 1985, c. S-19.

[10]   *Constitution Act, 1867*, (U.K.), 30 & 31 Vict., c. 3, s. 91(2), reprinted in R.S.C. 1985, App. II, No. 5.

[11]   S.C. 2000, c. 5.

[12]   See below, section (ii) Federal Legislation Governing Information for further discussion.

[13]   (U.K.), 30 & 31 Vict., c. 3, s. 91(11), reprinted in R.S.C. 1985, App. II, No. 5.

[14]   A term seldom used in common parlance, and which is undefined in Canadian legal dictionaries. *Black's Law Dictionary*, 8th ed. defines the term as: "Of, relating to, or assisted by charity; not-for-profit." *s.v.* "eleemosynary".

[15]   (U.K.), 30 & 31 Vict., c. 3, s. 92(7), reprinted in R.S.C. 1985, App. II, No. 5.

private nature.[16] However, this is not straightforward, but depends on the type of health issue being addressed by legislation. Thus, Estey J. for the Supreme Court of Canada indicates as follows:

> In sum "health" is not a matter which is subject to specific constitutional assignment but instead is an amorphous topic which can be addressed by valid federal or provincial legislation, depending in the circumstances of each case on the nature or scope of the health problem in question.[17]

In the area of public health, legislation concerning mandatory treatment and detention of heroin addicts, and that providing for detention of certain individuals with mental health problems, has been found to fall under provincial power.[18] Federal legislation prohibiting cigarette advertising is legitimate under the criminal law power.[19] In a case that arose in Québec shortly after Confederation, concerning the appointment of a local board of health to control an outbreak of smallpox, the Cour Supérieure ruled that a statute was *ultra vires* the federal government in that it:

> ... relates, not to quarantine or marine hospitals, but simply to the preservation of the public health within this Province, and thus concerns matters of a purely private and local nature; and therefore under the provisions of the British North America Act of 1867, does not fall within the jurisdiction of the said Dominion of Parliament.[20]

Thus, jurisdiction over public health other than quarantine historically rests primarily with the provinces as being of a private and local nature. One must question whether this will continue to be the primary head of power for public health, given the rapidity with which

---

[16] See *e.g.*, William Lahey, "Medicare and the Law: Contours of an Evolving Relationship" in Jocelyn Downie, Timothy Caulfield & Colleen Flood, eds., *Canadian Health Law and Policy*, 3d ed. (Markham, Ont.. LexisNexis Canada, 2007) 1 at 25.

[17] *Schneider v. British Columbia*, [1982] S.C.J. No. 64, [1982] 2 S.C.R. 112 at 142, 139 D.L.R. (3d) 417 (S.C.C.) ["*Schneider*" cited to S.C.R.] (Estey J. concurring with the majority in finding the *Heroin Treatment Act*, S.B.C. 1978, c. 24, *intra vires* the province of British Columbia).

[18] *Ibid.* (*Heroin Treatment Act*, S.B.C. 1978, c. 24, upheld as valid provincial law under ss. 92(7) and 92(13) of the *Constitution Act, 1867*); *Fawcett v. Ontario (Attorney-General)*, [1964] S.C.J. No. 39, [1964] S.C.R. 625, 45 D.L.R. (2d) 579 (S.C.C.) (*Mental Hospitals Act*, R.S.O. 1960, c. 236, upheld as valid provincial law under s. 92(7) of the *Constitution Act, 1867*).

[19] *RJR-MacDonald Inc. v. Canada (Attorney General)*, [1995] S.C.J. No. 68, [1995] 3 S.C.R. 199, 127 D.L.R. (4th) 1 (S.C.C.) ["*RJR-MacDonald*" cited to S.C.R.]. Although a majority of the Court found that the *Tobacco Products Control Act*, S.C. 1988, c. 20, was validly enacted under the federal criminal law power, numerous provisions within the statute were ultimately struck down on the grounds that they created unjustifiable limits on the right to freedom of expression as provided by s. 2(*b*) of the *Charter*.

[20] *Rinfret v. Pope* (1886) 12 QLR 303 at 305 (Qué. C.A.) (trial judgment unreported).

communicable disease now crosses borders and the difficulty in controlling its spread.

Thus far I have been discussing information and public health as separate entities. When reviewing jurisdictional issues as to public health information, an amalgam of the two, there is very little judicial interpretation of this overlap. A thorough analysis of this area is beyond the scope of this chapter. Suffice it to say that most statutory provisions concerning public health information are provincial. The federal government has been relatively non-interventionist thus far, asserting its jurisdiction in limited circumstances only. However, this role has been expanded with the enactment of *PIPEDA*. The next section examines federal legislation regarding information protection.

(ii) Federal Legislation Governing Information

This section discusses the major pieces of federal legislation governing information generally. The federal *Quarantine Act*[21] is reviewed later in the chapter in the sections dealing with the public health duty to self-report and mandatory reporting by third parties.

The federal *Privacy Act*[22] and *Access to Information Act*[23] in combination govern personal information collected, used, retained and disclosed by the federal public sector. These statutes were brought into force in 1983 in recognition that government departments were collecting ever-increasing volumes of personal information, and that there should be rules regarding its handling and disclosure. The *Privacy Act* has come under critique in recent years in that it has not been significantly updated despite major changes in the type and volume of information collected, it applies only to recorded information (thus, for example, live video feed is outside its scope), and it does not deal adequately with its interaction with other federal legislation touching upon information handling.[24]

---

[21]   S.C. 2005, c. 20.

[22]   R.S.C. 1985, c. P-21.

[23]   R.S.C. 1985, c. A-1.

[24]   Jennifer Stoddart, Privacy Commissioner of Canada, "Privacy in Canada in 2007: Where We've Been, Where We're Going" (Address given at second annual Ontario Bar Association Privacy Summit, 5 November 2007), online: <http://www.privcom.gc.ca/speech/2007/sp-d_071105_e.asp>; Jennifer Stoddart, Privacy Commissioner of Canada, "The Privacy and Security Partnership" (Address given at International Security Managers Association Conference, 25 June 2007), online: <http://www.privcom.gc.ca/speech/2007/sp-d_070625_e.asp>; Jennifer Stoddart, Privacy Commissioner of Canada, "Privacy Today and Tomorrow — Priorities for the Next Seven Years" (Address given at the Canadian Access and Privacy Association Annual General Meeting, 23 November 2004), online: <http://www.privcom.gc.ca/speech/2004/sp-d_041123_e.asp>; Heather Black, Assistant Privacy Commissioner of Canada, "Privacy Law Reform: Responding to a Networked

The Office of Privacy Commissioner was created under the *Privacy Act* to handle complaints under the statute, conduct audits, provide education services and engage in privacy-related research.[25] Decisions of the Privacy Commissioner are not binding on the public sector; in order to have an enforceable judgment, it is necessary that the aggrieved party proceed to Federal Court.[26]

The role of the federal government in the governance of personal information has expanded dramatically in recent years with the coming into force of *PIPEDA*.[27] Its genesis lay in two interrelated developments: the drafting of the Canadian Standards Association Model Code for the Protection of Personal Information[28] for proper collection, use, security and sharing of personal information; and a directive issued by the European Union that it would cease transferring personal information to countries that did not offer protections for such information that were substantially in conformance with its own standards.[29] Invoking the federal trade and commerce power, *PIPEDA* applies only to personal information collected, used or disclosed by the private sector in the course of commercial activity. *PIPEDA* came into force on January 1, 2002 *vis-à-vis* personal health information (whether electronic or not) which is disclosed outside the province for consideration, as well as to federally regulated businesses.[30] As of January 1, 2004, it also applies to any organization that collects, uses or discloses personal information in the course of commercial activity within provincial borders. Provinces have the option of enacting substantially similar legislation that supersedes *PIPEDA* for information within provincial borders.[31] To date, general private sector legislation in Québec[32] and British Columbia[33] has been declared substantially similar.[34] The situation in Alberta is somewhat more

World" (Address given as part of the McCarthy Tétrault Speaker Series, Halifax, Nova Scotia, 3 February 2005), online: <http://www.privcom.gc.ca/speech/2005/sp-d_050203_e.asp>.

[25] Office of the Privacy Commissioner of Canada, "About Us", online: <http://www.privcom.gc.ca/aboutUs/index_e.asp>.

[26] *Privacy Act*, R.S.C. 1985, c. P-21, ss. 35(1), 41-42.

[27] S.C. 2000, c. 5.

[28] Canadian Standards Association, "Model Code for the Protection of Personal Information" (1996), online: <http://www.csa.ca/standards/privacy/code/Default.asp?language=English>.

[29] EU Directive 95/46/EC of 24 October 1995, article 25(1), online: The European Union <http://eurlex.europa.eu/LexUriServ/LexUriServ.do?uri=CELEX:31995L0046:EN:HTML>.

[30] *Personal Information Protection and Electronic Documents Act*, S.C. 2000, c. 5, s. 30 (transitional provisions and various coming into force dates).

[31] *Ibid.*, s. 26(2)(*b*).

[32] *An Act respecting the protection of personal information in the private sector*, R.S.Q. c. P-39.1.

[33] *Personal Information Protection Act*, S.B.C. 2003, c. 63.

[34] *Organizations in the Province of Quebec Exemption Order*, S.O.R./2003-374; *Organization in the Province of British Columbia Exemption Order*, S.O.R./2004-220.

complex in that its general private sector legislation[35] has been declared substantially similar,[36] but health information is exempted from this statute and the *Health Information Act*[37] has not been declared substantially similar. This means that *PIPEDA* applies to health information in Alberta. The situation in Ontario is the reverse of that in Alberta. Ontario has not passed any general private sector legislation, but has passed the *Personal Health Information Protection Act, 2004*[38] which has been declared substantially similar and so exempts Ontario health care information from *PIPEDA*.[39] It should be noted that in provinces with legislation declared substantially similar, *PIPEDA* still applies to information being shared outside of the province and to federally regulated industries within the province. This has given rise to a challenge by the government of Québec as to its constitutionality.[40]

The reader may well query the applicability of *PIPEDA* to the health sector, given that its aim is to protect information collected, used or disclosed in the course of commercial activity. Indeed, in the nascent development of this legislation, it was thought not to apply to the health care/health services sectors. When it was realized that it would in fact apply, at least to certain types of activities, there was widespread opposition: "The Senate noted that there was a universal lack of support for PIPEDA in the health sector — albeit for different reasons ...".[41] It is now clear that *PIPEDA* applies in certain respects to personal health information when a commercial activity is occurring. Indeed, Industry Canada, under whose auspices *PIPEDA* falls, has developed a "Questions and Answers" document which indicates that in its view, the legislation does not apply in general to hospitals but does apply to physicians in private practice and to laboratories.[42] This interpretation is justified by Industry Canada on the basis that physicians and laboratories are engaging in commercial activity by virtue of billing for their services. On the other hand, they indicate, the core activity of a hospital is to provide patient care and not to make money; hence hospitals are not subject to *PIPEDA*.

[35] *Personal Information Protection Act*, S.A. 2003, c. P-6.5.
[36] *Organization in the Province of Alberta Exemption Order*, S.O.R./2004-219.
[37] R.S.A. 2000, c. H-5.
[38] S.O. 2004, c. 3, Sch. A.
[39] *Health Information Custodians in the Province of Ontario Exemption Order*, S.O.R./2005-399.
[40] *Renvoi à la Cour d'appel relatif à la Loi sur la protection des renseignements personnels et les documents électroniques* (L.C. 2000, ch. 5), O.I.C. 1368-2003, G.O.Q. 2003.II.184.
[41] M. Marshall & B. von Tigerstrom, "Health Information" in Jocelyn Downie, Timothy Caufield & Colleen Flood, eds., *Canadian Health Law and Policy*, 2d ed. (Markham, Ont.: Butterworths, 2002) 157 at 170.
[42] Industry Canada, "PIPEDA Awareness Raising Tools (PARTs) Initiative For The Health Sector", online: Industry Canada <http://ecom.ic.gc.ca/epic/internet/inecic-ceac.nsf/en/gv00235e.html>.

Ultimately it will be up to the courts to determine the overlap between the health sector and the applicability of *PIPEDA*. Given the newness of the legislation, to date there is little case law analyzing this issue.[43]

The apparent applicability of *PIPEDA* to physicians in private practice raises an important issue in those provinces where, under public health legislation, the individual with a communicable disease is mandated to provide to his or her physician the names of contacts for tracing. *PIPEDA* is based on a model of consent for the collection of personal information. While there are exceptions within the statute, public health is not one, and others do not appear to be applicable.[44] Thus, *PIPEDA* appears to require that a physician must have the patient's consent when collecting personal information about contacts, regardless as to provisions in public health legislation mandating the provision of information.

The federal *Statistics Act* provides that the federal government may collaborate with the provinces to collect, transmit and analyze health information.[45] There are no provisions in this statute mandating the provision of such information by individuals or by provinces; the power to compel information is confined to census and agriculture information.[46] The Act also provides for the sharing of information by Statistics Canada with the provinces, but states that this information must only go to the statistical agency of the province.[47] Further, the respondent (the subject of such information) is to be notified of such sharing.[48] Section 12 of the Act provides that Statistics Canada may enter into agreements with a federal or municipal department or corporation for the sharing of information; in this case, the respondent is to be informed of and may object to such sharing. Such objection results in the information not being shared unless

---

[43]   In *Rousseau v. Canada (Privacy Commissioner)*, [2008] F.C.J. No. 151, 2008 FCA 39 (F.C.A.), the Federal Court of Appeal found that an independent medical examination conducted at the behest of an insurer is a commercial activity. *PIPEDA* is therefore applicable to information gathered during such examinations.

[44]   See Mireille Lacroix *et al.*, "The Reporting and Management of Personal Information and Personal Health Information to Control and Combat Infectious Disease: An Analysis of the Canadian Statutory and Regulatory Framework" (2004) (Submitted to Health Canada, Centre for Surveillance Coordination, Population and Public Health Branch) at 38-39 for the argument that the ordering of tests without consent for a person suspected of having a communicable disease may be justified under s. 7(1)(*a*) as being clearly in the interests of the individual if consent cannot be obtained in timely fashion. It is my contention that provision of the names of contacts would not be similarly justifiable as in the interests of the patient; rather, it is the interest of third parties that is at stake.

[45]   R.S.C. 1985, c. S-19, s. 3(*b*).

[46]   *Ibid.*, s. 8.

[47]   *Ibid.*, s. 11.

[48]   *Ibid.*, s. 11(4).

another statute requires the provision of such information by the respondent.[49]

(iii) Provincial/Territorial Legislation

As stated above, public health falls mainly under provincial jurisdiction. Thus, every province/territory has one or more pieces of legislation governing public health, sexually transmitted infections and vital statistics.[50] Information aspects of public health legislation will be discussed in subsequent sections of this chapter. In this section, I review general legislation governing health information; information aspects of public health information will be discussed in subsequent sections of this chapter.

Just as the federal government has legislation governing access to and privacy of publicly held information, so too the provinces/territories have legislation regarding freedom of information and protection of privacy of information in the public sector.[51] Differences exist from

---

[49]   *Ibid.*, s. 12(2)(*b*).

[50]   *Public Health Act*, R.S.A. 2000, c. P-37; *Vital Statistics Act*, R.S.A. 2000, c. V-4 (Alberta). *Public Health Act*, S.B.C. 2008, c. 28 [not yet in force]; *Vital Statistics Act*, R.S.B.C. 1996, c. 479 (British Columbia). *Public Health Act*, C.C.S.M. c. P210 (as am. by S.M. 2006, c. 14); *Vital Statistics Act*, C.C.S.M. c. V60 (Manitoba). *Health Act*, R.S.N.B. 1973, c. H-2; *Venereal Disease Act*, R.S.N.B. 1973, c. V-2; *Vital Statistics Act*, S.N.B. 1979, c. V-3 (New Brunswick). *Communicable Diseases Act*, R.S.N.L. 1990, c. C-26; *Venereal Disease Prevention Act*, R.S.N.L. 1990, c. V-2; *Vital Statistics Act*, R.S.N.L. 1990, c. V-6 (Newfoundland and Labrador). *Public Health Act*, R.S.N.W.T. 1988, c. P-12; *Vital Statistics Act*, R.S.N.W.T. 1988, c. V-3 (Northwest Territories). *Health Act*, R.S.N.S. 1989, c. 195; *Vital Statistics Act*, R.S.N.S. 1989, c. 494 (Nova Scotia). *Public Health Act*, R.S.N.W.T. 1988, c. P-12, as duplicated for Nunavut by s. 29 of the *Nunavut Act*, S.C. 1993, c. 28; *Vital Statistics Act*, R.S.N.W.T. 1988, c. V-3, as duplicated for Nunavut by s. 29 of the *Nunavut Act*, S.C. 1993, c. 28 (Nunavut). *Health Protection and Promotion Act*, R.S.O. 1990, c. H.7; *Vital Statistics Act*, R.S.O. 1990, c. V.4 (Ontario). *Public Health Act*, R.S.P.E.I. 1988, c. P-30; *Vital Statistics Act*, R.S.P.E.I. 1988, c. V-4.01 (Prince Edward Island). *Public Health Act*, R.S.Q. c. S-2.2 (Québec). *Public Health Act, 1994*, S.S. 1994, c. P-37.1; *Vital Statistics Act*, S.S. 1995, c. V-7.1 (Saskatchewan). *Public Health and Safety Act*, R.S.Y. 2002, c. 176; *Vital Statistics Act*, R.S.Y. 2002, c. 225 (Yukon).

[51]   *Freedom of Information and Protection of Privacy Act*, R.S.A. 2000, c. F-25 (Alberta). *Freedom of Information and Protection of Privacy Act*, R.S.B.C. 1996, c. 165 (British Columbia). *Freedom of Information and Protection of Privacy Act*, C.C.S.M. c. F175 (Manitoba). *Protection of Personal Information Act*, S.N.B. 1998, c. P-19.1; *Right to Information Act*, S.N.B. 1978, c. R-10.3 (New Brunswick). *Access to Information and Protection of Privacy Act*, S.N.L. 2002, c. A-1.1. *Access to Information and Protection of Privacy Act*, S.N.W.T 1994, c. 20 (Northwest Territories). *Freedom of Information and Protection of Privacy Act*, S.N.S. 1993, c. 5 (Nova Scotia). *Access to Information and Protection of Privacy Act*, R.S.N.W.T 1994, c. 20, as duplicated for Nunavut by s. 29 of the *Nunavut Act*, S.C. 1993, c. 28 (Nunavut). *Personal Health Information Protection Act, 2004*, S.O. 2004, c. 3, Sch. A, s. 8(1). *Freedom of Information and Protection of Privacy Act*, R.S.O. 1990, c. F.31 (Ontario). *Freedom of Information and Protection of Privacy Act*,

province to province regarding the scope of coverage of the legislation; for instance, the inclusion of hospitals and universities.[52] There is also variation in the role of the privacy commissioner in that in British Columbia, for example, an order of the privacy commissioner is enforceable,[53] while in most jurisdictions the privacy commissioner's mandate is primarily educational and persuasive; similar to the federal legislation, only a court can make a binding order.[54]

The provinces of Québec, British Columbia and Alberta have enacted legislation governing the handling of personal information in the private sector generally.[55] Manitoba, Saskatchewan, Alberta and Ontario have enacted sector-specific health information legislation.[56] These statutes regulate the collection, use, disclosure and retention of personal health information. In addition, health services provider information is protected under the Alberta legislation.[57] A notable feature of this private sector legislation is the formalization of the role of holder of personal information as a custodian or trustee, with accompanying responsibilities and duties.

Provincial legislation governing specific aspects of the health sector, especially mental health and continuing care homes legislation, generally contains one or more provisions regarding confidentiality of patient records.[58]

R.S.P.E.I. 1988, c. F-15.01 (Prince Edward Island). *An Act respecting Access to documents held by public bodies and the Protection of personal information*, R.S.Q. c. A-2.1 (Québec). *Freedom of Information and Protection of Privacy Act*, S.S. 1990-91, c. F-22.01 (Saskatchewan). *Access to Information and Protection of Privacy Act*, R.S.Y. 2002, c. 1 (Yukon).

[52] The Nova Scotia *Freedom of Information and Protection of Privacy Act*, S.N.S. 1993, c. 5, s. 4(1) includes these entities, whereas they are not included under Saskatchewan's *Freedom of Information and Protection of Privacy Act*, S.S. 1990-91, c. F-22.01.

[53] *Freedom of Information and Protection of Privacy Act*, R.S.B.C. 1996, c. 165, s. 59. An application for judicial review of the Commissioner's order may be brought within days of its receipt.

[54] See *e.g.* Manitoba's *Freedom of Information and Protection of Privacy Act*, C.C.S.M. c. F175, s. 49. Section 66(4) of the Act allows the head of a public body to decline to implement the recommendations of the Ombudsman but written reasons for doing so must be provided. The Ombudsman or the initial complainant may appeal this decision under ss. 67 and 68, respectively.

[55] *An Act respecting the protection of personal information in the private sector*, R.S.Q. c. P-39.1; *Personal Information Protection Act*, S.B.C. 2003, c. 63; *Personal Information Protection Act*, S.A. 2003, c. P-6.5.

[56] *Personal Health Information Act*, C.C.S.M. c. P33.5; *Health Information Protection Act*, S.S. 1999, c. H-0.021; *Health Information Act*, R.S.A. 2000, c. H-5; *Personal Health Information Protection Act, 2004*, S.O. 2004, c. 3, Sch. A.

[57] *Health Information Act*, R.S.A. 2000, c. H-5, s. 1(1).

[58] See *e.g.*, *Hospitals Act*, R.S.N.S. 1989, c. 208, s. 71 (confidentiality of hospital records); *Continuing Care Act*, R.S.B.C. 1996, c. 70, s. 11 (confidentiality of client information).

Several provinces have enacted legislation, establishing a statutory tort of invasion of privacy. Saskatchewan's *Privacy Act*[59] was reviewed in *Peters-Brown v. Regina District Health Board,*[60] which involved the indiscriminate circulation within a penal institution of a list prepared by the Regina hospital identifying by name individuals around whom bodily fluid precautions were to be taken. The lawsuit was brought by an employee of the correctional institute whose name appeared on the list and who suffered humiliation among her colleagues as a result. No violation of the *Privacy Act* was found because the release by the hospital was not intentional. The employee also failed in her claim for defamation, but was successful in her claims for negligence and breach of contract.

(c) Common Law Protection of Information

As made clear in the last section, legislation governing information is not comprehensive in Canada. In jurisdictions and subject areas where no legislation has been enacted, and where there are gaps in the legislation, the common law operates. The duty of confidentiality has a long and venerable history in the health care context, finding one of its early manifestations in the Hippocratic Oath.[61] There are, however, a number of circumstances in which it may be appropriate or even mandatory to reveal information supplied in confidence in the absence of consent. In this section I elaborate on the duty of confidentiality and then discuss these exceptional circumstances.

Legal duties of confidentiality have arisen historically both at common law and within professional codes of ethics. In 1928, the Supreme Court of Canada described the duty of a physician as follows:

> Nobody would dispute that a secret ... is the secret of the patient, and, normally, is under his control, and not under that of the doctor. *Prima facie*, the patient has the right to require that the secret shall not be divulged; and that right is absolute, unless there is some paramount reason which overrides it.[62]

Therefore, contrary to our general societal presumption that what one is told may be conveyed to others in the absence of a request for secrecy, personal health information conveyed to a professional in the

---

[59]   R.S.S. 1978, c. P-24.

[60]   [1995] S.J. No. 609, [1996] 1 W.W.R. 337, 136 Sask. R. 126 (Sask. Q.B.) [*"Peters-Brown"* cited to W.W.R.], aff'd [1996] S.J. No. 761, [1997] 1 W.W.R. 638, 148 Sask. R. 248 (Sask. C.A.).

[61]   Hippocrates, "Oath" in *Hippocrates*, vol. 1, W.H.S. Jones, trans. (London: William Heinemann, 1928) at 301.

[62]   *Halls v. Mitchell*, [1928] S.C.J. No. 1, [1928] S.C.R. 125 at 136, [1928] 2 D.L.R. 97 (S.C.C.) [*"Halls"* cited to S.C.R.].

course of accessing health care services is treated in law as confidential in the absence of an indication otherwise.[63] Likewise, codes of ethics of healthcare professionals invariably contain one or more provisions laying out a duty of confidentiality.[64] The primary rationale for this approach is that if patients worry their information will not be kept confidential, they will be disinclined to seek medical care, especially if they suspect or know that their particular ailment is one about which they do not wish others to know due to potential for embarrassment, ridicule or discrimination.

(i)   Consensual Release

Health records are to be shared with the patient and with others if the patient consents to their release. If there is a substitute decision-maker, in the case of a mentally incompetent individual or an immature minor, that person is authorized to consent to release of information on behalf of the patient. Consent to the sharing of information for treatment purposes is to be inferred unless the patient has indicated to the contrary. These circumstances are discussed below.

(A) Patient Access and Authorization

Historically, the right of a patient to access his or her health records was unclear in law. In 1992, the Supreme Court of Canada settled this issue in the case of *McInerney v. MacDonald*.[65] The case arose from a situation where a woman sought access to her medical records created by her physician and also the records, x-rays and test results conveyed to her physician by other health care professionals. The Court ruled that while the physical records belong to the physician, the patient has a general right of access to the information contained therein, regardless as to who compiled the records — *i.e.*, the physician from whom the records are requested or other health care providers. The sole exception is in a circumstance where the health care provider believes on reasonable and

---

[63]   For discussion of this presumption in the context of physiotherapy records, see *R. v. Serendip Physiotherapy Clinic*, [2004] O.J. No. 4653, 245 D.L.R. (4th) 88 (Ont. C.A.), rev'g [2003] O.J. No. 2407, 65 O.R. (3d) 271 (Ont. S.C.J.), leave to appeal to S.C.C. refused [2004] S.C.C.A. No. 585 (S.C.C.A.).

[64]   See Canadian Medical Association, *CMA Code of Ethics* (update 2004) at ss. 31-37, online: <http://policybase.cma.ca/PolicyPDF/PD04-06.pdf>; Canadian Nurses Association, *Code of Ethics for Registered Nurses* at 14, online: <http://www.cna-nurses.ca/cna/documents/pdf/publications/CodeofEthics2002_e.pdf>; National Association of Pharmacy Regulatory Authorities, *Model Standards of Practice for Canadian Pharmacists* at standard 4, online: <http://www.napra.org/practice/standards.html>; Canadian Dental Association, *CDA Code of Ethics* at Art. 9, online: <http://www.cda-adc.ca/en/cda/about_cda/code_of_ethics/index.asp>.

[65]   [1992] S.C.J. No. 57, [1992] 2 S.C.R. 138, 93 D.L.R. (4th) 415 (S.C.C.) ["*McInerney*" cited to S.C.R.].

probable grounds that disclosure of the information carries "... a significant likelihood of a substantial adverse effect on the physical, mental or emotional health of the patient or harm to a third party".[66] A reasonable fee may be charged for the costs of permitting access or photocopying.[67]

The capacity of an adult to provide consent to use of personal information is presumed in law.[68] The parent of an immature minor is presumed in law to be the child's guardian and therefore qualified to make decisions concerning the child (and, by implication, information pertaining to the child) unless a court has ordered otherwise.[69] The situation regarding an incompetent adult is somewhat more complex. If he or she has while competent designated a surrogate decision-maker pursuant to provincial legislation, or if the court has designated a guardian, that designee is vested with authority to make decisions on behalf of the incompetent individual and, again by implication, decisions concerning access to the incompetent person's personal health information.[70] Mental health legislation in some provinces provides a hierarchy of substitute decision-makers for incompetent individuals.[71]

The individual or substitute decision-maker is in turn able to authorize the release of personal health information to third parties. It is necessary to ensure that only such information as falls within the authorization granted is released, and that the release is to the individual or organization specifically authorized to receive the information.

(B) Access by Other Healthcare Providers

Information has tended historically to flow among members of the healthcare team without hesitation. The era of electronic patient information, and heightened attention to privacy issues, has led to increased concerns regarding the free flow of information. The Canadian

---

[66]   *Ibid.*, at 158.

[67]   *Ibid.*, at 159.

[68]   D. Weisstub, chairman, *Enquiry on Mental Competency: Final Report* (Toronto: Queen's Printer for Ontario, 1990) at 35.

[69]   See *e.g.*, Ontario *Health Care Consent Act, 1996*, S.O. 1996, c. 2, Sch. A, s. 20; Nova Scotia *Maintenance and Custody Act*, R.S.N.S. 1989, c. 160, s. 18(4).

[70]   See *e.g.*, *Health Care Consent Act, 1996*, S.O. 1996, c. 2, Sch. A, ss. 20(1), 40(1), 57(1) (appointment of a surrogate decision-maker); *Dependent Adults Act*, R.S.A. 2000, c. D-11, s. 10(3) (broad powers which may be granted by the court to the guardian).

[71]   Patricia Peppin, "Informed Consent" in Jocelyn Downie, Timothy Caulfield and Colleen Flood, eds., *Canadian Health Law and Policy*, 3d ed. (Markham, Ont.: LexisNexis Canada, 2007) 189 at 213. Note that under the *Hospitals Act*, R.S.N.S. 1989, c. 208, s. 54(2), these provisions only apply in case of a hospitalized individual.

Medical Association has outlined the circumstances in which in their view information can be accessed or disclosed without specific consent:

> Consent to health information collection, use, disclosure and access for the primary therapeutic purpose may be inferred. Consent to subsequent collection, use, disclosure and access on a need-to-know basis by or to other physicians or health providers for this purpose, and for this purpose alone, may be inferred, as long as there is no evidence that the patient would not give express consent to share the information.[72]

Note that consent may be inferred solely for the primary therapeutic purpose and for no other purposes. Also note that the information released must be limited to that strictly required for the purposes of therapy. This concept is supported under the federal *PIPEDA*, which provides for implied consent in certain circumstances, interpreted by Industry Canada to include healthcare professionals within the "circle of care".[73]

Sharing of personal health information among professionals specifically within the public health system is covered in detail in the latter portion of this chapter.

(ii) Non-Consensual Release

Personal health information is to be maintained in confidence except as authorized or required by law. This section reviews the areas in which the common law or legislation has carved out exceptions to confidentiality. Releases specifically authorized in public health legislation will be discussed later in this chapter.

(A) Obligations Arising Under Statute

Some of the major reporting obligations in non-public-health-specific statutes are with regard to abuse. If a health professional (and in some provinces any individual) believes on reasonable grounds that a child is suffering or has in the past suffered from abuse, she or he is required to contact the child protection agency.[74] Note that abuse is

---

[72] Canadian Medical Association, "Health Information Privacy Code" (1998) at Art. 5.3, online: <http://www.cma.ca/index.cfm/ci_id/3216/la_id/1.htm>.

[73] Industry Canada, "PIPEDA Awareness Raising Tools (PARTs) Initiative For The Health Sector", online: <http://ecom.ic.gc.ca/epic/internet/inecic-ceac.nsf/en/gv00235e.html>.

[74] *Child, Youth and Family Enhancement Act*, R.S.A. 2000, c. C-12, s. 4 (Alberta); *Child, Family and Community Service Act*, R.S.B.C. 1996, c. 46, s. 14 (British Columbia); *Child and Family Services Act*, S.M. 1985-86, c. 8 (C.C.S.M. c. C80), s. 18 (Manitoba); *Family Services Act*, S.N.B. 1980, c. F-2.2, s. 30 (New Brunswick); *Child, Youth and Family Services Act*, S.N.L. 1998, c. C-12.1, s. 15 (Newfoundland and Labrador); *Child and Family Services Act*, S.N.W.T. 1997, c. 13, s. 8(1) (Northwest Territories); *Children and Family Services Act*, S.N.S. 1990, c. 5, ss. 23, 24, 25 (Nova Scotia); *Child and Family*

defined as including a failure to provide the child with required medical treatment.[75] The person reporting is protected from being sued for this disclosure unless the reporting is found to have been both false and malicious.[76]

In some provinces there is an obligation to report that an adult is in need of protection.[77] In others disclosure is permissive; in other words, the professional may at her or his discretion report that an adult is in need of protection.[78] In Nova Scotia, being "in need of protection" is defined as being subjected to physical or sexual abuse, or inadequate care, and further being incapable of protecting oneself due to physical or mental disability.[79] Where a person is suffering from a psychiatric disorder and poses a risk of harm to himself or herself or others, or a risk of serious deterioration, the treating physician may decide to refer the individual for further assessment and possible detention under provincial mental health legislation.[80]

There are a number of legislative provisions regarding reporting of medication prescriptions and adverse reactions. The federal *Narcotic Control Regulations* require that healthcare professionals keep a record of all prescriptions issued for narcotics and make these available to an inspector upon request.[81] At present, the reporting by health professionals to Health Canada of a suspected adverse reaction to a medication is voluntary.[82] Ontario's public health legislation requires the reporting of suspected adverse reactions to immunizing agents.[83]

(B) Other Obligations

A number of exceptions to the duty of confidentiality have been identified in common law and in legislation. These revolve around

---

Services Act, R.S.O. 1990, c. 11, s. 68 (Ontario); *Child Protection Act*, R.S.P.E.I. 1988, c. C5.1, s. 22 (Prince Edward Island); *Youth Protection Act*, R.S.Q. c. P-34.1, s. 39 (Québec); *Child and Family Services Act*, S.S. 1989-90, c. C-7.2, s. 12 (Saskatchewan); *Children's Act*, R.S.Y. 2002, c. 31, s. 117 (Yukon).

[75] *Ibid.*, at s. 22(2)(e).

[76] *Ibid.*, at s. 23(2).

[77] See *e.g.*, *Adult Protection Act*, R.S.N.S. 1989, c. 2, s. 5(1).

[78] See *e.g.*, *Adult Protection Act*, R.S.P.E.I. 1988, c. A-5, s. 4(1).

[79] *Adult Protection Act*, R.S.N.S. 1989, c. 2, s. 3(b).

[80] Gerald Robertson, *Mental Disability and the Law in Canada*, 2d ed. (Toronto: Carswell, 1994) at 383-96.

[81] C.R.C., c. 1041, s. 55, see online: <http://www.laws.justice.gc.ca/en/C-38.8/C.R.C.-c.1041/75957.html>.

[82] Health Canada, *Guidelines — Voluntary Reporting of Suspected Adverse Reactions to Health Products by Health Professionals and Consumers*, online: <http://www.hc-sc.gc.ca/dhp-mps/alt_formats/hpfb-dgpsa/pdf/medeff/ar-ei_guide-ldir-eng.pdf>.

[83] *Health Protection and Promotion Act*, R.S.O. 1990, c. H.7, s. 38(3).

emergency circumstances, protection of third parties from risk of significant harm, and subpoenas/search warrants.

First, a healthcare provider in an emergency situation is justified in providing necessary personal health information where imminently required to preserve the health or safety of a patient provided that the wishes of the patient are not known.[84] This common law principle has recently been supported by provisions under *PIPEDA*, which provide that an organization is entitled to use personal information without consent "for the purpose of acting in respect of an emergency that threatens the life, health or security of an individual".[85] Where necessary to disclose (as opposed to merely using) information in these emergency circumstances, if the individual whose information is being disclosed is alive, the organization must also notify him or her of the disclosure.[86]

Second, healthcare professionals are entitled to protect third parties by releasing information as necessary to avert a known threat to those third parties. This circumstance has been defined to exist where the risk is to an identifiable person or group of persons and the threat is serious and imminent.[87] It is important to note that this does not apply where a person is threatening self-harm; rather, it revolves around a threat to a third party.

Third, in the context of legal proceedings and criminal investigations, a search warrant or subpoena ordering the production of personal health information may be issued. A search warrant is issued by a Justice of the Peace in response to an application by legal counsel or by a peace officer. It orders that the bearer of the warrant be entitled to enter the premises identified in the document to search for information. A subpoena, on the other hand, may be issued by a member of the judiciary or by an administrative decision-maker (such as an arbitrator). Rather than authorizing entry, a subpoena orders that the named individual appear at a set time and location, and it may also order the accompanying production of specified documents. A healthcare professional faced with a subpoena should attend the hearing and identify the duty of confidentiality owed to the patient. The judge or hearing officer will then come to a determination as to whether the information must be provided. In the case either of a search warrant or a subpoena, the custodian of personal health information must ensure that the information provided is no more than that necessary to meet the terms of the order.

---

[84]   *Marshall v. Curry*, [1933] N.S.J. No. 6, [1933] 3 D.L.R. 260 (N.S.S.C.).

[85]   *Personal Information Protection and Electronic Documents Act*, S.C. 2000, c. 5, s. 7(2)(*b*).

[86]   *Ibid.*, at s. 7(3)(*e*).

[87]   *Smith v. Jones*, [1999] S.C.J. No. 15, [1999] 1 S.C.R. 455 at 486 (S.C.C.); L.E. Ferris *et al.*, "Defining the physician's duty to warn: consensus statement of Ontario's Medical Expert Panel on Duty to Inform" (1998) 158 C.M.A.J. 1473.

(d) Canadian Charter of Rights and Freedoms

The *Canadian Charter of Rights and Freedoms*[88] provides protection for individuals and, in certain respects, corporations against actions of the state that interfere with one's rights or freedoms. It operates at a level above statutory law in that if an unjustified violation is found in a provision of a federal or provincial statute or regulation, that provision is rendered of no force or effect.[89]

There is no right to privacy identified in the *Charter*; however, judicial interpretation has established that certain aspects of the individual's privacy interest are subject to *Charter* protection under s. 7 (right to life, liberty and security of the person), s. 8 (right to be secure against unreasonable search or seizure) and s. 15 (right to equality). If a violation of one of these rights is established, the state carries the onus of establishing that this violation is justified in a free and democratic society. In the public health context, individuals' privacy interests are balanced against the need for protection of the public by such measures as contact notification and posting of notices. As we shall see, the courts place a high value on protection, sometimes but not always at the expense of individual rights.

A majority of *Charter* cases establishing a right to privacy have been in the context of criminal proceedings.[90] Section 8 of the *Charter* states that "[e]veryone has a right to be secure against unreasonable search or seizure". Justice La Forest of the Supreme Court of Canada indicated that s. 8 protects a reasonable expectation of privacy, and that:

> [P]rivacy is at the heart of liberty in the modern state ... Grounded in man's physical and moral autonomy, privacy is essential for the well-being of the individual. For this reason alone, it is worthy of constitutional protection, but it also has profound significance for the public order.[91]

Section 8 of the *Charter* was under discussion in a case concerning charges laid under the Manitoba *Public Health Act*[92] against Mr. Van Wynsberghe regarding the operation of his restaurant.[93] An inspector

---

[88] Part I of the *Constitution Act, 1982*, being Schedule B to the *Canada Act 1982* (U.K.), 1982, c. 11 ["*Charter*"].

[89] *Ibid.*, s. 1.

[90] An exception is *Cheskes v. Ontario (Attorney General)*, [2007] O.J. No. 3515, 87 O.R. (3d) 581 (Ont. S.C.J.), in which Belobaba J. found a right to privacy under s. 7 in the context of adoption information.

[91] *R. v. Dyment*, [1988] S.C.J. No. 82, [1988] 2 S.C.R. 417 at 427, 55 D.L.R. (4th) 503 (S.C.C.) ["*Dyment*" cited to S.C.R.]. Justice La Forest was alluding to a passage from Alan F. Westin's *Privacy and Freedom* (New York: Atheneum, 1970) at 349-50.

[92] C.C.S.M. c. P210.

[93] *R. v. Van Wynsberghe*, [2001] M.J. No. 594 (Man. Prov. Ct.).

acquainted with Mr. Van Wynsberghe entered his property without asking permission and without showing identification. The statute permits entry without consent upon showing a certificate or other means of identification. Mr. Van Wynsberghe did not resist the entry. However, his passive acquiescence was insufficient to constitute consent. The entry of the inspector without consent was found to violate s. 8, and the evidence obtained pursuant to entry was not permitted to be used at trial.

The seizure of information by police in emergency rooms has also brought s. 8 into play.[94] When a physician hands over test results or bodily fluid samples to police, he or she becomes a "state actor" for purposes of the *Charter*.[95] The physician's duty of confidentiality to the patient results in a reasonable expectation of privacy on the part of the accused that information and samples provided in the course of treatment will not become part of a criminal investigation.[96]

Section 7 of the *Charter* states: "Everyone has the right to life, liberty and security of the person and the right not to be deprived thereof except in accordance with the principles of fundamental justice." This section was examined in the context of public health legislation in the case of *Canadian AIDS Society v. Ontario*.[97] Blood samples were collected from donors between December 1, 1984 and October 31, 1985 without requesting or getting informed consent to HIV testing. Ten years later, these samples were tested for presence of the HIV virus in order to trace tainted samples to the recipients for purposes of notification. At issue was whether 13 HIV-positive donors should be notified of their HIV status, and whether notice should go to the public health authorities in accordance with provisions in the *Health Protection and Promotion Act*.[98] The Canadian AIDS Society argued that this notification would violate the right to security of the person under s. 7 of the *Charter* in that the donors had not agreed to the testing of the blood samples. Justice Wilson of the Ontario Court of Justice (General Division) agreed that disclosure would constitute a violation of the donors' psychological integrity, and thus breach their right to security of the person.[99]

---

[94]   *R. v. Dersch*, [1993] S.C.J. No. 116, [1993] 3 S.C.R. 768 (S.C.C.) ["*Dersch*"].

[95]   *Ibid.*, 777 S.C.R.

[96]   *Ibid.*, 778 S.C.R.

[97]   [1995] O.J. No. 2361 (Ont. Gen. Div.), aff'd [1996] O.J. No. 4184, 31 O.R. (3d) 798 (Ont. C.A.), leave to appeal to S.C.C. refused [1997] S.C.C.A. No. 33 (S.C.C.). Note that the applicant also claimed a breach of *Charter* s. 8, but the court found that the "seizure" of blood was reasonable and therefore in the circumstances did not constitute a violation of the donor's s. 8 rights, "... having regard to the importance of public health" (at paras. 152, 159).

[98]   R.S.O. 1990, c. H.7.

[99]   *Canadian AIDS Society v. Ontario*, [1995] O.J. No. 2361 at para. 127 (Ont. Gen. Div.).

However, the analysis does not end here. Although a violation of the right to security had been found, in accordance with the latter part of the s. 7 test, the court went on to analyze whether the principles of fundamental justice had been violated. The court found that the reporting provisions of the *Health Protection and Promotion Act* set an appropriate balance between the privacy rights of the individual and the state interest in protecting and promoting public health.[100] Therefore the reporting was respectful of the principles of fundamental justice, and the s. 7 requirements were met. The application by the Canadian AIDS Society to prevent notification of the public health authorities and the donors failed. The court also made this crucial finding:

> In this civil suit, although due consideration will be given to the privacy rights of individuals, *the state objective of promoting public health for the safety of all will be given great weight.*[101]

This is an important signal: when the judiciary balances *Charter* values that protect the privacy rights of individuals against the public health interests of the collective, high priority will be given to the latter.

Finally, there is scope for analysis of the s. 15(1) *Charter* right, which guarantees:

> Every individual is equal before and under the law and has the right to the equal protection and equal benefit of the law without discrimination and, in particular, without discrimination based on race, national or ethnic origin, colour, religion, sex, age or mental or physical disability.

This *Charter* section has seldom been relied on in the context of health information. However, in *R. v. Mills*,[102] a case concerning the *Criminal Code* provisions restricting the availability to the accused of a sexual assault victim's medical and counselling records, the Supreme Court of Canada indicated that the s. 15(1) right to equality provides additional context (along with other *Charter* sections) for the protection of privacy of health information. This results from the fact that myths and stereotypes operate to the disadvantage of victims of sexual violence, and that discrimination on the basis of sex is prohibited under s. 15(1).[103]

The reader can anticipate further analysis of s. 15(1) in the public health context in the future. In *HIV Testing and Pregnancy: Medical and Legal Parameters of the Policy Debate*,[104] the authors conclude that

---

[100] *Ibid.*, at para. 133.

[101] *Ibid.*, at para. 133 [emphasis added].

[102] [1999] S.C.J. No. 68, [1999] 3 S.C.R. 668, 180 D.L.R. (4th) 1 (S.C.C.) ["*Mills*" cited to S.C.R.].

[103] *Ibid.*, at 727-28.

[104] L. Stoltz. & L. Shap, *HIV Testing and Pregnancy: Medical and Legal Parameters of the Policy Debate* (Ottawa: Health Canada, 1999).

"... a government policy that causes prejudice or disadvantage to pregnant women will be vulnerable to challenge under section 15(1) of the Charter".[105] Further, while aimed at protection of individuals, the Supreme Court of Canada has indicated that s. 15(1) also protects against "... discrimination against particular groups 'suffering social, political and legal disadvantage in our society'".[106] A group may be singled out for special treatment in public health legislation, as for example under recent changes to the Ontario *Health Protection and Promotion Act* that provide for orders against a "class of persons".[107] One has only to recall the discrimination experienced by the Asian community in Toronto when news was circulated as to the identity of the first known SARS case to understand that the impact of such an order on a particular group could be severe and problematic.[108]

If a violation of s. 7, 8 or 15(1) is found, the Court turns to s. 1 of the *Charter*, which states that:

> The *Canadian Charter of Rights and Freedoms* guarantees the rights and freedoms set out in it subject only to such reasonable limits prescribed by law as can be demonstrably justified in a free and democratic society.

The government bears the onus of establishing that a violation of the substantive *Charter* section is justified as a reasonable limit in society. The above discussion of the "principles of fundamental justice" is again relevant *vis-à-vis* the s. 1 analysis. The importance of protection of the public against the spread of communicable disease will weigh heavily in the balance when justifying state action. Nevertheless, the government cannot run roughshod over individual rights and freedoms unless it can demonstrate that its actions are necessary to protect the public. It must establish that its objective in taking such action is important enough to warrant overriding a constitutional right.[109] Further, it must demonstrate that its response/action is proportional to the issue with which it is dealing. An important part of the analysis is that the measure must impair as little as possible the right or freedom in question. Thus, in a *Charter* action, the government will need to justify limits on privacy of the individual or group as being an appropriate response to a threat to the health of the public.

---

[105]   *Ibid.*, at 51.

[106]   *Eldridge v. British Columbia (Attorney General)*, [1997] S.C.J. No. 86, [1997] 3 S.C.R. 624 at 667, 151 D.L.R. (4th) 577 (S.C.C.).

[107]   R.S.O. 1990, c. H.7, s. 22(5.0.1).

[108]   See *e.g.*, Ontario Human Rights Commission, News Release, "Commission urges tolerance and respect during the SARS health emergency" (4 April 2003), online: <http://www.ohrc.on.ca/en/resources/news/NewsRelease.2006-05-19.6813797222/view>; Caroline Alphonso, "Illness spawns some shunning of Asians" *The Globe and Mail* (3 April 2003) at NA9.

[109]   *R. v. Oakes*, [1986] S.C.J. No. 7, [1986] 1 S.C.R. 103 at 138-40 (S.C.C.).

III. PUBLIC HEALTH LEGISLATION

Each of the provinces and territories has enacted legislation governing public health. Also, the federal government has legislated in limited areas of public health. This portion of the chapter discusses the various major reporting obligations that arise under public health legislation, commencing with the duty on individuals to self-report the presence of a communicable disease, the duty on others to report, and the duty of confidentiality of medical officers of health. It then examines contact notification and notification of the public. The last two sections outline the uses of public health information for surveillance, epidemiology and research purposes, and the emergency context.

(a) Duty on Individuals to Self-Report

Depending on the province/territory of residence, and upon entering Canada, there may be a duty on individuals who think they have a communicable disease to report to a medical practitioner. This duty is separate and distinct from the obligation of a medical practitioner to convey information that an individual has or may have a communicable disease, which will be discussed in the next section. This obligation is in some jurisdictions restricted to sexually transmitted infections.

(i) Federal

The *Quarantine Act*[110] mandates the provision of health information by travellers arriving to or departing from Canada upon request by a quarantine officer.[111] It further requires that travellers who have reasonable grounds to suspect that they have or might have a communicable disease, or have recently been in close proximity to a person who has or may have a communicable disease, report this fact to a screening officer.[112] The same duty applies in the case of vector[113] infestation.

(ii) Provincial/Territorial

There is no duty on an individual to report that she or he may have a communicable disease in Nova Scotia, Ontario and Québec. In

---

[110]   S.C. 2005, c. 20.

[111]   *Ibid.*, s. 15(1). Travellers must provide the officer with any information or record in their possession that the officer may reasonably require in the performance of a duty under the Act.

[112]   *Ibid.*, s. 15(2).

[113]   *Ibid.* "Vector" is defined in s. 2 of the *Quarantine Act* as "... an insect or animal capable of transmitting a communicable disease".

Newfoundland and Labrador, a person suspecting that he or she has a venereal disease must report immediately either to a physician or to a Medical Officer of Health ("MOH").[114] Interestingly, there is no similar duty in the case of other communicable diseases. Instead, the individual who knows they have a communicable disease is constrained from being in a public conveyance or otherwise mingling with members of the public until advised by a health officer or medical practitioner that it is safe to do so.[115] Note that this does not apply where one merely suspects that she or he has a communicable disease.

Under law in Prince Edward Island, there is a duty on an individual who is infected, who is suspected of being infected or who suspects they are a carrier or contact of a regulated disease, to present to a physician.[116]

In New Brunswick, the suspicion that one is infected with a venereal disease is sufficient to create a duty on the part of that person to report to a medical practitioner.[117] New Brunswick places a duty on a "practitioner, nurse, householder or other person who recognizes or suspects the presence of a notifiable disease",[118] which could be interpreted as a duty on the individual to self-report. In the Northwest Territories, Nunavut and Yukon Territory, every person who has reason to believe he or she has a communicable disease generally, without limiting the duty to the context of sexually transmitted infections, must notify a medical practitioner or MOH.[119] Saskatchewan falls somewhere in the middle in terms of the duty to report a suspicion in that it has a restricted list which includes several sexually transmitted infections, tuberculosis, HIV/AIDS, and hepatitis B, C and D.

The individual is to report most of these diseases within 72 hours in Saskatchewan.[120] HIV is the sole exception; in this case one must see a healthcare professional within 30 days, unless diagnosed through an approved anonymous testing site, in which case no reporting is required.[121]

Finally, Alberta's legislation has the most stringent requirements for reporting. Similar to the three Territories, the obligation to consult a physician applies in the case of all prescribed communicable diseases and

---

[114] *Venereal Disease Prevention Act*, R.S.N.L. 1990, c. V-2, s. 3(1).
[115] *Communicable Diseases Act*, R.S.N.L. 1990, c. C-26, s. 16.
[116] *Notifiable and Communicable Diseases Regulations*, P.E.I. Reg. EC330/85, s. 4.
[117] *Venereal Disease Act*, R.S.N.B. 1973, c. V-2, s. 3.
[118] *General Regulation — Health Act*, N.B. Reg. 88-200, s. 94(2).
[119] *Communicable Diseases Regulations*, R.R.N.W.T. 1990, c. P-13, s. 2(a); *Communicable Diseases Regulations*, R.R.N.W.T. 1990, c. P-13, s. 2(a), as duplicated for Nunavut by s. 29 of the *Nunavut Act*, S.C. 1993, c. 28; *Regulations for the Control of Communicable Diseases in the Yukon Territory*, C.O. 1961/048, s. 3.
[120] *Public Health Act, 1994*, S.S. 1994, c. P-37.1, s. 33(1).
[121] *Disease Control Regulations*, R.R.S. c. P-37.1, Reg. 11, s. 11.

not just sexually transmitted infections.[122] The same duty is extended to persons with minor children under their custody, care or control if they suspect the child is infected.[123] And, uniquely, a MOH who believes on reasonable grounds that a person is engaging in, or has in the past engaged in, an activity that may threaten the health of the public may require that person to provide information as to the activity in question.[124]

(b) Mandatory Reporting by Third Parties

This section outlines the obligation of persons other than the potentially infected individual to report a suspicion that such individual has a communicable disease. Legislation in every province/territory as well as the federal *Quarantine Act* includes such an obligation. However, the provisions vary widely in terms of who bears an obligation and what information is to be provided.

(i) Federal

The *Quarantine Act* includes a number of reporting obligations. A quarantine officer who suspects that a traveller has a communicable disease or is infested with vectors, but does not believe this poses an immediate public health risk, may order the traveller to report to a specified public health authority.[125] The public health authority is to receive a copy of the report, and in turn is obliged to inform the quarantine officer as to whether or not the traveller does in fact report to them. Note that this raises a jurisdictional issue as to the entitlement of the federal government to place such an obligation on a local public health authority.[126]

The *Quarantine Act* also places an obligation upon the operator of a conveyance to report either a suspicion based on reasonable grounds that a person or item of cargo could cause a communicable disease to spread or that someone on the conveyance has died.[127] The operator also must answer questions asked by an officer and provide any information or records reasonably required by the officer.[128]

---

[122] *Public Health Act*, R.S.A. 2000, c. P-37, s. 20.
[123] *Ibid.*, s. 20(3).
[124] *Ibid.*, s. 18.
[125] *Quarantine Act*, S.C. 2005, c. 20, s. 25.
[126] Elaine Gibson, 18 November 2005, testimony before the Standing Committee on Health (38th Parl., 1st Sess.), online: House of Commons Committees <http://www.parl.gc.ca/committee/CommitteePublication.aspx?SourceId=92481>.
[127] *Quarantine Act*, S.C. 2005, c. 20, s. 34(2).
[128] *Ibid.*, s. 38.

(ii)   Provinces/Territories

(A) Who Bears the Obligation

Typically, a physician, registered nurse, the director of a laboratory or a person in charge of a hospital has a duty to report the likely presence of a communicable disease that comes to his or her attention. Québec circumscribes the duty more tightly by placing the obligation only on physicians and chief executive officers of laboratories and medical biology departments.[129] Others sometimes identified as subject to a reporting duty include a school principal or teacher, midwife, funeral director, embalmer, anyone requested to handle a dead body, ambulance operator, adult care facility licensee, daycare operator, and person in charge of a place of detention.[130] Worthy of note is a duty in Newfoundland and Labrador on a dairy person or milk vendor to report a case of communicable disease in himself or herself or a family member or employee.[131] Further, the proprietor, manager or person in charge of a laundry must immediately report a case of communicable disease "appearing on the premises".[132] Hotel and boarding house keepers must report a suspected carrier of a communicable disease.[133] Saskatchewan has included in the scope of its legislation a duty to report on the part of an operator of a food preparation or service establishment.[134]

The governments of New Brunswick, the Northwest Territories, Nunavut and Yukon Territory include broad duties in that all persons are required to report a suspicion that another person has a communicable disease.[135]

(B) Scope of Information to be Provided

The previous subsection outlined the differences from province to province in the range of persons on whom a duty to report is placed. There is also a divergence in terms of the amount and type of information that is

---

[129]   *Public Health Act*, R.S.Q. c. S-2.2, s. 82.

[130]   For example, in British Columbia numerous reporting duties are found not only in public health legislation but also in the *School Act*, R.S.B.C. 1996, c. 412, s. 91(5) (duty on teachers and principals), the *Adult Care Regulations*, B.C. Reg. 536/80, s. 10.6(2) (licensee of a community care facility), and the *Child Care Licensing Regulation*, B.C. Reg. 332/2007, s. 55(2) (licensee of a child care facility).

[131]   *Communicable Diseases Act*, R.S.N.L. 1990, c. C-26, s. 9.

[132]   *Ibid.*, s. 19.

[133]   *Ibid.*, s. 3.

[134]   *Public Health Act, 1994*, S.S. 1994, c. P-37.1, s. 32(1)(d).

[135]   *General Regulation — Health Act*, N.B. Reg. 88-200, s. 94(2); *Communicable Diseases Regulations*, R.R.N.W.T. 1990, c. P-13, s. 3; *Communicable Diseases Regulations*, R.R.N.W.T. 1990, c. P-13, s. 3, as duplicated for Nunavut by s. 29 of the *Nunavut Act*, S.C. 1993, c. 28; *Regulations for the Control of Communicable Diseases in the Yukon Territory*, C.O. 1961/048, s. 4.

to be included in the report. Generally, the reporting requirement for communicable diseases includes name, age, address, sex, name of disease, clinical and epidemiological details pertinent to diagnosis or follow-up, and name of the reporter.[136] This list is enhanced in a number of provinces. In Québec, for instance, reporting obligations include the telephone number and health insurance number of the infected individual as well as the date of onset and, in the case of specified diseases, all information concerning blood, organ or tissue donations made or received by the infected individual.[137] The Québec legislation also provides for the reporting of conditions or specific injuries resulting from environmental or occupational hazards.[138]

The government of Ontario requires, in addition to the general reporting requirements, the date of onset of symptoms, additional information considered necessary by the MOH, and the name and residence of the person who "refuses or neglects to continue the treatment in a manner and to a degree satisfactory to the physician".[139] In Saskatchewan, reporting obligations include the infected individual's phone number; the names, telephone numbers and addresses of contacts; known risk factors related to the individual; and any information considered by the public health officer to be necessary for control of the disease.[140]

(c) Duty of Confidentiality of Public Health Authorities

In addition to the duties developed at common law and in ethics for public health professionals to maintain confidentiality of patients' health information, provincial public health legislation uniformly contains one or more provisions explicitly prohibiting disclosure of personal information. Interestingly, the scope of the prohibition, to whom the duty of confidentiality applies, and the penalty for breaching the prohibition vary from province to province.

---

[136] See e.g., Forms Regulation, Alta. Reg. 193/1985, s. 1.

[137] Minister's Regulation under the Public Health Act, M.O. 011-2003, 5 November 2003, G.O.Q. 2003.II.3290, s. 6.

[138] Minister's Regulation under the Public Health Act, M.O. 011-2003, 5 November 2003, G.O.Q. 2003.II.3290, s. 3.

[139] Health Protection and Promotion Act, R.S.O. 1990, c. H.7, s. 34; see also Reports, R.R.O. 1990, Reg. 569, s. 1, enacted pursuant to the Health Protection and Promotion Act, R.S.O. 1990, c. H.7.

[140] Disease Control Regulations, R.R.S. 2000, c. P-37.1, Reg. 11, s. 14. Note, however, that this list does not apply in respect of HIV/AIDS where the test was conducted at an anonymous testing facility (s. 14(3)).

Legislation in Alberta,[141] British Columbia,[142] Ontario,[143] Québec[144] and Saskatchewan[145] places a duty to respect confidentiality with regard to all communicable disease information. Exceptions to this duty are relatively uniform, and include consent by the subject of the information, where required for the purpose of administering the Act, on court order, and where necessary in response to a public health threat. Saskatchewan legislation includes the release of de-identified information for "bona fide research or medical review".[146] Finally, the government of Ontario enacted a regulation in 1996 authorizing disclosure to Canadian Blood Services of information regarding a person who has donated or received blood with respect to certain enumerated diseases, most notably HIV and hepatitis C.[147]

Where the legislative provision concerning confidentiality has been breached, some of the statutes are silent as to penalty. In other statutes, the punishment ranges from a monetary penalty, imprisonment, forfeiture of one's office or dismissal from employment.

(d) Contact Notification

The laws concerning contact tracing constitute a veritable smorgasbord as to whether there is an obligation or discretion on the part of the infected individual to advise authorities as to the identity of contacts who may have been exposed to the disease. There is, in turn, wide variation as to who bears a duty to notify contacts, whether or not it is discretionary, who is to be notified, and what information is to be conveyed to the contacts.

The legislation varies widely; some statutes contain clear and detailed requirements about contact tracing, others are ambiguous, and others are silent on the topic. In the first instance, for Category II diseases, primarily sexually transmitted infections, the infected individual is required to supply the names of contacts in Saskatchewan.[148] Québec's legislation contains no provision compelling information to be provided

---

[141] *Public Health Act*, R.S.A. 2000, c. P-37, s. 53(1).

[142] *Public Health Act*, S.B.C. 2008, c. 28, s. 91 [not yet in force].

[143] *Health Protection and Promotion Act*, R.S.O. 1990, c. H.7, s. 39(1).

[144] *Public Health Act*, R.S.Q. c. S-2.2, s. 131.

[145] *Public Health Act, 1994*, S.S. 1994, c. P-37.1, s. 65(1).

[146] *Ibid.*, s. 65(2)(d)(ii).

[147] *Exemption — Subsection* 39(1) of *The Health Protection and Promotion Act*, O. Reg. 338/96.

[148] *Public Health Act, 1994*, S.S. 1994, c. P-37.1, s. 33(4). Note, however, that this requirement does not apply in respect of HIV and AIDS where the test was conducted at an anonymous testing facility.

by the individual.[149] In some provinces there is no clear duty on the individual to provide names.[150] In Alberta, names only are required;[151] in Prince Edward Island, the health officer may require the names and addresses of persons who might have been exposed to the disease.[152]

Secondly, even where there is no duty on the individual to provide information as to contacts, the physician may have a duty to notify others potentially infected if their identities are known. In the Yukon Territory, a medical practitioner is to advise any known contacts or carriers directly to adopt control measures and to carry out instructions; it is not clear whether he or she is also to reveal information as to the infected individual.[153] In New Brunswick, under legislation not yet in force, if a physician or nurse knows of contacts, this information is to be reported to the MOH.[154] Under New Brunswick's present legislation, the district medical health officer has a remarkably broad mandate:

> The district medical health officer may take all measures, which have proven practical in public health administration and which have been accepted by public health authorities, to carry out any preventive measure considered necessary to control and prevent the diffusion of a notifiable disease.[155]

The infected person may be required to contact others who might have been exposed.[156] In some provinces, in the case of specified diseases, the infected individual has the option of notifying others; if not, the physician or nurse is to do the notification.[157] Interestingly, in Saskatchewan, if the physician or nurse is notifying contacts, she or he is only to reveal the identity of the source individual if that individual has

---

[149]   *Public Health Act*, R.S.Q. c. S-2.2.

[150]   For example, Manitoba's legislation contains no explicit requirement for an individual to report their contacts, nor for the attending health practitioner to request such information. However, s. 24(1) of the *Diseases and Dead Bodies Regulation* (Man. Reg. 338/88R) authorizes a MOH to make orders with respect to contacts of a patient who has been placed in isolation.

[151]   *Public Health Act*, R.S.A. 2000, c. P-37, s. 31(2).

[152]   *Public Notifiable and Communicable Diseases Regulations*, P.E.I. Reg. EC330/85, s. 4(c).

[153]   *Regulations for the Control of Communicable Diseases in the Yukon Territory*, C.O. 1961/048, s. 5(1).

[154]   *Public Health Act*, S.N.B. 1998, c. P-22.4, s. 31 (assented to February 26, 1998 but not yet proclaimed in force).

[155]   *General Regulation — Health Act*, N.B. Reg. 88-200, s. 96.

[156]   *Health Protection Act*, S.N.S. 2004, c. 4, s. 33(1).

[157]   All category II diseases in Saskatchewan except where HIV testing was conducted at an anonymous testing site: *Public Health Act, 1994*, S.S. 1994, c. P-37.1, s. 33(4)(c); *Disease Control Regulations*, R.R.S. 2000, c. P-37.1, Reg. 11, s. 11(4); in Nova Scotia, this applies to both anonymous and non-anonymous HIV testing: *Reporting Requirements for HIV Positive Persons Regulations*, N.S. Reg. 197/2005, s. 13(a)-(b).

consented to this.[158] Further, duties of the contacted individual are specified to include seeking testing and care, and taking measures to significantly reduce the risk of infecting others in turn.[159]

Another range of duties applies in some of the Atlantic provinces. In Newfoundland and Labrador, the physician treating an individual with or suspected of having a communicable disease is obliged to report to a "hotel-keeper, keeper of a boarding house, or tenant within whose house or rooms the person lives" information, the content of which is unspecified.[160] In the case of sexually transmitted infections, a physician in Newfoundland and Labrador may also supply information to members of a household for purposes of protection of health.[161] Extending this latitude further, in Prince Edward Island, a physician or Chief Health Officer may notify family members (not confined to the household) of the suspicion of an infectious disease for the purposes of health protection.[162] The constitutionality of such broad provisions is questionable. Further, in Prince Edward Island, the health officer is mandated to report to the principal of the school where an infected individual *or any household member* is in attendance.[163]

The vast discrepancy in provisions for contact tracing from province to province is noteworthy. The reason for such differences is unclear. While mere variation is not sufficient ground for a *Charter* challenge, overstepping bounds necessary for protection of the public may well be. One of the fascinating elements of public health law is the paucity of constitutional challenges to state control of the area. Vulnerability of the infected individual, and sometimes corresponding lack of availability of legal resources to launch a challenge, may be the explanation.

(e) Public Notification

Most provincial/territorial legislation provides for notice to the public, or to a subset of the public, as to the presence of a communicable disease. Notification is in one of two general forms: traditionally, a placard could be placed at the residence of an individual to warn visitors

---

[158] *Disease Control Regulations*, R.R.S. 2000, c. P-37.1, Reg. 11, ss. 7-8 (specifying the information to be provided to the contacts); *Public Health Act, 1994*, S.S. 1994, c. P-37.1, s. 65 (providing for the confidentiality of all personal health information obtained under the Act or its regulations, subject to limited exceptions including where the subject of the information has consented to its release).

[159] *Disease Control Regulations*, R.R.S. 2000, c. P-37.1, Reg. 11, ss. 6(2)(b), 7(2)(b), 8(b).

[160] *Communicable Diseases Act*, R.S.N.L. 1990, c. C-26, s. 4(1).

[161] *Venereal Disease Prevention Act*, R.S.N.L. 1990, c. V-2, s. 14(3).

[162] *Notifiable and Communicable Diseases Regulations*, P.E.I. Reg. EC330/85, s. 14.

[163] *Public Health Act*, R.S.P.E.I. 1988, c. P-30, s. 12(1).

as to the presence of a communicable disease within its walls.[164] More recently, legislation in a number of provinces includes provision for class orders — *i.e.*, orders that pertain not to specified individuals but to members of a group.[165] In this case, it may be specified that the order may be communicated to the public and/or the media. The legislation on notification differs in terms of what may or must be included in the notice, how the notice is to be done and even who is to perform the notification. These topics are covered below.

As indicated earlier, most provinces and territories allow for some sort of notice to be provided at a place of isolation or quarantine, often referred to as placarding, as to the presence of a communicable disease. Saskatchewan and Québec are excemptions where legislation does not contain a provision permitting placarding. In Newfoundland and Labrador, the Minister may make regulations for placarding in case of the presence of a venereal disease; however, no such regulations exist at present.[166]

In Alberta, the notice must include particulars as to the disease in question unless considered not in the public interest.[167] In most provinces, the placard is to refer to the household being under quarantine or isolation, without naming individuals or specifying the disease. Manitoba's legislation states that in case of a tenement house or apartment building, the placard is to be placed outside the room or apartment, and there may also be signage at the entrance to the building which has "... printed on it in large letters the room or apartment number in which the diseased person resides ...".[168]

Recent legislative provisions in Saskatchewan, Ontario and Nova Scotia include class orders, and provide for communication of such orders directly to the public.[169] General public notification is to occur only where it is not practical to notify each member of the class of persons who are the subject of the order. This type of communication has particularly high potential to result in discrimination against both infected and uninfected members of the class in question, and should be utilized only in both rare and pressing circumstances.

A number of provinces provide for notification directly to the public where necessary for the protection of health. Thus, in Prince Edward

---

[164] See *e.g.*, *Diseases and Dead Bodies Regulation*, Man. Reg. 338/88R, s. 15.
[165] See *e.g.*, *Health Protection and Promotion Act*, R.S.O. 1990, c. H.7, s. 22(5.0.1).
[166] *Venereal Disease Prevention Act*, R.S.N.L. 1990, c. V-2, s. 20(h).
[167] *Public Health Act Forms Regulation*, Alta. Reg. 197/2004, s. 3.
[168] *Diseases and Dead Bodies Regulation*, Man. Reg. 338/88R, s. 15(3)-(4).
[169] *Public Health Act, 1994*, S.S. 1994, c. P-37.1, s. 45(5); *Health Protection and Promotion Act*, R.S.O. 1990, c. H.7, s. 22(5.0.3); *Health Protection Act*, S.N.S. 2004, c. 4, s. 33(5).

Island, the Chief Health Officer has the discretion to not only placard premises but to "authorize the dissemination of information regarding a quarantine order through any form of media".[170] New legislation in Nova Scotia is arguably the most permissive in allowing for direct communication of the identity of an individual with a communicable disease where required on reasonable belief to protect public health and where no less intrusive means appear to be available.[171]

Following the 2003 outbreak of SARS in Ontario, the identities of two individuals were provided to the public: the woman who returned home from Hong Kong to Toronto, apparently carrying the disease, and her son, who also contracted the disease. Both died, and Toronto Public Health released their names to media outlets in an attempt to prevent further spread of the disease by alerting those who might have been in contact with either person. This followed what has been described as "agonizing" over the decision and with the consent of relatives of the deceased.[172] Later in the outbreak, public health officials identified that they feared a nurse who had taken a commuter train may have contracted SARS. In this instance, the time and place of her travel was supplied to the media but not her name. No other individuals were named in Canada as carriers, but in Singapore, names of superspreaders were made public,[173] and radio frequency identification tags were used to track quarantined individuals.[174] In balancing the right of the individual to privacy against the need to protect the health of the public, there will be times when public health must take precedence; however, it is of critical importance that neither of these competing values be dispensed with lightly.

The appropriateness of public notification was under review in *P.G. Restaurant Ltd. v. Northern Interior Regional Health Board.*[175] A customer had vomited on one of the buffet tables at the Mama Panda restaurant, following which an outbreak of the Norwalk virus caused at least 13 people to become ill. A month and a half later, the Prince George Free Press published a front page article headed "Vomit serves up virus at buffet" and identified the restaurant by name. In the article, the Chief Environmental Health Officer of the Northern Interior Regional Health

---

[170]   *Public Health Act*, R.S.P.E.I. 1988, c. P-30, s. 5.1(5)(b).

[171]   *Health Protection Act*, S.N.S. 2004, c. 4, s. 15(3) (in force 1 November 2005).

[172]   Personal communication between author and Jane Speakman, Legal Division, City of Toronto.

[173]   L. Gostin *et al.*, "Ethical and Legal Challenges Posed by Severe Acute Respiratory Syndrome" (2003) 290 J.A.M.A. 3230.

[174]   See online: <http://www.nus.edu.sg/corporate/research/gallery/research54.htm>.

[175]   [2004] B.C.J. No. 424, 25 B.C.L.R. (4th) 242 (B.C.S.C.), rev'd as against the newspaper [2005] B.C.J. No. 751 (B.C.C.A.), leave to appeal to S.C.C. refused [2005] S.C.C.A. No. 270 (S.C.C.).

Board (the "Board"), Bruce Gaunt, was quoted as saying that the clean-up by the restaurant following the incident had been inadequate. The restaurant sued both the Board and the newspaper. While at trial the newspaper was found liable for defamation (overturned on appeal), the Board was found not to be liable in defamation nor in negligence. The facts and reasoning as to potential liability of the Board bears closer scrutiny.

At trial, Mr. Gaunt admitted to having made the quoted statements but testified that he had refused to identify the particular restaurant at which the incident had occurred. He indicated that he believed it served both the public and the food industry to disseminate information about the Norwalk virus and its ability to survive clean-up procedures. He did not believe the name of the restaurant was relevant to this public health story.

To establish defamation, the plaintiff must establish both that the comments were defamatory and that they identified the plaintiff. Justice Goepel of the British Columbia Supreme Court determined that the comments of Mr. Gaunt were defamatory in that they would tend to harm reputation.[176] However, he found that the words of Mr. Gaunt "... would not lead a reasonable person to conclude that the comments referred to the Restaurant".[177] Thus, the action against the Board failed.

Had they been found to have been defamatory, a number of defences were available and would have exonerated the Board. If what has been said is substantially true, the defence of justification operates as a complete defence to defamation. Justice Goepel found that Mr. Gaunt's quoted statements critical of the plaintiff were about the inadequacy of the clean-up, which he found to be substantially true and therefore met the test of justification.[178] Further, the defence of fair comment applied:

> Mr. Gaunt's comments were made in relation to a matter of public interest. The public of Prince George had an interest in being informed about an emerging food-borne illness that was extremely contagious and resistant to clean-up. The public also had an interest in knowing that individuals should not go out in public when they are feeling ill because this may result in their unknown illness being spread to others. The Board had a legitimate reason to educate the public about the Norwalk virus and various related health issues.[179]

Finally, the defence of qualified privilege applies when there is a legitimate reason on the part of the sender to communicate information and a corresponding interest on the part of the recipient part in receiving

---

[176]   *Ibid.*, at para. 123.
[177]   *Ibid.*, at para. 129.
[178]   *Ibid.*, at para. 151.
[179]   *Ibid.*, at para. 160.

the information. It is in reference to this defence that Justice Goepel provides the strongest support of the public health system in notifying the public of risks to their well-being. He found that:

> The Board had a statutory and legal duty to communicate health concerns to the general public. Awareness and education are significant factors that help protect the public from communicable diseases ... The Board had a similar moral and social duty to communicate information about the Norwalk virus in addition to its legal duty to do so.[180]

The court went on to find an interest in the public receiving this information:

> The public, in this case the readers of the *Free Press*, also had a legitimate interest in receiving the information. It was important for them to learn about Norwalk's contagious qualities and other related public health concerns.[181]

Thus, the defence of qualified privilege would operate to absolve the Board of liability had the comments of Mr. Gaunt been found to have been defamatory. If he had identified the restaurant, however, Justice Goepel notes that this defence would not have been available to the Board.[182]

The action in negligence failed on two grounds: First, it has generally not been found to apply in Canada to a claim based on a defamatory statement, especially where a municipal officer is responding to an issue of public interest. Second, the comments of Mr. Gaunt would have to have been untrue, but as noted above, they were found to have been substantially true. Thus, the Board was relieved of liability on the basis of negligence as well as defamation.[183]

It would appear that public health officials have a fairly wide degree of latitude in releasing information to the public concerning the outbreak of a communicable disease. Indeed, Justice Goepel identified both a legal and moral duty to do so. However, there is reason for caution in considering identifying individuals or establishments when discussing such an outbreak. Such drastic action should only be taken if revelation is considered clearly necessary in the interests of public health protection.

---

[180]   *Ibid.*, at paras. 163-66.
[181]   *Ibid.*, at para. 167.
[182]   *Ibid.*, at para. 168.
[183]   *Ibid.*, at 274-78 (B.C.L.R.).

(f)   Disease Prevention/Health Promotion Programs

Information is used in a variety of prevention, promotion and screening programs in public health. One example is that of programs initiated in a number of provinces to notify women of the results of their Pap test results. Cervical cancer is a pressing problem and regular screening is considered vital to prevention and early treatment. In 2003, the Saskatchewan Cancer Agency commenced a Prevention Program for Cervical Cancer (the "PPCC"). A testing laboratory would forward Pap test results to a woman's physician, as well as to the PPCC, which in turn would send letters to women advising them of their results.[184] The PPCC also was to send letters encouraging regular screening and follow up on adverse findings. Upon implementation of the program, more than 100 women complained to the Saskatchewan Privacy Commissioner that they were disturbed to receive letters from the PPCC (and, indeed, at times the information was received not by themselves but by ex-husbands or parents). Complaints included violation of privacy, lack of information about the program and an inability to opt out of participation in the program.[185] The Commissioner investigated the PPCC for compliance with the *Health Information Protection Act*[186] and determined that the statute permitted the information sharing involved with program, but noted this might well conflict with a right to privacy under the *Canadian Charter of Rights and Freedoms.*[187]

In light of this finding, the Commissioner recommended that the Saskatchewan government undertake a review of s. 27(2) of the *Health Information Protection Act* for *Charter* compliance, and that the matter be referred to the Court of Appeal.[188] He also recommended that the Agency provide an opt-out option for women.[189] He found that the Agency failed to meet the requirements of s. 9 in that they did not provide sufficient information to women about the program.[190]

The Saskatchewan Cancer Agency responded by increasing the quantity and availability of information on the program and by creating an

---

[184]   Saskatchewan, Office of the Information and Privacy Commissioner, *Investigation Report H-2005--002: Prevention Program for Cervical Cancer* (Saskatchewan Information and Privacy Commissioner: Gary Dickson) at 3, online: <http://www.oipc.sk.ca/Reports/H-2005-002.pdf>.
[185]   *Ibid.*, at 53-60.
[186]   *Ibid.*, at 1.
[187]   *Ibid.*, at 135 and 180-81.
[188]   *Ibid.*, at 16.
[189]   *Ibid.*, at 12.
[190]   *Ibid.*, at 112.

opt-out mechanism. To date there has not been a referral to the Court of Appeal.[191]

A similar program in Manitoba included an opt-out provision from the outset.[192] In Alberta, complaints were brought before the Privacy Commissioner regarding the provincial Cervical Cancer Screening Program and the absence of the ability to opt out.[193] Section 58(2) of the *Health Information Act*[194] reads as follows:

> In deciding how much health information to disclose, a custodian must consider as an important factor any expressed wishes of the individual who is the subject of the information relating to disclosure of the information, together with any other factors the custodian considers relevant.

The Office of the Privacy Commissioner found that there could not be consideration of one's wishes if opting out was not available. Thus, not having an opt-out provision was a violation of the statute.[195] However, during the course of the investigation the Cervical Cancer Screening Program brought in an amendment to allow for opting out.[196]

This example, and the different approaches taken in Manitoba, Saskatchewan and Alberta, draws into sharp relief the potential conflict between use of personal information in prevention/promotion programs and individual privacy. Such programs generally have the best of intentions, but it is imperative that health promotion be conducted without trampling on individual privacy. This serves as a strong reminder that the Canadian public is interested in making choices about use of personal information in the interests of health. At a bare minimum, proper notification of targeted individuals is necessary. Further, even where statutory compliance is found, there may be a higher standard developing in that individuals should be able to opt out of notification programs if they wish.

---

[191]   Personal correspondence with R. Gary Dickson, Saskatchewan Information and Privacy Commissioner, 9 June 2008.

[192]   Manitoba Cervical Cancer Screening Program, *Registry: Facts and Information*, online: <http://www.cancercare.mb.ca/cancercare_resources/MCCSP/pdfs/registry_english_06.pdf>.

[193]   Alberta, Information and Privacy Commissioner, *Report on the Collection, Use and Disclosure of Health Information for the Alberta Cervical Cancer Screening Program* (Investigation Report H2005-IR-002, 2005), online: <http://www.oipc.ab.ca/ims/client/upload/H2005_IR_002.pdf>.

[194]   R.S.A. 2000, c. H-5.

[195]   Alberta, Information and Privacy Commissioner, *Report on the Collection, Use and Disclosure of Health Information for the Alberta Cervical Cancer Screening Program* (Investigation Report H2005-IR-002, 2005) at 19, online: http://www.oipc.ab.ca/ims/client/upload/H2005_IR_002.pdf>.

[196]   *Ibid.*, at 22.

(g)   Surveillance, Epidemiology and Research

Information has long been an integral part of the protection of public health, in tracking health and disease trends and in seeking to understand their mechanisms. With the introduction and rapid growth of availability of electronic health information, accompanied by the increase in means of rapid travel of humans and vectors around the planet, the significance of and demand for health information has multiplied exponentially. The public health system in Canada has encountered difficulty in trying to keep up with these developments. The SARS crisis in Ontario brought to light an infectious disease information system that was described by Justice Archie Campbell as "inadequate",[197] plagued by "overwhelming and disorganized information demands",[198] with "blockages of vital information",[199] and rife with "legal confusion".[200] Further, he indicated, "[t]he lack of a single, effective, accessible information system, combined with a constant, intense demand for information from a number of different people and groups, resulted in chaos".[201] These problems reverberated up through the chain of reporting through the Ontario Ministry of Health and Long-Term Care to Health Canada and ultimately to the World Health Organization.[202] This section will touch on a few of the many reasons for this disarray.

First, what are the distinguishing features of surveillance, epidemiology, and research? The World Health Organization has defined surveillance as "the process of systematic collection, collation and analysis of data with prompt dissemination to those who need to know, for relevant action to be taken".[203]

Epidemiology is defined as "the study of the distribution of health and its determinants in specified populations, and the application of this study to control health problems".[204] Research is defined in the Tri-

---

[197]   Honourable Mr. Justice Archie Campbell, Commissioner, "The SARS Commission Interim Report: SARS and Public Health in Ontario" (2004) at 101, online: Ministry of Health and Long-Term Care <http://www.health.gov.on.ca/english/public/pub/ministry_reports/campbell04/campbell04.pdf>.

[198]   *Ibid.*, at 112.

[199]   *Ibid.*, at 122.

[200]   *Ibid.*, at 127.

[201]   *Ibid.*, at 119.

[202]   *Ibid.*, at 117.

[203]   World Health Organization Department of Communicable Disease Surveillance and Response, "Protocol for the Assessment of National Communicable Disease Surveillance and Response Systems: Guidelines for Assessment Teams" at 1, online: <http://whqlibdoc.who.int/hq/2001/WHO_CDS_CSR_ISR_2001.2_text_annexes1-11.pdf>.

[204]   *Ibid.*

Council Policy Statement[205] as "... a systematic investigation to establish facts, principles or generalizable knowledge".[206] The reader will note that there is potential for major overlap among the three concepts, such that the same activity could indeed constitute all three. It may not be necessary in all cases to categorize a project. However, the distinction between research and non-research is potentially significant in that research conducted in universities and other institutions in Canada that receive funding from the Tri-Councils must undergo research ethics review prior to commencement of the research, while non-research has no such requirement.[207]

An important concept regarding information usage is that of identifiability. As we have seen, much of the information collected by public health authorities in the first instance contains such identifiers as name, address, contact information and health insurance number. As well, less direct identifiers such as type of disease, postal code and gender may in combination result in positive identification of an individual. A decision of the English Court of Appeal has determined that where information being disclosed is properly anonymized, the individual who is the source of such information can no longer claim a privacy interest in the information.[208] This issue has not yet been squarely addressed in Canadian law, and therefore is open to debate.[209] It should be noted, however, that information legislation, while describing identifiability in differing ways, uniformly pertains only to information that constitutes "identifying information about an individual".[210] As we shall see below, provincial

---

[205]   Canadian Institutes of Health Research,   Natural Sciences and Engineering Research Council of Canada, Social Sciences and Humanities Research Council of Canada, "Tri-Council Policy Statement: Ethical Conduct for Research Involving Humans" (2003), online: Interagency Advisory Panel on Research Ethics <http://www.pre.ethics.gc.ca/english/policystatement/policystatement.cfm>. This document governs the conduct of research in Canadian institutions that receive funding from the three major national funding agencies: SSHRC, NSERC and CIHR (formerly the Medical Research Council of Canada).

[206]   *Ibid.*, at Art. 1.1.

[207]   The World Bank argues: "Surveillance is not research. Public health surveillance is essentially descriptive in nature. It describes the occurrence of injury or disease and its determinants in the population." World Bank Group, "Public Health Surveillance Toolkit", online: <http://survtoolkit.worldbank.org/docs/toolkit_part_a.pdf>. Amy L. Fairchild and Ronald Bayer, "Ethics and the Conduct of Public Health Surveillance" (2004) 303 Science 631, argue that the World Bank's position drawing a sharp demarcation between surveillance and research activities is based in economics and undermines the ethics mandate by avoiding research ethics review.

[208]   *R. v. Department of Health, Ex parte Source Informatics Ltd.*, [2001] Q.B. 424, [2000] 1 All E.R. 786, [2000] 2 W.L.R. 940, (sub nom. *Source Informatics Ltd., Re An Application for Judicial Review*) [1999] EWCA Civ 3011 (C.A.).

[209]   Elaine Gibson, "Is There a Privacy Interest in Anonymized Personal Health Information?" (2003) Health L.J. Special Edition 97.

[210]   *Personal Health Information Protection Act, 2004*, S.O. 2004, c. 3, Sch. A, s. 4(1).

public health legislation may or may not describe the type of information that can be disclosed in terms of identifiability. Nevertheless, this concept is important in that the less identifiable the item of information, the more reduced may be the privacy interest that surrounds it.

I will now discuss the specifics of information sharing by public health authorities as authorized by federal and provincial public health and vital statistics legislation.

(i)   Federal

The *Quarantine Act* permits the entering into an agreement between the Minister and a province or public health authority for purposes of administration and enforcement of the statute.[211] It authorizes the collection of health information to carry out the purposes of the statute.[212] Further, it provides for disclosure to other bodies as follows:

> The Minister may disclose confidential business information or personal information obtained under this Act to a department or to an agency of the Government of Canada or of a province, a government or public health authority, whether domestic or foreign, a health practitioner or an international health organization if the Minister has reasonable grounds to believe that the disclosure is necessary to prevent the spread of a communicable disease or to enable Canada to fulfill its international obligations.[213]

The *Public Health Agency of Canada Act* authorizes the Governor in Council to make regulations respecting the collection, use and distribution of information.[214] No such regulations have been enacted to date.

(ii)   Provincial

Legislation concerning vital statistics provides for the reporting of deaths, including cause of death. In a number of provinces, classification of cause of death is to be in accordance with the World Health Organization "International Statistical Classification of Diseases, Injuries and Causes of Death".[215] This standardization is useful in permitting the comparison of provincial statistics. However, not all provinces require this means of classification; for instance, the legislation of Newfoundland and

---

[211]   *Quarantine Act*, S.C. 2005, c. 20, s. 11.
[212]   *Ibid.*, s. 55.
[213]   *Ibid.*, s. 56(1).
[214]   S.C. 2006, c. 5, s. 15(1)(a).
[215]   See *e.g.*, *Vital Statistics Act*, R.S.A. 2000, c. V-4, s. 15(2); World Health Organization, "International Statistical Classification of Diseases and Related Health Problems, 10th Revision, Version for 2007", online: <http://www.who.int/classifications/apps/icd/icd10online>.

Labrador requires the reporting of deaths and their causes to the Registrar General, but is silent as to the system to be used.[216]

Provincial public health legislation often provides for the sharing of information within the province, sometimes with another health authority if an infected individual is known to be residing in another jurisdictional area[217] and generally to the Chief Medical Health Officer or co-ordinator of communicable disease control.[218] There is a lack of uniformity regarding sharing with other provinces and with the federal government. In some provinces the public health legislation is silent.[219] In others, such as Manitoba, the Minister or Chief Medical Officer of Health has broad authorization to provide to and obtain information from a department or agency of the government of Canada or of another province or territory "for the purpose of preventing, controlling or dealing with a threat to public health".[220] This may expressly include personal health information.[221] Unusually, Prince Edward Island's *Notifiable and Communicable Diseases Regulations* require reporting to the federal government "... a monthly compilation of all reports of notifiable diseases, with further information as may be required, ... to the appropriate agencies of the Government of Canada for the purposes of national disease surveillance".[222] The *Public Health Act* of Prince Edward Island provides broadly for disclosure deemed by the Chief Health Officer to be in the best interests of either the individual or the public.[223]

Québec's public health legislation specifically provides for ongoing surveillance of population health status and health determinants,[224] and authorizes the sharing of information to specific entities outside the province in limited circumstances:

> ... The national public health director may also communicate such information to any health authority outside Quebec if the communication is necessary to protect the health of that authority's population or forms part of the stipulations of an agreement with that health authority.[225]

---

[216] *Vital Statistics Act*, R.S.N.L. 1990, c. V-6.

[217] See *e.g.*, Saskatchewan *Disease Control Regulations*, S.S. 1994, P 37.1, Reg. 11, s. 13.

[218] See *e.g.*, *Public Health Act, 1994*, S.S. 1994, c. P-37.1, s. 37(1).

[219] *Public Health Act*, R.S.A. 2000, c. P-37. Note that Alberta's *Statistics Bureau Act*, R.S.A. 2000, c. S-18 does provide for arrangements being made with a Department of the Government of Canada for the sharing of information, but this is qualified by a provision on protection of identity (ss. 6 and 8(1)).

[220] *Public Health Act*, C.C.S.M. c. P210, s. 12.2(1).

[221] *Ibid.*, s. 12.2(2).

[222] P.E.I. Reg. 330/85, s. 9.

[223] *Public Health Act*, R.S.P.E.I. 1988, c. P-30, s. 22(2)(b).

[224] *Public Health Act*, R.S.Q. c. S-2.2, s. 33.

[225] *Ibid.*, s. 133.

The lack of consistency regarding circumstances under which information may be shared and utilized for purposes of surveillance, epidemiology and research has resulted in much consternation, especially in the context of outbreaks of newly emergent disease. SARS was a siren call to the nation. The major reviews conducted in its wake have all identified the need for attention to be devoted to this area. The National Advisory Committee on SARS and Public Health paraphrased T.S. Eliot in stating:

> [W]e can never build systems so perfect that people no longer need to be good. But the greatest lesson of SARS in Canada is arguably that there is no excuse for tolerating systems so imperfect that bad things happen unnecessarily to good people.[226]

Will our public health system be prepared for the next outbreak? The next and final section of this chapter reviews emergency powers under public health and emergency-specific legislation.

(h) Emergencies

Every province and territory, as well as the federal government, has legislation dealing specifically with emergencies, and there are often provisions in the public health legislation that authorize action in time of emergency. As we shall see, neither set of legislation tends to include emergency powers regarding the collection, use and disclosure of health information in time of crisis.

(i) Federal

The federal government has enacted an *Emergencies Act*[227] which replaces the former controversial *War Measures Act*.[228] Curiously, this statute does not address information sharing, and does not provide government with the power to compel the provision of information when a state of emergency has been declared.

The federal government also has legal authority to enter into agreements with the provinces to facilitate civil emergency preparedness. Section 6(1) of the *Department of Public Safety and Emergency Preparedness Act*[229] provides as follows:

> ... The Minister may

---

[226] National Advisory Committee on SARS and Public Health, *Learning from SARS: Renewal of Public Health in Canada* (Ottawa: Health Canada, 2003) (Chair: Dr. D. Naylor) at 97.

[227] R.S.C. 1985, c. 22 (4th Supp.).

[228] R.S.C. 1985, c. W-2, as rep. by R.S.C. 1985, c. 22 (4th Supp.), s. 80.

[229] S.C. 2005, c. 10.

(*a*) initiate, recommend, coordinate, implement or promote policies, programs or projects relating to public safety and emergency preparedness;

(*b*) cooperate with any province ...

......

(*d*) facilitate the sharing of information, where authorized, to promote public safety objectives.

This may authorize the entry into agreements with the provinces as to information sharing in a civil emergency, which is also sometimes permitted under provincial public health legislation.

(ii) Provincial

Every province and territory has specific emergency measures legislation that authorizes the declaration of a state of emergency in all or part of the jurisdiction and provides for added powers at such times — typically, warrantless entry and search, demolition of property, control or prohibition of travel, and conscription of services.[230] However, this legislation is silent as to the sharing of information. The Saskatchewan[231] and Yukon Territory[232] legislation do provide for the entry into agreements with the government of Canada or of any province or territory, which presumably would include the possibility of information sharing.

Clearly, emergency powers to deal with information sharing in a public health emergency fall primarily within the public health statutes if at all. Unfortunately, most of this legislation is also silent on the topic. Exceptions are Québec,[233] Alberta[234] and Saskatchewan,[235] each of which provide for the compelling of information from an individual where there is reason to believe that the individual has information relevant to a public health emergency. The Québec provision only pertains if a state of public health emergency has been declared by the government, and if so, it explicitly provides for the compelling of personal or confidential information.[236] British Columbia's new public health statute provides that, in an emergency as defined in the legislation, a health officer may "collect, use or disclose information, including personal information, (i) that could not otherwise

---

[230] See *e.g.*, New Brunswick's *Emergency Measures Act*, S.N.B. 1978, c. E-7.1.

[231] *Emergency Planning Act*, S.S. 1989-90, c. E-8.1, s. 13.

[232] *Civil Emergency Measures Act*, R.S.Y. 2002, c. 34, s. 4.

[233] *Public Health Act*, R.S.Q. c. S-2.2, s. 123(3).

[234] *Public Health Act*, R.S.A. 2000, c. P-37, s. 19.1(1)(b).

[235] *Public Health Act, 1994*, S.S. 1994, c. P-37.1, s. 45(2)(g).

[236] *Public Health Act*, R.S.Q. c. S-2.2, ss. 118, 123(3).

be collected, used or disclosed, or (ii) in a form or manner other than the form or manner required".[237]

In regard to emergency public health powers, the National Advisory Committee on SARS recommended that the federal government attempt to develop in collaboration with the provinces a "... legislative framework for disease surveillance and outbreak management in Canada, as well as harmonizing emergency legislation as it bears on public health emergencies".[238] It went on to state that if such a coordinated system could not be developed collaboratively, the federal government should unilaterally draft default legislation to cover these areas.[239] Today, further work to improve public health emergency preparedness is still required.

IV. CONCLUSION

If prevention and treatment are the twin pillars of our public health system, information is its bedrock. Without a strong and seamless foundation, the system may crumble, especially at times of greatest vulnerability. The Canadian experience of the SARS outbreak exposed not merely cracks but, in certain respects, chasms in the information structures of our public health system. In a 2008 report, the Auditor-General of Canada described aspects of the Canadian public health surveillance system as having "fundamental weaknesses",[240] and in particular stated that the system of sharing information with the provinces has "gaps" that disrupt the flow of "timely, accurate, and complete information".[241] An information-sharing agreement has been entered into between the federal government and the government of Ontario,[242] but not yet with the 12 other jurisdictions in Canada. It is essential that information structures be scrutinized closely and their imperfections addressed; only thus can we be confident that information will perform its proper functions in protecting health while providing appropriate respect for the privacy of Canadians.

---

[237] *Public Health Act*, S.B.C. 2008, c. 28, s. 54(1)(k) [not yet in force].
[238] National Advisory Committee on SARS and Public Health, *Learning from SARS: Renewal of Public Health in Canada* (Ottawa: Health Canada, 2003) (Chair: Dr. D. Naylor) at 216.
[239] *Ibid.*
[240] Canada, Auditor General of Canada, *2008 May Report*, Chapter 5 "Surveillance of Infectious Diseases — Public Health Agency of Canada", online: <http://www.oag-bvg.gc.ca/internet/English/parl_oag_200805_05_e_30701.html>.
[241] *Ibid.*
[242] *Ibid.*, at para. 5.37.

5

VACCINES AND EMERGING CHALLENGES FOR PUBLIC HEALTH LAW

Patricia Peppin[*]

The achievements of public health in eradicating contagious diseases have been stunning. By the end of the 20th century, programs of immunization, in combination with improved living conditions, had produced dramatic decreases in the incidence of significant contagious diseases in industrialized countries. Contagious diseases remain a threat in Canada as new diseases such as SARS emerge and as research for the purpose of biological warfare extends the possibilities of existing pathogens. Efforts to contain disease at the domestic level are inevitably affected by global conditions and Canada has a continuing role to play in contributing to international efforts at disease eradication.

Germs know no borders. David Fidler has argued that any legal analysis of global phenomena needs to be carried out at three levels: the level of domestic law, international law and global governance, which is the level of transnational actors such as international corporations and public health organizations like Médecins Sans Frontières and the World Health Organization ("WHO").[1] It is at the second level, where actors operate outside national boundaries and domestic legislation, that regulation of activities is weakest. Using this analytical framework, this chapter will analyze Canadian laws applying to vaccines and the consequences of these laws. At the same time, the analysis will take into account the transnational and international levels, as it focuses on actors

[*]   I am grateful for the invaluable research assistance of Joanna Harris, Sarah Viau and Kate Findlay at Queen's University and Heather Innes in Edmonton, Alberta.
[1]   David P. Fidler, "A Globalized Theory of Public Health Law" (2002) 30 J.L.M.E. 150.

such as pharmaceutical companies involved in vaccine production, public health organizations operating beyond domestic borders, and international organizations such as WHO.

The introduction provides an overview of the impact of public health measures on contagious disease in Canada, the United States and globally. It introduces the question of emerging contagious diseases and examines biological warfare as another means of transmission. Section II examines the issues of compensation and liability, beginning with the duties of care owed by vaccine manufacturers, government and health professionals, and the nature of litigation arising out of the adverse effects of vaccines. Alternative forms of compensation are examined, including proposals for a no-fault compensation fund. Section III focuses on mandatory and voluntary elements in the program of immunization in Canada. It begins with an examination of situations in which immunization is required by law, including statutory provision for immunization of school-age children, mandatory immunization of certain employees, military requirements, and quarantine. In Section IV, proposals for structural changes to improve the effectiveness and equity of the vaccine program are analyzed — a national immunization strategy, adverse event reporting, vaccine tracking and registries, equitable access to vaccines, and enhanced education of recipients and substitute decision-makers.

I.   INTRODUCTION

Reading historical accounts of the history of diseases such as smallpox and plague reveals the extent to which our lives have changed as a result of their containment and eradication. Hundreds of millions died from smallpox through history and two million died from it as recently as 1967.[2] In 18th century London, one in every ten deaths annually resulted from smallpox, with the death rate one in four for adults and 40 to 50 per cent for children.[3] Even those who survived "have only risen from their pillows frightfully scarred and disfigured by this malady".[4] In the middle of the 20th century, polio posed a real threat in Canada as 20,000 people contracted the debilitating disease each year;[5] anxious parents kept their children away from public places like swimming pools as the heat of summer descended. Measles (red measles) used to be responsible for

---

[2]   Jonathan B. Tucker, *Scourge: The Once and Future Threat of Smallpox* (New York: Atlantic Monthly Press, 2001) at 3.

[3]   Laurie Garrett, *Betrayal of Trust: The Collapse of Global Public Health* (New York: Hyperion, 2000) at 503, quoting Frank Fenner.

[4]   William Makepeace Thackeray, *The History of Henry Esmond.* 1852, quoted in Jonathan B. Tucker, *Scourge* (New York: Atlantic Monthly Press, 2001) at 13.

[5]   Council of Ontario Medical Officers of Health, *Position Paper on Public Funding of Immunisation in Ontario* (July 2003).

between 300 and 900 deaths in Canada each year, among 300,000 people who contracted the disease.[6] No cases of wild polio have been seen in the western hemisphere since 1991,[7] while diphtheria, mumps and measles are all virtually unknown. The success of the vaccination program can be seen in the data from Health Canada that compare highest annual disease incidence immediately prior to vaccine introduction with 2001 figures. These show declines for polio of 20,000 to 0; diphtheria of 9,000 to 0; rubella (German measles) of 69,000 to 23; mumps of 52,000 to 73; Haemophilus influenzae Type b (Hib) of 2,000 to 41; pertussis (whooping cough) of 25,000 to 2,477; and measles of 300,000 to 33.[8]

In the United States as well, the data indicate the extent to which these old forms of pestilence have been brought under control, diminishing the disabling conditions and suffering that they caused. The Centers for Disease Control data for the diseases above plus smallpox, tetanus and congenital rubella syndrome show the three-year average annual morbidity rates for vaccine-preventable diseases of children have dropped by 95 per cent for pertussis and 98 to 100 per cent for all the rest.[9]

Smallpox had been eradicated worldwide by 1980 through a monumental campaign undertaken by the World Health Organization and through the individual efforts of D.A. Henderson and many health workers over a decade.[10] Vaccines have contributed to the dramatic improvements in survival of children under the age of five on a global basis from 1990 to 2000, although the rates remained static in Sub-Saharan Africa.[11] A partnership to achieve higher child survival for children under five, in part through vaccination, has been formed by UNICEF, WHO, the Pan-American Health Organization, the Centers for Disease Control and Prevention ("CDC"), and the Global Alliance for Vaccines and Immunization. The Global Polio Eradication Initiative by UNICEF, WHO and Rotary International began in 1998 and reduced the number of cases from a daily rate of about 1,000 children to 483 cases in

---

[6]   Council of Ontario Medical Officers of Health, *Position Paper on Public Funding of Immunization in Ontario* (July 2003).

[7]   Kevin M. Malone & Alan R. Hinman, "Vaccination Mandates: The Public Health Imperative and Individual Rights" in Richard A. Goodman *et al.*, eds., *Law In Public Health Practice* (Oxford: Oxford University Press, 2003) 262-84 at 264, note 6.

[8]   Health Canada, Division of Immunization & Respiratory Diseases, Canadian Immunization Awareness Program, Provisional data, cited in a report prepared by Aventis Pasteur.

[9]   United States, Center for Disease Control, Provisional cases of selected notifiable diseases, week ending 23 December 2000. MMWR 2001; 49: 1164, 1167, 1173, cited in Malone and Hinman at 266, Table 13-1.

[10]   Jonathan B. Tucker, *Scourge* (New York: Atlantic Monthly Press, 2001).

[11]   Yves Bergerin (UNICEF), in Health Canada, Proceedings of the Canadian National Immunization Conference, *Canada's National Immunization Strategy: From Vision to Action* (December 2002) CCDR 2003; 29S4: 1-24, at 2.

the entire year in 2001,[12] a decrease of 99 per cent by 2000.[13] These significant achievements were placed at risk in northern Nigeria where some Muslim leaders refused to participate in immunization programs based on beliefs about the western-supplied vaccines.[14] The subsequent outbreak of polio in Nigeria spread to neighbouring countries in western and central Africa. Both international campaigns relied on mass participation to wipe out the disease at its source and to create sufficient immunity to protect the community from infection — a state referred to by epidemiologists as herd immunity. Both domestically and globally, eradication depends on the availability of vaccines and a public health network capable of reaching those who need the vaccines. Continuing protection against these diseases requires funding to maintain high immunization levels in the population, education to ensure that the risks and benefits are clearly understood, and sufficient quantities of high quality vaccines.

Even with many diseases seemingly brought under control, other contagious diseases remain uncontained. The influenza epidemic that ravaged the world as the First World War was being fought to a conclusion in 1918 took an unknown toll of lives. The number was 20 million as a low estimate and may have been as high as 100 million people worldwide, and it certainly exceeded the number of people killed by the Black Death, yet puzzlingly, this epidemic remains largely outside public consciousness.[15] The HIV/AIDS pandemic emerged in the last decades of the 20th century to claim lives, with a current estimate of 33.2 million (30.6 to 36.1 million) adults and children living with AIDS, and create devastating social consequences for communities across the globe.[16] In Africa, an entire generation of AIDS orphans has been created in the wake of the deaths of millions. An HIV vaccine is still on the horizon. Tuberculosis has re-emerged in the wake of HIV, and malaria and cholera are also making alarming reappearances. Laurie Garrett wrote in *The Coming Plague* that emerging diseases would create epidemics and pose significant challenges for public health systems both in the west and in

---

[12]   Andre Picard, "Sudanese polio case heightens fear" Toronto *The Globe and Mail* (23 June 2004) at A14.

[13]   Yves Bergerin (UNICEF), in Health Canada, Proceedings of the Canadian National Immunization Conference, *Canada's National Immunization Strategy: From Vision to Action* (December 2002) CCDR 2003; 29S4: 1-24.

[14]   Andre Picard, "Sudanese polio case heightens fear" Toronto *The Globe and Mail* (23 June 2004) at A14.

[15]   Gina Kolata, *Flu: The Story of the Great Influenza Pandemic of 1918 and the Search for the Virus That Caused It* (New York: Simon & Schuster, 1999) at 7-12.

[16]   Joint United Nations Programme on HIV/AIDS (UNAIDS), "2007 AIDS Epidemic Update" www.unaids.org/en/KnowledgeCentre/HIVData/EpiUpdate/EpiUpdArchive/2007/default.asp> (accessed 11 February 2008).

developing nations.[17] Her analyses of such diseases as Ebola fever, hemorrhagic fever, hantavirus, Lassa fever and AIDS provide compelling evidence of the continuing threat to human health of devastating diseases and the need for a global public health response. In 2000, Garrett's *Betrayal of Trust*[18] identified severe deficiencies in global public health capacity to respond to the threat of contagious diseases. SARS emerged in 2003 as the first new and puzzling 21st century disease, to remind us of the rapidity of transmission with transportation networks and of our global interdependence on domestic public health structures and on structures such as the World Health Organization operating at the transnational level.

Biological warfare — the deliberate use of contagious disease for political purposes by a state or other organized group — is another form of threat to armed forces and civilians. Vaccines are a defensive strategy against such warfare. History provides numerous examples of such germ warfare. In 1763, for example, smallpox was used as a weapon by the British forces against French loyalists in the form of contaminated blankets against Aboriginal people who had had no prior exposure to the disease.[19] North America's first germ warfare research was carried out by Frederick Banting in 1940, after obtaining funding from private investors; in 1942, Canada established a bacteriological production site for anthrax at Grosse Île, the former immigrant quarantine station in the St. Lawrence River to the east of Québec City.[20] Both the United States and the Soviet Union conducted research into biological weapons during the Cold War.[21] President Richard Nixon stopped American development of offensive uses in 1969[22] and, in 1972, the *Biological and Toxin Weapons Convention* was opened for signature. It declared germ warfare "repugnant to the conscience of mankind" and called a halt to all offensive research and

---

[17]   Laurie Garrett, *The Coming Plague: Newly Emerging Diseases in a World Out of Balance* (New York: Penguin Books, 1994).

[18]   Laurie Garrett, *Betrayal of Trust: The Collapse of Global Public Health* (New York: Hyperion, 2000).

[19]   Michael T. Osterholm & John Schwartz, *Living Terrors* (New York: Random House, 2000) at 69.

[20]   Ed Regis, *The Biology of Doom: The History of America's Secret Germ Warfare Program* (New York: Henry Holt and Company, 1999) at 22-24, 69-70, 104, 123.

[21]   Ed Regis, *The Biology of Doom* (New York: Henry Holt and Company, 1999); Michael T. Osterholm & John Schwartz, *Living Terrors* (New York: Random House, 2000); Judith Miller *et al.*, *Germs: Biological Weapons and America's Secret War* (New York: Simon & Schuster, 2001).

[22]   In two decades of production, almost 3 ½ tons of anthrax were produced in Building 470 at Fort Detrick. Ed Regis, "Our Own Anthrax: Dismantling America's weapons of mass destruction" *Harper's Magazine* (July 2004) 69 at 73.

required destruction of existing stockpiles.[23] Vaccine development for defensive purposes has the capacity to turn into offensive uses and policing suspected violations is clearly a difficult enterprise for international bodies.

Vaccines can provide protection against weaponized viruses and bacteria only if the use can be anticipated and if vaccines are available. The worst use of biological weapons took place during the Second World War, when the Japanese forces waged an extensive campaign of biological warfare in China and eventually throughout conquered Southeast Asia.[24] The Japanese campaign began with research into the contagious diseases under the direction of Shiro Ishii and proceeded in 1932[25] through lethal research on live victims, including vivisection, beginning in Beiyinhe and continuing in Unit 731 in Harbin, China,[26] and other such units. Plague-bombings were carried out using infested fleas dropped in grain from planes onto Chinese villages, leading to epidemics of bubonic plague, wells were deliberately contaminated with bacteria, and cholera epidemics were created, killing an estimated 580,000 people.[27] Over 9,000 incendiary balloons were sent out on the jet stream across the Pacific to attack North America.[28]

Little justice was achieved as many of the key researchers and leaders, a group that included more than 20,000 physicians and scientists, continued their research careers in universities and industry after the war.[29]

---

[23]   The *Biological and Toxin Weapons Convention* opened for signature in 1972, and was signed by 140 nations. Michael T.Osterholm & John Schwartz, *Living Terrors* (New York: Random House, 2000) at 70; Judith Miller *et al., Germs: Biological Weapons and America's Secret War* (New York: Simon & Schuster, 2001) at 69.

[24]   *Materials on the Trial of Former Servicemen of the Japanese Army Charged with Manufacturing and Employing Bacteriological Weapons* (partial transcript of the 1949 Soviet war crimes trial) (Moscow: Foreign Languages Publishing House, 1950); Daniel Barenblatt, *A Plague Upon Humanity* (New York: HarperCollins, 2004); Sheldon Harris, *Factories of Death* (London: Routledge, 1994).

[25]   Sheldon Harris, *Factories of Death* (London: Routledge, 1994) at 22-30, 59-67.

[26]   *Materials on the Trial of Former Servicemen of the Japanese Army Charged with Manufacturing and Employing Bacteriological Weapons* (partial transcript of the 1949 Soviet war crimes trial) (Moscow: Foreign Languages Publishing House, 1950), Indictment at 15-22; Russell Working & Bonna Chernyakova, "The Martyrs of Harbin: the 20th Century's Forgotten Villains" *Moscow Times* (27 April 2001).

[27]   Daniel Barenblatt, *A Plague Upon Humanity* (New York: HarperCollins, 2004) at 132, 164. Approximately 400,000 people were killed in cholera epidemics in China. Anthrax was also dispersed using animals and feathers, although with less lethal consequences (at 191-193). An International Symposium on the Crimes of Bacteriological Warfare held in 2002 in China agreed on this estimate (at xi, 173).

[28]   Russell Working, Special to the *Japan Times*, "The Trial of Unit 731" (5 June 2001).

[29]   Daniel Barenblatt, *A Plague Upon Humanity* (New York: HarperCollins, 2004) at 173, 233, xxiii.

The 1949 Soviet prosecution[30] of 12 doctors and military officers in Khabarovsk was highly significant since it demonstrated that crimes against humanity had been committed.[31] The Tokyo war crimes trials included no charges of biological warfare and evidence exists that the Americans entered into an agreement that resulted in the suppression of evidence, to obtain data from this research.[32] A recent class action commenced by relatives of Chinese victims was dismissed on the basis of the 1972 Japanese-Chinese agreement made when they re-established diplomatic relations, in which China renounced claims for war-related damages, although the judges ruled that the germ warfare allegations were true.[33] The Tokyo High Court rejected the appeal in April 2005, on the basis that states but not individuals were entitled to compensation.[34]

There are no simple answers to preventing genocidal atrocities. The Geneva Convention of 1925, the "Protocol for the Prohibition of the Use in War of Asphyxiating, Poisonous or Other Gases, and of Bacteriological Methods of Warfare" had been signed by 128 nations but was not signed by Japan until 1970 and by the United States until 1975. At the end of the Cold War it was revealed that the Soviet Union had been carrying on an extensive biological weapons program, created in 1973, "when the ink on the treaty banning germ weapons was barely dry", resulting in a stockpile of plague, smallpox, anthrax and other agents for their missiles and bombers at an annual cost of almost $1 billion.[35] Only with an effectively functional international security system will such protections be enforced and followed. The international norms on human subject experimentation that arose out of the Nuremberg trials were an essential step toward protecting the human rights of citizens in the face of such organized psychopathology. Efforts to strengthen international law on research on human subjects should continue and any strengthened law should deal with the ethics of states making use of the research resulting from the atrocities.

---

[30] *Materials on the Trial of Former Servicemen of the Japanese Army Charged with Manufacturing and Employing Bacteriological Weapons* (partial transcript of the 1949 Soviet war crimes trial) (Moscow: Foreign Languages Publishing House, 1950).

[31] Russell Working, Special to the *Japan Times*, "The Trial of Unit 731" (5 June 2001).

[32] Daniel Barenblatt, *A Plague Upon Humanity* (New York: HarperCollins, 2004) at 112-13, 176-236. See also Linda Hunt, *Secret Agenda: The United States Government, Nazi Scientists, and Project Paperclip, 1945 to 1990* (New York: St. Martin's Press, 1991).

[33] Russell Working, Special to the *Japan Times*, "The Trial of Unit 731" (5 June 2001).

[34] "Tokyo court rejects appeal of war victims" *China Daily* (20 April 2005).

[35] Judith Miller *et al.*, *Germs: Biological Weapons and America's Secret War* (New York: Simon & Schuster, 2001) at 167.

II. COMPENSATION AND LIABILITY

Canadian law provides a means for injured victims to sue manufacturers for harm caused by the defendant's negligence. Vaccine manufacturers owe a duty of care to the ultimate consumer.[36] Under the manufacturer's duty branch of *Donoghue v. Stevenson*,[37] a manufacturer owes a duty to take reasonable care in preparing, assembling, repairing, installing and inspecting the product. The standard of care in the vaccine area is likely to be very high since the product is one that is taken into the body. A manufacturer that fails to meet this standard in the manufacturing process, including the process of testing the product and inspecting it, would be found liable if a foreseeable type of injury was caused by this failure. Canadian law contains few examples of negligent drug or vaccine manufacturing. An allegation of negligent manufacturing was made in the rabies vaccine case of *Davidson v. Connaught Laboratories*[38] but there was no evidence of any defect or other negligence in its packaging or storage. In *Rothwell v. Raes*,[39] the plaintiff alleged that the pertussis vaccine had been negligently manufactured in that the manufacturer knew it was inherently dangerous and should have used current technological advances; the trial judge, Osler J., decided that there was no negligence since no tests had been done on the Japanese version that would lead the scientific community to accept that it was a superior product. In British Columbia, the court certified the class in *Harrington v. Dow Corning Corp.*,[40] for an action to determine whether silicone gel breast implants were reasonably fit for their intended purpose, or in effect that the breast implants should not have been on the market. Such an action permitted the class plaintiff to demonstrate the deficiency of the product without having to prove the subjective causation element, which the court thought required individual actions to resolve. The case was settled against the Dow defendants in 1999 as part of the global settlement which formed part of the U.S. bankruptcy proceedings[41] and against the remaining

---

[36]   Live vaccines may pose particular problems in this regard. For example, the live polio vaccine (Sabin vaccine) carries with it the risk of transmission to any person coming into contact with the bodily fluids of the vaccinated person — a parent or other caregiver of an infant, for instance. A court would want to examine whether a duty is owed to such third parties but should have little difficulty in reaching the conclusion that a duty is owed to such foreseeable plaintiffs.

[37]   [1932] A.C. 562 (H.L.).

[38]   [1980] O.J. No. 153 (Ont. H.C.J.).

[39]   [1988] O.J. No. 1847, 66 O.R. (2d) 449, 54 D.L.R. (4th) 193 (Ont. H.C.J.), aff'd [1990] O.J. No. 2298, 2 O.R. (3d) 332, 76 D.L.R. (4th) 280 (Ont. C.A.), leave to appeal to S.C.C. refused [1991] S.C.C.A. No. 58 (S.C.C.).

[40]   [1996] B.C.J. No. 734, 22 B.C.L.R. (3d) 97 (B.C.S.C.), aff'd [2000] B.C.J. No. 2237 (B.C.C.A.), leave to appeal to S.C.C. refused with costs [2001] S.C.C.A. No. 21 (S.C.C.).

[41]   *Harrington v. Dow Corning Corp.*, [2002] B.C.J. No. 1667 at para. 5 (B.C.S.C.).

corporate defendants in 2005.[42] The kind of action certified by the trial judge against the corporate defendants provides a means for plaintiffs to raise the issue of a manufacturer's testing of the product and the extent of the knowledge created during the pre- and post-marketing periods. Such a duty to test for product deficiencies seems integral to the *Donoghue v. Stevenson* manufacturer's principle of the duty to take reasonable care prior to the product reaching the ultimate consumer. Class certification proceedings have been commenced in four actions alleging various forms of negligence with respect to the presence of thimerosal in vaccines administered to young children in Ontario and British Columbia.[43]

The most common form of action in the prescription drug and vaccine area is the duty to warn action. A manufacturer owes a duty to the ultimate consumer to disclose the product risks of which it knows or should know.[44] The manufacturer knows of these risks in greater detail than the consumer and must increase the warning as the gravity of the harm increases.[45] When the product is a prescribed product, the prescribing professional is considered by the court to be a learned intermediary between the manufacturer and the consumer. The duty to disclose owed to the consumer may be discharged indirectly by warning the learned intermediary. Warnings must flow from the manufacturer to the prescribing health professional and from there to the patient/consumer or substitute decision-maker. Any prescribing professional owes a duty to inform the patient of the material risks and other factors at common law,[46] and, in provinces such as Ontario must meet the statutory standard of disclosure, which largely replicates the common law standard. Doctors and dentists have prescribing privileges and doctors are the professionals most often involved in prescribing drugs. As other health professionals acquire prescribing privileges, they too should become learned intermediaries.

---

[42] *Harrington v. Dow Corning Corp.*, [2007] B.C.J. No. 356 (B.C.S.C.).

[43] *East (Litigation Guardian of) v. Aventis Pasteur Limited/Aventis Pasteur Limitee* (unreported, 2002, Ont. S.C.J.) DPT, Td and DT vaccines; *White v. Merck Frosst*, [2004] O.J. No. 623 (Ont. S.C.J.), [2004] O.J. No. 1578 (Ont. S.C.J.), hepatitis B vaccines; *Chamberlain (Guardian ad Litem of) v. Aventis Pasteua Limited/Aventis Pasteur Limitee* (unreported, 2003 B.C.S.C.) DPT, TD and DT vaccines; and *Soursos (Guardian ad Litem of) v. Merck Frosst Canada & Co. and GlaxoSmithKline Inc.* (unreported, 2003, B.C.S.C.) hepatitis B vaccines.

[44] *Lambert v. Lastoplex Chemicals Co.*, [1971] S.C.J. No. 132, [1972] S.C.R. 569 (S.C.C.); *Hollis v. Dow Corning Corp.*, [1995] S.C.J. No. 104, [1995] 4 S.C.R. 634 (S.C.C.).

[45] *Buchan v. Ortho Pharmaceutical (Canada) Ltd.*, [1986] O.J. No. 2331, 54 O.R. (2d) 92 (Ont. C.A.).

[46] *Reibl v. Hughes*, [1980] S.C.J. No. 105, [1980] 2 S.C.R. 880 (S.C.C.); *Arndt v. Smith*, [1997] S.C.J. No. 65, [1997] 2 S.C.R. 539 (S.C.C.).

As Robins J. stated in *Buchan v. Ortho Pharmaceutical (Canada) Ltd.*[47] and La Forest J. in *Hollis v. Dow Corning Corp.*,[48] a fundamental inequality exists among these actors and a relationship of dependency and reliance exists for the patient as well as for the doctor. The knowledge disadvantage that exists among the three parties must be remedied by the manufacturer. As La Forest J. commented in *Hollis*:

> In light of the enormous informational advantage enjoyed by medical manufacturers over consumers, it is reasonable and just to require manufacturers, under the law of tort, to make clear, complete and current informational disclosure to consumers concerning the risks inherent in the ordinary use of their products. A high standard for disclosure protects public health by promoting the right to bodily integrity, increasing consumer choice and facilitating a more meaningful doctor-patient relationship. At the same time, it cannot be said that requiring manufacturers to be forthright about the risks inherent in the use of their product imposes an onerous burden on the manufacturers. As Robins J.A. explained in *Buchan*, *supra*, at p. 381, "drug manufacturers are in a position to escape all liability by the simple expedient of providing a clear and forthright warning of the dangers inherent in the use of their products of which they know or ought to know.[49]

The disclosure obligation is intended to ensure that the patient can make an informed decision about the product and also to ensure that the manufacturer is honest about the product.[50] In American cases involving mass immunization clinics and birth control pills, courts have found a duty on the manufacturer to warn the consumer directly in these situations rather than a duty to the consumer that may be discharged indirectly through warning the learned intermediary.[51] At mass immunization clinics, warnings may be posted so that consumers receive direct warnings. The five-member Court of Appeal in *Buchan* considered with some favour the indirect duty in birth control situations, *obiter*, but decided the case on the basis of the learned intermediary rule.

An action for failure to disclose product risks may pose significant causation difficulties for a plaintiff, particularly when the product is a scientific innovation such as a vaccine.[52] Several causation tests must be

---

47   [1986] O.J. No. 2331, 54 O.R. (2d) 92 (Ont. C.A.).
48   [1995] S.C.J. No. 104, [1995] 4 S.C.R. 634 (S.C.C.).
49   *Ibid.*, at para. 26.
50   James Britain, "Product Honesty is the Best Policy: A Comparison of Doctors' and Manufacturers' Duty to Disclose Drug Risks and the Importance of Consumer Expectations in Determining Product Defect" (1984) 79 Northwestern U.L. Rev. 342.
51   See the discussion in the final section of *Buchan v. Ortho Pharmaceutical (Canada) Ltd.*, [1986] O.J. No. 2331, 54 O.R. (2d) 92 (Ont. C.A.).
52   For comments on drug liability causation problems see Denis W. Boivin, "Factual Causation in the Law of Manufacturer Failure to Warn" (1998/99) 30 Ottawa L. Rev. 47; Jean Torrens, "Informed Consent and the Learned Intermediary Rule in Canada" (1994) 58

met simultaneously in a disclosure action. A plaintiff must prove factual causation on the balance of probabilities: that the vaccine more likely than not caused or contributed to the harm.[53] When a medical product is at issue, general scientific causation requires that the product in general be proved to be the cause in fact and particular scientific causation requires that the product has caused the injury to this particular plaintiff. For example, in *Rothwell v. Raes*,[54] the plaintiff, Patrick Rothwell, was unable to prove, using scientific evidence over the 74-day trial, that the pertussis vaccine more likely than not caused brain damage. In addition, Osler J. stated that even if he had been satisfied on that point, he would have found against the plaintiff in particular since he was not satisfied on the balance of probabilities that the particular damage suffered by Patrick Rothwell had been caused by the vaccine. Patrick Rothwell had shown early signs of neurological impairment and had a twin who had been stillborn. An early Québec decision in *Boilard v. City of Montreal*[55] involved a jury verdict that a vaccine used in compulsory immunization required by the city was infected; on appeal, this verdict was overturned as speculative and lacking any evidentiary basis.

The plaintiff in the disclosure action must also prove causation in relation to the decision. The Supreme Court of Canada in *Hollis* determined, as the Ontario Court of Appeal had found in *Buchan*, that the subjective test of causation should be used for this part of the action. If the manufacturer had disclosed the information adequately, would the plaintiff have proceeded with the vaccine? In contrast, in the action for inadequate disclosure by a physician to a patient, the Supreme Court of Canada has required the plaintiff to prove that the reasonable patient in his or her shoes would not have proceeded with the treatment. This modified objective test, established in *Reibl v. Hughes*, has been affirmed in the case of *Arndt v. Smith*.[56] The *Arndt* case gives weight to the subjective element in the analysis since three of the judges thought that the test should be subjective and the majority made the modified objective test more subjective by moving it from the decision's context, Mr. Reibl's pension entitlement, to the plaintiff's own values and beliefs, with the

---

Sask. L. Rev. 399; and my "Drug/Vaccine Risks: Patient Decision-Making and Harm Reduction in the Pharmaceutical Company Duty to Warn Action" (1991) 70 Can. Bar Rev. 473.

[53] *Snell v. Farrell*, [1990] S.C.J. No. 73, [1990] 2 S.C.R. 311 (S.C.C.); *Athey v. Leonati*, [1996] S.C.J. No. 102, [1996] 3 S.C.R. 458 (S.C.C.).

[54] [1988] O.J. No. 1847, 66 O.R. (2d) 449, 54 D.L.R. (4th) 193 (Ont. H.C.J.), aff'd [1990] O.J. No. 2298, 2 O.R. (3d) 332, 76 D.L.R. (4th) 280 (Ont. C.A.), leave to appeal to S.C.C. refused [1991] S.C.C.A. No. 58 (S.C.C.).

[55] (1914), 21 R.L. n.x. 58 (Qué. K.B.).

[56] *Reibl v. Hughes*, [1980] S.C.J. No. 105, [1980] 2 S.C.R. 880 (S.C.C.); *Arndt v. Smith*, [1997] S.C.J. No. 65, [1997] 2 S.C.R. 539 (S.C.C.).

caveat that they must be reasonably based.[57] A strong argument can be made on equitable grounds that a subjective test is *also* required, even when the modified objective test is used, since a plaintiff who would have proceeded with the treatment if she had had adequate information should not be able to win the action simply because the reasonable plaintiff in her shoes would not have proceeded.[58]

A causation problem may be posed by the relationship between the behaviour of the manufacturer and that of the prescribing doctor. In the *Hollis* case, the plaintiff sued both parties for breach of their respective duties of disclosure but two of three British Columbia Court of Appeal judges decided that the action against the doctor should be sent back for retrial. On appeal to the Supreme Court of Canada, the manufacturer attempted to argue that the action against them should not be heard in the absence of the findings against the doctor since, they argued, the doctor would not have disclosed the product risks to Hollis, even if the manufacturer had provided adequate information to the doctor. This argument is essentially an argument about intervening causation, with the manufacturer arguing that the doctor would have intervened to prevent the information from reaching the ultimate consumer even if the manufacturer had met its obligation. The argument is by definition a hypothetical one though, and both the *Buchan* court and the *Hollis* court decided that it would be unfair to require the plaintiff to prove that the doctor would have disclosed if the manufacturer had met its obligation. The Ontario Court of Appeal in *Buchan* created a rebuttable presumption that the doctor would have disclosed. They found that the manufacturer, Ortho Pharmaceutical (Canada) Ltd., had promoted the drug's safety so extensively that the doctor could not be considered an independent cause. The Supreme Court of Canada analyzed the issue in a similar manner, seeing an inequity in requiring a plaintiff to prove a hypothetical, identifying the problem of the defendant's actions undermining the plaintiff's power of proof, expressing concern about the plaintiff possibly losing both actions in a situation where the physician disclosed information actually possessed but wouldn't have disclosed the information that the manufacturer failed to disclose, and noting the ease of avoiding the dilemma through disclosing.[59]

---

[57]   Justice McLachlin concurred in the result but thought that the subjective test should be used and that the trial judge had used the subjective test. Justices Sopinka and Gonthier dissented, stating that the subjective test should be used but that the trial judge had used the objective test. These disagreements indicate the permeability of the boundary between subjective and modified objective determinations.

[58]   See the discussion in *Truman v. Thomas* (1980), 611 P.2d 902 (Cal. S.C.).

[59]   *Hollis v. Dow Corning Corp.*, [1995] S.C.J. No. 104, [1995] 4 S.C.R. 634 at paras. 53-61 (S.C.C.).

The earlier case of *Davidson v. Connaught Laboratories*[60] had raised an aspect of this issue. The plaintiff, Paul Davidson, had come into contact with a rabid cow at his family's farm in Ontario. By the time he became aware of the problem, he was in British Columbia where he obtained expert advice on the risks of rabies vaccine, including paralysis. When the plaintiff returned to his family physician to be vaccinated, the family physician did not disclose the risk of paralysis, although the trial judge thought that the standard of disclosure had been met because the 1/500 to 1/8,500 probability was so low. Davidson was considered to have been aware of the risk of death from rabies since it was common knowledge. Justice Linden found that the manufacturer, Connaught Laboratories, had failed to disclose the risks of the vaccine to the physician. Since the plaintiff had actual knowledge of the risks as a result of the consultation with the B.C. expert, disclosure by the physician would have made no difference and the action failed the but-for test of factual causation. The manufacturer was insulated from liability by the actual knowledge of the plaintiff. As well, the court reasoned, the plaintiff would have chosen the option of vaccination in any event, since the alternative was the risk of death from rabies. The causation problem in the *Davidson* case differs from that in *Buchan* and *Hollis* since Davidson possessed actual knowledge. The recent case of *Teubner v. Gasewicz*[61] had a similar result, finding that there was no causal connection between the failure of the lab to give nurses a refresher course on rubella vaccine risks and the plaintiff's harm, since the nurse and doctor were not negligent and the plaintiff had an awareness of the risk in any event.

Morgan v. Metropolitan Toronto (Municipality)[62] is another case that illustrates the problems created by insufficient knowledge at the time of vaccination. In 1994, the plaintiff, Lucia Morgan, was vaccinated against hepatitis B at a city clinic and after this vaccination suffered flu-like symptoms, which she did not discuss with the nurse, Ms. Jones, when she returned for the second shot. After this booster shot, Ms. Morgan experienced more severe and lasting symptoms and these were diagnosed the following year as chronic fatigue syndrome. Justice Sanderson examined extensive evidence as to the state of knowledge at the time of the vaccination and found that it did not include the risk of chronic fatigue syndrome.[63] As a result, the nurse had not breached the standard of disclosure. Justice Sanderson found that the causation element connecting any breach of disclosure to the harm had not been proved, applying a fairly subjective version of the decision causation test, since the plaintiff

[60]   [1980] O.J. No. 153 (Ont. H.C.J.).
[61]   [2001] O.J. No. 5216 (Ont. S.C.J.).
[62]   [2006] O.J. No. 4951 (Ont. S.C.J.), aff'd [2008] O.J. No. 3433 (Ont. C.A.) *[Morgan]*.
[63]   *Ibid.*, at paras. 125-148, 251, 326-332 (S.C.J.).

would have opted to receive the vaccine since she thought it was mandatory for her employment and because it was a rare risk whose adverse effects were considered temporary and not severe.[64] She made no finding on general causation but, for the purpose of appeal, included her observations indicating that she would have accepted the evidence indicating general causation and particular causation.[65] Since the plaintiff did not disclose to the nurse her flu-like symptoms following her first immunization, and since the standard of care in 1994 did not require Ms. Jones to ask clients about such reactions,[66] no breach of the standard of care was found in the administration of the second shot. The failure to report the adverse events following immunization, as required under the provincial legislation (the *Health Protection and Promotion Act*,[67]) was not causally linked to the injuries.[68] Thus, the action by Ms. Morgan, who suffered life-altering injuries from the hepatitis B vaccine, failed on the issues of disclosure of risks and on the issue of decision causation.

Vaccination cases arguably differ from other disclosure actions in those jurisdictions with a statutory requirement of vaccination for school entry (discussed in Section III). While it would not affect the existence of a manufacturer's duty of care to warn of product risks and a health professional's duty of disclosure, this statutory requirement could affect the causal relationship by minimizing the option of not having a child vaccinated. On the other hand, the possibility of obtaining an exemption, based on religion or conscience, recreates the real nature of the choice for those who claim these exemptions.

The *Lapierre*[69] case illustrates the problem faced by plaintiffs who suffer adverse reactions to vaccines. Nathalie Lapierre suffered acute viral encephalitis after vaccination with measles vaccine and became almost totally disabled. Her father sued the Québec government, basing their argument on the public benefit achieved at the expense of those few individuals who were susceptible to the vaccine's adverse effects, a risk estimated at one in a million vaccinated individuals.[70] The argument amounted to an affirmative use of the necessity defence, grounded in Québec civil law.[71] The Supreme Court of Canada denied the plaintiff's claim in spite of evident sympathy for her situation. The lack of success of

---

[64]   *Ibid.*, at para. 346.

[65]   *Ibid.*, at paras. 375-92.

[66]   *Ibid.*, at paras. 354-68.

[67]   R.S.O. 1990, c. H-7, s. 38.

[68]   *Morgan v. Metropolitan Toronto (Municipality)*, [2006] O.J. No. 4951 at paras. 372 75 (Ont. S.C.J.), aff'd [2008] O.J. No. 3433 (Ont. C.A.).

[69]   *Lapierre v. Québec (Attorney-General)*, [1985] S.C.J. No. 13, [1985] 1 S.C.R. 241 (S.C.C.).

[70]   *Ibid.*, at para. 22.

[71]   Art. 1057 C.C.

this action led to creation of a no-fault compensation fund in the province for individuals harmed by vaccines in Québec.

In a fault-based system like the Canadian negligence system, plaintiffs are unable to recover damages when their harm results from their inherent vulnerability to the vaccine rather than the negligence of a manufacturer, health professional or government. Causation tests are difficult for plaintiffs to meet and some rigour is appropriate to protect defendants from liability in the absence of factual causation. Because of the difficulties inherent in the legal process, many prospective plaintiffs do not sue.[72] No-fault compensation funds have received considerable support. In the *Davidson* case, Linden J. made an *obiter* comment recommending creation of a no-fault compensation scheme for persons injured through rare reactions to vaccines in the absence of fault.[73] Justice Krever made a similar recommendation in *Ferguson v. Hamilton Civic Hospital*,[74] saying that there was an urgent need to correct the lack of a remedy for a patient who suffers catastrophic disease without fault. At the end of *Rothwell v. Raes*, Osler J. expressed "the view, perhaps unbecoming to a trial judge, that the normal process of litigation is an utterly inappropriate procedure for dealing with claims of this nature" and advocated recovery in proceedings before a tribunal upon proof of prior good health, followed by the vaccine and catastrophic damage within a limited period.[75] In its recent Report, the Manitoba Law Commission recommended a public no-fault compensation fund for vaccine-related injury.[76]

Similarly, in *Morgan*, after finding against the plaintiff, Sanderson J. added additional comments,[77] stating that "[t]he road to protecting public

---

[72]   A Report to the Conference of Deputy Ministers of Health of the Federal/Provincial/ Territorial Review on Liability and Compensation Issues in Health Care, J. Robert Prichard (Chair), *Liability and Compensation in Health Care* (1990); Wendy Mariner, "Liability and Compensation for Adverse Reactions to HIV Vaccines" in Office of Technology Assessment, Congress of the United States, *Adverse Reactions to HIV Vaccines: Medical, Ethical and Legal Issues* (Washington, D.C.: U.S. Government Printing Office, 1995), 79-159 at 110-112.

[73]   *Davidson v. Connaught Laboratories*, [1980] O.J. No. 153 (Ont. H.C.J.).

[74]   Krever J. in *Ferguson v. Hamilton Civic Hospital*, [1983] O.J. No. 2497, 40 O.R. (2d) 577 at 618-19 (Ont. H.C.J.), aff'd [1985] O.J. No. 2538, 50 O.R. (2d) 754 (Ont. C.A.).

[75]   *Rothwell v. Raes*, [1988] O.J. No. 1847, 66 O.R. (2d) 449, 54 D.L.R. (4th) 193 (Ont. H.C.J.), aff'd [1990] O.J. No. 2298, 2 O.R. (3d) 332, 76 D.L.R. (4th) 280 (Ont. C.A.), leave to appeal to S.C.C. refused [1991] S.C.C.A. No. 58 (S.C.C.). Under these criteria, recovery would not have been possible for Rothwell who showed evidence of impairment prior to vaccination. Temporal association instead of causation would seem like a weak test.

[76]   Manitoba Law Commission, *Compensation of Vaccine-Damaged Children*, Report 104 (2000).

[77]   *Morgan v. Metropolitan Toronto (Municipality)*, [2006] O.J. No. 4951 at paras. 417-446 (Ont. S.C.J.) aff'd [2008] O.J. No. 3433 (Ont. C.A.).

health should not be paved with individual victims. Fair, meaningful, no-fault compensation should be made available to individuals suffering from serious adverse side effects of vaccines".[78] In support of this position, Sanderson J. identified the public benefits attributable to vaccines[79] and pointed to the difficulties faced by plaintiffs who are likely to be seriously ill and lacking in funds to pay the costs of such lengthy and complex litigation, adding that "[e]ven those able to afford such costs would likely be met (as here) with experts stridently touting vaccine safety".[80]

Justice Sanderson also identified problems created for the evidentiary process with the scientific evidence available to make reliable risk estimates and confidently rule out material risks. In her view, it was not sufficient to state that the evidence does not support a finding of risk when there have been inadequate data collected and analyzed to test the hypothesis.[81] Following on this assessment, she stated that we need active surveillance to provide sufficient data, investigation of each serious adverse reaction, adoption of standard scientific language, and registries with open access to the data.[82] The inclusion of these critical comments not only echoes those made by analysts of the system but also provides a view of how these failures to reduce scientific uncertainty diminish the lives of individuals and undermine justice.

The United States,[83] New Zealand, the United Kingdom[84] and Québec have established compensation funds for vaccine-injured recipients. The essential rationale is that set out in *Lapierre*: because the community benefits from high levels of vaccination, compensation should be paid to those who suffer on the community's behalf. Public benefits are achieved through improved overall health status, decreased health costs, and increased school, work and voluntary activity attendance, while most individuals benefit from better health as a result of the vaccine's protection from disease and herd immunity. Vaccines have risks, however, and some individuals suffer from seriously compromised health as a result of vaccination. When the benefits are demonstrably clear, vaccine risks may be less clearly articulated, lost in the benefits or not perceived. Nicole Kutlesa has argued that the extensive promotion of vaccination and its benefits, along with the related under-emphasis on vaccine risks, makes the system effectively mandatory because of the government's active

---

[78]   *Ibid.*, at para. 437 (S.C.J.).

[79]   *Ibid.*, at para. 436.

[80]   *Ibid.*, at para. 441.

[81]   *Ibid.*, at para. 420.

[82]   *Ibid.*, at para. 421.

[83]   United States, *National Childhood Vaccine Injury Act* (NCVIA; P.L. 99-660) of 1986 and the *Comprehensive Childhood Immunization Act* of 1993. The money for the compensation funds comes from an excise tax levied on vaccines.

[84]   United Kingdom, *Vaccine Damage Payments Act, 1979.*

promotion of vaccination, through funding, school attendance legislation, a "barrage" of ads and endorsements by government, monitoring of children's immunization histories and reminders of the need to keep vaccinations up-to-date.[85] As a result, she argues, a no-fault system should be established to provide compensation to "those individuals who, although selfishly motivated, nonetheless place themselves at risk of harm".[86]

Québec's no-fault compensation plan is found in the *Public Health Act*[87] and Regulations, which provides in s. 70 that the Minister shall compensate, "regardless of responsibility", any victim of bodily injury caused by a voluntary vaccination against identified diseases or infections or by a mandatory vaccination under the emergency powers provision in effect when the government declares an emergency, in either case administered in Québec. The Act preserves the right to sue.

The United States' National Vaccine Injury Compensation Program ("VICP") was established to provide no-fault compensation to individuals and families injured by vaccines covered by the fund.[88] The VICP is funded through money from the vaccine manufacturers in the form of a flat-rate excise tax on each vaccination dose sold, resulting in a surplus balance of $1.8 billion in 2002,[89] and more than $2 billion by 2007.[90] "Table" cases are those placed on the table list by the Department of Health and Human Services, and they require only proof of the vaccination, the nature of the claimant's injury found on the Injury Table, and the absence of other factors following immunization to demonstrate particular causation, with general causation presumed. "Non-table" cases require proof of general causation, according to the civil standard of proof accepted by the VICP, and not to scientific certainty.[91] Some limited possibilities exist for actions through the courts if a claim is denied; in the case of autism, some plaintiffs have gone directly to court, for example, by arguing that the suppliers of thimerosal are not vaccine

---

[85] Nicole J. Kutlesa, "Creating a sustainable Immunization System in Canada — The Case for a Vaccine-Related Injury Compensation Scheme" (2004) 12 Health L.J. 201 at 211, 206-207 and 241.

[86] *Ibid.*, at 201-202.

[87] R.S.Q. c. S-2.2, ss. 70-78.

[88] *National Childhood Vaccine Injury Act*, 42 U.S.C. (1986) ["NCVIA"].

[89] Nicole J. Kutlesa, "Creating a Sustainable Immunization System in Canada — The Case for a Vaccine-Related Injury Compensation Scheme" (2004) 12 Health L.J. 201 at 204-205, citing Advisory Commission on Childhood Vaccines, Minutes of 51st Meeting (6 June 2002).

[90] Stephen D. Sugarman, "Cases in Vaccine Court — Legal Battles over Vaccines and Autism" (2007) New Eng. J. Med. 1275-77 at 1276.

[91] *Ibid.*, at 1277. Justice Sanderson discusses the operation of the VICP and proof of causation in *Morgan v. Metropolitan Toronto (Municipality)*, [2006] O.J. No. 4951 at paras. 293-302 (Ont. S.C.J.), aff'd [2008] O.J. No. 3433 (Ont. C.A.).

manufacturers.[92] From 1988 to July 2006, claims under the VICP in 2,531 cases, not involving thimerosal/autism, led to payments of just over $902 million, with an average of about $850,000 for the 2,000 successful claims.[93] Over 5,000 claims have been filed alleging that autism resulted from vaccination with the measles-mumps-rubella ("MMR") vaccine and thimerosal-containing vaccines. The VICP announced in 2002 that a group of test cases would be heard on the issue of general causation in the Omnibus Autism Proceeding. The first three test cases, based on the theory that MMR vaccines and thimerosal-containing vaccines can combine to cause autism, were heard by the Special Masters in the U.S. Court of Federal Claims starting in the summer of 2007. The second group of three test cases, heard in May and July 2008, presented evidence of the theory that thimerosal-containing vaccines alone can cause autism, while the third theory, that MMR vaccines alone can cause autism, was presented as part of the first theory.[94]

Although a detailed examination of the public policy changes that could remedy the current deficiencies is beyond the scope of this chapter, it is worth noting that no-fault compensation funds have a sound basis in equitable principles and should be given serious consideration by the governments concerned. Issues such as eligibility criteria, compensation amounts, criteria for proof of causation and establishment of any presumptions need resolution in the creation and continuing evaluation of such public schemes. Compensation funds can produce additional benefits such as the Vaccine Adverse Event Reporting System ("VAERS"), mandating adverse event reporting by manufacturers, created under the NCVIA.[95] More limited reforms such as government-funded insurance, reform of the tort system or voluntary contracts would also have benefits, as well as disadvantages,[96] but the compensation fund is an idea that is more likely to serve the purpose of social justice and fit well with the public commitment to funding universally accessible health programs.

---

[92] Ibid.

[93] Ibid., at 1276.

[94] United States Court of Federal Claims, Office of Special Masters, In Re: Claims for Vaccine Injuries Resulting in Autism Spectrum Disorder or a Similar Neurodevelopmental Disorder, Various Petitioners v. Secretary of Health and Human Services. Omnibus Autism Proceeding, Autism Update (29 September 2008), online: <http://www.uscfc.uscourts.gov/sites/default/files/autism/autism_update_9_29_08.pdf>.

[95] Kevin M. Malone & Alan R. Hinman, "Vaccination Mandates: The Public Health Imperative and Individual Rights" in Richard A. Goodman et al., eds., Law In Public Health Practice (Oxford: Oxford University Press, 2003) at 267.

[96] Wendy Mariner, "Liability and Compensation for Adverse Reactions to HIV Vaccines" in Office of Technology Assessment, Congress of the United States, Adverse Reactions to HIV Vaccines: Medical, Ethical and Legal Issues (Washington: U.S. Government Printing Office, 1995) 79-159 at 119-125.

The perception that vaccines have unacceptable risks leads some to the decision not to have children vaccinated, and, as Hodge and Gostin have indicated, risk perception looks different from the individual and societal perspectives.[97] For example, vaccination rates declined after the swine flu vaccine seemed to show a causal link to the neurological disorder, Guillain-Barre syndrome.[98] It is difficult to estimate such effects in Canada because a fully developed network of registries is still under development, as discussed in Section IV. Ann Pierce commented that little knowledge exists about the perceptions of vaccine risks despite a large vaccine literature and active vaccine groups. The misconceptions include "beliefs about the disappearance of diseases regardless of vaccine use, the relative risks of vaccines and diseases, the potential existence of vaccine 'hot' lots, misunderstanding of base rate issues related to disease incidence among vaccinated and unvaccinated children, and concerns about overloading the immune system with multiple vaccinations given at the same time".[99] Anti-vaccination websites provide easily accessible information, express strong concerns about vaccine safety and rely extensively on emotional appeals for their messages.[100] Ross Silverman has noted that increasing numbers of parents are using American exemptions from mandatory immunization requirements and that because these are often clustered, the individuals themselves increase their own vulnerability and create a greater risk of spreading the contagious disease to others who have been vaccinated.[101]

If an unvaccinated person spreads a contagious disease to vaccinated persons, the injured person might bring an action against the unvaccinated person and any substitute decision-makers. Does an unvaccinated person owe a duty of care to others in the community to protect them from the harm of contagious diseases? Is an individual's choice not to engage in a preventive activity that would enhance protection for the community one that could lead to tort liability? The plaintiff would have high hurdles to

---

[97] James G. Hodge, Jr. & Lawrence O. Gostin, "School Vaccination Requirements: Historical, Social, and Legal Perspectives" (2001-2002) 90 Ky. L.J. 831 at 876-77.

[98] Gina Kolata, *Flu: The Story of the Great Influenza Pandemic of 1918 and the Search for the Virus That Caused It* (New York: Simon & Schuster, 1999), c. 6, "A Litigation Nightmare" at 151-95.

[99] Ann Pierce, "Vaccine Risk Communication: Lessons from Risk Perception, Decision Making and Environmental Risk Communication Research" (1997) 8 Risk 173. Her useful list of suggestions for research includes: targeting audiences; misconceptions and knowledge gaps; quantifying risk messages; communicating uncertainty; increasing information exchanges and input; evaluating the risk messages (at 199-200).

[100] R.M. Wolfe *et al.*, "Content and Design Attributes of Antivaccination Web Sites" (2002) 287(24) JAMA 3245-48.

[101] Ross D. Silverman, "No More Kidding Around: Restructuring Non-Medical Childhood Immunization Exemptions to Ensure Public Health Protection" (2003) 12 Annals of Health L. 277 at 285.

clear before a court would impose such liability. Tort law has a strong disinclination to require individuals to engage in affirmative action to rescue others. In a case involving social host liability, *Childs v. Desormeaux*,[102] the Supreme Court of Canada provided an analysis of the situations in which a positive duty of care have been found, noting that while these situations are not strict legal categories, they illustrate the factors that can lead to positive duties.[103] The first situation was described as one where the defendant invited persons to an obvious risk that they created or controlled, and the Court stated that "[t]hese cases are akin to the positive and *continuing* duty" of manufacturers to warn of product dangers.[104] The second situation is paternalistic relationships of supervision and control. The third situation involves the exercise of a public function or commercial enterprise including implied responsibilities to the public. The Court continued by stating that all these situations involve the defendant's material participation in the creation of the risk to which others have been invited.[105] Since the law is concerned about autonomy, the Court continued, it is only when such a special relationship exists that the law may impinge on the third party's autonomy, for example, by prohibiting a person who is unfit from participating in a sporting activity.[106] If we ask whether unvaccinated persons have participated in creating the risk of contagious disease, arguably they have, since other members of the community are dependent on a sufficiently high vaccination rate to diminish the naturally existing risk of the disease. Courts are reluctant to impose an obligation of difficult rescue, however, and would carefully scrutinize the level of risk to the defendant before concluding that any such duty to rescue existed. The court would make these assessments within its duty framework determining whether a special relationship of proximity and foreseeability existed, and whether there was any policy reason not to impose the duty, under the *Cooper v. Hobart* and *Kamloops*[107] tests, giving consideration in this case to autonomy and any religious or conscientious objections. The court would have to be satisfied that the plaintiffs were foreseeable victims or members of a class of foreseeable victims. Children in schools or day cares with the defendant would have a stronger case in this respect. In determining the standard of care, any court would have to assess the gravity of the harm and the probability of the risk, along with

---

[102]   [2006] S.C.J. No. 18 (S.C.C.).

[103]   *Ibid.*, at para. 34.

[104]   *Ibid.*, at para. 35 [emphasis in original].

[105]   *Ibid.*, at para. 38; See also Ernest Weinrib, "The Case for a Duty to Rescue" (1980) 90 Yale L.J. 247 at 256.

[106]   *Childs v. Desormeaux*, [2006] S.C.J. No. 18 at para. 39 (S.C.C.).

[107]   *Cooper v. Hobart*, [2001] S.C.J. No. 76, [2001] 3 S.C.R. 537 (S.C.C.); *Kamloops (City) v. Nielsen*, [1984] S.C.J. No. 29, [1984] 2 S.C.R. 2 (S.C.C.), adopting *Anns v. Merton London Borough Council*, [1978] A.C. 728 (P.C.).

consideration of cost and, in some cases, social utility. These factors would vary among vaccines and circumstances of contagion. At the duty stage, the plaintiff would have a very difficult case to make and would then have to prove both general causation, that the vaccine causes the disease in a general scientific sense, and particular causation, that the vaccine caused the plaintiff's condition. The harm caused to this plaintiff would have to be linked to the particular defendant,[108] and the foreseeability of the type of harm would need to be demonstrated.

Because many vaccination programs are directed at children, substitute decision-makers make the decisions, until the minor becomes capable of making the decision, in accordance with provincial law.[109] Differences between parents about the advisability of vaccines form the subject of litigation, particularly in situations where the parents are separated or divorced. *Di Serio v. Di Serio*[110] was a family law dispute in which the mother was given custody over the children for vaccination purposes on a best interests basis, in lieu of the father who was a vegan. *Chmiliar v. Chmiliar*[111] raised the issue of mature minors making their own decisions. The 13-year-old daughter was found generally capable of deciding but incapable because her irrational fear of vaccines, instilled by her mother, had removed the capacity to consent. Depending on the circumstances, this kind of parental pressure might appropriately be seen as an infringement on the voluntary nature of the decision. The father's application to have the vaccination ordered was dismissed because the vaccine was not seen as necessary for life and her fear outweighed the benefits. Religious objections to immunization were litigated in two earlier decisions: the 1968 *King v. King*[112] case in which religious objections did not bar the father from custody and *B.(C.R.) v. Newfoundland (Director of Child Welfare)*[113] in which the parents' religious objections were considered insufficiently harmful to justify state intervention on behalf of the three children. Parental concern about autism risk was litigated in *Children's Aid Society of the Region of Peel v. T.M.C.H.*,[114] in which medical evidence indicated that the newborn baby born to a woman who was a chronic carrier of hepatitis B needed immunization within 12 hours to prevent hepatitis B infection (which

---

[108]   See the indeterminate defendant problem in the DES cases, in particular: *Sindell v. Abbott Laboratories*, 607 P. 2d 924 (Calif. Sup. Ct., 1980).

[109]   The Ontario *Health Care Consent Act, 1996*, S.O. 1996, c. 2, Sch. A, as am. defines treatment in s. 2(1) as "anything that is done for a ... preventive ... purpose" and this definition would bring vaccination within the purview of the Act.

[110]   [2002] O.J. No. 5341 (Ont. S.C.J. Fm. Ct.).

[111]   [2001] A.J. No. 838 (Alta. Q.B.).

[112]   [1968] O.J. No. 470 (Ont. H.C.J.).

[113]   [1995] N.J. No. 389, 137 Nfld. & P.E.I.R. 1, 428 A.P.R. 1 (Nfld. S.C.).

[114]   [2007] O.J. No. 5084 (Ont. C.J.) and [2008] O.J. No. 217 (Ont. C.J.).

would have a 95 per cent chance of occurring otherwise) as well as other lifetime risks of liver cirrhosis and cancer. The baby's parents refused the treatment based on their research and belief that the hepatitis B vaccine might have caused their first child's autism. The motions judge decided that in spite of the noteworthy objections and their genuine concern for their child, the risk to the child that would be created by delay warranted an interim order to the Children's Aid Society with authority to consent to the treatment. The second hearing provided more time to consider the expert's evidence, which indicated the lack of evidence to support a link to autism.

III. MANDATORY IMMUNIZATION

Because public health has a community focus, it brings into sharp relief the role of the individual in relation to the state. Nancy Kass has analyzed trends in the ethics of public health,[115] starting in the 1970s and 1980s, with a focus on the issue of liberty and the "ethics of compelling behaviour". Voluntary approaches to public health were generally preferred and, to some, were the only permissible approaches. The problem with voluntary approaches to public health, however, is their limited effectiveness. Harm prevention, access and allocation issues began to be seriously considered in this period, while the HIV pandemic focused attention on screening, reporting, contact tracing and quarantine. Following this, she argued, concern among ethicists began to centre on allocation, health promotion and the right to health care. The inequalities that exist at the social level began to be seen as causally linked to health status,[116] and awareness of these social determinants of health has led to social justice becoming the central public health issue. Global justice, environmental ethics and public health research have most recently been the subjects of ethical analysis. The social justice emphasis that Kass has identified in the public health ethics literature is evident in the global health and human rights movement, which provided the driving force behind the two women's conferences of the 1990s, the Cairo and Beijing Conferences. In the context of vaccination, these debates come into focus in the area of mandatory vaccination, where public benefits are weighed against individual rights and where equal access to vaccination becomes be an issue.

In this section, the analysis of compulsory vaccines first examines legislative provisions mandating immunization for school-age children and the permissible exemptions under such schemes. It turns next to

---

[115]   Nancy E. Kass, "Public Health Ethics: From Foundations and Framework to Justice and Global Public Health" (2004) 32 J.L.M.E. 232.
[116]   *Ibid.*, citing Norman Daniels at note 62.

programs of mandatory immunization of employees, followed by the same issue in relation to military personnel. Finally, it looks at other Canadian public health legislation requiring immunization.

Immunization of school-age children has formed the keystone of the public health response to contagious diseases in North America. Once a sufficient number are vaccinated, protection against the disease is created for the group, an outcome referred to as herd immunity. When groups of individuals choose not to be vaccinated, this creates a pool within which the communicable disease may spread. If individuals are not vaccinated, they may pose a threat not only to themselves and others who have not been vaccinated, but also to the group of vaccinated individuals, who may still contract the disease. In the United States, mandatory immunization requirements prior to school entry have been created by all the states. In Canada, Ontario and New Brunswick require students to be vaccinated against designated diseases for school entry, with medical, religious or conscientious exemptions, and authorize exclusion from class in certain circumstances.[117] The designated diseases in Ontario and New Brunswick are diphtheria, tetanus, polio, measles, mumps and rubella[118] but not pertussis, hepatitis or human papillomavirus. Several other provinces provide for mandatory immunization orders or regulations to be made in particular circumstances, and permit exemptions on conscientious grounds,[119] while some provide for exclusion from school or other educational institutions.[120] The Ontario day care provisions place the onus on the day care operator to ensure that the child is immunized in accordance with the medical officer of health's recommendations, with a medical, religious or conscientious exemption available.[121]

Similar provisions in the United States have led to considerable litigation, focusing from the beginning on the compulsory nature of vaccination. In *Jacobson v. Massachusetts*, the United States Supreme Court decided in 1905 that compulsory vaccination was constitutional, as coming within the state's police powers, since the community was entitled

---

[117] *Immunization of School Pupils Act*, R.S.O. 1990, c. I.1, ss. 3, 4, as am. S.O. 2007, c. 10, Sch. E, s. 2; *General Regulation — Health Act*, N.B. Reg. 88-200, ss. 284-85; *Education Act*, S.N.B. 1997, c. E-1.12, s. 10.   Manitoba had such a provision in *The Public Schools Act* but repealed it in 1999: *The Public Schools Act*, R.S.M. 1987, c. P250, s. 261(1), as rep.; *The Public Schools Amendment Act*, S.M. 1999, c. 14, s. 5. See Manitoba Law Reform Commission, *Compensation of Vaccine-Damaged Children*, Report 104 (2000).

[118] *Immunization of Public School Pupils Act*, R.R.O. 1990, Reg. 645, s. 5; O. Reg. 299/96, s. 2; O. Reg. 443/03, s. 1.

[119] *Health Act*, R.S.B.C. 1996, c. 179, s. 13; *Public Health Act*, R.S.A. 2000, c. P-37, s. 38(3); *Public Health Act, 1994*, S.S. 1994, c. P-37.1, s. 64.

[120] *Public Health Act, 1994*, S.S. 1994, c. P-37.1, s. 45(2)(d)(ii); *Communicable Diseases Act*, R.S.N.L. 1990, c. C-26, s. 25.

[121] *Day Nurseries Act*, R.R.O. 1990, Reg. 262.

to protect itself against an epidemic threatening its members' safety. These powers must be used in accordance with the necessity of the case, reasonably, proportionately, and in order to avoid harm.[122] Although U.S. constitutional law has changed significantly in the direction of civil liberties in the past century, "the outcome would certainly reaffirm the basic power of government to safeguard the public's health".[123] All states have enacted laws conditioning school entry on vaccinations and grant exemptions on medical grounds, in accordance with the concern for harm avoidance in *Jacobson*; almost all states have religious exemptions and some permit conscientious grounds.[124] These religious and conscientious exemptions are not required constitutionally; however, they are also not prohibited under the U.S. Constitution.[125] Compulsory vaccination depends on public willingness and the exemptions make it more acceptable; at the same time, the responsibility to ensure vaccine safety arguably increases if vaccines are compulsory.[126]

If those provincial statutes that require childhood vaccination were challenged, the s. 1 argument would emphasize the compelling community and individual need for vaccination, the proportionality of the duty in relation to the harm that could occur to both, and the availability of provisions to protect s. 2 rights. The *Canadian Charter of Rights and Freedoms* explicitly provides protection for beliefs based on conscience and religion, and the exemptions provided on these grounds could be supported on this basis.[127] The strong judicial protections providing for individual autonomy in medical decision-making would need to be assessed in relation to community need for a mandatory program. In one Québec decision, *Charbonneau c. Poupart*, the trial judge found that individuals are entitled to make decisions about vaccination under the principle of the inviolability of the person and under the Canadian and Québec Charters.[128]

---

[122]   *Jacobson v. Massachusetts*, 197 U.S. 11 (S.C. 1905).
[123]   Lawrence O. Gostin, "*Jacobson v Massachusetts* at 100 Years: Police Power and Civil Liberties in Tension" (2005) 95 Am. J. Public Health 576 at 576.
[124]   James G. Hodge, Jr. & Lawrence O. Gostin, "School Vaccination Requirements: Historical, Social, and Legal Perspectives" (2001-2002) 90 Ky. L.J. 831 at 868, 874; Ross D. Silverman, "No More Kidding Around: Restructuring Non-Medical Childhood Immunization Exemptions to Ensure Public Health Protection" (2003) 12 Annals of Health L. 277.
[125]   James G. Hodge, Jr. & Lawrence O. Gostin, "School Vaccination Requirements: Historical, Social, and Legal Perspectives" (2001-2002) 90 Ky. L.J. 831 at 860.
[126]   Daniel A. Salmon *et al.*, "Compulsory vaccination and conscientious or philosophical exemptions: past, present, and future" (2006) 367(9508) The Lancet: 436.
[127]   Section 2(*a*) of the *Canadian Charter of Rights and Freedoms*, Part I of the *Constitution Act, 1982*, being Schedule B to the *Canada Act 1982* (U.K.), 1982, c. 11.
[128]   *Charbonneau c. Poupard*, [1990] R.J.Q. 1136 (Qué. S.C.).

The case of *R.B. v. Children's Aid Society of Metropolitan Toronto*[129] would provide an important precedent for consideration of the role of parents as medical decision-makers and the extent to which *Charter* protections apply to such substitute decisions. The issue in that case was whether the provision to declare a child in need of protection under the child protection legislation denied parents the right to choose medical treatment for their children, based on their religion, in a manner contrary to s. 7 and s. 2(*a*) of the *Canadian Charter of Rights and Freedoms*. The Supreme Court of Canada divided on all the issues although they decided unanimously to uphold the state action. Five judges found that s. 2(*a*) was breached but that the breach was saved by s. 1, while four judges found that s. 2(*a*) was not breached since freedom of religion does not include imposing practices that threaten the child's life, safety or health, and that section would not be applicable since the issue is the child's life and security of the person versus the parents' right to freedom of religion. The s. 7 decision was less clear-cut: four judges thought that the state may intervene when it considers it necessary to protect the autonomy or health of the child but only exceptionally, going on to find that liberty was breached but in accordance with the principles of fundamental justice; an additional judge agreed except with respect to the breach of the principles of fundamental justice; three judges thought the behaviour of the parents fell outside s. 7; and one that there was no infringement.

The situation of a child of Jehovah's Witness parents who deny blood transfusions on the basis of their religious belief, as in the preceding case, is often one with immediacy as the child requires blood in order to survive. The case would be weaker in a situation that did not involve such a clear threat to the health of the child. Some members of the Court clearly reasoned that parental decision-making that creates a threat for the individual and community did not engage *Charter* rights and this reasoning would apply in the mandatory immunization situation. However, assuming *Charter* rights were engaged, the proportionality of mandatory schemes would need to be assessed in relation to the degree of effectiveness of the voluntary mechanisms accepted in most provinces for children entering school. Arguments can be made that exempted children are free riders who secure the benefits of herd immunity while exposing others to the hazard of disease through contact with them.[130] On the other hand, the absence of a mandatory scheme creates a greater need for public

---

[129]   [1994] S.C.J. No. 24, [1995] 1 S.C.R. 315 (S.C.C.).
[130]   Ross D. Silverman, "No More Kidding Around: Restructuring Non-Medical Childhood Immunization Exemptions to Ensure Public Health Protection" (2003) 12 Annals of Health L. 277 at 284, note 43, outlining the argument in *Brown v. Stone*, 378 So. 2d at 223 (Miss. 1979), *Cert.* denied, 449 U.S. 887 (1980).

health care providers to inform people of the nature of the benefits and risks, and fulfillment of this responsibility can be beneficial to the entire system.

Healthcare workers and front-line staff working in particular types of group settings are required by law in some provinces to be vaccinated against communicable diseases. Public health measures empowering medical officers of health to isolate, quarantine or treat individuals in particular circumstances may provide support for these measures. In British Columbia, licensees in community care facilities under the *Adult Care Regulations* must require employees, "as a condition of employment, unless otherwise authorized by the medical health officer", to comply with the Ministry of Health immunization program and to participate in the TB control program, subject to s. 13 of the *Health Act*, which provides a conscientious belief exemption.[131] Alberta and Manitoba have provisions of more general application in their *Public Health Acts*, in Alberta authorizing cabinet to order immunizations in the event of an outbreak of a communicable disease[132] and in Manitoba empowering a medical officer of health to order a person to be vaccinated, inoculated or immunized in an epidemic or threatened epidemic.[133] Ontario's *Occupational Health and Safety Act* Health Care and Residential Facilities Regulation permits employers to create measures for immunization and inoculation against infectious diseases as part of its measures to protect the health and safety of workers, and requires that such measures be in writing.[134] Under the *Ambulance Act* in Ontario, paramedics and emergency medical attendants are required to be free from all communicable diseases set out in a Ministry standard.[135] Ontario's *Child and Family Services Act* Regulation, which applies to a broad range of group settings, requires licensees to ensure that employees have received such immunizations as are

---

[131]   *Community Care and Assisted Living Act*, S.B.C. 2002, c. 75, *Adult Care Regulations*, B.C. Reg. 536/80, s. 6.2, as am. B.C. Reg. 119/99, B.C. Reg. 457/2001, Sch. 1, s. 3, and B.C. Reg. 217/2004; the *Health Act*, R.S.B.C. 1996, c. 179, s. 13.   In British Columbia, unvaccinated employees may be excluded by a medical officer of health under their general power to isolate those known or suspected of suffering from a reportable communicable disease and to quarantine susceptible persons in contact with someone suffering from a reportable communicable disease. The *Health Act Communicable Disease Regulation*, Part 2 — Isolation and Quarantine, B.C. Reg. 4/83, as am.; and the *Public Health Act*, S.B.C. 2008, when it comes into force. See also B.C. Communicable Disease Policy Committee, Facility Influenza Immunization Policy (10 October 2007), online: <http://www.bcpublic service.ca/wphealth/employee/influenza/facilities_policies.pdf>.

[132]   *Public Health Act*, R.S.A. 2000, c. P-37.

[133]   *The Public Health Act*, C.C.S.M. c. P210, ss. 12(d)(iii), 19, as am. by S.M. 2002, c. 26, ss. 44, 49; S.M. 2005, c. 8, s. 12(e).

[134]   *Occupational Health and Safety Act*, Health Care and Residential Facilities Regulation, O. Reg. 67/93, ss. 8-9.

[135]   *Ambulance Act*, O. Reg. 257/00, s. 6(g), as am.

recommended by the local medical officer of health.[136] A similar provision applies to operators of day nurseries, who are required to ensure that each employee and, in the case of private home day care agencies, the operator and anyone ordinarily resident in the home, has received the immunizations recommended by the local medical officer of health, subject to exemptions on medical grounds or sincerely held convictions based on religion or conscience.[137]

Several court and arbitral decisions have upheld mandatory immunization requirements for employees both under statute and as measures put into place by employers themselves apart from any statutory obligation, while one decision has gone the other way. An Alberta employer's policy provided that staff who had not been immunized against influenza would not be permitted to work in the facility and would not be paid during an outbreak, although persons who were exempted on religious or medical grounds would also not be permitted to work, but would be paid.[138] The board found that Carewest's policy met the *KVP* test[139] and represented a "reasonable balance and compromise between the privacy interests of employees and the employer's legitimate concerns with respect to patient safety". In *Barkley v. Mohawk Council of Akwesasne*, the adjudicator reached a similar conclusion and upheld the dismissal of a casual health aide nurse, by applying the *KVP* test and finding that the Council's decision to require mandatory immunization at an adult care facility was reasonable and that they had a legitimate interest in the residents' health and well-being, which were at risk.[140] In another case, arguments by a food service worker against his union's withdrawal of the grievance by an employee who had not been vaccinated, contrary to the employer's mandatory program of hepatitis A vaccination for food service workers, were unsuccessful and his concerns about the vaccine were not considered to fall within the medical exemption.[141] Termination of a temporary employee, who had been vaccinated during an influenza epidemic but did not pick up the prescribed Tamiflu needed during the two weeks before the vaccination took effect, was considered appropriate, since she had not disclosed that she had not taken the Tamiflu and continued to work as a phlebotomist, travelling throughout the hospital

---

[136]   *Child and Family Services Act*, R.R.O. 1990, Reg. 70, s. 75.

[137]   *Day Nurseries Act*, R.R.O. 1990, Reg. 262, s. 62.

[138]   *Re Carewest and A.U.P.E.*, [2001] A.G.A.A. No. 76, 104 L.A.C. (4th) 240 (Smith) (Alberta Grievance Arbitration).

[139]   *Re KVP Co. and Lumber & Sawmill Workers' Union, Local 2537*, [1965] O.L.A.A. No. 2, 16 L.A.C. 73 (Robinson) (Ontario Labour Arbitration).

[140]   *Barkley v. Mohawk Council of Akwesasne*, [2000] C.L.A.D. No. 553 (Cantin) (Canada Labour Arbitration).

[141]   *Gordon v. Hotel, Restaurant & Culinary Employees & Bartenders Union, Local 40*, [2004] B.C.L.R.B.D. No. 138, [2004] L.V.I. 3468-9 (B.C. Labour Relations Board).

taking blood samples, contrary to the protocol which required employees not to enter if not protected by vaccine or Tamiflu.[142] In the *Kotsopoulos Grievance*, the issue was the paramedic's refusal to comply with the immunization requirement under the *Ambulance Act* Regulation, discussed above.[143] The Arbitrator upheld the firing on the basis of the legal requirement. Kotsopoulos commenced proceedings in the Ontario Divisional Court challenging the legislation under s. 7 of the *Charter*; he was unsuccessful in an attempt to obtain an interim injunction reinstating him pending disposition of the *Charter* challenge.[144]

In contrast, in the Ontario grievance involving a geriatric public hospital, St. Peter's Health Systems, the board supported the grievance of healthcare workers against the employer's flu vaccine policy, which required vaccination or treatment if there was a flu outbreak.[145] The board found that the employees were forced into medical treatment without consent, and without legislative or contractual authority, and that the employees' s. 7 rights were infringed. In the Alberta decision of *Chinook*, the board declined to follow the *St. Peter's Health Systems* decision in an unsuccessful grievance by nurses in ten long-term care facilities against the employer's flu vaccine policy, modelled on the *Carewest* policy.[146] In an outbreak, immunized staff could work as long as they were symptom-free, while non-immunized staff would be placed on unpaid leave, or could use vacation or leaves. Medical and religious grounds constituted exceptions. The board followed *Carewest* and an earlier Ontario decision in *Re Trillium Ridge*,[147] and decided that the policy met the *KVP* guidelines. The arbitrator in the British Columbia case of *Influenza Immunization Grievance*[148] considered these cases and distinguished *St. Peter's Health Systems* since it was premised on the absence of choice, while this case involved a choice between immunization and exclusion

---

[142] *North Bay General Hospital and O.P.S.E.U. (Anger)*, [2006] O.L.A.A. No. 533, 87 C.L.A.S. 169 (Ontario Randall) (Ontario Labour Arbitration).

[143] *North Bay General Hospital v. C.U.P.E., Local 139 (Kotsopoulos Grievance)*, [2003] O.L.A.A. No. 580 (Goodfellow) (Ontario Labour Arbitration). The regulation was amended in 2002 to provide an option for paramedics to participate in an educational review of influenza instead of being vaccinated. The educational opt-out does not fit within the usual parameters for exemption from vaccination requirements and lacks a constitutional basis. The rationale of educating people to induce them to participate is presumably at work.

[144] *Kotsopolous v. North Bay General Hospital*, [2002] O.J. No. 715 (Ont. S.C.J.).

[145] *Re St. Peter's Health Systems and C.U.P.E., Local 778*, [2002] O.L.A.A. No. 164, 106 L.A.C. (4th) 170 (Charney) (Ontario Labour Arbitation).

[146] *Re Chinook Health Region and U.N.A., Local 120*, [2002] A.G.A.A. No. 105, 113 L.A.C. (4th) 289 (Joliffe) (Alberta Labour Arbitration).

[147] *Re Trillium Ridge Retirement Home and S.E.I.U., Local 183*, [1998] O.L.A.A. No. 1046 (Emrich) (Ontario Labour Arbitration).

[148] *Interior Health Authority and B.C.N.U. Re: Influenza Immunization Grievance*, [2006] B.C.C.A.A.A. No. 167, 87 C.L.A.S. 216 (Burke) (B.C. Collective Agreement Arbitration).

from work without pay during an influenza epidemic — a choice, if unpalatable. The economic consequences were not severe enough to deny choice over one's own body, so as to constitute a *Charter* s. 7 infringement. The arbitrator also considered the issue of choice as analyzed in *Trillium Ridge* in which the arbitrator assessed whether consent was vitiated, taking into account the power imbalance, but still decided in favour of the employer. In *Loder v. Huron (County) Health Unit,*[149] the Ontario Health Services Appeal and Review Board confirmed an order by the Medical Officer of Health of Huron County to a nursing home to immediately exclude all non-immunized staff until steps were taken, finding that there were reasonable grounds to believe that an outbreak of influenza was present in the facility and the requirements in the order were necessary to deal with the risk, as required under s. 44 of the *Health Protection and Promotion Act.*[150]

Mandatory immunization of military personnel adds another dimension to the tension between the individual and the state. The *National Defence Act*[151] contains, in s. 126, the requirement that:

> Every person who, on receiving an order to submit to inoculation, re-inoculation, vaccination, re-vaccination, other immunization procedures, immunity tests, blood examination or treatment against any infectious disease, willfully and without reasonable excuse disobeys that order is guilty of an offence and on conviction is liable to imprisonment for less than two years or to less punishment.

The common law and co-extensive constitutional right to autonomous decision making in the area of medical treatment[152] come into tension with the power of the state to require immunization for the public good. In the case of military personnel, an individual's decision to opt out of a plan of vaccination has an additional risk for those who are in combat situations with that person and for the mission as a whole. Section 126 provides an exemption based on "reasonable excuse" but no guidelines indicate what constitutes a reasonable excuse and no process is provided to assess whether the exemption has been met in the circumstances. As a result, any individual wanting to decline immunization is forced to go through a Court Martial in order to defend his or her choice. Any *Charter* argument would consider whether the lack of guidelines and lack of a process for determining reasonable excuse, apart from charges, constitute a breach of fundamental justice under s. 7, and a reasonable and proportionate limitation under s. 1.

---

[149]   2005 CarswellOnt 10164 (Ont. H.S.A.R.B.).
[150]   R.S.O. 1990, c. H.7.
[151]   R.S.C. 1985, c. N-5.
[152]   *Malette v. Shulman*, [1990] O.J. No. 450 (Ont. C.A.); *Fleming v. Reid*, [1991] O.J. No. 1083, 4 O.R. (3d) 74 (Ont. C.A.).

If a vaccine has not been licensed, or if it is being used off-label for unapproved purposes, a presumption of a reasonable excuse should apply. Sergeant Michael Kipling was a flight engineer with a squadron deployed to Kuwait in 1998 as part of the multinational force attempting to induce Iraq to comply with the United Nations Security Council resolutions requiring weapons inspections.[153] Because of intelligence indicating that Iraq might use weaponized anthrax, the Commander ordered all members of the detachment to be vaccinated with anthrax vaccine. Sgt. Kipling refused to be vaccinated and was charged under s. 126 and sent back to Canada. Sgt. Kipling commented in a CBC interview that he refused the vaccination because of his concern about the possible adverse effects of the anthrax vaccine, due to the health problems experienced by Gulf War veterans, characterized as Gulf War Syndrome, that many thought were attributable to immunization.[154] It remains to be seen whether individual safety concerns, based on evidence, would constitute a reasonable excuse. The Court Martial Appeal Court did not decide this issue or the constitutionality of the mandatory immunization provision in s. 126, declining to decide the constitutional issue since the required notice had not been given to the attorneys general,[155] although it was their view that the trial court judge had not correctly applied s. 7 of the *Charter* to Sgt. Kipling's refusal.[156] Instead, the court decided to overturn the trial decision and send the matter back for retrial with a new judge, but the military subsequently decided not to proceed. It was the court's view that the issue of informed consent and whether the *Charter* applied to protect soldiers from being vaccinated without consent were not proper matters for a plea in bar of trial, under the pertinent regulations.[157] Had they decided differently, the effect would have been an end to the trial.

Mandatory immunization provisions also apply under the new federal *Quarantine Act*,[158] which was redrafted in response to SARS and the revised International Health Regulations (2005).[159] The Act applies to individuals entering or leaving Canada, and to conveyances such as planes and ships arriving or crossing into Canadian waters or airspace. Quarantine officers are authorized to screen for contagious diseases

---

[153]   *R. v. Kipling*, [2002] C.M.A.J. No. 1 at para. 3 (C.M.A.C.).

[154]   CBC, The Magazine, "That's An Order" (2002) Interview of Sgt. Mike Kipling by Hana Gartner. Transcript on file with the author. See also CBC News, "No vaccine for Canadian troops" (2001), online: <http://www.cbc.ca/story/canada/national/2001/10/12/vaccine011012.html>.

[155]   *R. v. Kipling*, [2002] C.M.A.J. No. 1 at paras. 30-32 (C.M.A.C.).

[156]   *Ibid.*, at paras. 28-29.

[157]   *Ibid.*, at paras. 23-27; The Queen's Regulations and Orders for the Canadian Forces, sub. 112.24(1).

[158]   *Quarantine Act*, S.C. 2005, c. 20.

[159]   World Health Organization, International Health Regulations (2005) 2d ed., at 17, online: <http://www.who.int/csr/ihr/IHR_2005_en.pdf>.

people entering or leaving Canada and, on the basis of a health assessment or medical examination, may order treatment or other measures, possibly including vaccination. In some circumstances an order to detain may be made, triggering an obligation to disclose the traveller's right to review. The quarantine officer may apply for a court order to comply with examination or treatment or other measures to prevent the spread of the disease.[160] The Act authorizes the Governor-in-Council to make certain kinds of emergency orders prohibiting or making entry into the country conditional in a situation posing an imminent and severe risk to public health.[161]

The broad powers of the federal government under the *Emergencies Act*[162] come into force on declaration of a designated national emergency, which includes a public welfare emergency. A national emergency is defined in s. 3 as an "urgent and critical situation" of a temporary nature that "seriously endangers the lives, health or safety of Canadians" and is beyond the capacity of a province to deal with or seriously threatens Canada's security, sovereignty or territorial integrity. Section 5 provides that a public welfare emergency is one caused by a real or imminent event, including disease in human beings that leads to danger to life that is so serious that it constitutes a national emergency. The *Emergencies Act* permits special temporary measures such as the regulation of travel, evacuation, the provision of essential services, and the distribution of products and services. Such measures might include the provision of vaccines where it could not be dealt with effectively under any other law of Canada. The *Emergency Management Act*[163] (enacted in 2007) and the *Department of Public Safety and Emergency Preparedness Act*[164] (enacted in 2005) specify structures and lines of responsibility for emergency preparation and response. Both statutes focus on coordination of activities, externally and internally with the provinces and territories. Provincial law may also be relevant.   For example, Québec's *Public Health Act* authorizes the government to declare a public health emergency within Québec and grants certain powers following the declaration, including the power to order compulsory vaccination of all or parts of the population against smallpox or any other contagious disease seriously threatening the health of the population.[165]

Federal jurisdiction rests on its power over matters of national concern and emergencies under the "peace, order and good government

---

[160]   *Quarantine Act*, S.C. 2005, c. 20, ss. 25, 26, 28-31.

[161]   *Ibid.*, ss. 58-61.

[162]   R.S.C. 1985, c. 22 (4th Supp.).

[163]   S.C. 2007, c. 15.

[164]   S.C. 2005, c. 10.

[165]   *Public Health Act*, R.S.Q. c. S-2.2, s. 123.

provision" of the *Constitution Act*, and on its powers over criminal law, trade and commerce, and quarantine. Since much constitutional authority over health is located at the provincial level under the "property and civil rights" power, the capacity to respond to international standards is fraught with difficulty, as the Naylor Report noted: "This [jurisdictional] situation is particularly problematic as the World Health Organization [WHO] moves to establish International Health Regulations that set expectations for member states as regards surveillance, reporting, and outbreak management".[166] The 2005 International Health Regulations ("2005 IHR") came into force 15 June 2007, marking the creation of a global legal framework "to prevent, protect against, control and provide a public health response to the international spread of disease in ways that are commensurate with and restricted to public health risks, and which avoid unnecessary interference with international traffic and trade".[167] By 21 December 2007, there were 193 state parties bound by the obligations in the 2005 IHR. The regulations are designed in recognition of the need for global coordination among various levels of government and other bodies to respond collectively to epidemics such as SARS, and to create requirements in the areas of disease surveillance, reporting and responding of states parties. The World Health Organization is empowered to gather relevant information and to declare a public health emergency of international concern and recommend steps, such as travel restrictions, to deal with the emergency. The Public Health Agency of Canada has the responsibility to comply with the international regulations, to support national preparedness, and co-ordinate federal activities to prevent and reduce public health risks.[168] Successful implementation of the 2005 IHR will depend on the ability of federal states to fulfill their responsibilities within their federal structures and constitutional arrangements.[169]

IV. STRUCTURAL CHANGES NEEDED TO ACHIEVE EFFECTIVE VACCINE POLICY

Public health structures have come under increasing scrutiny as the 1990s and 2000s have unfolded. The infected blood supply system, the

---

[166]   National Advisory Committee on SARS and Public Health, *Learning from SARS: Renewal of Public Health in Canada* (Ottawa: Health Canada, 2003) (Chair: Dr. D. Naylor) at 7, online: <http://www.phac-aspc.gc.ca/publicat/sars-sras/pdf/sars-e.pdf>.

[167]   World Health Organization, International Health Regulations (2005), 2d ed., Art. 2, at 17, online: <http://www.who.int/csr/ihr/IHR_2005_en.pdf>.

[168]   Public Health Agency of Canada, News Release, "International Health Regulations" (3 November 2004).

[169]   Kumanan Wilson, Christopher McDougall, Ross Upshur, the Joint Centre for Bioethics SARS Global Health Ethics Research Group, "The New International Health Regulations and the Federalism Dilemma" (January 2006) 3 PLoS Medicine 0030, available online: <www.plosmedicine.org>.

Walkerton water system, mad cow disease and SARS have revealed significant deficiencies in the capacity of the public health system to maintain health and to respond to the resulting crises. The Auditor-General's Report of 1999[170] pointed to serious problems in the surveillance of diseases and the framework to link the activities of government, and despite some improvements toward a national health surveillance framework, these problems were largely unresolved by the 2002 Status Report, compromising Health Canada's public health capacity.[171] The Naylor Report noted that the SARS experience underscored the problems of detection and communication of alerts.[172] Public health has none of the cachet of surgical waiting lists but, as the 19th and 20th century breakthroughs demonstrated, investments in hygiene, clean water and vaccines provide immense benefits for the community. Smallpox eradication is perhaps the best example of the cost effectiveness of public health investment. The total cost of the eradication campaign approximated $300 million, resulting in a saving of $2 billion a year over previous expenditures on vaccination, inspection and quarantine.[173] Public health expenditures for 2002–2003 were estimated by the Naylor Report to be in the range of $2-2.8 billion, depending on the definition of public health that was used.[174]

Although an established list of essential public health system functions does not exist, the national Advisory Committee on Population Health prepared a list consisting of health protection; health surveillance; disease and injury prevention; population health assessment; health promotion; and disaster response.[175] In the vaccine context, health protection includes the regulatory framework for approving vaccines, found in the *Food and Drugs Act*,[176] and administered through the Biologics and Genetic Therapies Directorate of Health Canada. The creation of the Public Health Agency of Canada in 2004 provided a central agency with designated public health responsibilities, including immunization. Health surveillance includes disease detection in addition to monitoring of adverse effects of vaccines. These functions are carried out primarily at the provincial/territorial level through local medical

[170]   Canada, *Report of the Auditor General of Canada to Parliament* (1999), c. 14.
[171]   Canada, *September Status Report of the Auditor General of Canada to Parliament* (2002), c. 2, online: <http://www.oag-bvg.gc.ca/internet/English/parl_oag_200209_e_1132.html>.
[172]   National Advisory Committee on SARS and Public Health, *Learning from SARS: Renewal of Public Health in Canada* (Ottawa: Health Canada, 2003) (Chair: Dr. D. Naylor) at 4G.5, online: <http://www.phac-aspc.gc.ca/publicat/sars-sras/pdf/sars-e.pdf>.
[173]   Jonathan B. Tucker, *Scourge* (New York: Atlantic Monthly Press, 2001) at 132.
[174]   National Advisory Committee on SARS and Public Health, *Learning from SARS: Renewal of Public Health in Canada* (Ottawa: Health Canada, 2003) (Chair: Dr. D. Naylor) at 4G.5, online: <http://www.phac-aspc.gc.ca/publicat/sars-sras/pdf/sars-e.pdf>.
[175]   *Ibid.*, at 3A.2.
[176]   R.S.C. 1985, c. F-27.

officers of health and at the federal level through reporting mechanisms and surveillance initiatives. The Centre for Infectious Disease Prevention and Control within PHAC is responsible for post-market vaccine surveillance.[177] Disease and injury prevention includes contact tracing and educational programs, both of which take place primarily at the provincial/territorial level, with some federal involvement. The final three functions take place through both levels of government. The federal government is also responsible for Aboriginal health. The federal government released two documents, *Blueprint* and *Blueprint II*, outlining a framework for change in the laws, regulations and structures governing drugs, vaccines and other products and recommending that a new regulatory framework be created for vaccines.[178] Bill C-51, legislation to amend the *Food and Drugs Act*, was introduced into the House of Commons in the spring of 2008.[179] If adopted in the new Parliament, the legislation will alter in fundamental ways the regulatory process for therapeutic products through progressive licensing, changing the standard for drug approval to a risk-benefit standard and heightened study in the post-marketing period, and will substantially enhance the powers of the Minister of Health throughout the process.

In this section, the analysis turns to those changes that could improve the structural capacity to respond to the threat of communicable diseases and create equitable access to its benefits. Recommendations for improvements in the Canadian vaccine structures have focused on the need for adverse events reporting, a national surveillance system, an immunization tracking system, even coverage across the country and a national vaccine strategy. A national immunization strategy has been advocated as a means to implement goals adopted by consensus conferences and to achieve a coordinated response to recommendations made by the National Advisory Committee on Immunization.[180] It would consist of five

---

[177]   Public Health Agency of Canada, *Canadian National Report on Immunization* (2006) 32S3 CCDR:1-44 at 29.

[178]   Health Canada, *Blueprint for Renewal: Transforming Canada's Approach to Regulating Health Products and Food* (2006), online: <http://www.hc-sc.gc.ca/ahc-asc/branch-dirgen/hpfb-dgpsa/blueprint-plan/blueprint-plan_e.html>. Health Canada issued a revised version, *Blueprint II*, after consultation on the initial document. Health Canada, *Blueprint for Renewal II: Modernizing Canada's Regulatory System for Health Products and Food* (2007), online: <http://www.hc-sc.gc.ca/ahc-asc/branch-dirgen/hpfb-dgpsa/blueprint-plan/blueprint-plan_ll_e.html>.

[179]   Bill C-51, *An Act to amend the Food and Drugs Act and to make consequential amendments to other Acts*, 2nd Sess., 39th Parl. (first reading: 8 April 2008).

[180]   Arlene King (Health Canada) & Greg Hammond (Manitoba Health), "Canada's National Immunization Strategy" in Proceedings of the Canadian National Immunization Conference, *Canada's National Immunization Strategy: From Vision to Action*. CCDR 2003; 2954: 1-24 at 3. See also Canadian Institutes of Health Research, "Research in

elements: a set of national goals and objectives; immunization safety; vaccine procurement; equitable access; and immunization registries.[181] Microbiologist Dr. Joanne Embree argued that a national immunization strategy would optimize protection by harmonizing childhood immunization schedules, efficiently introducing new vaccines, enabling enhanced monitoring of usage and adverse effects, and improving access, while opportunities for research and education would also be created.[182] The Romanow Report included a national immunization strategy as part of its recommendations,[183] and the Naylor Report highlighted the significance of "reinvigorating" such a strategy[184] by co-ordinating it under a new Canadian Agency for Public Health and earmarking $100 million per year for vaccine purchase and for improvements to the information systems. While the Kirby Report supported the Naylor Advisory Committee in its national immunization program recommendation, the Senate Report did not favour leaving immunization exclusively within provincial jurisdiction, and argued in favour of a national immunization strategy that would reduce costs dramatically.[185]

The National Immunization Strategy was accepted by the Deputy Ministers of Health[186] and the 2004 federal budget provided $45 million over five years to strengthen collaboration on immunization.[187] The 2006 Report on Immunization outlined progress in the areas of goal-setting and planning; vaccine safety through improvements to the surveillance and national storage guidelines; providing access harmonized across the

---

Infection & Immunity: Toward a National Immunization Strategy for Canada", online: <http://www.cihr-irsc.gc.ca/e/17777.html>.

[181]   Arlene King (Health Canada) & Greg Hammond (Manitoba Health), "Canada's National Immunization Strategy" in Proceedings of the Canadian National Immunization Conference, *Canada's National Immunization Strategy: From Vision to Action.* CCDR 2003; 2954: 1-24 at 4, Council of Ontario Medical Officers of Health, *Position Paper on Public Funding of Immunisation in Ontario* (July 2003).

[182]   Joanne Embree, "Pediatric Infectious Disease Notes" (2001) 6:6 Official Journal of the Canadian Paediatric Society.

[183]   Roy J. Romanow, Commission on the Future of Health Care in Canada, *Building on Values: the Future of Health Care in Canada* (Ottawa: 2002).

[184]   National Advisory Committee on SARS and Public Health, *Learning from SARS: Renewal of Public Health in Canada* (Ottawa: Health Canada, 2003) (Chair: Dr. D. Naylor) at 4G.5, pp. 87-88, online: <http://www.phac-aspc.gc.ca/publicat/sars-sras/pdf/sars-e.pdf>.

[185]   Canada, Senate (Standing Committee on Social Affairs, Science and Technology) (Chair: Michael J.L. Kirby) *Reforming Health Protection and Promotion in Canada: Time to Act* (Ottawa: 2003).

[186]   Public Health Agency of Canada, National Immunization Strategy, *Final Report 2003: A Report from the Federal/Provincial/Territorial Advisory Committee on Population Health and Health Security (ACPHHS) to the Conference of Federal/Provincial/Territorial Deputy Ministers of Health.*

[187]   Public Health Agency of Canada, *Canadian National Report on Immunization* (2006) 32S3 CCDR: 1-44 at 3.

country to four vaccines; establishment of the immunization registry network ("CIRN"); immunization research and education; and the vaccine-preventable disease surveillance working group, concluding that "[t]he NIS is a work in progress".[188]

Reporting of adverse events after vaccination is essential for the system to monitor and respond to problems associated with vaccines and to obtain a full picture of a drug's safety and efficacy. A passive reporting system, the Canadian Adverse Event Following Immunization Surveillance System ("CAEFISS", formerly "VAAES") is used for reporting by health professionals and people who have been vaccinated.[189] However, voluntary reporting is a notoriously unreliable means of obtaining information about the adverse effects of drugs. Ontario, Saskatchewan and Québec require such reporting. In Québec, the *Public Health Act* requires any physician or nurse who observes "an unusual clinical manifestation, temporally associated with vaccination" in a vaccine recipient or person in contact with them, and suspects a link, to report to the appropriate public health director as soon as possible, and, if the person has agreed to participate in the vaccine registry, record the information in the registry.[190] The Ontario *Health Protection and Promotion Act*[191] provides in s. 38 that, if consent to administering an immunizing agent, as defined, has been given in accordance with the *Health Care Consent Act*,[192] the physician or other person authorized to immunize the patient shall inform the consenting person of the importance of immediately informing a physician or registered nurse of any reaction that might be a "reportable event", as defined in the Act, following the vaccination. Physicians, nurses and pharmacists providing professional services to a person are required to report such a reportable event that may be related to an immunization to the medical officer of health. In addition to providing a mandatory reporting obligation for the physician, nurse or pharmacist, which supersedes any obligation of confidentiality, this provision is also designed to ensure that the person consenting to the immunization is aware of the conditions, such as anaphylactic shock, persistent screaming, arthritis or encephalitis, that might indicate an adverse reaction to the vaccine, and of the importance of reporting to a physician or nurse any such event. The Saskatchewan *Public Health Act*

[188] Public Health Agency of Canada, *Canadian National Report on Immunization* (2006) 32S3 CCDR: 1-44 at 5.
[189] Joanne Embree, "Assessing Immunization Programs" (2002) 7:9 Official Journal of the Canadian Paediatric Society; Public Health Agency of Canada, *Canadian National Report on Immunization* (2006) 32S3 CCDR: 1-44, s. 5.
[190] *Public Health Act*, R.S.Q. c. S-2.2, ss. 68, 69.
[191] R.S.O. 1990, c. H.7, s. 38, as am. S.O. 2007, c. 10, Sch. F, s. 11(1), (2).
[192] S.O. 1996, c. 2, Sch. A.

Disease Control Regulations[193] provide a mandatory reporting obligation on a person providing an immunization to report to a designated public health officer any serious adverse reactions to a vaccine within 48 hours of becoming aware of the reaction and any reactions that are not serious within two weeks. Legitimate concerns about privacy of information have created reluctance to report test results and adverse effects of medications, particularly in the area of HIV/AIDS.[194] However, mandatory reporting of HIV tests on blood donated ten years earlier was challenged in *Canadian AIDS Society v. Ontario*[195] as an infringement of a constitutional right to privacy, and to life, liberty and security of the person, and was found not to have breached either right, with the further finding that any infringement would have been saved under s. 1 because of public safety and the donors' right to know about their HIV status.

Yves Robert of the Québec Ministry of Health and Social Services made a series of recommendations about this issue: that each jurisdiction have a passive reporting system; that adverse events resulting from vaccines be reportable by all persons carrying out vaccinations; that such reporting be internationally standardized; that databases be compatible, linked and accessible at all levels; that databases be created by immunization registries and product inventories; that safety assessment be continuous from the prelicensure stage; that passive and active surveillance systems be improved, including creating active systems for adults; that adverse event data be used in decision-making; that such data be linked to surveillance and investigational resources so that warning signals are followed up; and that surveillance and community resources be linked so that the public can be kept well-informed and controversies can be dealt with through information.[196]

A surveillance system for vaccines is an active and comprehensive way of monitoring adverse events and collecting data about them. For example, Lawrence Gostin has noted that surveillance provided the foundation for malaria control and the eradication of smallpox, and surveillance data were essential to discovering why an outbreak of polio among early polio vaccine recipients had taken place, enabling tracing to a

---

[193]   *Disease Control Regulations*, R.R.S. 2000, c. P-37.1, Reg. 11, s. 23.

[194]   Barbara von Tigerstrom, "Public Health" in Jocelyn Downie, Timothy Caulfield & Colleen Flood, eds., *Canadian Health Law and Policy*, 3d ed. (Markham, Ont.: LexisNexis Canada, 2007) at 484-86.

[195]   [1995] O.J. No. 2361 (Ont. Gen. Div.), aff'd [1996] O.J. No. 4184 (Ont. C.A.), leave to appeal denied [1997] S.C.C.A. No. 33 (S.C.C.A.); see Barbara von Tigerstrom, "Public Health" in Jocelyn Downie, Timothy Caulfield & Colleen Flood, eds., *Canadian Health Law and Policy*, 3d ed. (Markham, Ont.: LexisNexis Canada, 2007) at 485.

[196]   Yves Robert, Health Canada, Proceedings of the Canadian National Immunization Conference, *Canada's National Immunization Strategy: From Vision to Action*, CCDR 2003; 2954: 1-24 at 11.

single manufacturer and avoiding undermining the entire vaccine effort.[197] The Canadian Paediatric Society administers IMPACT, Immunization Monitoring Program ACTive, an active surveillance network operating in 12 paediatric hospitals nationwide.[198] The data provided through this network make it possible to determine the incidence of severe adverse reactions and the severity of infections such as pertussis, meningitis, Hib and chickenpox, to assess the risks and benefits of new vaccines, and to determine the need for new immunization programs. Such a system is a significant improvement over relying on reporting obligations or voluntary reporting. The Canadian Paediatric Surveillance Program gathers data from paediatricians who have reported rare illnesses and can also monitor rare events following immunizations.[199] Québec has implemented central databases for vaccine preventable disease surveillance, adverse event reporting and immunization coverage.[200]

An immunization tracking system was recommended as "urgently needed" by the Canadian Immunization Conference in 1996, and the goal of a national network was developed to assist jurisdictions in delivering immunizations to all children and measuring coverage rates.[201] At this time, only Ontario, Manitoba and Prince Edward Island have such systems. In 2004, the Canadian Immunization Registry Network survey found that five jurisdictions had fully functioning registries (British Columbia, Saskatchewan, Manitoba, Prince Edward Island and New Brunswick); three were in the process of developing them (Alberta, Ontario, Newfoundland and Labrador); two were considering it (Québec and the Northwest Territories); and three had no registry (Nova Scotia, Yukon and Nunavut).[202] Registries form an important component of such tracking systems as they can provide comprehensive data to monitor the extent of vaccination in the population for each disease, vaccine risks and effectiveness, and disease incidence. Unless comprehensive data exist

---

[197]   Lawrence Gostin, *Public Health Law: Power, Duty, Restraint* (Berkeley: University of California Press, 2000) at 116.

[198]   Canadian Paediatric Society, IMPACT, online: <http://www.cps.ca/english/surveillance/ IMPACT/IMPACT.htm>; Joanne Embree, "Assessing Immunization Programs" (2002) 7:9 Official Journal of the Canadian Paediatric Society. Funding for 11 centres is provided by the Immunization Division of Health Canada and for one Alberta centre by Alberta Health.

[199]   Joanne Embree, "Assessing Immunization Programs" (2002) 7:9 Official Journal of the Canadian Paediatric Society.

[200]   Richard Masse (Québec), Proceedings of the Canadian National Immunization Conference, *Canada's National Immunization Strategy: From Vision to Action*, CCDR 2003; 2954: 1-24 at 4.

[201]   Health Canada, *Canada Communicable Disease Report* (September 1998), vol. 24-17; Public Health Agency of Canada, Canadian Immunization Registry Network <http://www. phac-aspc.gc.ca/im/cirn-rcri/index-eng.php>.

[202]   Public Health Agency of Canada, *Canadian National Report on Immunization* (2006) 32S3 CCDR: 1-44 at para. 1.5.

about levels of vaccination in the population, who has been vaccinated and the vaccination dates, follow-up cannot be made to individuals and safety data cannot be calculated accurately, because no denominator exists to calculate the rate of adverse effect incidence (even if an accurate numerator existed, based on the leaky reporting system). Particular legal problems are created by registries and care needs to be taken in their establishment in order to minimize infringement of individual privacy.[203] Creation of a registry can also minimize later problems with the handling of records by ensuring that disclosure has been made to individuals and an informed decision has been made prior to information gathering.

Equal access to vaccines is an important aspect of health promotion, while barriers to vaccine accessibility lead to under-vaccination.[204] Access to vaccines against nine diseases is consistently provided across Canada. Between 1998 and 2003, the National Advisory Committee on Immunization ("NACI") added four vaccines to its list of recommended vaccines, for a total of 13, but coverage for these additional vaccines was not provided evenly across the country.[205] These expensive new vaccines — conjugate pneumococcal vaccine, conjugate meningococcal vaccine, varicella vaccine and acellular pertussis vaccine — were estimated to rise to a steady cost of about $200 million per year.[206] The 2004 federal budget provided $300 million to support the introduction of the four new childhood and adolescent vaccines and the 2006 Report documented the significant impact of public funding from 2003 to 2006 in harmonizing access across the country.[207]

The gathering of reliable and valid information is essential to the effective operation of this area of the public health system. The legal protection of autonomy for persons making decisions about their own and others' health care relies on the provision of accurate information and judgment about the risks, benefits and alternatives to vaccines. Simply put, if the information is unavailable, then it can't be disclosed to the patient. This result diminishes the autonomy and efficacy of decision-makers and may create a problem of trust. If adverse effects become

---

[203] Ellen Wright Clayton *et al.*, "Informed Consent for Genetic Research on Stored Tissue Samples" (1995) 274 JAMA 1786; Lawrence O. Gostin & Zita Lazzarini, "Childhood Immunization Registries: A National Review of Public Health Information Systems and the Protection of Privacy" (1995) 274 JAMA 1793.

[204] James G. Hodge, Jr. & Lawrence O. Gostin, "School Vaccination Requirements: Historical, Social, and Legal Perspectives" (2001-2002) 90 Ky. L.J. 831 at 882.

[205] Barbara Sibbald, "One Country, 13 Immunization Programs" (2003) 168:5 C.M.A.J. 598.

[206] National Advisory Committee on SARS and Public Health, *Learning from SARS: Renewal of Public Health in Canada* (Ottawa: Health Canada, 2003) (Chair: Dr. D. Naylor) at 4G.5, p. 87, online: <http://www.phac-aspc.gc.ca/publicat/sars-sras/pdf/sars-e.pdf>.

[207] Public Health Agency of Canada, *Canadian National Report on Immunization* (2006) 32S3 CCDR: 1-44 at Table 1.

evident subsequently, individuals may suffer harm in the meantime and others may lose confidence in the vaccine structures. Drugs and vaccines are both produced by the multinational and domestic pharmaceutical companies and a rising awareness of the limits of regulation in controlling pharmaceutical company shortcomings in the disclosure of information may also harm confidence in the vaccine system. The Internet is a powerful educational tool that may also project speculation or misinformation. The vaccine structure needs to have the capacity to respond to questions about vaccine safety with reliable information. Concerns about the safety of vaccines need to be addressed through careful federal assessment of vaccines in the regulatory licensing process and wide distribution of reliable information in a comprehensible form.

The need for capacity to assess product risks is seen in the concerns that have arisen about the presence of thimerosal, a mercury-based preservative used during the manufacturing process and in some vaccines, and whether thimerosal causes neurological damage, autism in particular. The Institute of Medicine released a 2004 review of thimerosal safety in which the immunization safety committee rejected a causal connection between thimerosal-containing vaccines and autism.[208] Health Canada concluded in 2004 that: "The best available science to date has shown that there is no link between vaccines containing thimerosal and autism or other behaviour disorders."[209] They noted that this opinion was held by the World Health Organization, the FDA and the Institute of Medicine. The Global Advisory Committee on Vaccine Safety ("GACVS") created by WHO has a mandate to review vaccine safety issues and determine whether causal relationships exist between vaccines and adverse events.[210] In Canada, NACI found that such a causal link had "never been substantiated" but recommended taking the precaution of using vaccines without thimerosal to reduce lead exposure.[211] NACI, which advises the Public Health Agency of Canada, issued an updated statement on thimerosal in 2007. In its 2007 update, NACI reviewed the studies and concluded that "the weight of evidence to date clearly refutes an

---

[208]   Institute of Medicine, *Immunization Safety Review: Vaccines and Autism* (Washington, D.C.: National Academy Press, 2004).

[209]   Health Canada, "Questions and Answers: Thimerosal in Vaccines and Autism" (May 2004).

[210]   Philippe Duclos (WHO), Public Health Agency of Canada, Proceedings of the Canadian National Immunization Conference, Canada Communicable Disease Report (CCDR) 2003; 29S4: 1-24 at 18, online: <http://www.phac-aspc.gc.ca/publicat/ccdr-rmtc/03vol29/29s4/index.html>.

[211]   National Advisory Committee on Immunization "Statement on Thimerosal" (2003) at <http://www.phac-aspc.gc.ca/publicat/ccdr-rmtc/03vol29/acs-dcc-1/index.html>.

association between thimerosal and neurodevelopmental disorders".[212] Because preservatives play an important role in ensuring that vaccines are free from contaminants, NACI noted the need to support the development of alternative preservatives and set out the long-term goal of removing thimerosal from vaccines to decrease total mercury exposure and maintain public confidence.[213] Canada's routine childhood vaccines are almost all thimerosal-free except for some multi-dose influenza and hepatitis B vaccines that might be offered as part of routine childhood immunizations, although these vaccines are also available in thimerosal-free forms.[214]

Many of the issues raised above have emerged in the controversy over the human papillomavirus ("HPV") vaccine. The vaccine, Gardasil, was approved for marketing in Canada in July 2006[215] and was licensed by the FDA for use in girls and women aged 9-26 years, acknowledging the manufacturer's commitments to safety and efficacy studies in the post-marketing period.[216] Its use in this age group was recommended by NACI, the U.S. Centers for Disease Control Advisory Committee on Immunization Practices,[217] and the British Department of Health Joint committee on vaccination and immunization, subject to independent cost-benefit analysis.[218] One month after the NACI recommendation in February 2007, the federal government announced in the budget that $300 million would be given to the provinces to carry out an immunization program. Four provinces — Nova Scotia, Prince Edward Island, Newfoundland and Labrador, and Ontario — implemented a program of vaccination for girls while other provinces planned to bring it in later. This included Québec, Manitoba and British Columbia who planned to introduce it in the fall of

---

[212]   National Advisory Committee on Immunization, "Thimerosal: Updated Statement" (1 July 2007) 33 CCDR, ACS 6, online: <http://www.phac-aspc.gc.ca/publicat/ccdr-rmtc/07vol33/acs-06/index_e.html>.

[213]   *Ibid.*, at 7-8.

[214]   *Ibid.*, at 7.

[215]   Public Health Agency of Canada, "Human Papillomavirus (HPV) Prevention and HPV Vaccine: Questions and Answers", online: <http://www.phac-aspc.gc.ca/std-mts/hpv-vph/hpv-vph-vaccine_e.html>.

[216]   Lawrence O. Gostin & Catherine D. DeAngelis, "Mandatory HPV Vaccination: Public Health vs Private Wealth", Editorial (2 May 2007) 297 JAMA 1921, citing U.S. Food and Drug Administration, *Product Approval Information — Licensing Action* (8 June 2006), online: <http://www.fda.gov/cber/approvltr/hpvmer060806L.htm>.

[217]   Lawrence O. Gostin & Catherine D. DeAngelis, "Mandatory HPV Vaccination: Public Health vs Private Wealth", Editorial (2 May 2007) 297 JAMA: 1921 at 1921.

[218]   Angela E. Raffle, "Challenges of Implementing Human Papillomavirus (HPV) Vaccination policy" (25 August 2007) 335 BMJ 375 at 375-377. She noted that it had not been recommended in a report by the Vaccine European New International Collaboration Effort which questioned the assumed benefit, although four European countries had proceeded to provide it.

2008.[219] The HPV vaccine builds on research demonstrating a link between HPV and cervical cancer and is considered a breakthrough as a vaccine to prevent cancer. The vaccine acts against four common types of HPV, a sexually transmitted infection, that lead to cervical cancer and anogenital warts.[220] Girls aged 9 to 15 are the primary target of the vaccine since the vaccine works preventively on those who have not been exposed to HPV through sexual contact. The clinical trials in the 16 to 25 age group demonstrated a very high rate of efficacy, in the range approaching 100 per cent, in preventing cervical cancer among the sample groups.[221] Few 9 to 15-year-olds were included in the studies and they were followed for only 18 months — "thin information" on which to base the NACI recommendation, in the opinion of Abby Lippman and co-authors.[222] The vaccine's efficacy in the 9 to 15 age group has not been assessed.[223] The studies have been carried out over relatively short periods of time and researchers have identified the need for longer-term efficacy and safety studies among a larger group. Angela Raffle has stated that it is still unknown how long immunity lasts since there was only a five-year follow-up period.[224] The vaccine does not protect against the other types of HPV that cause approximately 30 per cent of cervical cancers.[225]

Licensing of the HPV vaccine has led researchers to raise important questions in the medical and public health literature. Some questions focused on whether the vaccine should be made available on a mandatory basis (a question posed in the American literature); whether the vaccine should be made available universally and be publicly funded as part of a national vaccine strategy (a question posed in the Canadian literature); and what combination of vaccination and other public health measures would be best to meet the goals. Dimensions of the question that have been raised address the following concerns.

---

[219]   The Canadian Women's Health Network, "The HPV Vaccine, One Year Later" (2008) 10:2 *Network Magazine*, online: <http://www.cwhn.ca/network-reseau/10-2/10-2pg4.html>.

[220]   Public Health Agency of Canada, "Human Papillomavirus (HPV) Prevention and HPV Vaccine: Questions and Answers", online: <http://www.phac-aspc.gc.ca/std-mts/hpv-vph/hpv-vph-vaccine_e.html>.

[221]   National Advisory Committee on Immunization "Statement on Human Papillomavirus Vaccine" (2007) 33 CCDR 12; Lawrence O. Gostin & Catherine D. DeAngelis, "Mandatory HPV Vaccination: Public Health vs Private Wealth", Editorial (2 May 2007) 297 JAMA: 1921 at 1921, citing U.S. Food and Drug Administration. Gardasil.

[222]   Abby Lippman *et al.*, "Human Papillomavirus, Vaccines and Women's Health: Questions and Cautions" (28 August 2007) 177 C.M.A.J. 484.

[223]   Lawrence O. Gostin & Catherine D. DeAngelis, "Mandatory HPV Vaccination: Public Health vs Private Wealth", Editorial (2 May 2007) 297 JAMA 1921 at 1921.

[224]   Angela E. Raffle, "Challenges of Implementing Human Papillomavirus (HPV) Vaccination Policy" (25 August 2007) 335 BMJ 375 at 376.

[225]   Public Health Agency of Canada, "Human Papillomavirus (HPV) Prevention and HPV Vaccine: Questions and Answers" at 2, online: <http://www.phac-aspc.gc.ca/std-mts/hpv-vph/hpv-vph-vaccine_e.html>.

First, what role should vaccination play in relation to screening through Pap smears? Screening has been extremely successful in reducing the rate of cervical cancer, with the incidence rate, adjusted for age, declining from 15 per cent per 100,000 women in 1978 to 3 per cent per 100,000 women in 2004.[226] Screening has been found to provide 80 per cent protection while the quadrivalent vaccine will not reach the one-third of cancers caused by other types or reach girls who were sexually abused as children and exposed prior to vaccination.[227] Careful assessment of the implications of introducing the vaccine must be done in relation to screening and other public health measures in place. As part of this assessment, consideration must be given to the potential impact of vaccination on participation in screening, including the possibility that a misunderstanding of the vaccine might lead to less safe-sex practices and lowered Pap screening results.[228]

Any proposed immunization plan needs to be considered in light of the full range of medical and public health questions, such as those developed into a framework of analysis by Erickson and colleagues, which includes "the burden of the disease, vaccine characteristics and immunization strategy, cost-effectiveness, acceptability, feasibility, and evaluability of program, research questions, equity, ethical, legal and political considerations".[229] The cost effectiveness of any mass immunization program requires assessment, a step not carried out in Canada before funding was announced.[230] If funds are made available for vaccination, particularly for an expensive vaccine such as this one, what other health priorities will not receive funding?[231] Because the incidence of cervical cancer is relatively low and the disease develops over time, there is not the same urgency, while time is available to consider the implications of various options before proceeding to mass immunization and public funding. As Abby Lippman has stated, questions and cautions exist and the decision needs to be based on reliable evidence-based research. There is a need for examination of current health inequities to make sure that the

---

[226] B.L. Johnston & J.M. Conly, "The Human Papillomavirus: The Promise of Cervical Cancer Prevention" (2007) 18 Can. J. Infect. Dis. Med. Microbiol 229 at 229 and note 13.

[227] Angela E. Raffle, "Challenges of Implementing Human Papillomavirus (HPV) Vaccination Policy" (25 August 2007) 335 BMJ 375 at 376; Raffle's reply to letter from Nick Hallam <http://www.bmj.com/cgi/eletters/335/7616/375>.

[228] Abby Lippman et al., "Human Papillomavirus, Vaccines and Women's Health: Questions and Cautions" (28 August 2007) 177 C.M.A.J. 484, noting that these questions were raised at the NACI workshop on the vaccine.

[229] L.J. Erickson, P. De Wals, & L. Farand, "An Analytical Framework for Immunization Programs in Canada" (March 2005) 13 Vaccine 2470 at 2470.

[230] Abby Lippman et al., "Human Papillomavirus, Vaccines and Women's Health: Questions and Cautions" (28 August 2007) 177 C.M.A.J. 484.

[231] Lawrence O. Gostin & Catherine D. DeAngelis, "Mandatory HPV Vaccination: Public Health vs Private Wealth", Editorial (2 May 2007) 297 JAMA 1921.

vaccine won't make those inequities worse, along with information gathering through registries, public education, a definition of goals and a review of current policies. The Canadian Women's Health Network has argued recently that a review of the decision to proceed with mass immunization programs should occur and if not, that a delay or a full education program at least should take place.[232] The Réseau québecois d'action pour la santé des femmes ("RQASF"), which had called for a moratorium in 2007, with support from numerous other groups, has recently pressed for increased public education, government action to counter the manufacturer's promotional activities, measures to improve access to and monitoring of Pap test screening, improved sex education programs, and consideration of investment in other STDs.[233] NACI identified the need for a Pap smear screening database, cervical cancer registries and vaccine registries to be developed and linked, in addition to networks of people working in the various fields involved.[234]

Canada has developed decision-making structures for immunization policy, including NACI and the Canadian Immunization committee, a federal-provincial-territorial body with the responsibility to make recommendations on effective vaccinations to be made available on an equitable basis, and for cancer prevention policy.[235] What was the decision-making process that led the Canadian government to fund the HPV vaccine without following the processes established to provide sound scientific and health policy advice for immunization policy and cancer prevention? Public trust, an essential component of successful vaccination programs, may be undermined if conflicts of interest become apparent or if political decision-making supersedes considerations of expertise and social goals.

Merck & Co., the manufacturer of Gardasil, the licensed vaccine, lobbied for the vaccine to be made mandatory in the United States and stopped only when this role was identified publicly.[236] As Larry Gostin and Catherine DeAngelis commented, this lobbying effort in the interests

---

[232] The Canadian Women's Health Network, "The HPV Vaccine, One Year Later" (2008) 10:2 *Network Magazine*, online: <http://www.cwhn.ca/network-reseau/10-2/10-2pg4.html>.

[233] Nathalie Parent, The Fédération du Québec pour le planning des naissances, "Quebec groups call for a moratorium on HPV vaccination campaign" (2008) 10:2 *Network Magazine*, online: <http://www.cwhn.ca/network-reseau/10-2/10-2pg4.html>.

[234] National Advisory Committee on Immunization "Statement on Human Papillomavirus Vaccine" (2007) 33 CCDR 12 at 20.

[235] André Picard, "How politics pushed the HPV vaccine" *The Globe and Mail* (11 August 2007).

[236] Lawrence O. Gostin & Catherine D. DeAngelis, "Mandatory HPV Vaccination: Public Health vs Private Wealth", Editorial (2 May 2007) 297 JAMA 1921 at 1922 and note 18; Saul S. Pollack, "Lobbying for vaccine to be halted" *The New York Times* (21 February 2007).

of the company's profits is inappropriate, especially in the period closely following the product's licensing.[237]

Joanna Erdman has addressed the issue of a gap in health equity, pointing to the significant disparity in cervical cancer incidence and mortality rates among marginalized groups of girls and women, women with low incomes and literacy skills, Aboriginal women and new immigrants suffering and dying in disproportionate numbers from cervical cancer. Health inequity needs to be addressed in the area of the HPV vaccine policy, she has argued, so that the HPV vaccine doesn't make the situation worse for vulnerable groups of women. Further, she notes, health policy that fails to ensure that disadvantaged persons may participate in its benefits is challengeable on constitutional grounds. She concludes that the Canadian HPV strategy promotes equity as it is publicly funded and accessible in being school-based. At the same time, the program raises other health equity issues such as promotion of the vaccine through creating perceptions of universal high levels of cervical cancer risk and locating responsibility for sexual health on a gendered basis.[238] Immaculada de Melo-Martin has raised similar equity concerns, noting that "[e]vidence shows that morbidity and mortality for this disease vary according to socioeconomic status, level of education, and ethnicity. Worldwide, women with lower socioeconomic status and less education suffer from a higher incidence of this cancer".[239] Melo-Martin has argued that if Pap smears are widely used in a population then the vaccine may contribute only marginally to cancer rates, while in a population which has received less screening, the benefit of the vaccine may be lost because of limited access to the vaccine.[240] At the same time, any school delivery system needs to be assessed for its likely success in reaching adolescent girls. In developing countries, many girls have left school or have low attendance rates.[241]

Vaccines are vital to the health of people around the globe. If we consider the number of people who have died as a result of contagious diseases, we can see that the capacity to immunize people against contagious diseases is a powerful tool on behalf of humanity. Safe and efficacious vaccines, effectively assessed and regulated as they begin to be used, given with full information, and accessible to those who need them, have a significant role to play in the achievement of global public health.

---

[237]   Lawrence O. Gostin & Catherine D. DeAngelis, "Mandatory HPV Vaccination: Public Health vs Private Wealth", Editorial (2 May 2007) 297 JAMA 1921 at 1922.

[238]   Joanna N. Erdman, "Health Equity, HPV and the Cervical Cancer Vaccine" (2008) Health L.J. (forthcoming).

[239]   Immaculada de Melo-Martin, "The Promise of the Human Papillomavirus Vaccine Does Not Confer Immunity Against Ethical Reflection" (April 2006) 11 The Oncologist 393 at 394.

[240]   Ibid.

[241]   Ibid.

6

HIV/AIDS AND PUBLIC HEALTH LAW

Mary Anne Bobinski[*]

I. INTRODUCTION

The Human Immunodeficiency Virus ("HIV") was first recognized in the early 1980s as reports of unusual infections and immune system suppression in some gay men began to appear in medical journals and in public health reports.[1] The struggle to find the causes and methods of treating these conditions is nearly three decades old, yet each phase of society's effort to grapple with this relatively new disease still resonates with lessons learned and unlearned. This chapter highlights the ways in which HIV infection has focused attention on the close relationship between public health practice and the legal system. The chapter begins with a brief summary of the medical aspects of HIV infection, the current data on the scope of infection in Canada and around the world, and an overview of the key public health law debates sparked by HIV. The remaining sections of the chapter will focus on the legal aspects of two major types of public health policies and objectives: case identification and the prevention of transmission.

---

[*] The author is grateful to Holly Harlow, Rachael Manion and Brenda Osmond for research assistance. The author also wishes to recognize the excellent resources on the legal and policy aspects of HIV/AIDS developed by the Canadian HIV/AIDS Legal Network, online: <http://www.aidslaw.ca>; these resources provide an in-depth analysis of many of the issues summarized in this chapter. This chapter largely focuses on the public health implication of HIV/AIDS in common law Canada.
[1] See for example U.S. Centers for Disease Control and Prevention, "A Cluster of Kaposi's Sarcoma and Pneumocystis carinii Pneumonia among Homosexual Male Residents of Los Angeles and Orange Counties, California" (18 June 1982) 31 MMWR 305.

II.   MEDICAL ASPECTS OF HIV/AIDS

(a)   Understanding HIV/AIDS

HIV is a retrovirus transmitted when virus-laden body fluids or tissues from an infected person come into contact with a portal of entry (such as an open wound or mucosal membrane) of another individual.[2] The major routes of transmission over the history of the disease have included: blood transfusions or tissue transplants, sexual activity such as vaginal or anal intercourse, perinatal transmission through childbirth or breastfeeding, transmission through sharing needles used for injections, and accidental exposures to blood or other infected body fluids in occupational settings.[3] The probability of transmission depends on a number of factors including the type of exposure and the concentration of viral particles.[4] Once transmission occurs, the virus can be found in a wide range of different body tissues although it creates a home base or reservoir of infected cells in lymphatic tissue.[5] The virus preferentially infects CD4 T-lymphocytes, key actors in the body's immune system.[6]

Untreated HIV infection follows a relatively long course that can last a decade or more. During the acute phase, the virus invades host cells and causes those cells to assist in the creation and dissemination of new viral particles. Two to three weeks after infection, many individuals experience a transitory fever, swollen lymph glands, a rash and other mild symptoms; these might be the only outward manifestation of HIV infection for many years.[7] The infected person creates antibodies in response to the virus but the immune response is not effective in clearing

---

[2]   A retrovirus is one which uses RNA to encode its basic genetic instructions rather than DNA. Researchers have made great progress in understanding the process of infection at the cellular level. See generally Warner C. Greene & B. Matija Peterlin, "Molecular Insights into HIV Biology" (February 2006) in Laurence Peiperl, Susa Coffey, Oliver Bacon & Paul Volberding, eds., *HIV InSite Knowledge Base* (online textbook from the UCSF Center for HIV Information), online: <http://hivinsite.ucsf.edu/InSite?page=kb-00&doc=kb-02-01-01>. The HIV InSite Knowledge Base offers medical reference material about HIV infection in an online format which allows for updates to incorporate recent research results.

[3]   Health Canada, "HIV and AIDS in Canada: Surveillance Report to December 31, 2003" (April 2004) at 66-67, online: Public Health Agency of Canada <http://www.phac-aspc.gc.ca/publicat/aids-sida/haic-vsac1203/pdf/haic-vsac1203.pdf>. See also C. Bradley Hare, "Clinical Overview of HIV Disease" (January 2006) in Laurence Peiperl, Susa Coffey, Oliver Bacon & Paul Volberding, eds., *HIV InSite Knowledge Base*, online: <http://hivinsite.ucsf.edu/InSite?page=kb-00&doc=kb-02-01-01>.

[4]   See, *e.g.*, Melissa Pope & Ashley T. Hasse, "Transmission, acute HIV-1 infection and the quest for strategies to prevent infection" (2003) 9 Nat. Med. 847.

[5]   *Ibid.*, at 847.

[6]   Mario Stevenson, "HIV-1 pathogenesis" (2003) 9 Nat. Med. 853 at 853.

[7]   Melissa Pope & Ashley T. Hasse, "Transmission, acute HIV-1 infection and the quest for strategies to prevent infection" (2003) 9 Nat. Med. 847.

the viral infection.[8] The window between infection and the creation of detectable antibodies (a process called seroconversion) can be three or more months. A person is capable of transmitting the virus to others during this window period but may nonetheless test negative in standard antibody tests used to determine exposure to HIV.

The infection then enters what has been misnamed the latent phase or latency period. While it is true that the infected individual may not exhibit clear signs and symptoms of infection, the virus itself remains very active. Researchers have demonstrated that the virus continues to interact with the immune system, eventually destroying it.[9] The demise of the immune system is then associated with advanced HIV infection. The patients who first came to the attention of public health officials in the early 1980s had advanced HIV infection; they had suppressed immune systems and a wide range of opportunistic infections.[10] This constellation of symptoms was given the name "Acquired Immunodeficiency Syndrome (AIDS)" even before the viral cause was identified in 1983 and long before the first tests for HIV antibodies became available in 1985.[11]

The distinction between HIV infection and a diagnosis of AIDS might be thought of as meaningless in some respects and misleading in others. It is meaningless because an individual can transmit the virus to others throughout the course of infection, whether or not there has been an AIDS diagnosis. It is misleading because AIDS statistics necessarily underestimate the true incidence and prevalence of HIV infection. The distinction nonetheless has retained its vitality, in part because of history and the clinical significance of an AIDS diagnosis. The distinction also

---

[8] Norman L. Letvin & Bruce D. Walker, "Immunopathogenesis and immunotherapy in AIDS virus infections (2003) 9 Nat. Med. 861.

[9] *Ibid.*

[10] An "opportunistic infection" is one which is more frequently observed in individuals with depressed immune function and which is more rarely observed in persons with healthy immune systems; it can also be called an "indicator disease".

[11] U.S. CDC, U.S. Dep't Health and Human Services, "CDC Guidelines for National Human Immunodeficiency Virus Case Surveillance, Including Monitoring for Human Immunodeficiency Virus Infection and Acquired Immunodeficiency Syndrome" (10 December 1999) 48 MMWR Recomm Rep. (RR13) 1 (detailing most recent surveillance guidelines and summarizing historical changes in diagnostic criteria). The case definition for "AIDS" in the United States is slightly broader than the case definition used across Canada and many other countries because it includes persons with HIV infection and evidence of depressed immune function (CD4 T-lymphocyte counts of less than 200 cells per microliter) who may not yet have experienced an "indicator" disease. Compare Canadian AIDS Society (CAS) and Health Canada, "A Guide to HIV/AIDS Epidemiological and Surveillance Terms" (2002) 10-11, online: Public Health Agency of Canada <http://www.phac-aspc.gc.ca/publicat/haest-tesvs/pdf/hiv_glossary_e.pdf> with U.S. CDC, "1993 Revised Classification System for HIV Infection and Expanded Surveillance Case Definition for AIDS Among Adolescents and Adults" (18 December 1992) 41 MMWR Recomm Rep. (RR17) 1.

reflects practical differences in the ability to gather data about HIV infection as opposed to AIDS diagnoses. Individuals with the symptoms necessary for an AIDS diagnosis are quite sick; they are more likely to come to the attention of health care professionals and to be correctly diagnosed than individuals with asymptomatic HIV infection. This was certainly true in the early years of the pandemic, before the introduction of medical tests indicative of HIV infection, and remains true today to the extent that HIV surveillance data depends on voluntary HIV testing.

(b) HIV Testing

The early HIV-related tests searched for antibodies to the HIV virus in blood samples and results took weeks to obtain.[12] Rapid HIV antibody tests can yield results from blood samples within minutes.[13] Other new tests look for antibodies in saliva and urine.[14] Tests that probe directly for HIV rather than for antibodies can be used to identify cases of infection before an individual has developed antibodies; public health officials are exploring cost-effective and efficient methods of using these tests to reduce the risk of "false negative" results for persons tested during the "window period".[15]

Once an individual has been diagnosed with HIV infection, health care providers and researchers rely on more elaborate tests to make clinical assessments about the stage of infection and the effectiveness of therapy. One testing methodology measures viral load, or the amount of HIV virus found in a sample.[16] Another focuses on the level of CD4 T-lymphocytes as a measure of the status of the infected person's immune system.[17] The most recently developed tests attempt to measure the drug

---

[12]   C. Bradley Hare, "Clinical Overview of HIV Disease" in Laurence Peiperl, Susa Coffey, Oliver Bacon & Paul Volberding eds., *HIV InSite Knowledge Base*, online: <http://hivinsite.ucsf.edu/InSite?page=kb-00&doc=kb-02-01-01>.

[13]   *Ibid.* See also, Canadian HIV/AIDS Legal Network, "Rapid HIV testing" in *HIV Testing* (2007) (series of 12 information sheets on HIV testing in Canada), online: <http://www.aidslaw.ca/publications/publicationsdocEN.php?ref=713>; Public Health Agency of Canada, "Point-of-Care HIV Testing Using Rapid HIV Test Kits: Guidance for Health-Care Professionals" (2007) 33:S2 CCDR 1, online: <http://www.phac-aspc.gc.ca/publicat/ccdr-rmtc/07pdf/33s2-eng.pdf>.

[14]   C. Bradley Hare, "Clinical Overview of HIV Disease" in Laurence Peiperl, Susa Coffey, Oliver Bacon & Paul Volberding, eds., *HIV InSite Knowledge Base*, online: <http://hivinsite.ucsf.edu/InSite?page=kb-00&doc=kb-02-01-01>.

[15]   Public Health Agency of Canada, "HIV Testing and Counselling: Policies in Transition?" (2007) (research paper prepared for the International Public Health Dialogue on HIV Testing and Counseling, Toronto, 17 August 2006), online: <http://www.phac-aspc.gc.ca/aids-sida/publication/hivtest/index-eng.php>.

[16]   *Ibid.*

[17]   *Ibid.*

resistance of the viral strains infecting a particular individual; these tests can improve medication management for the individual and are also an important source of data on the overall rates of viral resistance to particular antiretroviral therapies.[18]

(c) Treatment for HIV Infection and Associated Illnesses

The early years of the HIV pandemic were characterized by the complete absence of treatments directly addressing the infection itself. Treatment instead focused on combatting the opportunistic infections which caused morbidity and mortality for persons with advanced HIV infection.[19] The first drug to directly combat HIV replication in infected individuals was introduced in 1987.[20] This drug, and the few other single-agent drug therapies developed during the early 1990s, were an important but incomplete advance. These "monotherapies" had significant side effects and their effectiveness was rapidly diminished by the emergence of drug-resistant viral strains. Researchers continued to develop new drugs designed to target different parts of the virus's life cycle.[21]

Researchers also discovered that the antiretroviral drugs could be used to reduce the risk of HIV transmission from a woman to her child during pregnancy and birth. The North American rate of perinatal transmission is approximately 25-30 per cent without treatment.[22] The risk of HIV transmission can be reduced to single digit percentages if the pregnant woman takes even a short course of antiretroviral therapy.[23] Antiretroviral therapy can also be used to reduce the risk of HIV transmission arising from other types of exposure incidents.

By 1995, researchers began to recommend combination drug therapies to patients. This approach, often called highly active

---

[18] *Ibid.* Specialized tests may also be able to link cases of HIV infection by studying the genetic variation of the virus; however, linking cases does not demonstrate the direction of transmission. See, *e.g.*, Gary Blick *et al.*, "The Probable Source of Both the Primary Multidrug-Resistant (MDR) HIV-1 Strain Found in a Patient with Rapid Progression to AIDS and a Second Recombinant MDR Strain Found in a Chronically HIV-1–Infected Patient" (2007) 195 J. Infect. Dis. 1250.

[19] Public Health Agency of Canada, "HIV Testing and Counselling: Policies in Transition?" (2007) (research paper prepared for the International Public Health Dialogue on HIV Testing and Counseling, Toronto, 17 August 2006), online: <http://www.phac-aspc.gc.ca/aids-sida/publication/hivtest/index-eng.php>. See also Roger J. Pomerantz & David L. Horn, "Twenty years of therapy for HIV-1 infection" (July 2003) 9 Nat. Med. 867.

[20] Pomerantz & Horn, *ibid.* (zidovudine or AZT).

[21] *Ibid.*, at 868.

[22] Ronald O. Valdiserri, Lydia L. Ogden & Eugene McCray, "Accomplishments in HIV prevention science: implications for stemming the epidemic" (July 2003) 9 Nat. Med. 881 at 884.

[23] *Ibid.*

antiretroviral therapy ("HAART") was very effective in reducing viral load and mortality rates in many persons with HIV infection.[24] The new therapeutic regime still could not eliminate the viral infection, but researchers, care providers and the public began to contemplate a future in which HIV infection might be considered to be a serious chronic illness rather than an inevitably fatal condition. This enthusiasm soon was tempered by many factors including the continued development of drug resistant strains of HIV, the severe and debilitating drug side effects experienced by many patients, and the significant social, practical and economic barriers to successfully accessing and maintaining adherence to this complex and expensive form of care.[25]

(d)   HIV/AIDS Statistics and Special Populations

HIV is now a global pandemic.[26] According to the Joint United Nations Programme on HIV/AIDS ("UNAIDS"), "an estimated 33.2 million people (range 30.6–36.1 million) were living with HIV in 2007".[27] Global HIV prevalence rates have remained level since 2001; however, the numbers of people living with HIV have continued to rise, due to population growth and the life-prolonging effects of antiretroviral therapy.[28] The prevalence and incidence of HIV infection varies from country to country and, often, from population group to population group within a particular geographic region.[29]   Sub-Saharan Africa has the highest levels of HIV infection globally: "[m]ore than two thirds (68%) of all people HIV-positive live in this region where more than three quarters (76%) of all AIDS deaths in 2007 occurred"; the disease is the leading cause of death in that region.[30] While HIV prevalence has been declining

---

[24]   Roger J. Pomerantz & David L. Horn, "Twenty years of therapy for HIV-1 infection" (July 2003) 9 Nat. Med. 867 at 868.

[25]   *Ibid.*, at 869-72.

[26]   A "pandemic" is a disease that is widespread across many countries or around the world; an "epidemic" can occur in a narrower geographic location. See Oxford English Dictionary, *s.v.* "pandemic" and "epidemic", online: <http://dictionary.oed.com>.

[27]   UNAIDS, "AIDS Epidemic Update: December 2007" at 1, online: <http://data.unaids.org/pub/EPISlides/2007/2007_epiupdate_en.pdf>.

[28]   *Ibid.*, at 4.

[29]   "Incidence is the number of *new* events of a specific disease during a specified period of time in a specified population." Canadian AIDS Society (CAS) and Health Canada, "A Guide to HIV/AIDS Epidemiology and Surveillance Terms" (2002) at 31 (emphasis in original), online: Public Health Agency of Canada <http://www.phac-aspc.gc.ca/publicat/haest-tesvs/pdf/hiv_glossary_e.pdf>. "Prevalence is the total number of people with a specific disease or health condition living in a defined population at a particular time." It is often useful to express incidence or prevalence as a "rate" or as a proportion of the total population at risk for the condition (*ibid.*, at 39).

[30]   UNAIDS, "AIDS Epidemic Update: December 2007", online: <http://data.unaids.org/pub/EPISlides/2007/2007_epiupdate_en.pdf> at 4, 15.

or leveling off in some regions in Africa, HIV prevalence in southern Africa remains high, with eight countries in that region registering adult HIV prevalence rates over 15 per cent.[31] Outside Sub-Saharan Africa, the HIV epidemic is "primarily concentrated among populations most at risk, such as men who have sex with men, injecting drug users, sex workers, and their sexual partners".[32]

The major routes of transmission have varied from region to region and over time. This has had a significant impact on the populations affected by the disease. For example, despite the early association in North America between HIV transmission and unprotected sexual activities between males, over half of all people living with HIV worldwide are women.[33] Young people are also disproportionately affected, accounting for 40 per cent of all new HIV infections world wide.[34]

Although gaps and errors in reporting make it difficult to know the precise date for HIV/AIDS prevalence and incidence in any society, the statistics for HIV/AIDS in Canada make clear that the prevalence of infection is significant and that it is not uniformly spread throughout society. As of December 31, 2006, over 20,000 cases of AIDS had been diagnosed in Canada since the beginning of the epidemic; there were more than 13,000 reported deaths during this same time period.[35] The incidence and prevalence of HIV infection is even more difficult to determine because of variability in the rates of testing, the degree of reporting, and the rates of risky behaviour or activities. Within these constraints, public health researchers have produced reasonable estimates:

> The Public Health Agency of Canada (PHAC) produced estimates of HIV prevalence to the end of 2005 and HIV incidence in 2005 ... It was estimated that at the end of 2005 there were approximately 58,000 ... people in Canada living with HIV (including those living with AIDS), of whom approximately 27% were undiagnosed. The number of people in Canada newly infected with HIV in 2005 was estimated to be 2,300-4,500.[36]

---

[31] *Ibid.*, at 15.

[32] *Ibid.*, at 4.

[33] *Ibid.*, at 8.

[34] *Ibid.*, at 21.

[35] Health Canada, "HIV and AIDS in Canada: Surveillance Report to December 31, 2006" (2007) at 7 and 59 (due to reporting delays, omissions and errors, these figures cannot be compared to deduce the number of individuals currently living with an AIDS diagnosis in Canada), online: Public Health Agency of Canada <http://www.phac-aspc.gc.ca/aids-sida/publication/survreport/pdf/survrep1206.pdf>.

[36] *Ibid.*, at 1 (reference omitted). Note that this figure represents the number of persons *living* with HIV infection, not the number of Canadians who have acquired HIV infection since the beginning of the epidemic. Incidence and prevalence rates are subject to error.

The number of HIV diagnoses declined from 1996 to 2000, increased in 2001, and then remained stable at about 2,500 new diagnoses per year beginning in 2002.[37]

Researchers organize data in "exposure categories" according to the likely mode of transmission. There have been significant changes in the routes of HIV transmission for new infections over time. Sexual activity between men accounted for over 60 per cent of the cases of HIV infection reported from 1985–2000 but accounted for less than 40 per cent of the new infections reported in 2006.[38] Exposure to HIV through intravenous drug use ("IDU") also has varied over time, rising to over 28 per cent in 1998–1999 before beginning to drop.[39] This exposure category still accounted for nearly 20 per cent of the newly reported infections in 2006.[40] Meanwhile, the percentage of cases associated with heterosexual contact has increased from about 12 per cent in 1985–2000 to just over 30 per cent in 2006.[41]

The same Canadian data can also be analyzed using gender and ethnic categories. The percentage of new HIV infection reports in adult women has more than doubled since the early years of the epidemic, rising from about 11 per cent of the positive test results recorded from 1985–1996 to approximately 28 per cent of the positive test results in 2006.[42] HIV infection data cannot currently be used to track ethnicity because of inconsistent reporting across provinces. Ethnicity data is available for reported AIDS cases and shows significant ethnic variations.[43] About 11 per cent of AIDS diagnoses in 2006 were recorded

---

Researchers reported in 2008 that HIV incidence rates in the United States were 40 per cent higher than had been thought. Lawrence K. Altman, "HIV Study Finds Rate 40% Higher Than Estimated" *The New York Times* (3 August 2008).

[37] Health Canada, "HIV and AIDS in Canada: Surveillance Report to December 31, 2006" (2007) at 2 (Figure 1), online: Public Health Agency of Canada <http://www.phac-aspc.gc.ca/aids-sida/publication/survreport/pdf/survrep1206.pdf>.

[38] *Ibid.*, at 17 (Table 5A). There is a separate exposure category for men who have sex with men and who are also involved in injection drug use. Only a small (and relatively constant) percentage of HIV test reports are found in this combined exposure group (*ibid.*).

[39] Health Canada, "HIV and AIDS in Canada: Surveillance Report to December 31, 2006" (2007), online: Public Health Agency of Canada <http://www.phac-aspc.gc.ca/aids-sida/publication/survreport/pdf/survrep1206.pdf> at 17 (Table 5A); and Health Canada, "HIV and AIDS in Canada: Surveillance Report to December 31, 2003" (April 2004) at 16 (Table 5A), online: Public Health Agency of Canada <http://www.phac-aspc.gc.ca/ publicat/aids-sida/haic-vsac1203/pdf/haic-vsac1203.pdf>.

[40] Health Canada, "HIV and AIDS in Canada: Surveillance Report to December 31, 2006" (2007), online: Public Health Agency of Canada <http://www.phac-aspc.gc.ca/aids-sida/publication/survreport/pdf/survrep1206.pdf> at 17 (Table 5A).

[41] *Ibid.*

[42] *Ibid.*, at 13 (Table 3).

[43] *Ibid.*, at 56 (Table 20). Ethnicity data is not available for AIDS cases in Ontario beginning in 2005.

in Black Canadians.[44] The percentage of AIDS cases diagnosed in Aboriginal Canadians moved from low single digits in the period from 1979–2000 to nearly 25 per cent of diagnoses reported in 2006.[45] These increases are cause for significant concern as they might reflect changes in the distribution of risky behaviours and/or differences in access to medical treatments that slow or prevent the movement from HIV infection to an AIDS diagnosis.

(e) HIV/AIDS and Public Health

The medical aspects of HIV lead inexorably into a range of issues for public health officials, judges and politicians. Confronted with an apparently new life-threatening disease, members of each of these groups have struggled to establish policies that would protect the public's health while also protecting the individual liberty, lives and dignity of those infected with the virus. Several characteristics of HIV have arguably driven the public policy debate. Unlike other serious illnesses such as smallpox or pandemic influenza, HIV is relatively difficult to transmit. The routes of transmission involve exposure to blood or body fluids through typically voluntary activities. The activities associated with transmission — sex, needle-sharing and childbearing — are value-laden and sometimes controversial. Persons infected with the virus can live for decades in relatively good health, able to participate in employment and their communities without posing any threat to public health.

Public health policies seek to match the threat of disease with the required response.[46] HIV presented a new challenge when it emerged in the 1980s. While similar to other sexually transmitted diseases in its mode of transmission and its association with socially stigmatized behaviours, it was decidedly dissimilar in the severity of the consequences and the absence of effective treatments. While similar to other life threatening diseases such as tuberculosis (TB) or smallpox, it was quite dissimilar in its degree of infectiousness, its mode of transmission, the absence of a vaccine, and the length of time during which infected and contagious

---

[44]   *Ibid.* By comparison, only 2.5 per cent of Canadians identified themselves as Black in the 2006 Census: "2006 Census: Ethnic origin, visible minorities, place of work and mode of transportation", online: Statistics Canada <http://www.statcan.ca/Daily/English/080402/d080402a.htm>.

[45]   Health Canada, "HIV and AIDS in Canada: Surveillance Report to December 31, 2006" (2007), online: Public Health Agency of Canada <http://www.phac-aspc.gc.ca/aids-sida/publication/survreport/pdf/survrep1206.pdf> at 56 (Table 20).

[46]   See generally Lawrence O. Gostin, *Public Health Law: Power, Duty, Restraint* (Berkeley: University of California Press, 2008); Lawrence O. Gostin, Scott Burris & Zita Lazzarini, "The Law and the Public's Health: A Study of Infectious Disease Law in the United States" (1999) 99 Colum. L. Rev. 59.

persons remained capable of contributing to society. How should society respond to this new disease? The emergence of HIV infection prompted policy makers to begin to re-examine long-neglected aspects of public health policy and law.

The ensuing debates focused on three broad areas: (1) the proper locus of public health authority and responsibility; (2) the extent to which HIV-specific policies or laws were warranted; and (3) the balance between the exercise of public health authority and the protection of individual liberty.

The first issue is a familiar one for societies, like Canada, operating within a federal form of government. The Constitution of 1867 gives health-related responsibilities to both the federal government and the provinces. Provinces have the primary authority and responsibility for the protection of local public health.[47] Provinces also maintain jurisdiction over "Property and Civil Rights in the Province", including common law claims arising in torts and contracts.[48] The federal government has direct jurisdiction over preventing the transmission of disease over international borders.[49] The federal government also controls criminal law, trade and commerce, and retains the authority "to make Laws for the Peace, Order, and good Government of Canada in relation to all Matters not coming within the Classes of Subjects by this Act assigned exclusively to the Legislatures of the Provinces".[50] The end result is a complex web of interlocking responsibilities for the management of the challenges posed by HIV.

Based in part on studies of Canada's response to emerging infectious diseases such as SARS, Canada established a new federal Public Health Agency with a newly created position for a Chief Public Health Officer in 2006.[51] The legislation suggests that the federal government hopes to take more affirmative steps to promote public health while recognizing and

---

[47]   *Constitution Act, 1867* (U.K.), 30 & 31 Vict., c. 3, s. 92(7), reprinted in R.S.C. 1985, App. II, No. 5.

[48]   *Ibid.*, s. 92(13). See also National Advisory Committee on SARS and Public Health, "Learning from SARS: Renewal of Public Health in Canada" (October 2003) at 166, online: <http://www.phac-aspc.gc.ca/publicat/sars-sras/pdf/sars-e.pdf>.

[49]   *Constitution Act, 1867* (U.K.), 30 & 31 Vict., c. 3, s. 92(7), reprinted in R.S.C. 1985, App. II, No. 5. See also National Advisory Committee on SARS and Public Health (*ibid.*, at 166).

[50]   *Constitution Act, 1867, ibid.*, s. 91(2) (criminal law power); s. 91(27) (trade and commerce); s. 91 preamble (Peace, Order and good Government).

[51]   *Public Health Agency of Canada Act, 2006*, S.C. 2006, c. 5.

respecting jurisdictional complexities.[52] The implications of this reorganization for Canada's response to HIV are not yet clear.

The second major debate focuses on "HIV exceptionalism": whether HIV infection presents unique characteristics that require an individualized legal or social response or whether it would be more appropriate to rely on general principles applicable to a wide range of other diseases or health conditions.[53] Advocates for people with HIV infection or for communities considered to be at risk for infection noted the special problems of fear and discrimination surrounding HIV and sometimes argued for specific new legal protections. Critics of exceptionalism argued that HIV should be treated like any other potentially fatal transmissible condition. These critics of special policies for HIV-infection contended that the emphasis on the rights of persons with HIV-infection prevented the implementation of traditional public health strategies, such as testing, reporting and contact tracing.

At a more general level, the debate about "exceptionalism" grew out of concerns about the capacity of the public health and legal systems to respond to a wide range of diseases or conditions. Policy-makers in countries around the world reacted to the unique problems presented by HIV infection with a host of tailored policies and laws governing discrete areas of concern ranging from the use of HIV-antibody testing to the creation of specific criminal offences related to the intentional or reckless transmission of HIV.[54] Critics of this approach argued that the existing

---

[52]   The Preamble establishes five major goals for the federal government: (1) "to take public health measures, including measures relating to health protection and promotion, population health assessment, health surveillance, disease and injury prevention, and public health emergency preparedness and response"; (2) "to foster collaboration within the field of public health and to coordinate federal policies and programs in the area of public health"; (3) "to promote cooperation and consultation in the field of public health with provincial and territorial governments"; (4) "to foster cooperation in that field with foreign governments and international organizations, as well as other interested persons or organizations"; and (5) to "contribute to federal efforts to identify and reduce public health risk factors and to support national readiness for public health threats" (*ibid.*). See also Amir Attaran & Kumanan Wilson, "A Legal and Epidemiological Justification for Federal Authority in Public Health Emergencies" (2007) McGill L.J. 381 (advocating expansion of federal legislation regarding epidemics); Kumanan Wilson & Christopher MacLennan, "Federalism and Public Health Law in Canada: Opportunities and Unanswered Questions" (2005) 14:2 Health L. Rev. 3.

[53]   Ronald Bayer & Amy L. Fairchild, "Changing the Paradigm for HIV Testing — The End of Exceptionalism" (2006) 355 N. Eng. J. Med. 647; Ronald Bayer, "Public health policy and the AIDS epidemic: An end to HIV exceptionalism?" (1991) 324 N Engl. J. Med. 1500.

[54]   The trend toward HIV-specific legislation was particularly pronounced in the United States. See for example, "State Statutes Dealing with HIV and AIDS: A Comprehensive State-by-State Summary" (2004 Edition) 13 Law & Sexuality 1. For a summary of HIV-related statutes in the United States see also online: <http://www.law.tulane.edu/tlsjournals/tlas/aids_statutes.aspx>.

framework of public health laws and policies should not be abandoned in response to new threats like HIV but that the system should be adjusted to take into account the lessons learned from the encounter. Thus, the proper response to fears about the disclosure of HIV-related information would be to re-examine the adequacy of confidentiality protections generally rather than enacting a completely new law to protect HIV-related information.

The third major debate involves the balance between protection of the public and protection of the individual. A public health policy strictly focused on risk identification and elimination theoretically could include highly intrusive measures, such as mandatory testing, treatment or quarantine, designed to identify and to reduce the risk of transmission. At the other extreme, rigid protection of individual liberties could render public health authorities powerless to address real risks posed by individuals with highly contagious and dangerous diseases. The correct path clearly lies somewhere between these two extremes, and the debates surrounding HIV infection provided an important opportunity to consciously chart a new course. The result was a new conceptualization of public health and individual liberty that values both as essential to a safe society. The protection of individual liberty began to be viewed as an important public health tool rather than as a conflicting obligation.[55] Protection of individual liberties might encourage persons at risk for HIV infection to present themselves for HIV testing and counseling, for example.

The remaining sections of this chapter will explore how Canada's public health and legal systems have responded to the problems presented by HIV. This chapter will focus on two categories of public health interventions: (1) identifying cases of infection through HIV testing and reporting; and (2) using law to reduce the risk of transmission. The chapter will conclude with a brief discussion of the implications of HIV-related policies for the future.

III. CASE IDENTIFICATION: HIV TESTING AND CONFIDENTIALITY

(a) Overview

Gathering information about a possible health threat is an important precondition to mounting an effective response. Authorities need to know that an illness is present in a population to effectively manage public

---

[55]   See generally Lawrence O. Gostin, Scott Burris & Zita Lazzarini, "The Law and the Public's Health: A Study of Infectious Disease Law in the United States" (1999) 99 Colum. L. Rev. 59.

health policies. Health care providers must know a person is infected to properly direct that person's health care. Individuals also have an interest in knowing their own health status in order to seek proper treatment and to ensure the safety of others. Although every member of society should take steps to reduce risky activities, individuals who discover they are infected with HIV have a particularly powerful basis for changing their behaviour to reduce the risk of transmission to others.[56] These issues are particularly important for HIV infection, given the dramatic consequences of infection.

The introduction of HIV antibody tests in 1985 presented an opportunity to gather information about the incidence and prevalence of HIV infection and to use that information for the benefit of the individual and society. Two key questions must be answered about HIV testing programs: (1) Under what circumstances can the tests be administered?; and (2) What use can be made of the results? Section III (b) will focus on the implementation of HIV testing. Section III (c) will explore the implications of privacy and confidentiality for the use of test results and then will relate the debate to the specific issue of HIV/AIDS reporting rules.

(b) HIV Testing

One key issue for HIV testing programs involves the degree of voluntariness associated with the testing program.[57] "Mandatory" testing programs are those in which the testing is imposed whether or not the person to be tested consents. "Conditional" testing programs are those associated with participation in a voluntary activity (such as donating

---

[56]   Public Health Agency of Canada, "HIV Testing and Counselling: Policies in Transition?" (2007) (research paper prepared for the International Public Health Dialogue on HIV Testing and Counseling, Toronto, 17 August 2006), online: <http://www.phac-aspc.gc.ca/aids-sida/publication/hivtest/index-eng.php> at 58-63 ("In numerous studies, people change their behaviour after learning they are HIV-positive" at 58).

[57]   This typology is adapted from Mark A. Hall, Mary Anne Bobinski & David Orentlicher, *Health Care Law & Ethics* (New York. Aspen Publishing, 2007) at 923-24. The Canadian HIV/AIDS Legal Network offers a slightly different formulation. In its view, "mandatory testing" includes "requiring HIV testing as a condition of obtaining a certain status, service or benefit, such as employment or health services". Canadian HIV/AIDS Legal Network, "Mandatory and compulsory testing for HIV" in (2007) *HIV Testing* (series of 12 information sheets on HIV testing in Canada), online: <http://www.aidslaw.ca/publications/publicationsdocEN.php?ref–713>. "Compulsory testing" is deemed to be "compelling or forcing a person or group of people to be tested, such that the person cannot choose to refuse testing and cannot legally avoid it" (*ibid.*). See also, Ralf Jürgens, "Mandatory or Compulsory HIV Testing" in *HIV Testing and Confidentiality: Final Report*, (2001) online: <http://www.aidslaw.ca/publications/interfaces/downloadFile.php?ref=282>.

blood): an individual can avoid testing by choosing not to participate in the activity. "Routine" HIV testing is not well defined. For some, it involves treating HIV testing like a wide range of other medical tests and procedures for which a general consent to care and treatment is sufficient to authorize the test. Two other approaches to routine testing preserve a more specific informed consent process. Under the "opt-out" approach an individual is told that HIV testing is routine but the person can still "opt-out" or decline testing. Under the "opt-in" approach, individuals are told that HIV testing is routinely offered and they are given an opportunity to agree or to refuse. Opt-in routine testing programs thus resemble more traditional voluntary testing programs, except all persons in a particular group are offered testing.

The UNAIDS/WHO issued a policy statement on HIV testing in 2004 that sought to reinforce the continued necessity for HIV testing to follow the "three C's" with a focus on confidentiality, counseling, and informed consent.[58] "Client-initiated", voluntary counseling and testing programs "remain[ed] critical to the effectiveness of HIV prevention".[59] The policy recommended that "routine offer[s] of HIV testing by health care providers" be limited to three populations: to persons being assessed or treated for sexual transmitted diseases, to pregnant women in order to offer treatment designed to reduce the risk of HIV transmission to their offspring, and to patients "seen in clinical and community based health service settings where HIV is prevalent and antiretroviral treatment is available...".[60] The policy recommended that systematic, provider-initiated tests falling into these three categories be offered on an "opt-out" basis.[61]

The United States pushed routine testing well beyond these recommendations in 2006 when the U.S. Centers for Disease Control ("U.S. CDC") issued a major new set of recommendations supporting routine, "opt-out" HIV testing for all adults.[62] The new recommendations gained the support of many health law policy experts and researchers for

[58]   UNAIDS and WHO, "UNAIDS/WHO Policy Statement on HIV Testing" (June 2004), online: <http://www.who.int/ethics/topics/en/hivtestingpolicy_who_unaids_en_2004.pdf>. To be minimally acceptable, the policy provides that the informed consent process include information about "the clinical benefit and the prevention benefits of testing ... the right to refuse ... the follow-up services that will be offered and ... in the event of a positive test result the importance of anticipating the need to inform anyone at ongoing risk who would otherwise not suspect they were being exposed to HIV infection" (ibid., at 2).
[59]   Ibid.
[60]   Ibid.
[61]   Ibid.
[62]   Bernard M. Branson et al., "Revised Recommendations for HIV Testing of Adults, Adolescents, and Pregnant Women in Health-Care Settings" (2006) 55:RR-14 MMWR 1. The recommendations "are intended for all health-care providers in the public and private sectors" (ibid.).

several reasons.[63] First, opt-out testing would maintain a voluntary approach to HIV testing. Second, the stringent specific informed consent procedures associated with HIV exceptionalism arguably were no longer warranted given existing strong legal protections from discrimination for HIV-positive persons. Third, the movement of HIV into "low risk" populations meant that many people with HIV infection were unaware they were at risk and were unlikely to seek out testing, making routine screening an important public health tool. Fourth, early identification of HIV infection could be coupled with early medical intervention to improve health care outcomes for persons found to be infected with HIV.

The reactions to the U.S. CDC recommendations were not uniformly positive. Some argued that the move to routine testing was based on a false premise: that the specific informed consent process created a bureaucratic barrier to the expansion of voluntary testing.[64] Critics also expressed fears about the dilution of voluntariness and suggested that targeted counseling and testing programs would be more efficient and effective.[65]

The U.S. CDC recommendations were followed the next year by new guidelines from UNAIDS/WHO recommending that HIV testing be routinely offered on an opt-out basis to a wider range of populations:

> 1) for all patients … whose clinical presentation might result from underlying HIV infection; 2) as a standard part of medical care for all patients attending health facilities in generalized HIV epidemics; and 3) more selectively in concentrated and low-level epidemics.[66]

---

[63] See, e.g., Douglas J. Koo et al., "HIV Counseling and Testing: Less Targeting, More Testing" (2006) 96 Am. J. Public Health 962; Thomas R. Frieden et al., "Applying Public Health Principles to the HIV Epidemic" (2005) 353 N. Eng. J. Med. 2397; Samuel A. Bozzette, "Routine Screening for HIV Infection — Timely and Cost Effective" (2005) 352 N. Eng. J. Med. 620; A. David Paltiel et al., "Expanded Screening for HIV in the United States — An Analysis of Cost-Effectiveness" (2005) 352 N. Eng. J. Med. 586.

[64] Ann Hilton Fisher, Catherine Hanssens & David I. Schulman, "The CDC's routine HIV testing recommendation: legally, not so routine" (2006) 11:2/3 Canadian HIV/AIDS Pol'y & L. Rev. 17 at 18.

[65] Ronald Bayer and Amy L. Fairchild, "Changing the Paradigm for HIV Testing — The End of Exceptionalism" (2006) 355 N. Eng. J. Med. 647 at 949; David R. Holtgrave, "Costs and Consequences of the U.S. Centers for Disease Control and Prevention's Recommendations for Opt-Out HIV Testing" (2007) 4 PLOS Medicine 1011; Canadian HIV/AIDS Legal Network, "Outcomes of the Symposium on HIV Testing and Human Rights" (Briefing paper, Montréal, 24-25 October 2005), online: Canadian HIV/AIDS Legal Network <http://www.aidslaw.ca/publications/interfaces/downloadFile.php?ref=273>.

[66] UNAIDS/WHO, "Guidance on Provider-Initiated HIV Testing and Counselling in Health Facilities" (2007) at 5, online: <http://www.who.int/hiv/pub/guidelines/9789241595568_en.pdf>; and Madhavi Swamy, "UN agencies issue new guidelines for HIV testing" (2007) 12:2/3 Canadian HIV/AIDS Pol'y & L. Rev. 39.

The new guidelines continued to reject the expansion of routine, opt-out testing into lower risk populations: "[h]ealth care providers should *not* recommend HIV testing and counseling to all persons attending all health facilities in settings with low-level and concentrated epidemics, since most people will have a low risk of exposure to HIV".[67] The new guidelines recognize that the expansion of HIV screening might require offering pre-test counseling in a modified form, but still retain the general requirements of adherence to the "'three C's — informed consent, counseling and confidentiality".[68]

Canadian public health authorities generally have supported voluntary HIV testing programs meeting the "three C's", with a few exceptions that will be discussed below. The current Canadian testing guidelines provide that "[t]esting should only be carried out with the consent of the person being tested", and that "Provider-Initiated Testing and Counselling (PITC)" "should be offered to any person with risk behaviour or at risk, any person with clinical or laboratory clues suggestive of HIV infection, or any person who requests it".[69]

It is estimated that 23-30 per cent of people with HIV infection in Canada are unaware of their status.[70] Canadian public health authorities have studied the development of policies designed to reach people unaware of their HIV infection but as of early 2008 had not yet joined the U.S. CDC in recommending expansion of routine testing for all adults.[71]

---

[67]   UNAIDS/WHO, *ibid.*, at 8 (emphasis in original).

[68]   *Ibid.*, at 19.

[69]   Public Health Agency of Canada, "HIV Testing and Counselling: Policies in Transition?" (2007) (research paper prepared for the International Public Health Dialogue on HIV Testing and Counseling, Toronto, 17 August 2006), online: <http://www.phac-aspc.gc.ca/aids-sida/publication/hivtest/index-eng.php> at 22. The Public Health Agency is studying the possible expansion of routine PITC on an opt-in or opt-out basis (*ibid.*, at 53-57) (discussing benefits and risks of expanded PITC on either an opt-in or opt-out basis).

[70]   *Ibid.*, at 30-32; and Sally Murray and Erica Weir, "HIV Screening" (2005) 173 C.M.A.J. 752.

[71]   In 2006, the Public Health Agency of Canada commissioned a research paper focusing on HIV testing and counseling policy related to persons unaware of their HIV infection because they had never been tested or because they had received a false negative result. Public Health Agency of Canada, "HIV Testing and Counselling: Policies in Transition?" (2007) (research paper prepared for the International Public Health Dialogue on HIV Testing and Counseling, Toronto, 17 August 2006), online: <http://www.phac-aspc.gc.ca/aids-sida/publication/hivtest/index eng.php>. The study identified "gaps in knowledge" related to HIV testing, the informed consent process, and other areas (*ibid.*, at 69-71). For an article arguing against the expansion of routine testing in Canada, see Joanne Csete & Richard Elliott, "Scaling up HIV testing: human rights and hidden costs" (2006) 11:1 Canadian HIV/AIDS Pol'y & L. Rev. 1.

The Public Health Agency is expected to release new recommendations regarding HIV testing at some point during 2008.[72]

Policy recommendations and medical practice guidelines constitute one important determinant of practices regarding HIV testing; however, these policies must operate within a legal framework. The law governing testing programs therefore is another very important determinant of the HIV testing practices in any given jurisdiction. The next sections of this chapter will focus on the legal rules governing testing and the interaction of law and policy in the area of HIV testing in Canada.

(i)   Voluntariness as the General Legal Requirement

Debates about the proper scope of voluntariness or involuntariness in HIV testing programs are ultimately a combined question of public health policy and law. HIV testing implicates legal rights and obligations at both the provincial and federal levels.[73] The first source of legal authority rests with the provinces because of their control of the delivery of health care and the protection of public health.[74] Whether or not an HIV test can be administered will depend on provincial rules governing public health and regulation of health professions. Common law rules also play an important role, particularly given the informed consent requirement imposed on physicians.

Federal law is relevant in some areas as well, particularly where the testing program intersects with federal authority over international borders or over criminal law. Finally, the rights guaranteed under the *Canadian Charter of Rights and Freedoms* provide significant protections from intrusive testing programs.[75] Under s. 7 of the *Charter*, "Everyone has the right to life, liberty and security of the person and the right not to be deprived thereof except in accordance with the principles of fundamental

[72]   Public Health Agency of Canada, "Point-of-Care HIV Testing Using Rapid HIV Test Kits: Guidance for Health-Care Professionals" (2007) 33:S2 CCDR 1, online: <http://www.phac-aspc.gc.ca/publicat/ccdr-rmtc/07pdf/33s2-eng.pdf> at 2 (noting "[f]urther analysis of legal, ethical, and human rights considerations will be provided in a policy framework to address HIV testing in Canada to be published by the Public Health Agency of Canada (PHAC) in 2008").

[73]   See Ralf Jürgens, "Mandatory or Compulsory HIV Testing" in *HIV Testing and Confidentiality: Final Report* (2001), online: <http://www.aidslaw.ca/publications/interfaces/downloadFile. php?ref=282>; Joanne Csete & Richard Elliott, "Prevention and Protection: Enhancing Both HIV Testing and Human Rights in Canada" (2007) at 5, online: Canadian HIV/AIDS Legal Network <http://www.aidslaw.ca/publications/interfaces/downloadFile. php?ref=1065>.

[74]   See *supra*, text accompanying notes 47-50.

[75]   *Canadian Charter of Rights and Freedoms*, Part I of the *Constitution Act, 1982*, being Schedule B to the *Canada Act 1982* (U.K.), 1982, c. 11.

justice."[76] Section 8 provides that "Everyone has the right to be secure against unreasonable search or seizure."[77] These rights are "subject only to such reasonable limits prescribed by law as can be demonstrably justified in a free and democratic society".[78]

All of these sources of law, along with public health guidelines and professional practice standards, point generally to the presumption that HIV testing in Canada should be performed only with the informed consent of the person to be tested. Indeed, HIV testing policies ordinarily involve a relatively elaborate process of pre-test counseling, consent, and post-test counseling.[79] These policies have not been rooted in specific judicial decisions[80] or legislation and therefore occasionally spark controversy.

Advances in testing technology now permit both rapid HIV screening and home testing for HIV. Rapid testing is generally considered to provide significant advantages over older screening methods.[81] Yet rapid testing also creates the risk of an expansion of testing to new situations in which truly voluntary testing and counseling may be more difficult to achieve.[82] The Public Health Agency of Canada recommendations for health care professionals on rapid HIV tests note the importance of adhering to the "three C's" but recognize the difficulties of

---

[76]   *Ibid.*, s. 7.

[77]   *Ibid.*, s. 8.

[78]   *Ibid.*, s. 1.

[79]   Public Health Agency of Canada, "HIV Testing and Counselling: Policies in Transition?" (2007) (research paper prepared for the International Public Health Dialogue on HIV Testing and Counseling, Toronto, 17 August 2006), online: <http://www.phac-aspc.gc.ca/aids-sida/publication/hivtest/index-eng.php> at 22-26.

[80]   *Ibid.* See also *Canadian AIDS Society v. Ontario*, [1996] O.J. No. 4184, 31 O.R. (3d) 798 (Ont. C.A.), leave to appeal to S.C.C. refused [1997] S.C.C.A. No. 33 (S.C.C.) (court assumes without deciding an issue involving informed consent and HIV testing, noting, "It is better that the issue whether this sense of moral obligation is a legal one be decided in a case which depends upon this issue for its result" (at para. 3)).

[81]   See Canadian HIV/AIDS Legal Network, "Rapid HIV testing" in *HIV Testing* (2007) (series of 12 information sheets on HIV testing in Canada), online: <http://www.aidslaw.ca/publications/publicationsdocEN.php?ref=713> at 1 (noting possible benefits of rapid testing include great client satisfaction and increased likelihood that clients will receive results).

[82]   *Ibid.* (noting in particular the risks of rapid HIV testing during labour and delivery); Joanne Csete & Richard Elliott, "Prevention and Protection: Enhancing Both HIV and Human Rights in Canada" (2007) at 5, online: Canadian HIV/AIDS Legal Network <http://www.aidslaw.ca/publications/interfaces/downloadFile.php?ref=1065> at 20-27 (detailed description of risks, benefits and recommendations for rapid screening); Public Health Agency of Canada, "HIV Testing and Counselling: Policies in Transition?" (2007) (research paper prepared for the International Public Health Dialogue on HIV Testing and Counseling, Toronto, 17 August 2006), online: <http://www.phac-aspc.gc.ca/aids-sida/publication/hivtest/index-eng.php> at 50-51.

achieving this standard for tests used in some circumstances, such as during labour and delivery.[83]

Home testing presents a different set of issues. Should Canadians have access to home tests for HIV infection available in other jurisdictions even though pre- and post-test counseling might be conducted through written materials or phone counselors rather than through face-to-face counseling? Canada's Therapeutic Products Program has not yet approved any home HIV test, in part because of significant concerns about the accuracy of positive or negative results and the suitability of telephone counseling.[84] Some HIV policy commentators contend that the benefits of expanded testing might outweigh the risks of home testing, at least within a carefully regulated framework.[85]

An even more complex set of issues have been raised by arguments that testing should be expanded and perhaps even mandated when testing will protect health and safety or when the testing will be imposed on individuals whose liberties are restricted, such as prisoners. These issues will be considered in the next section of this chapter.

(ii)   Limits on Voluntariness

Countries around the world have considered a wide range of HIV testing programs since 1985. Canadian policy-makers have generally resisted calls to make HIV testing mandatory, with only a few exceptions. Proposals to limit the detailed counseling and consent process for HIV testing typically have at least one of three objectives: (1) eliminating "exceptionalism"; (2) protecting health and safety, particularly for third parties; and (3) protecting Canada from the costs and risks of infectious disease. The inclination to expand HIV testing into new spheres is fuelled

---

[83]   Public Health Agency of Canada, "Point-of-Care HIV Testing Using Rapid HIV Test Kits: Guidance for Health-Care Professionals" (2007) 33:S2 CCDR 1, online: <http://www.phac-aspc.gc.ca/publicat/ccdr-rmtc/07pdf/33s2-eng.pdf> at 4. See also Joanne Csete & Richard Elliott, "Prevention and Protection: Enhancing Both HIV Testing and Human Rights in Canada 5" (2007), online: Canadian HIV/AIDS Legal Network <http://www.aidslaw.ca/publications/interfaces/downloadFile.php?ref=1065> at 20-25.

[84]   Public Health Agency of Canada, "HIV Testing and Counselling: Policies in Transition?" (2007) (research paper prepared for the International Public Health Dialogue on HIV Testing and Counseling, Toronto, 17 August 2006), online: <http://www.phac-aspc.gc.ca/aids-sida/publication/hivtest/index-eng.php> at 49-50; Canadian HIV/AIDS Legal Network, "Home HIV testing information sheet" in *HIV Testing* (2007) (series of 12 information sheets on HIV testing in Canada), online: <http://www.aidslaw.ca/publications/publications docEN.php?ref=713>.

[85]   Canadian HIV/AIDS Legal Network, "Home HIV testing information sheet" in *HIV Testing* (2007) (series of 12 information sheets on HIV testing in Canada), online: <http://www.aidslaw.ca/publications/publicationsdocEN.php?ref=713>; "Home HIV testing: Why not in Canada?" (2000) 162 C.M.A.J. 1545.

as well by advances in technology that can reduce the time between test and result to a matter of minutes.[86] Rapid test results could be used immediately by decision-makers in a broad range of contexts, such as in altering the course of care for women in labour or for guiding the decision of whether to undergo post-exposure prophylactic treatment to reduce the risk of transmission.

Opponents of HIV exceptionalism argue that HIV tests should be treated much like any other test that can provide important information about the health needs of the individual to be tested. HIV testing should be made "routine" whenever administration would be medically appropriate. The definition of "routine" varies. To some, testing could be performed whenever an individual has given a general consent for care and treatment. Others favour routine programs using the "opt-out" or "opt-in" procedures described above. Advocates for making HIV tests routine note the benefits to be derived by the individual and to society from the early identification and possible treatment of HIV infection. Opponents of routine HIV testing note that HIV testing carries special emotional, social and financial risks due to the stigma and discrimination still associated with the disease. Opponents also express skepticism about the benefits of testing in the absence of counseling, support services, and adequate medical treatment.

There has been a shift toward making HIV testing programs more routine in at least some circumstances over the past decade. One example involves the routine screening of pregnant women and/or newborns. Public health authorities and legislatures in the United States moved toward opt-out routine HIV screening for pregnant women and routine or mandatory screening for newborns once therapies became available to reduce the risk of perinatal transmission.[87] Most Canadian provinces have implemented some version of routine perinatal HIV screening program, most often via guidelines issued by public health officials or physician groups.[88] Provinces differ in offering either "opt-in" or "opt-out" routine

---

[86]   See generally Canadian HIV/AIDS Legal Network, "Rapid HIV testing" in *HIV Testing* (2007) (series of 12 information sheets on HIV testing in Canada), online: <http://www. aidslaw.ca/publications/publicationsdocEN.php?ref=713>; and Public Health Agency of Canada, "Point-of-Care HIV Testing Using Rapid HIV Test Kits: Guidance for Health-Care Professionals" (2007) 33:S2 CCDR 1, online: <http://www.phac-aspc.gc.ca/ publicat/ccdr-rmtc/07pdf/33s2-eng.pdf>.

[87]   See, *e.g.*, U.S. CDC, "Revised Recommendations for HIV Screening in Pregnant Women" (9 November 2001) 50 MMWR Recomm Rep. (RR19) 59. Some jurisdictions in the U.S. began to require HIV screening for newborns, with or without parental consent. U.S. CDC, "HIV Testing Among Pregnant Women — United States and Canada, 1998-2001" (15 November 2002) 51 MMWR 1013.

[88]   See David R. Burdge *et al.*, "Canadian consensus guidelines for the management of pregnant HIV-positive women and their offspring" (24 June 2003) 168 C.M.A.J. 1683,

perinatal screening.[89] The "opt-out" programs are generally thought to result in higher levels of HIV testing but public health officials in Ontario have been able to achieve similar rates in an "opt-in" testing program.[90] A study of Alberta's "opt-out" program demonstrates high rates of testing but also raises concerns given that only two-thirds of respondents "always informed women that they have a choice to decline" testing.[91]

The second challenge to the principle of voluntariness has come in cases where it has been argued that less-than-totally-voluntary testing will protect the health and safety of third parties. Proponents of routine HIV screening note that individuals receiving positive results can change their behaviour to avoid transmitting the virus to others. The clearest and least controversial example of testing to protect third parties occurs during the blood donation process in Canada and elsewhere.[92] Screening programs

online: Canadian Medical Association Journal <http://www.cmaj.ca/cgi/data/168/13/1671/DC1/1> (note that appendix is available only online); U.S. CDC, "HIV Testing Among Pregnant Women — United States and Canada, 1998-2001" (15 November 2002) 51 MMWR 1013 (reporting higher rates of HIV testing in Provinces with "opt-out" than in "opt-in" testing programs); Gayatri C. Jayaraman, Jutta K. Preiksaitis & Bryce Larke, "Mandatory reporting of HIV infection and opt-out prenatal screening for HIV infection: effect on testing rates" (18 March 2003) 168 C.M.A.J. 679 (increase in testing rates associated with opt-out prenatal testing program).

[89]   Public Health Agency of Canada, "HIV Testing and Counselling: Policies in Transition?" (2007) (research paper prepared for the International Public Health Dialogue on HIV Testing and Counseling, Toronto, 17 August 2006), online: <http://www.phac-aspc.gc.ca/aids-sida/publication/hivtest/index-eng.php> at 26-27. Seven provinces and territories offer opt-out testing. Public Health Agency of Canada, "HIV/AIDS Epi Updates, November 2007" at 43-44 (Alberta, Manitoba, New Brunswick, Newfoundland and Labrador, Québec, the Northwest Territories and Nunavut). Three provinces use the opt-in strategy (British Columbia, Yukon, Saskatchewan, Nova Scotia, Ontario and Prince Edward Island) (ibid.).

[90]   "Opt-in" programs generally have lower rates of testing than "opt-out" programs; however, Ontario demonstrated that "a high rate of HIV testing for pregnant women can be achieved through voluntary opt-in testing using multiple approaches to promote the intervention ... [O]verall the rates currently being achieved are as high as some jurisdictions using the opt-out approach". Public Health Agency of Canada, "HIV Testing and Counselling: Policies in Transition?" (2007) (research paper prepared for the International Public Health Dialogue on HIV Testing and Counseling, Toronto, 17 August 2006), online: <http://www.phac-aspc.gc.ca/aids-sida/publication/hivtest/index-eng.php> at 26-27.

[91]   Ibid., at 27.

[92]   See for example Canadian Blood Services, "HIV and AIDS", online: <http://www.bloodservices.ca/CentreApps/Internet/UW_V502_MainEngine.nsf/page/E_HIV+and+AIDS?OpenDocument> (discussing testing policy). There appears to be little debate about the necessity for and validity of HIV testing for donors or blood or other tissues/organs capable of transmitting HIV. Ralf Jürgens, "Consent" in HIV Testing and Confidentiality: Final Report (2001), online: Canadian HIV/AIDS Legal Network <http://www.aidslaw.ca/publications/interfaces/downloadFile.php?ref=282>. Unlinked anonymous screening ("UAS") of blood and tissue samples is also conducted without specific informed consent of individual though within a carefully reviewed ethical framework (ibid.); D. Coburn, "Guidelines on ethical and legal considerations in anonymous unlinked HIV seroprevalence research" (1991) 144 C.M.A.J. 1603.

for pregnant women and newborns, discussed above, could be justified on this basis. Other, more controversial proposals advanced but not broadly accepted include mandatory HIV-testing for health care patients, health care providers, or prisoners.[93]

One form of testing to protect third parties — post-exposure testing — has gained legislative and judicial support in Canada. In general, post-exposure testing involves allowing a person exposed to the blood or body fluids of another to require the "source" individual to undergo testing for HIV or other bloodborne pathogens. Those favouring post-exposure testing argue that it can provide important information that could be used to make decisions about whether to undergo prophylactic anti-retroviral treatment to reduce the risk of HIV transmission.[94] The availability of rapid testing has increased the strength of this justification because prophylactic treatment must be started quickly to maximize effectiveness. Critics of post-exposure testing argue that the results usually are ambiguous and often useless by the time they are obtained;[95] they

---

[93]   Some health care providers have argued that routine HIV screening should be employed before patients undergo surgical procedures that might present a risk of HIV exposure to their caregivers. See Canadian HIV/AIDS Legal Network, "Mandatory and compulsory testing for HIV" in *HIV Testing* (2007) (series of 12 information sheets on HIV testing in Canada), online: <http://www.aidslaw.ca/publications/publicationsdocEN.php?ref=713> at 1 (discussing proposals to test health care patients); K. Chapman *et al.*, "Testing patients for HIV before surgery: the views of doctors performing surgery" (1995) 7 AIDS Care 125 (significant percentage of anonymously surveyed doctors at two London teaching hospitals favoured some sort of mandatory screening). Publicity surrounding an HIV-infected surgeon in Montréal led the Québec Medical Association to adopt a policy requiring physicians to know their HIV status and for HIV-positive physicians to disclose the information to their employers. Canadian HIV/AIDS Legal Network, "Mandatory and compulsory testing for HIV" in *HIV Testing* (2007) (series of 12 information sheets on HIV testing in Canada), online: <http://www.aidslaw.ca/publications/publicationsdocEN.php?ref =713> at 1-2 (noting policy and disputing rationale). A correctional officers union proposed amending federal legislation to permit "compulsory testing of inmates in federal prisons for HIV and other infectious diseases" (*ibid.*) (noting 2006 proposal and disputing the rationale).

[94]   Post-exposure prophylactic ("PEP") treatment to prevent HIV infection should be started within hours of the exposure to be effective: U.S. CDC, "Updated U.S. Public Health Service Guidelines for the Management of Occupational Exposures to HIV and Recommendations for Postexposure Prophylaxis" (30 September 2005) 54 MMWR Recomm Rep. (RR9) 1, 8.

[95]   If common antibody tests are used, a negative test result does not mean that the source individual is uninfected; the person could have a recent HIV infection without having detectable HIV antibodies, resulting in a false negative test result. Critics of post-exposure testing argue that the unreliability of a negative test eliminates the utility of testing; persons exposed to the blood or body fluids of another might just proceed on the assumption that they might have been exposed to HIV. Proponents of post-exposure testing argue that a positive antibody test result would be meaningful to a person deciding whether to undergo PEP and that directly testing for viral RNA would be even more effective. See, Canadian HIV/AIDS Legal Network, "Mandatory and compulsory testing for HIV" in *HIV*

therefore contend any benefits from testing are greatly outweighed by the intrusion on individual liberty associated with a mandatory test.

The post-exposure testing debate in Canada involves many different types of possible exposure to HIV. Some persons may have been exposed to HIV during a sexual assault or other crime involving exposure to bodily substances. Other people may have been exposed to HIV when providing emergency medical care, such as the scene of accidents. Police officers or correctional employees are sometimes exposed to bodily fluids from suspects or prisoners in their custody. More broadly, health care providers may be exposed to the bodily fluids of patients due to exposure incidents in proving non-emergency care, such as through needle-sticks.

The early debate arose in the courts when survivors of sexual offences asked that the accused or convicted sex offender undergo testing for HIV. Until relatively recently, there was no statutory authorization for this type of testing in Canada.[96] Post-exposure testing of persons convicted or accused of sexual offences was permitted in other jurisdictions such as in the United States.[97] Concerns about the true benefits of testing are particularly acute in these cases as the time lag between exposure and testing is likely to be quite long. A Québec court rejected a request for testing where the source individual was merely accused of committing the offence.[98] In *R. v. J.P.B.*, the court entered an order requiring HIV testing of a defendant convicted of sexual assault.[99] The case is only of narrow applicability because the order was based on a general authorization for judicial orders under the *Young Offenders Act*.[100] An Ontario trial court

---

Testing (2007) (series of 12 information sheets on HIV testing in Canada), online: <http://www.aidslaw.ca/publications/publicationsdocEN.php?ref=713> at 2-3. In a few reported decisions, criminal defendants have agreed to undergo HIV testing. See, *e.g.*, *R. v. Luu*, [2006] O.J. No. 1083, 2006 CarswellOnt 1689 (Ont. C.J.); and *R. v. T. (J.E.)*, [2005] B.C.J. No. 206, 2005 BCPC 26, [2005] B.C.W.L.D. 2843, [2005] W.D.F.L. 1885 (B.C. Prov. Ct.).

[96] Canadian HIV/AIDS Legal Network, "Mandatory and compulsory testing for HIV" in *HIV Testing* (2007) (series of 12 information sheets on HIV testing in Canada), online: <http://www.aidslaw.ca/publications/publicationsdocEN.php?ref=713> at 2-3.

[97] William E. Adams, Jr. *et al.*, *AIDS: Cases and Materials* (Durham: Carolina Academic Press, 2002) at 90-97.

[98] Canadian HIV/AIDS Legal Network, "Rapid HIV Screening at the Point of Care: Legal and Ethical Questions" (2000) at 61, online: <http://www.aidslaw.ca/publications/publicationsdocEN.php?ref=284> (citing *R. v. Beaulieu*, [1992] J.Q. no 2046, [1992] R.J.Q. 2959, (Que. Ct.))

[99] *R. v. J.P.B.*, [1992] N.W.T.J. No. 207, [1993] N.W.T.R. 65, [1993] 2 W.W.R. 414 (N.W.T. Terr. Ct.) [*J.P.B.* cited to N.W.T.R.]. See also Canadian HIV/AIDS Legal Network, "Rapid HIV Screening at the Point of Care: Legal and Ethical Questions" (2000), online: <http://www.aidslaw.ca/publications/publicationsdocEN. php?ref=284> at 61.

[100] The court noted that "pursuant to the *Young Offenders Act*, s. 20(1), an Order may be made which is in the best interest of the young person and the public" and may "impose on the young person such other reasonable and ancillary conditions as it deems advisable and in the best interest of the young person and the public" (*J.P.B.*, *ibid.* at para. 10).

also issued an order compelling a person convicted of sexual assault to undergo HIV testing, but the same judge later refused to enter a new testing order involving the same parties, noting that "[i]n the absence of statutory authority, the court must proceed with caution".[101] What little case law there is thus suggests that courts in Canada would be reluctant to authorize post-exposure testing in sexual assault cases without statutory authorization.

The Uniform Law Conference of Canada issued a report and a model act governing post-exposure testing in 2004.[102] The Model Act represents an effort to balance "[s]ource individuals' *Charter*-protected rights to privacy and security" against "the interests of exposed individuals, the interests of other individuals, and the public interest in their health and well being".[103] The Act broadly covers individuals exposed to the source individual's bodily substances "as a result of being a victim of crime"; "while providing emergency health services or emergency first aid to that individual"; or "while performing any prescribed function in relation to that individual".[104] The Act requires evidence in the form of a physician's report that there is a significant

---

[101]   *C. (D.) v. 371148 Ontario Ltd.*, [1997] O.J. No. 2367, 13 C.P.C. (4th) 132 (Ont. Gen. Div.), Macdonald J. The case involved Paul Bernardo. The original order was unpublished but the court reproduced the terms in a subsequent proceeding (at para. 1):

> In September 1996, I ordered that the Defendant, Paul Bernardo, submit himself for testing for AIDS and other sexually transmitted diseases by providing a sufficient quantity of blood samples for that purpose. I reproduce paragraphs 1 and 2 of the September order. ...
>
> THIS COURT ORDERS that the Defendant Paul Bernardo presently in the custody of Correctional Services, Canada submit himself for testing for aids [*sic*] and other sexually transmitted diseases and provide a duly qualified medical person appointed by Correctional Services, Canada with a sufficient quantity of his blood for that purpose. ...

[102]   Uniform Law Conference of Canada (Mandatory Testing and Disclosure Working Group), *Uniform Mandatory Testing and Disclosure Act (Draft and Commentary)*, n.d., online: <http://www.ulcc.ca/en/us/Uniform_Mandatory_Testing_and_Disclosure_Act_Draft_En.pdf> [*Uniform Mandatory Testing and Disclosure Act*]. The report notes that

> [u]nder current law, an individual exposed to the risk of communicable disease infection ... does not have an efficacious means to compel the source individual to provide a bodily sample for assessment and treatment purposes. The lack of this type of legal mechanism is a particular concern for emergency services providers, peace officers, and correctional officers ... [who] may be exposed to risks of communicable disease infection in the course of their work ...

Ibid., at 1. For a discussion of the Model Act and related legislative initiatives, see Richard Elliott, "Undue Force: An Overview of Provincial Legislation on Forced Testing for HIV" (2007), online: Canadian HIV/AIDS Legal Network <http://www.aidslaw.ca/publications/interfaces/downloadFile.php?ref=1210>.

[103]   *Uniform Mandatory Testing and Disclosure Act*, *ibid.*, at 1.

[104]   *Ibid.*, at 5-6 (s. 3).

health risk to the exposed person.[105] The Act gives an exposed individual the right to seek a testing order from a provincial superior court requiring that a medical officer ensure that a sample is taken and analysed by appropriate personnel.[106] The Act puts in place restrictions on the use of the test result.[107]

Four provinces — Alberta, Nova Scotia, Ontario and Saskatchewan — now have legislation based on the Model Act.[108] These provinces have followed the basic structure of the Act while modifying the group of exposed persons, the application procedures and the penalties for offences. For example, Alberta's statute focuses on persons who "ha[ve] come into contact with a bodily substance of a source individual ... while providing emergency assistance" or "while performing duties as a firefighter, paramedic or peace officer".[109] It does not expressly cover persons who might have been exposed to bodily substances as the result of criminal conduct. The Alberta legislation is unique in that it authorizes issuance of a testing order that requires the medical officer to check the "communicable diseases databases", which might mean that the source individual is never required to provide a sample.[110]

Ontario covers the categories of exposed persons identified in the Model Act but then adds a new category: a person exposed "[i]n the course of his or her duties, if the person belongs to a prescribed class".[111] The regulations provide that the "prescribed class" includes correctional employees, employees of police forces, firefighters, paramedics and paramedic students, nurses, physicians, and medical students.[112] Ontario thus appears to have greatly expanded the scope of mandatory testing to cover a wide range of occupational exposures.

---

[105] *Ibid.*, at 8 (s. 4).

[106] *Ibid.*, at 1-2. Under the Act, "[d]isobeying a testing order is an offense". *Ibid.*, at 2.

[107] *Ibid.*, at 2.

[108] Some of these jurisdictions now also have issued regulations under the Acts. See, *e.g.*, *Mandatory Testing and Disclosure Act*, S.A. 2006, c. M-3.5; *Mandatory Testing and Disclosure Regulation*, Alta. Reg. 190/2007; *Mandatory Testing and Disclosure Act*, S.N.S. 2004, c. 29; *Mandatory Testing and Disclosure Regulations*, O.I.C. 2006-246, N.S. Reg. 75/2006; *Mandatory Blood Testing Act, 2006*, S.O. 2006, c. 26; O. Reg. 449/07; *Mandatory Testing and Disclosure (Bodily Substances) Act*, S.S. 2005, c. M-2.1. See also Richard Elliott, "Undue Force: An Overview of Provincial Legislation on Forced Testing for HIV" (2007), online: Canadian HIV/AIDS Legal Network <http://www.aidslaw.ca/publications/interfaces/downloadFile.php?ref=1210> (analyzing the legislation).

[109] *Mandatory Testing and Disclosure Act*, S.A. 2006, c. M-3.5, s. 3(1). The Act also covers individuals "while being involved in a circumstance or activity described in the regulations", but the regulations are silent on this point (*ibid.*): Alta. Reg. 190/2007 (*Mandatory Testing and Disclosure Regulation*).

[110] *Mandatory Testing and Disclosure Act*, S.A. 2006, c. M-3.5, s. 4(3).

[111] *Mandatory Blood Testing Act, 2006*, S.O. 2006, c. 26, s. 2.

[112] Reg. 449/07, s. 3.

There are also significant differences in the provincial rules governing the timeline for applications and orders, the strength of the rules protecting the confidentiality of the sample and test results, and the penalties for violation of the mandatory testing schemes.[113] Critics of post-exposure testing argue that it violates the *Charter*;[114] given the often-limited benefits of post-exposure testing for the person exposed, courts may be unwilling to find the intrusion on bodily integrity or the search and seizure of blood samples to be reasonable or necessary.[115]

The final justification for the expansion of HIV testing involves the protection of countries from the "importation" of disease as well as from the expenses associated with providing medical treatment. These HIV testing programs have been repeatedly rejected in international guidelines.[116] The United States recently moved to amend its immigration law to permit persons with HIV to obtain visas.[117]

---

[113]   Richard Elliott, "Undue Force: An Overview of Provincial Legislation on Forced Testing for HIV" (2007), online: Canadian HIV/AIDS Legal Network <http://www.aidslaw.ca/publications/interfaces/downloadFile.php?ref=1210> (analysing the legislation).

[114]   See for example Richard Elliott, "Undue Force: An Overview of Provincial Legislation on Forced Testing for HIV" (2007), online: Canadian HIV/AIDS Legal Network <http://www.aidslaw.ca/publications/interfaces/downloadFile.php?ref=1210> at 19-20; Canadian HIV/AIDS Legal Network, "Rapid HIV Screening at the Point of Care: Legal and Ethical Questions" (2000), online: <http://www.aidslaw.ca/publications/publicationsdoc EN.php?ref=284> at 51-52; Theodore de Bruyn, "Occupational Exposure to HIV and Forced HIV Testing: Questions and Answers" (2002), online: Canadian HIV/AIDS Legal Network <http://www.aidslaw.ca/publications/publicationsdocEN.php?ref=278>.

[115]   Richard Elliott, "Undue Force: An Overview of Provincial Legislation on Forced Testing for HIV" (2007), online: Canadian HIV/AIDS Legal Network <http://www.aidslaw.ca/publications/interfaces/downloadFile.php?ref=1210> at 19-20. See also Richard Elliott, "Legislation to Authorize Forced Testing for HIV in the Event of Occupational Exposure: An Unjustified and Unnecessary Rights Violation: A submission to the Government of Manitoba" (April 2008) at 17-26, online: Canadian HIV/AIDS Legal Network, <http://www.aidslaw.ca/publications/publicationsdocEN.php?ref=849>. The *Charter*'s protection of privacy will be considered in Section III (c), below.

[116]   Joint United Nations Programme on HIV/AIDS (UNAIDS) and International Organization for Migration (IOM), "UNAIDS/IOM Statement on HIV/AIDS-Related Travel Restrictions" (June 2004) at 3 (citing statements of other international organizations), online: UNAIDS <http://www.unaids.org/en/PolicyAndPractice/KeyPopulations/PeopleHIV/mobility_technical_policies.asp>. Continuing concerns about the issue led UNAIDS to establish a new International Task Team on HIV-related Travel Restrictions charged with drafting new recommendations "toward the elimination of HIV-specific restrictions". See "Third meeting of the International Task Team on HIV-related Travel Restrictions" (18 July 2008) (noting that recommendations expected to be finalized and submitted in November/December 2008), online: UNAIDS <http://www.unaids.org/en/KnowledgeCentre/Resources/FeatureStories/archive/2008/20080718_travel_restrictions.asp>.

[117]   Associated Press, "House Passes Broader Plan to Fight AIDS" *The New York Times* (2 July 2008), online: *The New York Times* <http://www.nytimes.com/2008/07/25/washington/25aids.html?ref=world> (House sending bill to President for signature amending 8 U.S.C.A. §1182 (West 2007) which provided that aliens ineligible for a visa or admission

Under Canada's federal *Immigration and Refugee Immigration Act*[118] and regulations, various categories of visitors and immigration applicants are required to undergo a medical examination, which can include routine testing for HIV infection.[119] Canada no longer argues that HIV testing is necessary to protect public health, except for visitors intending to work in certain jobs which are likely to present the risk of exposure to their blood or body fluids.[120] The immigration testing rules are instead justified as necessary to implement the Act's provisions making inadmissible certain categories of applicants who are "reasonably ... expected to cause excessive demand on health or social services".[121] Limits on the *Charter*'s applicability[122] restrict legal challenges to HIV testing in this area.

---

included those "who ... [were] determined (in accordance with regulations prescribed by the Secretary of Health and Human Services) to have a communicable disease of public health significance, which shall include infection with the etiologic agent for acquired immune deficiency syndrome").

[118] *Immigration and Refugee Protection Act*, S.C. 2001, c. 27.

[119] Citizenship and Immigration Canada, *Designated Medical Practitioner Handbook*, online: <http://www.cic.gc.ca/english/resources/publications/dmp-handbook/index.asp>. See also Canadian HIV/AIDS Legal Network, "Canada's immigration policy as it affects people living with HIV/AIDS" (February 2007), online: <http://www.aidslaw.ca/publications/publicationsdocEN.php?ref=97>.

[120] *Immigration and Refugee Protection Regulations*, S.O.R./2002-227, s. 30(1)(*b*). See also Canadian HIV/AIDS Legal Network, "Canada's immigration policy", *ibid.*

[121] *Immigration and Refugee Protection Act*, S.C. 2001, c. 27 ("IRPA"), s. 38(1)(*c*). See also, Tim Fankin, "Supreme Court clarifies immigration medical inadmissibility provision" (2006) 11:1 Canadian HIV/AIDS Pol'y & L. Rev. 37 (discussing whether S.C.C. decision requiring individualized determination in case of business-class immigrants involving excessive demand on social services might be applied to cases involving claims of excessive demand on the public health system due to HIV infection).

[122] For an extensive commentary, see Canadian HIV/AIDS Legal Network, "HIV/AIDS and Immigration: Final Report" (2001), online: <http://www.aidslaw.ca/publications/publicationsdocEN.php?ref=103>. See also *Chiarelli v. Canada (Minister of Employment & Immigration)*, [1992] S.C.J. No. 27, [1992] 1 S.C.R. 711, 90 D.L.R. (4th) 289 (S.C.C.) (discussing interaction of s. 6 of the *Charter*, governing mobility rights, with the *Immigration Act, 1976*, S.C. 1976-77, c. 52), *Chesters v. Canada (Minister of Citizenship & Immigration)*, [2002] F.C.J. No. 992, [2003] 1 F.C. 361 (F.C.T.D.) (examining application of *Charter* to case involving medical examination; noting that entry into Canada by persons who are not citizens or permanent residents "is a privilege and its grant lies within the purview of the Canadian government ..." (*ibid.*, at para. 120)). See also *Covarrubias v. Canada (Minister of Citizenship and Immigration)*, [2006] F.C.J. No. 1682, 2006 FCA 65, [2007] 3 F.C.R. 169 (F.C.A.) (*in dicta* dealing with statutory interpretation, noting that "where a country makes a deliberate attempt to persecute or discriminate against a person by deliberately allocating insufficient resources for the treatment and care of that person's illness or disability, as has happened in some countries with patients suffering from HIV/AIDS, that person may qualify under ... [subparagraph 97(1)(*b*)(iv) of the *IRPA*], for this would be refusal to provide the care and not inability to do so" (*ibid.*, at para. 39)).

(c)   Privacy, Confidentiality and Reporting to Public Health Authorities

(i)   Privacy and Confidentiality

An HIV test involves more than an invasion into one's bodily integrity and revelation of personal information. The value (and potential harm) of testing is closely related to the use made of the test results. A test on its own is useless; the result must be given to someone — such as the person tested — for the test to be meaningful. Different testing techniques yield different amounts of information about the person tested. Anonymous testing reveals the least information as the person undergoing testing uses a code to retrieve their result. "Non-nominal" testing also uses a code system rather than the individual's name, but the physician ordering the test will know the identity of the person tested. Under "nominal" testing, the identity of the person being tested is readily linked to the test result. Anonymous testing is sometimes controversial: anonymity may encourage some to undergo testing but this same characteristic might make it difficult for health care providers to provide follow-up or to collect accurate data about the spread of the infection in a population.[123]

Information about positive test results theoretically could be made available for use in everything from individual medical decisions to government budget planning. Individuals infected with HIV generally seek to limit disclosure of the information to prevent stigma and discrimination.[124] The release of HIV-related information is subject to legal constraints at both the provincial and federal levels of government.[125]

---

[123]   Public Health Agency of Canada, "HIV Testing and Counselling: Policies in Transition?" (2007) (research paper prepared for the International Public Health Dialogue on HIV Testing and Counseling, Toronto, 17 August 2006), online: <http://www.phac-aspc.gc.ca/aids-sida/publication/hivtest/index-eng.php> at 24-26.

[124]   Public Health Agency of Canada, "HIV Testing and Counselling: Policies in Transition?" (2007) (research paper prepared for the International Public Health Dialogue on HIV Testing and Counseling, Toronto, 17 August 2006), online: <http://www.phac-aspc.gc.ca/aids-sida/publication/hivtest/index-eng.php> at 46-47 (discussing issues of stigma and discrimination for people living with HIV infection); and Canadian HIV/AIDS Legal Network, "Confidentiality" in *HIV Testing* (2007) (series of 12 information sheets on HIV testing in Canada), online: <http://www.aidslaw.ca/publications/publicationsdocEN.php?ref=713>. See also Richard Elliott & Jennifer Gold, "Protection against discrimination based on HIV/AIDS status in Canada: the legal framework" (2005) 10:1 Canadian HIV/AIDS Pol'y & L. Rev. 20.

[125]   See generally Canadian HIV/AIDS Legal Network, "Privacy Protection and the Disclosure of Health Information: Legal Issues for People Living with HIV/AIDS in Canada" (2004), online: <http://www.aidslaw.ca/publications/publicationsdocEN.php?ref=189>; and Canadian HIV/AIDS Legal Network, "Confidentiality" in *HIV Testing* (2007) (series of 12 information sheets on HIV testing in Canada), online: <http://www.aidslaw.ca/

Once again, some of the key debates involve determining the proper level of governmental regulation; balancing the individual's liberty interests with the need to protect health and safety; and promoting or avoiding HIV exceptionalism. The remainder of this subsection will review the scope of legal protection for the confidentiality of HIV-related information. Subsection III (c) (*ii*) in this chapter will apply these principles to a key public health strategy focused on case identification: names-based reporting of HIV infection to public health authorities in Canada.

There are many potential sources of an obligation to limit the disclosure of HIV test results. The Canadian HIV/AIDS Legal Network, in its extensive report on privacy protections for persons with HIV infection, suggests distinguishing between an individual's right to privacy, a duty owed by some persons in some circumstances to maintain confidentiality, and the evidentiary rules of privilege.[126] Despite the number of sources protecting the privacy of some types of information, an individual with HIV infection does not have the absolute right to control the disclosure of information about his or her status. Each source of protection has limits and exceptions.

Canadian courts have found a constitutionally-protected right of privacy in the *Charter*, particularly ss. 7 and 8.[127] (For further discussion, see Chapter 4, "Public Health Information Privacy and Confidentiality".) In contrast to the relatively robust constitutional protection of privacy interests, privacy has not been well-protected at common law in Canada.[128] In *Caltagirone v. Scozzari-Cloutier*, the court considered whether a plaintiff's aunt could be held liable for disclosing his HIV status to other

publications/publicationsdocEN.php?ref=713>. See also, Special Issue: Privacy Law (2006) 43:3 Alta. L. Rev. 549-551.

[126] Canadian HIV/AIDS Legal Network, "Privacy Protection and the Disclosure of Health Information: Legal Issues for People Living with HIV/AIDS in Canada" (2004), online: <http://www.aidslaw.ca/publications/publicationsdocEN.php?ref=189> at 2-3.

[127] Section 7 of the *Charter* gives "[e]veryone ... the right to ... liberty and security of the person and the right not to be deprived thereof except in accordance with the principles of fundamental justice": *Canadian Charter of Rights and Freedoms*, s. 7, Part I of the *Constitution Act, 1982*, being Schedule B to the *Canada Act 1982* (U.K.), 1982, c. 11. Section 8 gives "[e]veryone the right to be secure against unreasonable search or seizure" (*ibid.*). See also Richard B. Bruyer, "Privacy: A Review and Critique of the Literature" (2006) 43 Alta. L. Rev. 553 (critiquing grounding of privacy in liberty).

[128] Canadian HIV/AIDS Legal Network, "Privacy Protection and the Disclosure of Health Information: Legal Issues for People Living with HIV/AIDS in Canada" (2004), online: <http://www.aidslaw.ca/publications/publicationsdocEN.php?ref=189> at 17. See also Russell Brown, "Rethinking Privacy: Exclusivity, Private Relation and Tort Law" (2006) 43 Alta. L. Rev. 589; Robyn M. Ryan Bell, "Tort of Invasion of Privacy — Has its Time Finally Come?" in Todd Archibald & Michael Cochrane, eds., *Annual Review of Civil Litigation* (Toronto: Thomson Carswell, 2005) at 225.

relatives of the plaintiff during a "heated argument".[129] The court rejected a claim for intentional infliction of emotional distress because the defendant did not have the requisite intent to cause the plaintiff any mental distress.[130] The court noted the lack of guidance regarding the principles to be used in common law breach of privacy claims[131] and offered its own analysis of the essential elements.[132] The court concluded that the aunt's conduct constituted an actionable breach of privacy but that the plaintiff had failed to prove that the breach caused his injuries.[133]

Some types of relationships — such as the physician-patient relationship — give rise to specific confidentiality duties,[134] as may standards of care applicable to health care professionals and facilities.[135]

The balance between individual liberty and other public needs noted in the constitutional analysis is repeated under the common law. The common law duty to maintain confidentiality typically includes a series of exceptions designed to protect the patient, other individuals, and society at

---

[129]   *Caltagirone v. Scozzari-Cloutier*, 2007 WL 3077446, 2007 CarswellOnt 6753 (Ont. S.C.J.).

[130]   *Ibid.*, at paras. 6-9.

[131]   *Ibid.*, at paras. 10-13.

[132]   According to the court:

[T]he tort could be structured through answers to the following questions:

1.   Is the information acquired, collected, disclosed or published of a kind that a reasonable person would consider private?

2.   Has the Plaintiff consented to acquisition or collection of the information?

3.   If not, has the information been acquired or collected for a legal process or public interest reason? If so, what is that reason?

4.   Has the Plaintiff consented to disclosure or publication of the information?

5.   If not, has the information been disclosed or published for a legal process or public interest reason? If so, what is that reason?

6.   Is the legal process or public interest reason put forward for acquisition, collection, disclosure or publication one that a reasonable person would consider outweighs the interest of the individual in keeping the information private? …

If, at the end of the analysis, one finds either no legal process or public interest reason for acquisition, collection, disclosure or publication of the information, or the legal process or public interest reason is outweighed by the private interest, then an actionable breach of privacy has occurred.

Ibid., at paras. 21-22.

[133]   *Ibid.*, at paras. 23-33.

[134]   Canadian HIV/AIDS Legal Network, "Privacy Protection and the Disclosure of Health Information: Legal Issues for People Living with HIV/AIDS in Canada" (2004), online: <http://www.aidslaw.ca/publications/publicationsdocEN.php?ref=189> at 18-19. See also *McInerney v. MacDonald*, [1992] S.C.J. No. 57, [1992] 2 S.C.R. 138, 93 D.L.R. (4th) 415 (S.C.C.).

[135]   See, *e.g.*, *Peters-Brown v. Regina District Health Board*, [1995] S.J. No. 609, 136 Sask. R. 126 (Sask. Q.B.), aff'd [1996] S.J. No. 761, 148 Sask. R. 248 (Sask. C.A.).

large.[136] There is little Canadian case law on the existence or scope of exceptions to the common law duty of physicians or others to maintain the confidentiality of information. The leading case actually involves the evidentiary privilege attached to solicitor-client communications.

Evidentiary privileges differ from the traditional duty to protect confidentiality because they arise only in the specialized setting of judicial proceedings. Common law jurisdictions in Canada provide the strongest privilege to solicitor-client and spousal communications; "communications between a health professional and a patient" are subject to a "case-by-case" privilege analysis.[137] The fact that the existence and scope of the privilege is determined on a case-by-case basis creates uncertainty about the scope of evidentiary protection for patient information.[138]

Canadian jurisdictions, unlike those in the United States, have not enacted special HIV confidentiality statutes and thus avoided the HIV exceptionalism debate in this area. Canadians have focused on improving general privacy protections, but concerns about the disclosure of HIV-related information have not fuelled the debate. Instead, interest in privacy protection has been driven by the perception that computerized medical records and the electronic transmission of data have created a greater threat to the confidentiality of sensitive information.[139] Medical information stored electronically is potentially subject to broader dissemination than the information contained in the traditional patient medical file. In addition, the information may be accessible to a broad range of persons or institutions, limiting the utility of the narrow confidentiality protections found within the physician-patient relationship.

---

[136] See generally Mark A. Hall, Mary Anne Bobinski & David Orentlicher, *Health Care Law & Ethics* (New York: Aspen Publishing, 2007) at 185-96.

[137] Canadian HIV/AIDS Legal Network, "Privacy Protection and the Disclosure of Health Information: Legal Issues for People Living with HIV/AIDS in Canada" (2004), online: <http://www.aidslaw.ca/publications/publicationsdocEN.php?ref=189> at 20-21.

[138] *Ibid.*, at 20-21 (discussing application of "Wigmore criteria" in determining existence and scope of the privilege).

[139] See for example Nola M. Ries, "Patient Privacy in a Wired (and Wireless) World: Approaches to Consent in the Context of Electronic Health Records" (2006) 43 Alta. L. Rev. 681 (reviewing developments in electronic records and trends that may reduce privacy and consent constraints while increasing the need to focus on records security); Nola M. Ries & Geoff Moysa, "Legal Protections of Electronic Health Records: Issues of Consent and Security" (2005) 14:1 Health L. Rev. 18 (reviewing development of electronic records, the risks and benefits of these records, and the regulatory framework); Public Health Agency of Canada, "HIV Testing and Counselling: Policies in Transition?" (2007) (research paper prepared for the International Public Health Dialogue on HIV Testing and Counseling, Toronto, 17 August 2006), online: <http://www.phac-aspc.gc.ca/aids-sida/publication/hivtest/index-eng.php> at 8 (noting that confidentiality "has required continuous reinforcement in agency and institutional policies as well as education of health care workers and communities because confidentiality is often breached both within institutions and communities").

Privacy therefore is increasingly subject to protection by federal and provincial legislation — so much so that it is sometimes difficult to determine which slightly different sets of rules will apply to a particular situation.

The ever-expanding array of privacy-related legislation can be roughly analyzed according to several criteria: federal or provincial enactment; the types of entities/individuals given an obligation to maintain confidentiality; the types of information protected; the expansiveness of exceptions or exclusions from protection; and the strength of the enforcement system.[140] Professor Gibson's chapter in this volume provides a more detailed discussion of the intricacies of privacy legislation.

This section began with the observation that HIV testing carries with it a series of questions about the use of test results. The analysis of the wide range of legal doctrines and rules governing the disclosure of HIV-related information suggests that individuals have a general right to control the disclosure of health information, including information about HIV infection. Yet there are significant exceptions to this principle. The *Charter* protects individuals from invasions of privacy, except where permitted by s. 8 or where disclosure is necessary to serve a "substantial" interest,[141] so long as the infringement on privacy is "reasonable and demonstrably justified".[142] Common law protections are relatively weak and contain exceptions for disclosures required by law or related to the need to protect public health or safety. Statutory and regulatory provisions at the federal and provincial levels have expanded the scope of protection to a broader range of actors but continue to include significant exceptions. Section III (c) (*ii*) will focus on a key debate, which pits individual privacy interests against the governmental interest in collecting information about cases of HIV infection.

(ii)   Names-Based HIV Reporting to Public Health Authorities

As noted in Section III (b) (*i*), HIV testing carries with it the risk that test results might be made available to others. The clearest risk comes during conditional or mandatory testing programs; after all, the very fact that the test is mandated suggests there is a strong interest in the test result. Blood and tissue donors are routinely screened for HIV infection; donors who test positive for HIV are placed on an indefinite deferral list

---

[140]   This analytical framework is adapted from Mark A. Hall, Mary Anne Bobinski & David Orentlicher, *Health Care Law & Ethics* (New York: Aspen Publishing, 2007) at 180.

[141]   *R. v. Oakes*, [1986] S.C.J. No. 7, [1986] 1 S.C.R. 103, 26 D.L.R. (4th) 200 (S.C.C.).

[142]   *Ibid.*

to prevent use of their blood or tissue.[143] This use of HIV test results has not been particularly controversial; indeed the major dispute has involved how to improve the collection and use of information on a nationwide scale.[144]

Post-exposure testing rules also inherently involve the disclosure of HIV-related information to third parties — it is, after all, the disclosure of the information to the person who might have been exposed to HIV which is the core justification for the testing itself. Yet post-exposure testing programs attempt to limit the intrusion on the privacy of the person who is forced to undergo testing. The Ontario *Mandatory Blood Testing Act*, for example, provides that the analyst of the sample should make reasonable efforts to deliver the results to the physician of the exposed person (the "applicant") and, where requested, to the source individual's ("respondent's") physician.[145] The statute prohibits the use of the test result or the disclosure of the test result for any other purpose.[146]

These disclosure policies focus on the protection of the health and safety of third parties. A strong interest in protecting health and safety might justify the intrusion into individual privacy interests, but may the government require the disclosure of HIV-related information for other reasons, such as to improve the collection of data regarding the incidence and prevalence of HIV infection within a population? Which level of government should take responsibility for the collection and distribution of surveillance data? These issues were hidden in this chapter's discussion of the collection of HIV/AIDS statistics in Section II (d), above.[147]

The answer to these questions implicates two of the major strands of debate about HIV-related policies: finding the proper balance between individual liberty and public health objectives and struggling with whether HIV should be treated differently because of the social stigma associated with the disease. For HIV, the debate has gone through two stages. In the early days of the pandemic, Canadian and American jurisdictions made AIDS diagnoses reportable to public health authorities in a form which included the name or other identifiable information about the person

---

[143] See for example Canadian Blood Services, "Indefinite Deferrals", online: <http://www. bloodservices.ca/CentreApps/Internet/UW_V502_MainEngine.nsf/page/Indefinite%20Deferral ?OpenDocument>.

[144] See generally Library and Archives Canada, "Commission of Inquiry on the Blood System of Canada, Final Report" (1997) ("Krever Report"), online: Library and Archives Canada <http://epe.lac-bac.gc.ca/100/200/301/hcan-scan/commission_blood_final_rep-e/ index.html>.

[145] *Mandatory Blood Testing Act, 2006*, S.O. 2006, c. 26, s. 5(2).

[146] *Ibid.*, ss. 7, 8.

[147] See generally UNAIDS, "The Role of Name-Based Notification in Public Health and HIV Surveillance" (2000) at 6-10 (brief history of disease reporting), online: UNAIDS <http://www.who.int/hiv/strategic/surveillance/en/unaids_00_28e.pdf>; Lawrence O. Gostin, Scott Burris & Zita Lazzarini, "The Law and the Public's Health: A Study of Infections Disease Law in the United States" (1999) 99 Colum. L. Rev. 59.

diagnosed.[148] Although this identifying information is collected at the state or provincial level, only the case report without identifying information is conveyed on to the national government in Canada and the United States.[149]

The introduction of HIV antibody testing in 1985 created a new source of information about the prevalence and incidence of HIV infection, yet government authorities have faced considerable controversy in crafting policies regarding HIV reporting. For many public health officials, HIV reporting was a logical extension of existing policies on AIDS reporting.[150] For others and for advocates of civil liberties, the risks of HIV reporting outweighed the benefits. Critics of HIV reporting noted the long period during which persons with HIV infection could remain healthy and capable of working, the absence of effective treatments for the infection, the risk that HIV reporting might deter people from undergoing testing, and the injuries that could follow from breaches in

---

[148]   In the United States, for example, all 50 states listed AIDS as a reportable diagnosis in the 1980s. See Dennis H. Osmond, "Epidemiology of HIV/AIDS in the United States" (March 2003) in Laurence Peiperl, Susa Coffey, Oliver Bacon, & Paul Volberding, *HIV Insite Knowledge Base* (online textbook from the UCSF Center for HIV Information), online: <http://hivinsite.ucsf.edu/InSite?page=kb-00&doc=kb-02-01-01>.

[149]   See Canadian AIDS Society (CAS) and Health Canada, "A Guide to HIV/AIDS Epidemiology and Surveillance Terms" (2002) 6, 8 ("AIDS case report" & "notifiable disease"), online: Public Health Agency of Canada <http://www.phac-aspc.gc.ca/publicat/haest-tesvs/pdf/hiv_glossary_e.pdf>; UNAIDS, "The Role of Name-Based Notification in Public Health and HIV Surveillance" (2000), online: UNAIDS <http://www.who.int/hiv/strategic/surveillance/en/unaids_00_28e.pdf> at 6-11 (AIDS reporting more controversial in Canada than in the United States). National data collection is formally voluntary. See *e.g.*, U.S. CDC, "CDC Guidelines for National Human Immunodeficiency Virus Case Surveillance, Including Monitoring for Human Immunodeficiency Virus Infection and Acquired Immunodeficiency Syndrome" (10 December 1999) 48 MMWR Recomm Rep. (RR13) 1 (detailing most recent surveillance guidelines and summarizing historical changes in diagnostic criteria); and Elaine Gibson, "Public Health Information, Federalism, and Politics" (2007) 16:1 Health L. Rev. 5 (arguing that federal government should increase collaboration with Provinces, and potentially consider legislation, to improve information-sharing about infectious diseases).

[150]   UNAIDS, "The Role of Name-Based Notification in Public Health and HIV Surveillance" (2000), online: UNAIDS <http://www.who.int/hiv/strategic/surveillance/en/unaids_00_28e.pdf> at 12:

> In the United States ... some public health officials ... made the claim that the very justification for AIDS reporting extended logically to HIV. Concerns about the accuracy of epidemiological surveillance and the capacity to intervene with infected individuals confirmed this view. Name reporting, advocates asserted, could alert public health agencies to the presence of individuals infected with a lethal virus; would permit such agencies to ensure that such persons were properly counseled; would permit those responsible for disease surveillance to better execute their tasks; would permit partner notification; and would permit officials to notify infected individuals when effective therapeutic agents became available.

confidentiality.[151] As a result, many jurisdictions in the United States and Canada either did not require reporting of HIV test results or did not require reporting by name or unique identifier. This policy led to charges of HIV exceptionalism and to concerns that public health authorities were being denied access to information that could be important in policy responses to infection.

The balance began to shift as new antiretroviral treatments became available; these treatments reduced the incidence of AIDS diagnoses[152] and also made it more likely that individuals would be motivated to seek out HIV testing as a precursor to treatment. The trend accelerated in 1999, when the U.S. CDC recommended that states establish HIV case surveillance systems modeled on those used for AIDS diagnoses, which included the name of the person testing positive for HIV.[153] All states in the U.S. were to move to nominal HIV reporting by the end of 2007.[154]

The debate also unfolded in Canada during this time period with a steadily expanding number of provinces and territories requiring the reporting of HIV test results, most often by name, to a designated public health official. According to the Public Health Agency of Canada:

> By 2003, positive HIV test results and AIDS diagnoses had been designated as notifiable in all Canadian provinces and territories. In most testing situations, laboratories and physicians are responsible for reporting HIV infection, but this varies by province or territory.

> When HIV infection is notifiable, "nominal/name-based" or "non-nominal/non-identifying" information about an individual who tests positive for HIV infection is forwarded to provincial or territorial public health officials. This includes demographic data, such as the person's age and gender; risks associated with the transmission of HIV; and laboratory data, such as the date of the person's first positive HIV test.

---

[151]   See generally *ibid.*, at 12-13; Lawrence O. Gostin & James G. Hodge, Jr., "The 'Names Debate': The Case for National HIV Reporting in the United States" (1998) 61 Alb. L. Rev. 679.

[152]   The U.S. CDC noted the impact of this change: "With the advent of more effective therapy that slows the progression of HIV disease, AIDS surveillance data no longer reliably reflect trends in HIV transmission and do not accurately represent the need for prevention and care services." U.S. CDC, "CDC Guidelines for National Human Immunodeficiency Virus Case Surveillance, Including Monitoring for Human Immunodeficiency Virus Infection and Acquired Immunodeficiency Syndrome" (10 December 1999) 48 MMWR Recomm Rep. (RR13) 1.

[153]   *Ibid.* ("CDC has concluded that confidential name-based HIV/AIDS surveillance systems are most likely to meet the necessary performance standards ... as well as to serve the public health purposes for which surveillance data are required. Therefore, CDC advises that state and local surveillance programs use the same confidential name-based approach for HIV surveillance as is currently used for AIDS surveillance nationwide.")

[154]   Richard Pearshouse, "U.S.: All states to move to names-based HIV reporting in 2007" (2007) 12:1 Can. HIV/AIDS Pol'y & L. Rev. 37.

HIV infection is not legally notifiable at the national level, yet notification to PHAC is voluntarily undertaken by all provinces and territories. Positive HIV test reports and reported AIDS cases are provided non-nominally to PHAC.[155]

Some provinces also continue to offer the option of anonymous HIV testing.[156] The end result is that Canada has retained a mixed system under which individuals in many provinces/territories retain access to non-nominal/non-identifiable testing programs. The availability of anonymous and non-identifiable testing probably is an important factor in encouraging members of at-risk groups to seek out HIV testing.[157]

IV. STRATEGIES TO REDUCE TRANSMISSION

(a) Law and the Transmission of Disease

This chapter has been primarily concerned with the medical, social and legal aspects of identifying and tracking cases of HIV infection. The prevention of new cases of HIV transmission is undoubtedly at least an equally important objective. The remaining sections of this chapter will focus on whether and how the legal system should foster public health objectives by reducing the risk of HIV transmission. These sections will focus on three different sources of law: public health law, tort law and criminal law.

---

[155] Public Health Agency of Canada, "HIV/AIDS Epi Updates, November 2007" at 13. The report suggests but does not discuss the perennial dispute about whether public health data should be gathered at the provincial or federal level in Canada. Provincial public health legislation or regulations typically require reporting of certain identified communicable diseases by identified categories of persons (typically physicians and laboratories) to an identified provincial public health authority. See for example British Columbia Centre for Disease Control, "List of Reportable Communicable Diseases in BC" (April 2008), online: <http://www.bccdc.org/content.php?item=7>. Although public health primarily is a matter of provincial concern, the federal government also plays an important role in encouraging the collection and distribution of data on a nationwide basis. The SARS epidemic focused renewed attention on the need to create a national public health infrastructure. The new federal Public Health Agency of Canada is charged with a number of important tasks, including helping to coordinate data collection about communicable diseases such as HIV/AIDS. Public Health Agency of Canada, "HIV/AIDS Epi Updates, November 2007".

[156] Ibid., at 14-15 (Table 1) (five provinces continue to offer anonymous testing; two offer anonymous testing but positive test results are reported nominally).

[157] Ibid., at 14-15.   But see James M. Tesoriero et al., "The Effect of Name-Based Reporting and Partner Notification on HIV Testing in New York State" (2008) 98 Am. J. Public H. 728 (HIV testing rates in NY did not decline after adoption of nominal reporting and contact tracing; high-risk individuals not aware of law and few expressed concerns about policy).

(b) Traditional Public Health Law

(i) Introduction

The testing and reporting regimes described above provide an important foundation for the public health response by giving information about the existence and prevalence of a particular disease. Public health authorities use a wide range of strategies to reduce the risks associated with communicable diseases, including contact tracing and partner notification; mandatory treatment; vaccination; and isolation/quarantine.[158] Many of these strategies are simply inapplicable to the problem of HIV infection: there is (as yet) no treatment capable of eliminating the virus from an infected person,[159] no vaccine to prevent transmission, and the costs of isolation/quarantine would greatly outweigh the benefits given the long course of HIV infection and the relative difficulty of transmitting the virus. The debate about whether and how to employ traditional public health strategies to prevent infection has therefore focused on contact tracing and partner notification. This section will focus on whether and how to employ three specific public health strategies to prevent infection: post-exposure prophylaxis for sexual or needle-sharing incidents, contact tracing and public health orders.

(ii) Post-Exposure Prophylaxis after Sexual Activity or Injection Drug Use

Soon after the development of antiretroviral drug therapies, researchers began to explore whether the drugs could be used to reduce the risk of HIV transmission after an exposure incident.[160] The early focus was on occupational transmission in health care settings and public health authorities in the United States and Canada quickly developed and regularly updated protocols for post-exposure prophylaxis ("PEP") in these settings.[161] Studies indicated that PEP significantly reduced the risk

---

[158] See generally Lawrence O. Gostin, *Public Health Law: Power, Duty, Restraint* (Berkeley: University of California Press, 2008); Lawrence O. Gostin, Scott Burris & Zita Lazzarini, "The Law and the Public's Health: A Study of Infectious Disease Law in The United States" (1999) 99 Colum. L. Rev. 59.

[159] Current therapies cannot "cure" HIV infection, but they can be applied to reduce the risk of HIV infection arising from an exposure incident. See *supra*, text accompanying notes 94-117.

[160] David K. Henderson & Julie L. Gerberding, "Prophylactic zidovudine after occupational exposure to the human immunodeficiency virus: an interim analysis" (1989) 160 J. Infect. Dis. 321.

[161] See, *e.g.*, "An Integrated Protocol to Manage Health Care Workers Exposed to Bloodborne Pathogens" (1997) 23:S2 CCDR 1 (Table 4 and Appendix), online: Public Health Agency of Canada <http://www.phac-aspc.gc.ca/publicat/ccdr-rmtc/97vol23/23s2/index.html>; Adelisa

of HIV transmission following needlestick and other percutaneous exposures in the health care settings.[162] PEP was also considered and implemented for other types of occupational exposures, such as for police officers and firefighters, as well as for survivors of sexual assault.[163]

Despite the efficacy of PEP, there was considerable controversy about whether PEP should be made available to persons who were exposed or potentially exposed to HIV through voluntary sexual activity or injection drug use.[164] The controversy included expressions of concern about whether moral judgments about certain types of behaviour might be colouring the public health response. Public health officials defended the delay in expanding nonoccupational PEP ("nPEP"), noting that nPEP's effectiveness had not been demonstrated for other types of exposure incidents, that broadly available nPEP might indirectly encourage risky conduct, that antiretroviral drugs had significant side effects and expense, and that persons receiving nPEP might be a future source of drug-resistant virus in the community.[165]

After several years of additional study and consultation, the U.S. Department of Health and Human Services found that these concerns did not outweigh the benefits of offering nPEP to persons with nonoccupational exposures.[166] Under the new recommendations, persons who present themselves within 72 hours after a sufficiently risky exposure

[162] L. Panlilio et al., "Updated U.S. Public Health Service Guidelines for the Management of Occupational Exposures to HIV and Recommendations for Postexposure Prophylaxis" (2005) 54 MMWR Recomm Rep. (RR09) 1

[163] See, e.g., D.M. Cardo et al. "A case-control study of HIV seroconversion in health care workers after percutaneous exposure" (1997) 337 N. Eng. J. Med. 1485 (ten-fold reduction in transmission rate).

[164] See, e.g., Ellen R. Wiebe et al., "Offering HIV Prophylaxis to People Who Have Been Sexually Assaulted: 16 Months' Experience in a Sexual Assault Service" (2000) 162 C.M.A.J. 641 (study of Vancouver-based program; the first North American PEP program to be offered in a sexual assault service). Study results found low rates of PEP adherence and resulted in guideline revision to target highest risks of HIV infection (ibid., at 641).

[165] Dawn K. Smith et al., "Antiretroviral Postexposure Prophylaxis After Sexual, Injection-Drug Use, or Other Nonoccupational Exposure to HIV in the United States: Recommendations from the U.S. Department of Health and Human Services" 54 MMWR Recomm Rep (RR2) 1, 2 (citing history of consultation on the topic).

[166] Ibid., at 2-5 (reporting results of research and consultation related to each of these concerns).

Ibid., at 12. See also, James O. Kahn et al., "Feasibility of Postexposure Prophylaxis (PEP) against Human Immunodeficiency Virus Infection after Sexual or Injection Drug Use Exposure: The San Francisco PEP Study" (2001) 183 J. Inf. Dis. 707; Jeffrey N. Martin et al., "Use of Postexposure Prophylaxis Against HIV Infection Following Sexual Exposure Does Not Lead to Increase in High-Risk Behavior" (2004) 18 AIDS 787; Mauro Schechter et al., "Behavioral Impact, Acceptability, and HIV Incidence Among Homosexual Men With Access to Postexposure Chemoprophylaxis for HIV" (2004) 35 J. Acquir. Immune Defic. Syndr. 519.

incident with a known HIV-infected person should be given access to the therapy.[167] The guidelines do not recommend for or against nPEP where the exposure incident involves a person of unknown HIV status.[168] Finally, "[f]or persons whose exposure histories represent no substantial risk for HIV transmission or who seek care >72 hours after potential nonoccupational exposure, the use of antiretroviral nPEP is not recommended".[169] The guidelines offer additional commentary on the use of nPEP for "vulnerable populations", including inmates and injection drug users. The guidelines support the use of nPEP for both these groups, noting in particular that "injection-drug use should not deter clinicians from prescribing nPEP if the exposure provides an opportunity to reduce the risk for consequent HIV infection".[170]

Access to nPEP in Canada is somewhat more complex. There are no national guidelines affirming the appropriateness of nPEP. There is evidence of great variability in the availability of nPEP across Canada, with little or no access in some areas and limited access in others.[171] Ironically, given Canada's commitment to publicly funded health care, part of the difficulty with access may be financial: "In Britain, if a physician concludes treatment is necessary, the cost ... is covered by the National Health Service. For Canadians whose drug costs are not covered

---

[167] Dawn K. Smith *et al.*, "Antiretroviral Postexposure Prophylaxis After Sexual, Injection-Drug Use, or Other Nonoccupational Exposure to HIV in the United States: Recommendations from the U.S. Department of Health and Human Services" 54 MMWR Recomm Rep. (RR2) 1 at 8 (text and "Figure 1. Algorithm for evaluation and treatment of possible nonoccupational HIV exposures"). nPEP should be administered as soon as possible after exposure, ideally within hours, but not later than 72 hours after exposure to be effective, and must be continued for four weeks. The therapy can have debilitating side effects and that costs are not insignificant. *Ibid.*, at 8-11.

[168] *Ibid.*, at 9 ("Clinicians should evaluate the risk for and benefits of this intervention on a case-by-case basis"). The recommendations note the desirability of obtaining the source's HIV status voluntarily, ideally through a rapid HIV test (*ibid.*).

[169] *Ibid.*

[170] *Ibid.*, at 15. The guidelines implicitly suggest that clinicians can take into account whether the exposure incident is "an exceptional occurrence" or part of ongoing conduct in determining whether nPEP is appropriate (*ibid.*). ("In judging whether exposures are isolated, episodic, or ongoing, clinicians should consider that persons who continue to engage in risk behaviors (*e.g.*, commercial sex workers or users of illicit drugs) might be practicing risk reduction ... Therefore a high risk exposure might represent an exceptional occurrence for such persons despite their ongoing risk behavior" (*ibid.*).)

[171] See, *e.g.*, Ann Silversides, "HIV Prophylaxis Expensive and Sometimes Difficult to Obtain" (2006) 175 C.M.A.J. 1360 ("the delivery of PEP for accidental sexual exposure has received the least policy attention"); and Canadian AIDS Treatment Information Exchange (CATIE), "PEP: Post-Exposure Prophylaxis (Treatment After Exposure to HIV)" (March 2005) ("Policy and practices of providing PEP may vary in different cities"), online: <http://www.catie.ca/acasfs_e.nsf/dfac88ab9edb2ab485256cc2006448f6/b2d401786c9de2b0852571b400638a4b!OpenDocument>.

by a public or private drug plan, the $1000 to $1500 price tag can be a major deterrent to treatment."[172]

There is evidence that provincial drug programs are unwilling to cover the costs of nPEP. British Columbia's Centre for Excellence in HIV/AIDS offers extensive and detailed "Accidental Exposure Guidelines", to "[provide] a framework for a program of expert advice and prompt anti-retroviral prophylaxis for accidental exposures in the health care setting and community"; however, the B.C. Centre's guidelines note that "[t]his program does not provide coverage for events which arise in the individual's personal life such as consensual adult sex or incidents arising in drug using environments".[173] The B.C. Centre notes that "individuals who feel they have been exposed in these situations can purchase drugs".[174]

The gap in access to nPEP for Canadians is troubling. The medical and public health benefits of nPEP have been recognized by leading public health organizations, including the U.S. Department of Health and Human Services.[175] It is not clear why a medically beneficial treatment that also promotes public health objectives should be excluded from public coverage when other therapies related to the consequences of our "personal lives" remain publicly funded. The funding gap creates a

---

[172] Silversides, *ibid.*, at 1360.

[173] British Columbia Centre for Excellence in HIV/AIDS, "Management of Accidental Exposure to HIV Guidelines" (as of September 2007), online: <http://www.cfenet.ubc.ca/content.php?id=86>.

[174] *Ibid.* The B.C. Centre notes that "a guideline for this eventuality [possible exposure through consensual adult sex or drug using environments] is available", citing Dawn K. Smith *et al.*, "Antiretroviral Postexposure Prophylaxis After Sexual, Injection-Drug Use, or Other Nonoccupational Exposure to HIV in the United States: Recommendations from the U.S. Department of Health and Human Services" 54 MMWR Recomm Rep. (RR2) 1. This program's position on nPEP is reinforced in another portion of its guidelines:

It is not the intention of this program to provide provincially funded drugs to persons exposed to HIV as part of their personal lives, *e.g.*, consensual adult sex or sharing injection equipment. The principles enunciated here may be applicable to some of those exposures, and the exposed person and their physician may choose to obtain the medications through another source.

Ibid., at 4. (Physicians considering nPEP are instructed to review the U.S. guidelines.) See also Ann Silversides, "HIV prophylaxis expensive and sometimes difficult to obtain" (2006) 175 C.M.A.J. 1360 (quoting a medical resident with two patients who had inquired about nPEP: "The [drug] cost would have been covered if I had a needle-stick [injury] ... it didn't seem fair that they would have to pay. This seems to me to be an anomaly in the health care system").

[175] Dawn K. Smith *et al.*, "Antiretroviral Postexposure Prophylaxis After Sexual, Injection-Drug Use, or Other Nonoccupational Exposure to HIV in the United States: Recommendations from the U.S. Department of Health and Human Services" 54 MMWR Recomm Rep. (RR2) 1. See also Martin Fisher *et al.*, UK Guideline for the Use of Post-Exposure Prophylaxis for HIV Following Sexual Exposure" (2006) 17 Int'l J. of STD & AIDS 81.

significant barrier to the use of a proven method of reducing HIV transmission.

The next issue beyond nPEP may well be "prEP": pre-exposure prophylaxis, or using antiretroviral therapies before potential exposures to reduce the risk of transmission. Researchers are exploring whether pre-exposure use of antiretroviral therapies can reduce the risk of HIV transmission.[176] Some gay men in the United States reportedly have begun to use prEP.[177] Many of the same concerns about indirectly encouraging risky behaviour and the potential for drug resistant strains of HIV have been raised along with the obvious ethical, financial and practical challenges to providing pre-exposure antiretroviral access when many already infected with the virus around the world are unable to access treatment.[178]

(iii) Contact Tracing and Partner Notification

The terms "contact tracing" and "partner notification" tend to be used interchangeably along with the broader concept of "partner counseling and referral services (PCRS)".[179] Whatever term is issued, contact tracing has several benefits. Persons who have been exposed to the risk of HIV transmission are given vitally important information that allows them to seek testing and counseling about methods of reducing the risk of transmission in the future. Persons who discover they are infected have an opportunity to change their behaviour to prevent transmitting the virus to others and to seek early medical care.

---

[176] See, e.g., P. Denton et al., "Antiretroviral Pre-Exposure Prophylaxis Prevents Vaginal Transmission of HIV-1 in Humanized BLT Mice" (2008) 15 PLoS Med. e13. See also, online: PrEP Watch <http://www.prepwatch.org/trials.htm>.

[177] Albert Liu et al., "Limited Knowledge and Use of HIV Post- and Pre-Exposure Prophylaxis Among Gay and Bisexual Men" (2008) 47 JAIDS 241.

[178] See, e.g., Greg Szekeres & Thomas Coates, "Policy and Practice Implications of HIV Pre-Exposure Prophylaxis (PrEP) in the United States" (November 2006) (summarizing clinical trials, concerns, and recommendations), online: UCLA Program in Global Health <http://globalhealth.med.ucla.edu/publications/prep_nov06.pdf>. See also, Roxanne Nelson, "Study Reports Benefit of HIV Pre-Exposure Chemoprophylaxis" (2007) 7 Lancet Infect. Dis. 706; and Aranka Anema, Evan Wood & Julio S.G. Montaner, "The Use of Highly Active Retroviral Therapy to Reduce HIV Incidence at the Population Level" (2008) 179 C.M.A.J. 13 (focusing on impact of expanded access to antiretrovirals for persons with clinical indications rather than prEP).

[179] Matthew Hogben et al., "The Effectiveness of HIV Partner Counseling and Referral Services in Increasing Identification of HIV-Positive Individuals" (2007) 33:2S Amer. J. Prev. Med. S89 ("Partner counseling and referral services (PCRS) comprise a range of services intended to support HIV-positive individuals and their partners in making health choices and receiving appropriate health care as well as to promote healthier communities by reducing the spread of HIV" at S89).

Contact tracing generally involves gathering information from a source individual (typically called the "index case"), who is infected with a communicable disease, about people ("contacts") who might have been exposed to the illness.[180] Successful contact tracing requires the source individual's cooperation in identifying contacts.[181] For HIV infection, this process can include identifying sexual partners, needle-sharing partners, the recipients of blood or tissue donations, or others who might have been exposed to the blood or body fluids of the source individual under circumstances which could present the risk of infection. Occasionally, a health professional or public health official already knows the identity of possible contacts.[182]

In traditional contact tracing programs, also termed "provider referral" programs, once the index case identifies one or more possible contacts, then public health authorities alert the contacts to the risk that they might have been exposed to the disease.[183] Contacts are counselled about the need to undergo testing and, if they test positive, are encouraged to disclose the identities of their contacts and to seek medical care.

The standard approach toward communicating with contacts includes safeguarding the identity of the source individual.[184] This protection might prove illusory, however, where a contact has only a few — or even one — possible sources of risk.[185] Contact tracing can be

[180]   See generally Ralf Jürgens, "Partner Notification" in "*HIV Testing and Confidentiality: Final Report*" (2001), online: Canadian HIV/AIDS Legal Network <http://www.aidslaw.ca/publications/interfaces/downloadFile.php?ref=282>; Lawrence O. Gostin & James G. Hodge, "Piercing the Veil of Secrecy in HIV/AIDS and Other Sexually Transmitted Diseases: Theories of Privacy and Disclosure in Partner Notification" (1998) 5 Duke J. Gender L. & Pol'y 9; William. E. Adams, Jr. *et al.*, *AIDS: Cases and Materials* (Durham: Carolina Academic Press, 2002) at 112-13.

[181]   But see *F. (I.) v. Peel (Region) Health Department*, 2006 WL 4752624 (Ont. H.S.A.R.B.), 2006 CarswellOnt 9249 (Dkt HP.7321) (public health authorities seek order requiring husband to disclose wife's name for partner notification in case involving gonorrhea).

[182]   The index case may be accompanied by a sexual or needle sharing partner, for example.

[183]   See Canadian HIV/AIDS Legal Network, "Confidentiality" in *HIV Testing* (2007) (series of 12 information sheets on HIV testing in Canada), online: <http://www.aidslaw.ca/publications/publicationsdocEN.php?ref=713> at 2 (discussing types of partner notification). See also M. Golden *et al.*, "Support Among Persons Infected with HIV for Routine Health Department Contact for HIV Partner Notification" (1 February 2003) 32 J. Acquir Immune Defic Syndr. 196 (study suggests that a majority of persons with HIV infection favour health department-facilitated contact notification programs).

[184]   Lawrence O. Gostin & James G. Hodge, "Piercing the Veil of Secrecy in HIV/AIDS and Other Sexually Transmitted Diseases: Theories of Privacy and Disclosure in Partner Notification" (1998) 5 Duke J. Gender L. & Pol'y 9.

[185]   A contact individual is likely to be able to identify a source individual when the contact has only had one sexual partner, no needle sharing partners, and no other possible sources of exposure. See also Timothy K.S. Christie & Perry R.W. Kendall, "The Science of Partner Notification: A Review of Available Evidence" (April 2003) 45 B.C. Med. J. 124, online:

intrusive or embarrassing for the source individual and may inadvertently result in the disclosure of the identity of the source individual.[186] The process can be labour intensive and expensive if carried out by public officials. Contact tracing techniques continue to evolve; new methods of contact tracing take into account the impact of the Internet on facilitating sexual encounters, for example, by using e-mail to make contact with otherwise anonymous sexual contacts.[187]

Professors Gostin and Hodge identify two variations on traditional contact tracing programs.[188] One type of program relies on the index case to disclose the risk of infection to their contacts while public health officials provide support and reminders to the index case.[189] The second variation on traditional contact tracing programs is a "hybrid" approach, often called "conditional referral".[190] These contact tracing programs combine aspects of the provider and patient referral strategies: index cases are to be told, for example, that the disclosure will be made by public health officials unless the index case makes the disclosure within a set time frame.[191]

In the early years of the HIV epidemic, there was considerable debate about whether and how contact tracing should be employed for

---

<http://www.bcmj.org/science-partner-notification-review-available-evidence>.

[186] See, e.g., F. (I.) v. Peel (Region) Health Department, 2006 WL 4752624 (Ont. H.S.A.R.B.), 2006 CarswellOnt 9249 (Drt. HP. 7321) (husband resists disclosing name of wife for purposes of partner notification in case involving gonorrhea).

[187] Matthew J. Mimiaga et al., "Acceptability of an Internet-Based Partner Notification System for Sexually Transmitted Infection Exposure Among Men Who Have Sex With Men" (2008) 98 Amer. J. Public H. 1009; U.S. CDC, "Using the Internet for Partner Notification of Sexually Transmitted Diseases — Los Angeles County, California, 2003" (20 February 2004) 53 MMWR 129.

[188] Lawrence O. Gostin & James G. Hodge, "Piercing the Veil of Secrecy in HIV/AIDS and Other Sexually Transmitted Diseases: Theories of Privacy and Disclosure in Partner Notification" (1998) 5 Duke J. Gender L. & Pol'y 9. See also Canadian HIV/AIDS Legal Network, "Confidentiality" in HIV Testing (2007) (series of 12 information sheets on HIV testing in Canada), online: <http://www.aidslaw.ca/publications/publicationsdocEN.php?ref= 713>; Janet S. St. Lawrence et al., "STD Screening, Testing, Case Reporting, and Clinical and Partner Notification Practices: A National Survey of US Physicians" (2002) 92 Amer J. Public Health 1784-88 (noting that most physicians relied on patients to follow up on partner notification on their own or with the health department).

[189] Gostin and Hodge express concerns that "[p]atient referral programs provide no assurance that contacts are notified, little control over the quality of the information conveyed, and no confidentiality protection for the identity of the index patient" (ibid., at 26-27).

[190] Ibid., at 27.

[191] Ibid. See also A. Carballo-Dieguez et al., "Intention to Notify Sexual Partners about Potential HIV Exposure Among New York City STD Clinic's Clients" (29 August 2002) 29 Sex. Transm. Dis. 465.

HIV infection.[192] Proponents argued that this traditional public health strategy should be used to inform potential contacts about the risk of infection so they could undergo testing and modify their behaviour to reduce the risk of infection to others. Some suggested the failure to employ PCRS was a form of HIV exceptionalism that gave greater weight to individual privacy than to the preservation of life.[193] Opponents of contact tracing argued that the cost of contact tracing outweighed the benefits.[194] The U.S. CDC was an early and strong proponent of contact tracing in the United States yet implementation proved difficult.[195]

---

[192] See generally Lawrence O. Gostin & James G. Hodge, "Piercing the Veil of Secrecy in HIV/AIDS and Other Sexually Transmitted Diseases: Theories of Privacy and Disclosure in Partner Notification" (1998) 5 Duke J. Gender L. & Pol'y 9 at 25-26; and Ralf Jürgens, "Partner Notification" in *HIV Testing and Confidentiality: Final Report* (2001), online: Canadian HIV/AIDS Legal Network <http://www.aidslaw.ca/publications/interfaces/down loadFile.php?ref=282>.

[193] See *New York State Society of Surgeons v. Axelrod*, 77 N.Y.2d 677 (1991) (medical organizations bring suit against Commissioner of Health in effort to force state government to include HIV on list of communicable diseases subject to contact tracing; state law subsequently amended).

[194] Lawrence O. Gostin & James G. Hodge, "Piercing the Veil of Secrecy in HIV/AIDS and Other Sexually Transmitted Diseases: Theories of Privacy and Disclosure in Partner Notification" (1998) 5 Duke J. Gender L. & Pol'y 9 at 78. Recent studies suggest a favorable cost/benefit ratio. See, *e.g.*, Matthew Hogben *et al.*, "The Effectiveness of HIV Partner Counseling and Referral Services in Increasing Identification of HIV-Positive Individuals" (2007) 33:2S Amer. J. Prev. Med. S89; Devon D. Brewer, "Case-Finding Effectiveness of Partner Notification and Cluster Investigation for Sexually Transmitted Diseases/HIV" (2005) Sexually Transmitted Diseases 78. Some jurisdictions have employed a modified approach which focuses scarce public health resources on finding contacts from "low risk groups" who might be thought to have less reason to be aware of the risk of exposure. See U.S. CDC, "Current Trends Partner Notification for Preventing Human Immunodeficiency Virus (HIV) Infection — Colorado, Idaho, South Carolina, Virginia" (1 July 1988) 37 MMWR 393. In the early days of the pandemic in the United States, this meant focusing on the heterosexual contacts of persons with HIV infection. The Royal Society of Canada adopted a similar analysis in the 1980s. Ralf Jürgens, "Partner Notification" in *HIV Testing and Confidentiality: Final Report* (2001), online: Canadian HIV/AIDS Legal Network <http://www.aidslaw.ca/publications/interfaces/downloadFile. php?ref=282>.

[195] U.S. CDC, "Incorporating HIV Prevention into the Medical Care of Persons Living with HIV: Recommendations of the CDC, the Health Resources and Services Administration, the National Institutes of Health, and the HIV Medicine Association of the Infectious Disease Society of America" (18 July 2003) 52 MMWR Recomm Rep. (RR12) 1; U.S. CDC, *Technical Guidance for HIV/AIDS Surveillance Programs, Volume III: Security and Confidentiality Guideline* (2006) (Attachment G focuses on Using HIV Surveillance Data to Document Need and Initiate Referrals"), online: <http://www.cdc.gov/hiv/ surveillance.htm>; M. Golden *et al.*, "Partner Notification for HIV and STD in the United States: low coverage for gonorrhea, chlamydial infection, and HIV" (June 2003) 30 Sex. Transm. Dis. 490 (study suggests that barely over 50 per cent of persons testing positive for HIV in high prevalence areas of the U.S. have been interviewed for partner notification).

Contact tracing was rejected by influential groups in Canada early in the epidemic, but became an accepted part of public health practice in the 1990s.[196] In 1997, the Federal/Provincial/Territorial Advisory Committee on AIDS produced general guidelines on partner notification.[197] The Committee affirmed the utility of partner notification and established principles, such as confidentiality and voluntariness.[198] The guidelines suggest that the precise form of contact tracing program might vary from province to province based on a variety of factors.[199]

The contact tracing programs developed across Canada were established through public health policy and professional guidelines, sometimes without any specific legislative action.[200] In 2001, four provinces or territories required partner notification, legal authorities in three provinces appeared to permit contact tracing, and four provinces lacked any relevant legislation.[201] More provinces now have enacted or are considering specific legislative authorization for contact tracing as a part

---

[196]   See generally UNAIDS, "The Role of Name-Based Notification in Public Health and HIV Surveillance" (2000), online: UNAIDS <http://www.who.int/hiv/strategic/surveillance/en/ unaids_00_28e.pdf> at 36 (citing rejection of contact tracing in 1984 by the National Advisory Committee on AIDS); Public Health Agency of Canada, "Supplement: Point of Care HIV Testing Using Rapid HIV Test Kits: Guidance for Health-Care Professionals" (November 2007) 33:S2 CCDR 1, 10 ("HCPs are required ... to assist in contact tracing and counseling of the patient"); Public Health Agency of Canada, "HIV Testing and Counselling: Policies in Transition?" (2007) (research paper prepared for the International Public Health Dialogue on HIV Testing and Counseling, Toronto, 17 August 2006), online: <http://www.phac-aspc.gc.ca/aids-sida/publication/hivtest/index-eng.php> at 23, 63-64 ("Partner notification must be undertaken in all cases of AIDS and HIV infection. Local public health authorities are available to assist with partner notification and help with referral. The treating physician is responsible for ensuring that partner notification is initiated" at 23); Ralf Jürgens, "Partner Notification" in HIV Testing and Confidentiality: Final Report (2001), online: Canadian HIV/AIDS Legal Network <http://www.aidslaw.ca/ publications/interfaces/downloadFile.php?ref=282>.

[197]   Ralf Jürgens, "Partner Notification" in HIV Testing and Confidentiality: Final Report (2001), online: Canadian HIV/AIDS Legal Network <http://www.aidslaw.ca/publications/ interfaces/downloadFile.php?ref=282>; Canadian HIV/AIDS Legal Network, "Confidentiality" in HIV Testing (2007) (series of 12 information sheets on HIV testing in Canada), online: <http://www.aidslaw.ca/publications/publicationsdocEN.php?ref=713> at 2-3.

[198]   Ralf Jürgens, "Partner Notification" in HIV Testing and Confidentiality: Final Report (2001), online: Canadian HIV/AIDS Legal Network <http://www.aidslaw.ca/publications/ interfaces/downloadFile.php?ref=282>.

[199]   Ibid.

[200]   Ralf Jürgens, "Mandatory or Compulsory HIV Testing" in HIV Testing and Confidentiality: Final Report (2001), online: <http://www.aidslaw.ca/publications/interfaces/downloadFile. php?ref=282> ("Legislation differs substantially from province to province, but these differences are often not reflected in the provinces' partner notification practices").

[201]   Ibid. (citing Ontario, Saskatchewan, the Northwest Territories and Yukon as jurisdictions requiring partner notification; Prince Edward Island, New Brunswick and Alberta as authorizing contact tracing; and Newfoundland, Nova Scotia, Québec and British Columbia as failing to have applicable legislation).

of efforts to bolster public health preparedness for a wide range of infectious diseases such as SARS.[202] A range of partner notification options are offered to HIV infected persons, including patient, provider, and conditional referral.[203] Contact tracing would now appear to have become a mainstream public health policy for HIV infection.

(iv) Public Health Orders

Most public health law and policy initiatives focused on HIV have stressed individual rights and voluntary cooperation rather than coercion. Yet the state's power to invade individual liberty where necessary to protect the public health is well established.[204] When should public health authorities use coercion instead of persuasion to reduce the risk of HIV transmission?

There have been hints of the coercive powers of the provincial and federal governments in previous sections. Mandatory reporting requirements, post-exposure testing provisions, and orders requiring the disclosure of contact represent a few examples. The public health laws also provide authority for even more substantial restrictions on individual liberty designed to protect others from the risk of disease transmission. Public health officials may consider coercive measures when HIV-infected individuals who know their status and the risks continue to engage in conduct that places others at risk for infection.[205]

---

[202]   See, *e.g.*, Bill 23, B.C. *Public Health Act*, 2008, s. 29 (legislative proposal, third reading) ("a medical health officer may order a person to do one or more of the following: ... provide to the medical health officer or a specified person ... information respecting persons who may have been exposed to an infectious agent ... by the person"), online: B.C. Ministry of Health <http://www.health.gov.bc.ca/phact/>.

[203]   See for example P.R.W. Kendall, "Provincial Health Officer's Report of HIV Reportability" (February 2002) at 22-24 (discussing options), online: Health Services <http://www.healthservices.gov.bc.ca/pho/pdf/hivreportability.pdf>; I. Rasooly *et al.*, "A survey of public health partner notification for sexually transmitted diseases in Canada" (July-August 1994) 85 Can. J. Pub. Health S48 (Supplement 1) (physicians often considered responsible for partner notification for HIV).

[204]   See generally, Lawrence O. Gostin, *Public Health Law: Power, Duty, Restraint* (Berkeley: University of California Press, 2008).

[205]   According to some researchers, "it appears clear that at least a substantial minority of people with HIV do not disclose their seropositivity to all of their sex partners." O. Kenrik Duru *et al.*, "Correlates of Sex Without Serostatus Disclosure Among a National Probability Sample of HIV Patients" (2006) 10 AIDS Behav. 495. Researchers have focused on trying to understand more about the determinants of disclosure versus non-disclosure among HIV-infected individuals. See also Jeffrey T. Parsons *et al.*, "Consistent, Inconsistent, and Non-Disclosure to Casual Sexual Partners Among HIV-Seropositive Gay and Bisexual Men" (2005) 19:S1 AIDS S87; P.M. Gorbach *et al.*, "Don't Ask, Don't Tell: Patterns of HIV Disclosure Among HIV Positive Men Who Have Sex with Men with Recent STI Practicing High Risk Behavior in Los Angeles and Seattle" (2004) 80 Sex.

Many provinces and territories have specific legislation authorizing certain public health officials to issue orders restricting individual liberty to protect public health.[206] Alberta's *Public Health Act* includes specific provisions giving certain public heath authorities the power to issue orders compelling persons with HIV to refrain from engaging in conduct putting others at risk of transmission:

> 29(1) A medical officer of health who knows of or has reason to suspect the existence of a communicable disease . . . may initiate an investigation to determine whether any action is necessary to protect the public health.
>
> (2) Where the investigation confirms the presence of a communicable disease, the medical officer of health . . .
>
> (b)   may . . .
>
>   (i)   take whatever steps the medical officer of health considers necessary . . .
>
>   (B)   to protect those who have not already been exposed to the disease,
>
>   (C)   to break the chain of transmission and prevent spread of the disease, and
>
>   (D)   to remove the source of infection;
>
>   (ii)   by order . . . .
>
>   (C)   prohibit a person from having contact with other persons or any class of persons
>
> for any period and subject to any conditions that the medical officer of health considers appropriate, where the medical officer of health determines that the person's engaging in that activity could transmit an infectious agent . . . .[207]

Transm. Inf. 512; Daniel H. Ciccarone *et al.*, "Sex Without Disclosure of Positive HIV Serostatus in a US Probability Sample of Persons Receiving Medical Care for HIV Infection" (2003) 93 Amer. J. Public H. 949; Michael D. Stein *et al.*, "Sexual Ethics: Disclosure of HIV-Positive Status to Partners" (1998) 158 Arch. Intern. Med. 253; Robert Klitzman and Ronald Bayer, *Mortal Secrets: Truth and Lies in the Age of AIDS* (Baltimore, MD: John Hopkins University Press, 2003).

[206] Canadian HIV/AIDS Legal Network, "Disclosure of HIV Status After Cuerrier: Resources for Community Based AIDS Organizations" (2004) at 5-1 to 5-34 online; <http://www.aidslaw.ca/publications/publicationsdocEN.php?ref=36>; and Canadian HIV/AIDS Legal Network, "Public health laws and HIV prevention" in *Criminal Law and HIV* (2008 information sheets), online: <http://www.aidslaw.ca/publications/publicationsdocEN.php?ref=847>.

[207] Under the *Communicable Diseases Regulation*, HIV-infected persons are prohibited from "engag[ing] in any activity that may transmit disease": Alta. Reg. 238/85, Sch. 4.

Alberta's *Public Health Act* also gives additional power to address "recalcitrant patients" with certain diseases such as HIV infection or AIDS:[208]

> 39(1) Where a physician, community health nurse, midwife or nurse practitioner knows or has reason to believe that a person
>
> (a)   is infected with a disease prescribed in the regulations for the purposes of this section, and
> (b)   refuses or neglects . . .
>
>> (ii)   to comply with any other conditions that have been prescribed by a physician as being necessary to mitigate the disease or limit its spread to others,
>
> the physician, community health nurse, midwife or nurse practitioner shall immediately notify the medical officer of health in the prescribed form.
>
> (2) Where the medical officer of health is satisfied as to the sufficiency of the evidence that the person may be infected, the medical officer of health shall issue a certificate in the prescribed form. . . .[209]

The "certificate" gives authority for peace officers to seize the recalcitrant patient for commitment in a facility and for a physician to make additional orders designed to prevent the transmission of disease.[210] Persons subject to a certificate can apply to the Court of Queen's Bench for the cancellation of the certificate.[211] A patient can also be released if the physician certifies that he or she is satisfied that the patient will comply with any conditions necessary to protect public health.[212]

In 2005, an expert working group convened by the Federal/Provincial/Territorial Advisory Committee on HIV/AIDS issued recommendations regarding the response to risky behaviour by HIV-infected persons.[213] The working group endorsed "a graduated response":

[208]   Alberta *Communicable Diseases Regulation*, Alta. Reg. 238/85, Sch. 3.
[209]   Alberta *Public Health Act*, R.S.A. 2000, c. P-37, s. 39.
[210]   *Ibid.*, at s. 40. ("(1) A certificate is authority (a) for any peace officer to apprehend the person named in it and convey the person to any facility specified by the medical officer of health within 7 days from the date the certificate is issued ... and (d) for a physician to prescribe any other conditions necessary to mitigate the disease or limit its spread to others.")
[211]   *Ibid.*, at s. 39. ("(5) A person in respect of whom a certificate is issued may apply by originating notice to a judge of the Court of Queen's Bench at any time for cancellation of the certificate. ... (9) The judge may grant or refuse the order applied for and may make any other order the judge considers appropriate.")
[212]   *Ibid.*, at s. 41. The patient can be re-apprehended if he or she fails to adhere to these conditions: *ibid.*, at s. 43. An isolation order is also possible: *ibid.*, at ss. 44-46.
[213]   "Persons Who Fail to Disclose Their HIV/AIDS Status: Conclusions Reached by an Expert Working Group" (2005) 31:5 CCDR 53 (no author listed).

The first level focuses on counselling and education [which might include mandating that an infected person use protection during sexual activity]. The second level consists of assisting the HIV-positive person to access support services. The third level involves issuing public health orders to regulate the person's behaviour. The fourth level involves issuing apprehension and isolation orders under public health law, while the final level involves criminal prosecution.[214]

The working group's recommendations were based in large part on a system of graduated intervention adopted by the Calgary Health Region under Alberta's public health legislation, described above.[215] The working group noted that "Due process and *Charter* rights must be respected in ... [coercive governmental interventions]. This includes advance notice of the intervention, the right to counsel, timely reviews of decisions rendered, the right to a fair hearing, and the right to appeal decisions."[216]

Public health orders are often compared and contrasted with the use of criminal law, as discussed in Section IV (d).[217] Commentators generally suggest that the use of public health law is preferable to the use of criminal law, in part because of factors such as the ability to tailor the coercive intervention to the specific risk and the reduced stigma.[218] Ultimately, though, it is important to recognize that public health law orders can be enforced with some of the same sanctions found in criminal law, such as with fines or imprisonment.[219] In addition, unless carefully

---

[214] Glenn Betteridge, "Recommendations published concerning non-disclosure of HIV status" (2005) 10:2 Canadian HIV/AIDS Pol'y & L. Rev. 18, 18 (citing "Persons Who Fail to Disclose Their HIV/AIDS Status", *ibid.*, at 57-60).

[215] "Persons Who Fail to Disclose Their HIV/AIDS Status", *ibid.*, at 57-60.

[216] *Ibid.*, at 54. See also, Canadian HIV/AIDS Legal Network, "Public health laws and HIV prevention" in *Criminal Law and HIV* (2008 information sheets), online: <http://www.aidslaw.ca/publications/publicationsdocEN.php?ref=847>; and Nola M. Ries, "Legal Issues in Disease Outbreaks: Judicial Review of Public Health Powers" (2007) 16:1 Health L. Rev. 11.

[217] See, *e.g.*, UNAIDS, "Criminal Law, Public Health and HIV Transmission: A Policy Options Paper" (2002) (authored by Richard Elliott), online: <http://data.unaids.org/publications/IRC-pub02/JC733-CriminalLaw_en.pdf>.

[218] See, *e.g.*, *ibid.*, at 29 ("[i]n the very small number of cases where involuntary measures are reasonably and demonstrably essential, the use of carefully controlled involuntary public health measures is generally to be preferred over criminal sanction") (citing National Advisory Committee on AIDS, "HIV and Human Rights in Canada" (1992)).

[219] *Ibid.*, at 28. According to the UNAID report,

At the most coercive extreme, public health laws take on a quasi-criminal character. Health officials may have the power to compel examination and medical treatment of people suspected of being infected with a transmissible disease. They may also order an infected person to conduct themselves in such a manner as to avoid, or reduce the likelihood of, infecting others. An example would be an order prohibiting a HIV-positive person from having unprotected sex and/or ordering that person to disclose his or her HIV infection to sexual partners. Depending on the legislation in question, breaches of such public health orders could result in penalties such as fines

implemented, public health orders can result in perpetual restrictions on liberty.[220] The next two sections turn to the use of tort and criminal law to address risky behaviour.

(c) Tort Liability

(i) Introduction

Tort law formally has several purposes, including establishing the standard of care expected in society, deterring wrongful conduct that deviates from this standard of care, and compensating persons injured by wrongful conduct. Tort law duties generally are established through individual cases brought by claimants seeking compensation for injuries allegedly caused by the wrongful conduct of the defendants. A finding of liability serves to compensate the plaintiff and to establish a deterrent for others engaging in similar behaviour. Tort law might therefore be an important source of a duty to protect others from HIV infection.

There are, however, two barriers to this use of tort law. First, it is not always clear whether and how to apply the basic elements of tort claims to problems involving HIV infection. Second, behind the formal structure and functions of tort law, reality is more complex. Many people are completely unaware of tort standards of conduct and tort duties probably do not really shape the behaviour of individuals as much as judges or lawyers might want. Moreover, tort claims are not likely to be brought against impecunious, uninsured defendants. This is likely to be a factor in the use of tort law to shape the behaviour of persons infected with HIV to the extent that HIV infection has disproportionately impacted socially and economically marginalized communities. Thus both the formal elements and informal realities of tort law have affected the types of HIV-related claims made in Canada.

---

or imprisonment; or such orders could be backed up by court orders, with similar penalties for breaching a court-issued order. Health officials also generally have the power to detain a person if this is demonstrably justified as necessary to prevent the transmission of disease (generally and preferably in a health-care setting, although again legislation and practice may vary across jurisdictions). The law may authorize the use of the state's police powers to enforce detention orders by public health officials.

Ibid. See also, Canadian HIV/AIDS Legal Network, "Public health laws and HIV prevention" in Criminal Law and HIV (2008 information sheets), online: <http://www. aidslaw.ca/publications/publicationsdocEN.php?ref=847>.

[220] See, Canadian HIV/AIDS Legal Network, "Public health laws and HIV prevention" in Criminal Law and HIV (2008 information sheets), online: <http://www.aidslaw.ca/publications/ publicationsdocEN.php?ref=847>; Isabel Grant, "The Boundaries of Criminal Law: The Criminalization of the Nondisclosure of HIV" (2008) Dal. L.J. (forthcoming) (manuscript on file with author).

This chapter will focus on four different types of potential HIV-related tort duties: the duty of blood banking organizations to protect recipients; the duty of HIV-infected health care providers to protect their patients from infection; the duty of an HIV-infected person to protect his or her sexual or needle sharing partners; and the duty of physicians or other professionals to warn third parties of the risk of infection.

(ii) Blood Banking Litigation

Blood and tissue banking organizations faced the spectre of tort liability in the early years of the epidemic after it became clear that AIDS could be transmitted by exposure to blood but before implementation of HIV-antibody screening tests in 1985.[221] Blood banking organizations struggled to protect the safety of the blood supply, using a range of methods including asking those believed to be at high risk of infection to refrain from donation.[222] They considered using surrogate testing and screening methods, keenly aware that these blunt instruments might cause unintended injuries by limiting the supply of blood. Once the HIV antibody test became available, officials had to determine whether and how to test past donations.[223]

The Commission of Inquiry on the Blood System of Canada conducted an extensive investigation of the blood system's response to HIV, issuing a three-volume final report in 1997.[224] The Report, commonly referred to as the Krever Report after the Commissioner of the Inquiry, criticizes many of the choices made by persons involved in securing the blood supply from the risks of HIV and other diseases. Indeed, the Commission's activity generated litigation reaching the Supreme Court of Canada on the authority of a Commission of Inquiry to publish statements that might be misconstrued as findings of criminal or civil liability.[225] Blood banking organizations and others have been found

---

[221] The connection to blood was drawn relatively early in the pandemic by the high rates of disease among hemophiliacs.

[222] For more background on the history of HIV and the blood supply, see E. Feldman & Ronald Bayer, *Blood Feuds: AIDS, Blood, and the Politics of Medical Disaster* (New York: Oxford University Press, 1999); Lauren B. Leveton, Harold C. Sox, Jr. & Michael A. Stoto, *HIV and the Blood Supply: An Analysis of Crisis Decisionmaking* (Washington, D.C.: National Academies Press, 1995), online: The National Academic Press <http://www.nap.edu/catalog/4989.html>.

[223] See for example *Canadian AIDS Society v. Ontario*, [1996] O.J. No. 4184, 31 O.R. (3d) 798 (Ont. C.A.), leave to appeal to S.C.C. refused [1997] S.C.C.A. No. 33 (S.C.C.).

[224] See generally Library and Archives Canada, "Commission of Inquiry on the Blood System of Canada, Final Report" (1997) ("Krever Report"), online: Library and Archives Canada <http://epe.lac-bac.gc.ca/100/200/301/hcan-scan/commission_blood_final_rep-e/index.html>.

[225] *Canada (Attorney General) v. Canada (Commission of Inquiry on the Blood System-Krever Commission)*, [1997] S.C.J. No. 83, [1997] 3 S.C.R. 400 (S.C.C.), Cory J. [*Canada*

liable for failing to exercise due care and for failing to warn individuals of the risk of infection.[226] In *Walker Estate v. York-Finch General Hospital*, the Supreme Court of Canada found that the defendants were negligent in the manner in which they screened donors to reduce the risk of HIV before the implementation of HIV testing.[227]

(iii) HIV-Infected Health Care Providers

HIV infection can be transmitted by exposure to blood or other infected body fluids. These fluids are common in health care settings and health care providers have adopted the use of "universal precautions" to minimize the risk of exposure for health care providers and patients.[228] Because of lapses or failures in the use of universal precautions, the provision of some types of health care involving persons with HIV infection may involve very small risks.

There are a few cases of documented HIV transmission from HIV-infected patients to health care providers, but the risk of transmission is considered to be quite low.[229] Patients generally do not have a tort duty to inform their health care provider of their infection. Furthermore, HIV infection is considered to be a protected disability in Canada and health

---

(Attorney General) cited to S.C.R.]. The Court held that the Commission did not have the authority to establish civil or criminal liability but found that it had not exceeded its authority; in addition, the Commission had provided adequate procedural and notice protections for the complainants.

[226] See for example *Pittman Estate v. Bain*, [1994] O.J. No. 463, 112 D.L.R. (4th) 257 (Ont. Gen. Div.). Blood banking organizations and other defendants have also been found to have observed the standard of care and therefore shielded from liability. See for example Collin Smith & Grant Holly, "Court strikes out latest action in contaminated blood litigation" (December 2003) 8 Can. HIV/AIDS Pol'y and L. Rev. 1 at 56 (citing *Robb v. St. Joseph's Health Centre; Rintoul v. St. Joseph's Health Centre; Farrow v. Canadian Red Cross Society*, [2001] O.J. No. 4605 (Ont. C.A.), leave to appeal to S.C.C. refused [2002] S.C.C.A. No. 44 (S.C.C.)).

[227] *Walker Estate v. York-Finch General Hospital*, [2001] S.C.J. No. 24, [2001] 1 S.C.R. 647, 198 D.L.R. (4th) 193 (S.C.C.).

[228] Health Canada, "Preventing the Transmission of Bloodborne Pathogens in Health Care and Public Service Settings" (May 1997) 23:S3 CCDR 1, online: Public Health Agency of Canada <http://www.phac-aspc.gc.ca/publicat/ccdr-rmtc/97pdf/cdr23s3e.pdf>.

[229] See, *e.g.*, B. Stringer, C. Infante-Rivard & J. Hanley, "Quantifying and Reducing the Risk of Bloodborne Pathogen Exposure" (2001) 73 AORN J. 1142; Theodore de Bruyn, "Occupational Exposure to HIV and Forced HIV Testing: Questions and Answers", online: Canadian HIV/AIDS Legal Network, <http://www.aidslaw.ca/publications/publications docEN.php?ref=278>; Canadian AIDS Society, "Position Statement, Occupational Exposure, June 2007" (risk of HIV transmission following needlestick injury approximately 0.3 per cent; two probable and one definite case of HIV transmission from patients to providers in Canada), online: Canadian AIDS Society <http://www.cdnaids.ca/web/ setup.nsf/ActiveFiles/Occupational+Exposure+colour/$file/Occupational%20Exposure%20 colour.pdf>.

care providers therefore are prohibited from discriminating against HIV-infected patients.[230]

Although the level of risk is similar, the rights and duties of HIV-infected health care providers have been more controversial.[231] Should HIV-infected health care providers be permitted to continue to treat patients? If they do, should they be required to disclose their status to patients so that patients can knowingly agree or refuse to accept the admittedly very small risks?

There is little regulation and no reported litigation involving the duties of HIV-infected health care providers in Canada. The Québec College of Physicians recommends that physicians know their HIV status and that HIV-infected physicians consult with their employers before performing certain types of medical procedures.[232] The policy does not require an infected provider to disclose his or her status to patients.[233]

It is not clear whether HIV-infected physicians must disclose their HIV status to their patients under tort or fiduciary principles.[234] The

[230]   Theodore de Bruyn, "A Plan of Action for Canada to Reduce HIV/AIDS-Related Stigma and Discrimination" (2004) at 15-19 (summarizing anti-discrimination regulatory framework). Discrimination against patients persists. See, e.g., Brad Sears & Deborah Ho, "HIV Discrimination in Health Care Services in Los Angeles County: The Results of Three Testing Studies" (reporting that 46 per cent of skilled nursing facilities, 26 per cent of plastic surgeons, and 55 per cent of obstetricians surveyed refused services to HIV-infected patients), online: Williams Institute at UCLA, <http://www.law.ucla.edu/williamsinstitute/publications/Discrimination%20in%20Health%20Care%20LA%20County.pdf>.

[231]   See, e.g., Mary Anne Bobinski, "Patients and Providers in the Courts: Fractures in the Americans with Disabilities Act" (1998) 61 Alb. L. Rev. 785 (noting issue of physician disclosure under U.S. law); Mary Anne Bobinski, "Autonomy and Privacy: Protecting Patients from Their Physicians" (1994) 51 U. Pitt. L. Rev. 291 (analyzing disclosure obligations under U.S. law).

[232]   Collège des Médecins du Québec, "Le Médecin et les Infections Transmissible par le Sang" (2004), online: Collège des Médecins du Québec <http://www.cmq.org/DocumentLibrary/UploadedContents/CmsDocuments/Position_infections_transmissibles_sang.pdf>.

[233]   Ibid. The policy is similar to that adopted by the U.S. CDC, "Recommendations for Preventing Transmission of Human Immunodeficiency Virus and Hepatitis B Virus to Patients During Exposure-Prone Invasive Procedures" (12 July 1991) 40 MMWR Recomm Rep. (RR8) 1, in that affected physicians who perform procedures presenting a risk of infection must be evaluated by an expert review panel to determine whether and how they may continue to practice.

[234]   McInerney v. MacDonald, [1992] S.C.J. No. 57 at para. 20, [1992] 2 S.C.R. 138, 93 D.L.R. (4th) 415 (S.C.C.), per LaForest J. See also, Mary Anne Bobinski, "Patients and Providers in the Courts: Fractures in the Americans with Disabilities Act" (1998) 61 Alb. L. Rev. 785; Mary Anne Bobinski, "Autonomy and Privacy: Protecting Patients from Their Physicians", (1994) 51 U. Pitt. L. Rev. 291. See also U.S. CDC, "Recommendations for Preventing Transmission of Human Immunodeficiency Virus", ibid. ("HCWs [health care workers] who are infected with HIV... should not perform exposure-prone procedures unless they have sought counsel from an expert review panel and been advised under what circumstances, if any, they may continue to perform these procedures ... Such circumstances

Québec College of Physicians policy and a similar approach adopted by the U.S. CDC both suggest that HIV-infected health care providers may pose a significant risk to patients during some "exposure prone" medical procedures.[235] A court might take the view that traditional informed consent rules or fiduciary principles require that infected health care workers seeking to perform these procedures inform their patients of the significant risks.[236]

On the other hand, the Alberta Court of Queen's Bench decision in *Halkyard Estate v. Mathew* suggests that the HIV-infected physician does not have a duty to disclose this information to patients. In *Halkyard*, the court considered a claim that a surgeon with epilepsy had a duty to disclose his condition to his patient as a "material risk" under the informed consent process.[237] The court rejected the claim, finding that any issues about the ability of the defendant to continue to practice should be dealt with by his medical providers and the hospital in which he practiced rather than through the doctrine of informed consent. The Court of Appeal, in affirming the judgment, noted that the result might have been different if the plaintiff had been able to demonstrate harm caused by the failure to disclose. It is not clear how this would apply in the case of an HIV-infected health care worker. Presumably a patient who could prove that he or she acquired HIV from his or her health care provider during an exposure-prone procedure might be able to bring an informed consent claim. What should be the result if the patient learns of the possible risk after a procedure and suffers anxiety and repeated HIV testing as a result without ever becoming infected?[238]

---

would include notifying prospective patients of the HCW's seropositivity before they undergo exposure-prone invasive procedures").

[235] For discussion of other provincial policies and approaches, see Tyler Oswald, "Healthcare Workers Infected with Bloodborne Illnesses in Canada" (2007) 10:4 Healthcare Quarterly 64.

[236] See *supra*, note 234; Canadian HIV/AIDS Legal Network, "Criminalization of HIV exposure: current Canadian law" at 2, in *Criminal Law and HIV* (2008 information sheets), online: <http://www.aidslaw.ca/publications/publicationsdocEN.php?ref=847>.

[237] *Halkyard Estate v. Mathew*, [1998] A.J. No. 986, [1999] 5 W.W.R. 643 (Alta. Q.B.) ["*Halkyard Estate* (Q.B.)" cited to A.J.]; aff'd [2001] A.J. No. 293, 2001 ABCA 67 (Alta. C.A.) ["*Halkyard Estate* (C.A.)" cited to A.J.].

[238] *Halkyard Estate* (Q.B.), *ibid.*, at paras. 6-19. The case may have turned on the absence of evidence linking the failure to disclose with the death of the patient. The Court of Appeal, in affirming the judgment, noted that "[w]hen harm is caused by the lack of disclosure, liability in negligence may arise": *Halkyard Estate* (C.A.), *ibid.*, at para. 11. A patient might learn of the risk during a "look back" investigation conducted by a health institution that discovers that one of its health care workers was infected with HIV. See, *e.g.*, U.K. Dep't of Health, "HIV Infected Health Care Workers: Guidance on Management and Patient Notification" (2005) online: <http://www.advisorybodies.doh.gov.uk/eaga/pdfs/hiv_workers_280705.pdf>. The issues raised by "fears of HIV" claims are considered *supra*, text accompanying notes 256-64.

(iv) Tort Duties and Sexual Partners

What about the use of tort rules to promote safer behaviour by those who are or might be infected with HIV? Do persons diagnosed with HIV infection or those who are at risk for infection have a duty to refrain from conduct that could put others at risk? Should it be sufficient to inform others of the risk of infection? This section will focus on tort litigation involving sexual partners and the patients of HIV-infected health care providers.

Courts in the United States have considered claims brought under tort theories such as assault and battery; misrepresentation, fraud and deceit; and negligence.[239] Although there are few references in reported case law, some Canadian commentators believe our courts will impose tort damages where an infected person fails to disclose his or her status to a potential sexual or needle sharing partner.[240] The Supreme Court of Canada's decisions in two HIV-related criminal law cases, to be discussed below, might lend support to the application of tort law.

(v) Physicians and the Duty to Warn Third Parties

Health care providers who breach the standard of care in failing to protect patients from HIV infection, such as through failing to order appropriate testing or perinatal prophylactic treatment to prevent HIV transmission, can be held liable in tort.[241] Physicians who know or should know of a patient's HIV infection clearly have a duty to inform an infected patient and can be held liable for the reasonably foreseeable

---

[239] Deanna A. Pollard, "Sex Torts" (2007) 91 Minn. L. Rev. 769; Gregory G. Sarno, "Tort Liability for Infliction of Venereal Disease" (1985-2008) 40 A.L.R. (4th) 1089. Plaintiffs in the United States generally prefer negligence-based claims because intentional torts are often excluded from coverage under homeowners and other insurance policies.

[240] Nicolas Bala, "Tort Remedies and the Family Law Practitioner" (March 1999) 16 Can. Fam. L.Q. 423 (internal citations omitted):

The Supreme Court of Canada has indicated that a person who knows, or should reasonably know, that he or she has AIDS or another sexually transmitted disease may be liable in negligence to a partner who is not warned of the risk of infection and contracts the disease. This principle could be used to impose liability on an unfaithful spouse who negligently or knowingly infects his or her spouse as a result of a sexually transmitted disease.

See also Neo J. Tuytel, "Sexual Misconduct Claims: A Primer for Insurers on Liability and Coverage Issues Involving Sexual Assault, Abuse and Harassment (Part I)" (1998) 16 Can. J. Ins. L. 61 (focusing on sexual misconduct cases rather than disease transmission cases).

[241] See, e.g., M. (G.) v. Alter, [2006] O.J. No. 2762, 2006 WL 1903331, 2006 CarswellOnt 4190 (Ont. S.C.J.) (discussing settlement dispute in case arising from physician's alleged failure to offer appropriate HIV testing and treatment to prevent transmission to pregnant woman, whose child was infected with HIV).

consequences of failing to do so.[242] Assume that a physician has correctly diagnosed a patient's HIV infection and has informed the patient of his or her status and the necessary precautions to avoid further transmission of the disease. Does the physician have any further duties?

Studies demonstrate that a significant percentage of HIV-infected persons will continue to engage in behaviour that presents a risk to others without disclosing their status.[243] Some commentators and litigants argue that physicians should have an additional duty to warn third parties when the health professional knows that an HIV-infected person is placing others at risk for infection. The proposed duty is controversial for several reasons.[244] First, the duty may conflict with the physician's duty to maintain patients' confidences. Second, it is not always clear what actions will meet the duty — must a physician contact the third party directly or will a notice to public health authorities or other officials suffice? Third, the proposed rules are often fairly vague in establishing the scope of third parties (typically called "identifiable victims") subject to protection. Finally, the doctrine is controversial because it imposes a duty on physicians to a third party who is not the physician's patient.

The duty to warn is most famously associated with the California Supreme Court's decision in *Tarasoff v. University of California Regents*.[245] In *Tarasoff*, the court found that psychiatrists could be held liable to non-patients for "failing to exercise reasonable care to protect a third party where the therapists know or should know that their patient presents a serious danger of violence" to the third party, non-patient.[246] The case provides a somewhat unstable foundation upon which to build a duty to warn third parties, given that it has been rejected or limited in many jurisdictions in the United States.[247] Other American cases more clearly focus on a physician's duty to breach patient confidentiality when

---

[242] See, *e.g.*, *Healey v. Lakeridge Health Corp.*, [2006] O.J. No. 4277, 2006 CarswellOnt 6574 (Ont. S.C.J.) (physician who fails to diagnose patient's TB might be held liable to third parties infected by the patient); and *Pittman Estate v. Bain*, [1994] O.J. No. 463, 112 D.L.R. (4th) 257 (Ont. Gen. Div.) (husband infected wife with HIV before being informed of his infection).

[243] See note 205 at 3.

[244] Canadian HIV/AIDS Legal Network, "Confidentiality" in *HIV Testing* (2007) (series of 12 information sheets on HIV testing in Canada), online: <http://www.aidslaw.ca/ publications/publicationsdocEN.php?ref=713>. See also Mark A. Hall, Mary Anne Bobinski & David Orentlicher, *Health Care Law & Ethics* (New York: Aspen Publishing, 2007) at 185-98.

[245] *Tarasoff v. University of California Regents*, 551 P.2d 334 (Cal. S.C. 1976).

[246] See *e.g.*, Mark A. Hall, Mary Anne Bobinski & David Orentlicher, *Health Care Law & Ethics* (New York: Aspen Publishing, 2007) at 185-98.

[247] *Ibid.*

the patient has a contagious disease that poses a threat to identifiable third parties.[248]

Physicians in many Canadian provinces or territories have either the legal duty or the permissive authority to warn third parties:

> [A]t least six provinces or territories (Alberta, Manitoba, Saskatchewan, Ontario, Prince Edward Island and the Yukon) have legislation that requires or permits physicians to disclose confidential information without a patient's consent if there are reasonable grounds to believe that this will avoid or minimize danger to another person. Where such statutes do not exist, health professionals must be guided by any other relevant legislation that governs medical confidentiality, court decisions regarding confidentiality and its limits, and professional codes or guidelines.[249]

One commentator has suggested that physicians in Canadian jurisdictions without specific legislation authorizing or requiring disclosure should refrain from making disclosures to protect third parties.[250]

There is a significant difference between being "required" or "permitted" to disclose otherwise confidential patient information. Canadian courts have not yet directly confronted the question of whether there is a common law duty to disclose a patient's HIV status to protect third parties.[251] The legal duty might be drawn from professional and ethical guidelines. In 1998, Ontario's Medical Expert Panel on Duty to Inform adopted a consensus statement that explicitly recommended a duty to warn third parties "when a patient threatens to cause serious harm to another person or persons and it is more likely than not the threat will be

---

[248]   *Ibid.*, at 192-93; Tracey A. Bateman, "Liability of Doctor or Other Health Practitioner to Third Party Contracting Contagious Disease from Doctor's Patient" (1993-2008) 3 A.L.R. (5th) 370.

[249]   Canadian HIV/AIDS Legal Network, "Confidentiality" in *HIV Testing* (2007) (series of 12 information sheets on HIV testing in Canada), online: <http://www.aidslaw.ca/publications/publicationsdocEN.php?ref=713> at 3. See also M. Carey, "The Limits of Doctor-Patient Confidentiality in Canada" (1998) 19 Health L. Can. 52, 1998 C.H.L. Lexis 24 at 26-28. Carey cites as one example a case involving liability for a failure to disclose syphilis to the known partner of someone when both parties were patients (citing *C. v. D.*, [1924] O.J. No. 113, 56 O.L.R. 209 (Ont. H.C.J.)); and *supra*, Section III (c) (i) of this chapter (discussing common law and statutory exceptions).

[250]   Donald G. Casswell, "Disclosure by a Physician of AIDS-Related Patient Information: An Ethical and Legal Dilemma" (1989) The Can. B. Rev. 225.

[251]   In *Pittman Estate v. Bain*, [1994] O.J. No. 463, 112 D.L.R. (4th) 257 (Ont. Gen. Div.) the court did not reach the issue of whether the physician had a duty to disclose the patient's risk for HIV to his wife because liability could be predicated on the fact that the physician had not informed the patient of the risk: *Pittman Estate v. Bain, ibid.* ("It was unnecessary to determine whether an independent duty was owed to KP's wife, because there was a duty to inform KP himself, and, on the evidence, if KP had been told, he would certainly have alerted his wife.")

carried out".[252] However, the Ontario panel's recommendations conflict with the privacy code adopted by the Canadian Medical Association during the same time period. The CMA code focuses strongly on the need to preserve confidentiality and limits disclosures to those required by law or court order.[253] The law in this area continues to remain unclear as there are no reported Canadian cases finding a health care professional liable for breaching a duty to warn in a case involving HIV.[254]

Even where courts have recognized tort-based obligations to prevent harm, plaintiffs face substantial obstacles in proving injury and causation. Where a plaintiff has HIV infection, it is often difficult to prove that the defendant was the source of the infection. The litigation can involve potentially embarrassing testimony about possible alternative sources of infection.[255]

---

[252] Lorraine E. Ferris *et al.*, "Defining the Physician's Duty to Warn: Consensus Statement of Ontario's Medical Expert Panel on Duty to Inform" (2 June 1998) 158 C.M.A.J. 1473. See also Christopher Zinn, "Wife Wins Case Against GPs Who did not Disclose Husband's HIV Status" (2003) 326 BMJ 1286 (reporting on US$473,400 award to woman under negligence and breach of contract theories; GPs had told man she was about to marry of his positive test result but "fail[ed] to ensure that . . . [he] told his wife about the result").

[253] Canadian Medical Association, *Health Information Privacy Code*, online: <http://www.cma.ca/index.cfm/ci_id/3216/la_id/1.htm#prin5>. See also John Hoey, "The CMA's Health Information Privacy Code: Does it Go Too Far?" (1998) 159 C.M.A.J. 953, 954 (noting possible conflict); and Canadian HIV/AIDS Legal Network, "Confidentiality" in *HIV Testing* (2007) (series of 12 information sheets on HIV testing in Canada), online: <http://www.aidslaw.ca/publications/publicationsdocEN.php?ref=713> at 3.

[254] *Ibid.*, at 3.

[255] See, *e.g.*, *supra* note 18 (discussing use of HIV testing to identify common sources of infection); and *John B. v. Superior Court*, 38 Cal.4th 1177, 137 P.3d 153 (Cal. Sup. Ct. 2006). In *John B.*, the California Supreme Court weighted the competing interests and permitted discovery of sensitive personal information in case involving possible HIV transmission from husband to wife:

> Here, defendant has invoked his constitutional right to privacy as justification for refusing to answer questions concerning his HIV status or his sexual history. Bridget, in turn, has identified not only ... [the state's interest in truthful fact-finding in legal proceedings], but also the state's compelling interest in preventing the spread of AIDS, a communicable and dangerous disease ... [Various provisions in the criminal code] ... are strong statements by the Legislature that the spread of HIV is a serious public health threat and that its control is of paramount importance. ...
> In balancing these competing concerns, we note at the outset that. ... [b]oth parties have admitted they are HIV positive, informally and in court filings. John thus has a diminished privacy interest in his HIV status. ... Moreover, not only does the complaint allege sufficient facts to permit the inference that John infected Bridget with HIV, but John has alleged that Bridget infected him.   By thus putting his own medical condition at issue, John has "substantially lowered" his expectation of privacy even further. ... After balancing the competing interests in this case, we are persuaded that Bridget is entitled to discovery concerning John's sexual history and HIV status.

Ibid., 38 Cal.4th at 1199, 137 P.3d at 167 (citations omitted).

In many cases, plaintiffs are not able to demonstrate they have acquired HIV infection. In these cases, plaintiffs have sought to recover for the fear of acquiring HIV. These HIV phobia cases can be problematic, given the difficulty of drawing a line between compensable mental anguish and non-compensable, irrational fear.[256] In *Garner v. Blue & White Taxi Co-operative Ltd.*, for example, a passenger sustained a needle-stick from a syringe while sitting in a cab.[257] The court found the defendant was not liable for the injury because the cab driver had observed the required standard of care.[258] The court nonetheless considered the plaintiff's damage claims. The court noted that although the passenger repeatedly tested negative for HIV infection and was told "that there was a 99 percent chance that he had not contracted HIV virus as of ... [a date] six months after the accident ... [he] continued to be fearful".[259] The court found that the plaintiff suffered this anxiety for three years and assessed the proper damage for suffering at $5,000.[260]

Most U.S. courts that have considered the issue attempt to limit HIV phobia claims to circumstances which involved a real risk of transmission (called "actual exposure") and to the time period during which a reasonable person might suffer from the fear of infection.[261] In *Fitzgerald v. Tin*, the British Columbia trial court considered and rejected this trend in another case involving a needle-stick injury to a passenger in a taxicab.[262] The court held:

> I am satisfied that the "Possible Exposure" approach should be adopted in Canada. Until it can be shown with reasonable certainty that a plaintiff is not HIV positive, that plaintiff suffers the mental anguish of having a reasonable fear that they have become HIV positive. It was not

---

[256] These cases also raise interesting procedural questions about the appropriate statute of limitations period: see, *e.g.*, *Birrell v. Providence Health Care Society*, [2008] B.C.J. No. 53, 2008 BCCA 14, 73 B.C.L.R. (4th) 223, 2008 CarswellBC 41 (B.C.C.A.) (granting leave to appeal on question whether statute of limitations should begin to run from the time notice given of possible exposure); and the appropriate range of damages in cases where no disease has been transmitted: see, *e.g.*, *Rideout v. Health Labrador Corp.*, [2007] N.J. No. 292, 2007 NLTD 150, 2007 CarswellNfld 268 (N.L.T.D.) (reviewing proposed settlement including adequacy of awards to plaintiffs who received notice that they might have been exposed to HIV and other diseases due to failure to sterilize equipment in gynecological clinic).

[257] *Garner v. Blue & White Taxi Co-operative Ltd.*, [1995] O.J. No. 2636 (Ont. Gen. Div.).

[258] *Ibid.*, at paras. 22-25.

[259] *Ibid.*, at para. 29.

[260] *Ibid.* The damages were not awarded because of the determination that the defendant was not liable.

[261] See Kimberly C. Simmons, "Recovery for Emotional Distress Based on Fear of Contracting HIV or AIDS" (1998-2003) 59 A.L.R. (5th) 535; *Shumosky v. Lutheran Welfare Services of Northeastern PA, Inc.*, 784 A.2d 196 (Pa. Super. 2001) (collecting cases; noting majority use actual exposure rule).

[262] *Fitzgerald v. Tin*, [2003] B.C.J. No. 203, 11 B.C.L.R. (4th) 375 (B.C.S.C.).

unreasonable for Ms. Fitzgerald to fear HIV infection after being exposed to a syringe. A syringe is clearly a medically viable channel of transmission of the HIV virus. The applicable standard of care requires that a person such as Ms. Fitzgerald conduct her life as if she had been actually exposed to HIV-positive fluids until such time as a blood test reveals ... that she is not HIV positive.[263]

Fitzgerald tested negative at seven months; the court awarded $15,000 in damages for her mental distress during this time period.[264]

This brief overview of the relation between tort law and the risk of HIV transmission suggests that tort has been relatively underutilized to establish norms of conduct in Canada compared to the United States. This may reflect a general aversion to establishing standards of care via litigation or the relative paucity of damages available to tort claimants in Canada. In any event, it does not appear that tort liability has been constrained by charges of HIV exceptionalism.

(d) Criminal Law

As noted above, a small but significant percentage of HIV-infected persons continue to engage in conduct that could present a risk of transmission to others. There are ranges of behaviours and risks. Some HIV-infected persons always disclose their status and/or engage in safer practices while some do so much of the time; a very small percentage of persons with HIV infection actively seek to transmit the virus to others.[265] The general category of "risky behaviour" includes a wide range of actual risks, for the probability of HIV transmission depends on factors such as the type of activity (from low to higher risk sexual or needle sharing activities), the "role" of the HIV-infected person (as a man or woman,

---

[263]   *Ibid.*, at para. 50.

[264]   *Ibid.*, at paras. 50-52 and Conclusion. Michael P. Busch & Glen A. Salten, "Time Course of Viremia and Antibody Seroconversion Following Human Immunodeficiency Virus Exposure" (1997) 102 Am. J. Med. Supp. 2 177. About 95 per cent of persons infected with HIV will produce antibodies to the virus within six months of exposure if they have been infected with the virus. Testing directly for the presence of the virus could reduce the time period of reasonable anxiety significantly. See *supra*, note 15.

[265]   Dennis H. Osmond *et al.*, "Changes in Prevalence of HIV Infection and Sexual Risk Behavior in Men Who Have Sex with Men in San Francisco: 1997-2002" (2007) 97 Amer. J. Pub. H. 1677 (noting increase in sexually risky activities); David A. Moskowitz & Michael E. Roloff, "The Existence of a Bug Chasing Subculture" (2007) 9 Culture, Health & Sexuality 347 (documenting existence of "bug chasers": persons seeking to become HIV-infected); Christian Grov & Jeffrey T. Parsons, "Bug Chasing and Gift Giving: The Potential for HIV Transmission Among Barebackers on the Internet" (2006) 18 AIDS Educ. & Prev. 490 ("bug chasing" and "gift giving" exist in "barebacking" culture (men who seek unprotected anal sex) but the percentage of men actively seeking to transmit or to receive HIV is small).

participating in "receptive" or "penetrative" sexual activities of different types), the HIV-infected person's viral load and the presence or absence of skin irritations or abrasions.[266]

Criminal law generally is used to deter and to punish wrongful conduct. As an instrument of public health policy, criminal law standards constitute society's strongest statement regarding morally blameworthy conduct. The use of criminal law to address the risks of HIV transmission raises difficult legal issues and policy questions. How well does the criminal law framework respond to the complexities of risky activities and intentions noted above? Does the use of criminal law further the goal of protecting public health?

Criminal prosecutions have been quite common in the United States, particularly for members of the Armed Forces who are governed by the Military Code of Justice.[267] Defendants have been convicted of HIV-related criminal offences for conduct ranging from spitting on another person to repeated sexual acts. Prosecutors have been successful in using traditional criminal offences ranging from attempted murder to assault with a deadly weapon. Many states also have specific laws making it a criminal offence to expose others to the risk of HIV transmission.[268] Ironically, this type of HIV exceptionalism has frustrated some prosecutors, who argue they were able to invoke more substantial criminal penalties using traditional general offences such as attempted murder.[269]

In Canada, prosecutions for HIV-infected persons who place others at risk seem increasingly common and the sanctions seem increasingly severe.[270] Canadian prosecutions are based on one or more of several theories: common nuisance;[271] criminal negligence;[272] and assault,[273] including

---

[266] Scott Burris *et al.*, "Do Criminal Laws Influence HIV Risk Behavior? An Empirical Trial" (2007) 39 Ariz. St. L. J. 467, 476-77.

[267] See generally, Alan Stephens, "Annotation, Transmission or Risk of Transmission of Human Immunodeficiency Virus (HIV) or Acquired Immunodeficiency Syndrome (AIDS) as Basis for Prosecution or Sentencing in Criminal or Military Case" (1993-2008) 13 A.L.R. (5th) 628.

[268] *Ibid.*; Michael L. Closen *et al.*, "Criminalization of an Epidemic: HIV-AIDS and Criminal Transmission Laws" (1994) 46 Ark. L. Rev. 921-83 (annotated panel discussion).

[269] Closen *et al.*, "Criminalization of an Epidemic", *ibid.*

[270] Canadian HIV/AIDS Legal Network, "Prosecutions under the *Criminal Code*" in *Criminal Law and HIV* (2008 information sheets), online: <http://www.aidslaw.ca/publications/publicationsdocEN.php?ref=847>; Isabel Grant, "The Boundaries of Criminal Law: The Criminalization of the Nondisclosure of HIV" (2008) Dal. L.J. (forthcoming).

[271] Under the *Criminal Code*, R.S.C. 1985, c. C-46, provisions on common nuisance:

    180. (1) Every one who commits a common nuisance and thereby
        (a) endangers the lives, safety or health of the public, or
        (b) causes physical injury to any person, is guilty of an indictable offence and liable to imprisonment for a term not exceeding two years.
    (2) For the purposes of this section, every one commits a common nuisance who does an unlawful act or fails to discharge a legal duty and thereby

aggravated assault;[274] and sexual assault.[275] The key criminal prosecutions under assault involve questions about the interpretation of the *Criminal Code* provisions regarding consent.[276] The consent issue first made its way up to the Supreme Court of Canada in *R. v. Cuerrier.*[277]

    (*a*) endangers the lives, safety, health, property or comfort of the public; or

    (*b*) obstructs the public in the exercise or enjoyment of any right that is common to all the subjects of Her Majesty in Canada.

The provision has been applied to the knowing donation of HIV-infected blood without disclosure of HIV status, *R. v. Thornton*, [1991] O.J. No. 25, 3 C.R. (4th) 381 (Ont. C.A.), aff'd [1993] S.C.J. No. 62, [1993] 2 S.C.R. 445 (S.C.C.), as well as to sexual activity by an HIV-infected person, *R. v. Williams*, [2003] S.C.J. No. 41, [2003] 2 S.C.R. 134 at para. 71, 230 D.L.R. (4th) 39 (S.C.C.) ["*Williams* (S.C.C.)" cited to S.C.R.]; *R. v. Williams*, [2004] N.J. No. 140, 2004 NLCA 24 at para. 5, 184 C.C.C. (3d) 193 (N.L.C.A.) ["*Williams* (C.A.)" cited to NLCA] (sentencing).

272   Under the *Criminal Code*, *ibid.*, provisions governing criminal negligence:

    219. (1) Every one is criminally negligent who (*a*) in doing anything, or (*b*) in omitting to do anything that it is his duty to do, shows wanton or reckless disregard for the lives or safety of other persons.

    (2) For the purposes of this section, "duty" means a duty imposed by law . . . .

273   The *Criminal Code*, *ibid.*, defines general assault in s. 265:

    265. (1) A person commits an assault when (*a*) without the consent of another person, he applies force intentionally to that other person, directly or indirectly . . .

    (2) This section applies to all forms of assault, including sexual assault, sexual assault with a weapon, threats to a third party or causing bodily harm and aggravated sexual assault.

    (3) For the purposes of this section, no consent is obtained where the complainant submits or does not resist by reason of ... (*c*) fraud. ...

274   Under s. 268 of the *Criminal Code*, *ibid.*: "(1) Every one commits an aggravated assault who wounds, maims, disfigures or endangers the life of the complainant."

275   Aggravated sexual assault is defined in s. 273 of the *Criminal Code*, *ibid.*: "(1) Every one commits an aggravated sexual assault who, in committing a sexual assault, wounds, maims, disfigures or endangers the life of the complainant."

276   Under s. 273.1 of the *Criminal Code*, *ibid.*:

    273.1 (1) Subject to subsection (2) and subsection 265(3), "consent" means, for the purposes of section [ ] ... 273, the voluntary agreement of the complainant to engage in the sexual activity in question.

    (2) No consent is obtained, for the purposes of section [ ] 273, where ... (*b*) the complainant is incapable of consenting to the activity; (*c*) the accused induces the complainant to engage in the activity by abusing a position of trust, power or authority ...

    (3) Nothing in subsection (2) shall be construed as limiting the circumstances in which no consent is obtained.

    273.2 It is not a defence to a charge under section ... 273 that the accused believed that the complainant consented to the activity that forms the subject-matter of the charge, where (*a*) the accused's belief arose from the accused's ... (ii) recklessness or willful blindness; or (*b*) the accused did not take reasonable steps, in the circumstances known to the accused at the time, to ascertain that the complainant was consenting.

277   [1998] S.C.J. No. 64, [1998] 2 S.C.R. 371, 162 D.L.R. (4th) 513 (S.C.C.). Justice Cory delivered the judgment joined by Justices Major, Bastarache and Binnie. Justice

In *Cuerrier,* the defendant was instructed by a public health nurse to "use condoms every time he engaged in sexual intercourse and to inform all prospective sexual partners that he was HIV-positive".[278] The defendant had unprotected sex with two complainants without informing them of his status.[279] Cuerrier "was charged with two counts of aggravated assault".[280] Neither complainant tested HIV positive at the time of trial.[281] Trial court entered a verdict of acquittal which was upheld by the Court of Appeal.[282] The Supreme Court allowed the appeal and ordered a new trial.

The Court found that Cuerrier had endangered the lives of the complainants.[283] The remaining issue involved the consent provision of the statute. Justice Cory, writing for the majority, found that it was "no longer necessary when examining whether consent in assault or sexual assault cases was vitiated by fraud to consider whether the fraud related to the nature and quality of the act".[284] "[T]raditional requirements for fraud, namely dishonesty and deprivation" would also suffice to vitiate consent.[285] According to the judgment, "[t]he actions of the accused must be assessed objectively to determine whether a reasonable person would find them to be dishonest" through deceit or non-disclosure.[286] Deprivation could be shown either by "actual harm or simply a risk of harm" so long as the dishonesty "had the effect of exposing the person consenting to a significant risk of serious bodily harm".[287] In addition, "the Crown will still be required to prove beyond a reasonable doubt that the complainant would have refused to engage in unprotected sex with the accused" if she had knowledge of his HIV status.[288]

L'Heureux-Dubé wrote separately. Justice McLachlin submitted reasons with Gonthier J. joining.

[278]   *Ibid.,* at para. 78.

[279]   *Ibid.,* at paras. 79-82.

[280]   *Ibid.,* at para. 83.

[281]   *Ibid.*

[282]   *Ibid.*

[283]   *Criminal Code,* R.S.C. 1985, c. C-46, s. 273.

[284]   *R. v. Cuerrier,* [1998] S.C.J. No. 64 at para. 108, [1998] 2 S.C.R. 371, 162 D.L.R. (4th) 513 (S.C.C.).

[285]   *Ibid.,* at para. 125.

[286]   *Ibid.,* at para. 126.

[287]   *Ibid.,* at para. 128.

[288]   *R. v. Cuerrier,* [1998] S.C.J. No. 64 at para. 130, [1998] 2 S.C.R. 371, 162 D.L.R. (4th) 513 (S.C.C.). Madam Justice L'Heureux-Dubé would have adopted a more expansive view of fraud, permitting dishonesty to vitiate consent to sexual activity whenever the dishonesty was about a matter important enough to affect consent (*ibid.,* at para. 16). Madam Justice McLachlin would have adopted a narrower understanding of the fraud provision, limiting fraud to cases where "there was (a) a deception as to the sexual character of the act; (b) deception as to the identity of the perpetrator; or (c) deception as to the presence of a sexually transmitted disease giving rise to a serious risk or probability of infecting the complainant" (*ibid.,* at para. 70).

The interveners in *Cuerrier* argued that criminalization of HIV exposure was unnecessary because other public health measures already were available to address the conduct of HIV infected persons and because the risk of criminal liability might deter some individuals from undergoing testing.[289] Justice Cory firmly rejected these arguments, expressing skepticism about the effectiveness of other public health law measures and noting that people were likely to undergo HIV testing because it was in their best interest to get treatment.[290]

The Supreme Court of Canada revisited the issue of criminal liability for persons with HIV infection in *R. v. Williams*.[291] In *Williams*, the accused discovered that he was HIV-infected and then continued to have sexual relations with the complainant without telling her of his infection.[292] The problem for the Crown was that there was no proof as to when the complainant acquired HIV infection. She might have been infected by Williams before he was aware of his HIV status. Justice Binnie, writing for the majority, found that the accused could not be convicted of aggravated assault because of the lack of proof that he had endangered the complainant's life after he knew that he had HIV.[293] The accused was properly convicted of attempted aggravated assault and common nuisance.[294]

The Supreme Court's rulings in *Williams* and *Currier* confirmed the validity of the criminal law approach in Canada. Courts are continuing to

---

[289]   *Ibid.*, at paras. 140-46. See *supra*, Section IV (b) (iv) (public health orders).

[290]   *R. v. Cuerrier*, [1998] S.C.J. No. 64 at paras. 140-46, [1998] 2 S.C.R. 371, 162 D.L.R. (4th) 573.

[291]   [2003] S.C.J. No. 41, [2003] 2 S.C.R. 134 (S.C.C.).

[292]   *Ibid.*, at paras. 3-10.

[293]   *Ibid.*, at paras. 25, 46. Justice Binnie notes that criminal liability could apply even to cases in which the defendant was never officially informed of his or her HIV status:

The critical date for the purpose of establishing fraud to vitiate consent (*Criminal Code*, s. 265(3)(c)) is when the respondent had sufficient awareness of his HIV-positive status that he can be said to have acted "intentionally or recklessly, with knowledge of the facts constituting the offence, or with willful blindness toward them" (*R. v. Sault Ste. Marie (City)*, [1978] 2 S.C.R. 1299 (S.C.C.), at p. 1309) . . . Once an individual becomes aware of a risk that he or she has contracted HIV, and hence that his or her partner's consent has become an issue, but nevertheless persists in unprotected sex that creates a risk of further HIV transmission without disclosure to his or her partner, recklessness is established (*ibid.*, at paras. 27-28).

[294]   *Ibid.*, at paras. 60-66 (affirming conviction for attempted aggravated assault; noting *mens rea* and more than preparatory step toward *actus reus*); *R. v. Williams*, [2004] N.J. No. 140, 2004 NLCA 24 at para. 73, 184 C.C.C. (3d) 193 (N.L.C.A.) (conviction for common nuisance affirmed). Professor Isabel Grant notes that the Court's reasoning in *Williams* leads to the ironic result that prosecutors will find it easier to prosecute defendants for aggravated assault when the defendants' sexual contacts remain uninfected: Isabel Grant, "The Boundaries of Criminal Law: The Criminalization of the Nondisclosure of HIV" (2008) Dal. L.J. (forthcoming).

work through the implications of the criminal law approach in different areas. For example, Binnie J.'s suggestion in *Williams* that a defendant could not use willful ignorance of his or her HIV status as a defence has reduced concerns that criminal liability would simply encourage people to refuse testing. Yet questions remain about when a defendant will be deemed to have sufficient knowledge of the risk of HIV infection to be subject to the duty to disclose.[295] Should previous participation in high risk activities be sufficient to impose a duty to warn? What about the degree of endangerment to life necessary for an assault conviction: how should this be mapped against the broad range of risks for different types of activities? Should a defendant's use of safer sex or needle-sharing practices or low viral load be sufficient to avoid criminal liability, at least for assault? What if an HIV-infected person informs a sexual contact of his or her status immediately after a sexual encounter and urges the contact to obtain post-exposure prophylaxis in order to greatly reduce any risk of harm?[296] The answers are unclear.[297] Finally, how should the criminal law respond to the admittedly rare problem of "bug chasing"? Should a person who knowingly transmits HIV to a willing recipient be held criminally responsible for murder or assisted suicide?

From a policy perspective, the trend toward the greater use of criminal law in Canada and elsewhere runs counter to substantial and growing concerns about whether the approach is misguided and perhaps even counterproductive to public health goals. A recent empirical study found that the behaviours and beliefs of HIV-infected people about

---

[295]   Canadian HIV/AIDS Legal Network, "Criminalization of HIV exposure: current Canadian law"; Isabel Grant, "The Boundaries of Criminal Law: The Criminalization of the Nondisclosure of HIV" (2008) Dal. L.J. (forthcoming).

[296]   See C. Dodds, "Positive Benefits: Preventive Impact of Post-Exposure Prophylaxis Awareness Among Those Diagnosed with HIV" (2007) 84 Sex. Transm. Infect. 92 (significant percentage of sample of men seeking post-exposure prophylaxis learned that a sexual partner was HIV positive following sexual contact). This example raises a potential conflict between criminal law and public health objectives. While pre-sexual activity disclosure of status might be preferred, even a post-exposure disclosure can give a sexual contact information that could be used to secure treatment and to avoid transmission. The optimal criminal law rule might therefore be to take an immediate post-exposure disclosure into account in reducing the severity of the offense or punishment.

[297]   Compare *R. v. Edwards*, [2001] N.S.J. No. 221, 2001 NSSC 80 (N.S.S.C.) (safer sex practices might reduce risk of harm below point justifying criminal liability) with *R. v. Mabior*, [2008] M.J. No. 277 at paras. 99-117 (Man. Q.B.) (endangerment of life proven even where condom used but broken during act, where protections used and when viral load low). See also, Canadian HIV/AIDS Legal Network, "Criminalization of HIV exposure: current Canadian law" in *Criminal Law and HIV* (2008 information sheets), online: <http://www.aidslaw.ca/publications/publicationsdocEN.php?ref=847> at 1-2 ("the law is unclear about whether a person living with HIV has a duty to disclose his or her status when engaging in other sexual acts with a lower risk of HIV transmission than unprotected anal or vaginal sex").

disclosure or sexual activity were unrelated to the nature of the criminal law rules in their particular jurisdiction.[298] Some critics argue that criminal sanctions can injure public health if the spectre of criminal liability discourages people from undergoing HIV testing. In addition, criminal liability standards might have unintended consequences if responsibility for protecting against HIV infection is distributed unevenly across society, such as when it is placed on people with HIV infection and not on those who believe they are uninfected. These concerns are echoed in a UNAIDS policy brief issued in 2008:

> There are no data indicating that the broad application of criminal law to HIV transmission will achieve either criminal justice or prevent HIV transmission. Rather, such application risks undermining public health and human rights. Because of these concerns, UNAIDS urges governments to limit criminalization to cases of intentional transmission, *i.e.*, where a person knows his or her HIV positive status, acts with the intention to transmit HIV and does in fact transmit it.[299]

It remains to be seen whether Canada, or indeed any country, will step back from the use of criminal law in response to these recommendations.

V.   LESSONS FOR THE FUTURE

It is commonplace to note that many citizens and health care providers in the 1980s were quaintly confident about medicine's inevitable triumph over infectious diseases. The recognition of widespread illness and the discovery of the HIV virus was the first of many tests to this confidence. The virus's unique characteristics made plotting a response difficult for health care providers, public health officials, policy-makers, and judges. The course of the HIV pandemic over the past 28 years sparked the re-examination of long neglected aspects of public health policy and law.

This chapter's treatment of the public health law aspects of HIV infection highlighted two major areas: (1) the public health aspects of case identification; and (2) the role of the legal system in addressing the risk of transmission. Although the legal response to HIV infection has been diverse and complex, three major thematic debates emerged: (1) What level(s) of government should be involved in the protection of public health? (2) Should HIV's unique characteristics inspire exceptional legal

---

[298]   Scott Burris *et al.*, "Do Criminal Laws Influence HIV Risk Behavior? An Empirical Trial" (2007) 39 Ariz. St. L.J. 467. See also Scott Burris & Edwin Cameron, "The Case Against Criminalization of HIV Transmission" (2008) 300 JAMA 578 (setting out the "case against criminalization").

[299]   UNAIDS, "Policy Brief: Criminalization of HIV Transmission" (2008), online: <http://data.unaids.org/pub/BaseDocument/2008/20080731_jc1513_policy_criminalization_en.pdf>.

strategies or should the response to HIV be "mainstreamed" into public health law and practice? and (3) What is the proper balance between the protection of individual liberties and the promotion of public health and safety?

Canada's approach to the problems presented by HIV infection has largely been consistent with international norms and evolving public health norms. Jurisdictional issues — always present in a federal system of government — have resulted from time to time in complex overlapping systems of regulation. Canada's approach to protecting privacy and preserving the confidentiality of medical information is one example of this difficulty. The impact of the still relatively new Public Health Agency of Canada on HIV policies remains to be seen.[300]

Canada has adopted many public health strategies that are informed by experience with HIV but has tended to avoid HIV exceptionalism. Unlike the United States, Canada never adopted special HIV testing and confidentiality statutes or HIV-specific criminal statutes. Canadian jurisdictions instead tended to incorporate the special concerns arising from the social stigma and discrimination associated with HIV into the pre-existing legal framework for informed consent, confidentiality, public health measures, and criminal law. In many areas, this mainstreaming of HIV issues appears to have succeeded in both promoting public health and protecting individual liberty. Criminal law is an important exception, given the increasingly frequent use of the relatively blunt instrument of criminal law to address the complex and nuanced questions of risk in sexual and needlesharing activity.

Finally, Canada has an excellent record of developing public health policies that incorporate the protection of individual liberty as a fundamental component of public health rather than an opposing goal. Yet Canada's focus on individual rights arguably is fading. The emergence of moderately effective therapies to prolong life for persons infected with HIV appears to have played major role in changing this dynamic. Given the availability of life-extending treatment, people with HIV infection may now be motivated to seek testing and treatment even without continued focus on individual rights. The whittling away of the "three C's" approach to HIV testing in favour of "routine" testing may be an important example of this phenomenon.

---

[300]   New policies on HIV testing expected to be released by PHAC in 2008 may provide an important signal.

7

TOBACCO CONTROL AND THE LAW IN CANADA

Barbara von Tigerstrom[*]

I. INTRODUCTION

Tobacco-related disease is the leading cause of preventable death in Canada and in the world.[1] One third to one half of all habitual smokers will die of tobacco-related disease, losing an estimated average of 15 years of life expectancy.[2] Tobacco-related diseases include cardiovascular and respiratory diseases, lung cancer and other cancers.[3] The U.S. Surgeon General has recently expanded the list of diseases caused by smoking, and stated that smoking harms nearly every organ of the body.[4] It has also been established that the health effects of tobacco are shared to a significant extent by non-smokers who are exposed to second-hand smoke ("SHS", also known as environmental tobacco smoke, passive smoking or

[*]   Acknowledgements: The author would like to thank Nola M. Ries (Health Law Institute) and Dr. Neil Boister (University of Canterbury School of Law) for their input and assistance on the first edition of this chapter, and Erin Schroh (College of Law, University of Saskatchewan) for providing research assistance for the second edition.

[1]   Eva M. Makomaski Illing & Murray J. Kaiserman, "Mortality Attributable to Tobacco Use in Canada and its Regions, 1998" (2004) 95 Can. J. Public Health 38 at 42-43; WHO, *The World Health Report 2003* (Geneva: WHO, 2003) at 91.

[2]   WHO, *WHO Report on the Global Tobacco Epidemic, 2008* (Geneva: WHO, 2008), online: <http://www.who.int/tobacco/mpower/mpower_report_full 2008.pdf> at 14.

[3]   Dolly Baliunas *et al.*, "Smoking-attributable Mortality and Expected Years of Life Lost in Canada 2002: Conclusions for Prevention and Policy" (2007) 27 Chronic Diseases in Canada 154 at 154.

[4]   U.S. Department of Health and Human Services, *The Health Consequences of Smoking: A Report of the Surgeon General* (Georgia: U.S. Department of Health and Human Services, Centers for Disease Control and Prevention, National Center for Chronic Disease Prevention and Health Promotion, Office on Smoking and Health, 2004), online: CDC <http://www.cdc.gov/tobacco/data_statistics/sgr/sgr_2004/index.htm>.

involuntary smoking). SHS has been established as a cause of lung cancer and linked to other cancers and a range of other health problems.[5] In Canada, it is estimated that just under 5 million people, approximately 19 per cent of the population aged 15 and older, are current smokers.[6] Although smoking prevalence is steadily decreasing,[7] the number of deaths due to smoking ("smoking attributable mortality" or "SAM") remains high and is declining more slowly that smoking prevalence, due to the latent period between smoking and SAM.[8] A study based on 1998 data found that SAM accounted for more than 47,000 deaths in Canada, representing 22 per cent of all deaths (six times the number of deaths from car accidents, alcohol, murder and suicides combined).[9] A more recent study found that in 2002, almost 40,000 deaths (16.6 per cent of all deaths) were attributable to smoking.[10]

The economic cost associated with tobacco use is also significant. The main economic costs are from direct health care costs and lost productivity; other costs include an increase in fire insurance premiums, property damage and environmental damage (from fires and packaging materials).[11] Some industry reports have attempted to counter these cost estimates by suggesting that SAM is actually economically beneficial because the premature deaths of smokers relieves the state of the "burden"

---

[5]   International Agency for Research on Cancer, *Tobacco Smoke and Involuntary Smoking* (IARC Monographs, vol. 83) (Lyon: IARC, 2002); summary available online: IARC <http://monographs.iarc.fr/ENG/Monographs/vol83/volume83.pdf>; U.S. Department of Health and Human Services, *Reducing Tobacco Use: A Report of the Surgeon General* (Georgia: U.S. Department of Health and Human Services, Centers for Disease Control and Prevention, National Center for Chronic Disease Prevention and Health Promotion, Office on Smoking and Health, 2000) at 195-96, online: <http://www.cdc.gov/tobacco/data_ statistics/sgr/sgr_2000/>.

[6]   Health Canada, "Canadian Tobacco Use Monitoring Survey ("CTUMS"): Summary of Results for the First Half of 2007 (February-June)", online: <http://www.hc-sc.gc.ca/hl-vs/tobac-tabac/research-recherche/stat/_ctums-esutc_2007/wave-phase-1_summary-sommaire_e. html>.

[7]   Health Canada, "Canadian Tobacco Use Monitoring Survey ("CTUMS"): Smoking Prevalence 1999-2007", online: <http://www.hc-sc.gc.ca/hl-vs/tobac-tabac/research-recherche/ stat/_ctums-esutc_prevalence/prevalence_e.html>.

[8]   Dolly Baliunas *et al.*, "Smoking-attributable Mortality and Expected Years of Life Lost in Canada 2002: Conclusions for Prevention and Policy" (2007) 27 Chronic Diseases in Canada 154 at 160.

[9]   Eva M. Makomaski Illing & Murray J. Kaiserman, "Mortality Attributable to Tobacco Use in Canada and its Regions, 1998" (2004) 95 Can. J. Public Health 38 at 42-43.

[10]   Dolly Baliunas *et al.*, "Smoking-attributable Mortality and Expected Years of Life Lost in Canada 2002: Conclusions for Prevention and Policy" (2007) 27 Chronic Diseases in Canada 154 at 159.

[11]   See *e.g.*, Rob Cunningham, *Smoke & Mirrors: The Canadian Tobacco War* (Ottawa: International Development Research Centre, 1996) at 12.

of caring for elderly individuals.[12] Even if this is true in a certain sense, it is not the sort of cost-benefit analysis that most would accept as a proper guide for public policy. The economic costs associated with tobacco consumption have been one motivator for tobacco control measures, and these measures are likely to be very cost-effective.[13] In addition, as we will see below in the discussion of tobacco litigation, some governments have sought to recover the health care costs attributable to tobacco-related disease from the industry.

Looking beyond our borders, it is clear that the health impact of tobacco consumption is also a major global issue. Tobacco-related disease is the leading cause of preventable death worldwide, with an annual death toll of over five million — approximately one in ten adult deaths, or one death every six seconds; the annual death toll is expected to reach eight million by 2030 without effective and widespread intervention.[14] Furthermore, the human and economic costs of tobacco use and tobacco-related disease are borne disproportionately by developing states and by lower socioeconomic groups within states.[15]

Given the profound impact of tobacco consumption on the health of their populations, many governments have designed and implemented a broad range of measures to reduce this consumption and the harm it causes. Early anti-smoking advocates emphasized economic and moral harms, although there was some awareness of the potential harm to health.[16] Modern tobacco control policies developed as a response to the growing body of medical evidence:

> The evolution in medical knowledge since the 1950s has radically altered the social and political landscape, producing a growing consensus, both nationally and internationally, that tobacco consumption is a *sui generis* problem that can only be properly addressed with an array of innovative and multifaceted legislative responses.[17]

---

[12]   For discussion, see *e.g.*, Cunningham, *ibid.*, at 14 (referring to a 1994 study commissioned by Imperial Tobacco); Melissa E. Crow, "Smokescreens and State Responsibility: Using Human Rights Strategies to Promote Global Tobacco Control" (2004) 29 Yale J. Int'l L. 209 at 209-10 (referring to a 2001 study by Philip Morris).

[13]   See *e.g.*, Murray M. Finkelstein, "Obesity, Cigarette Smoking and the Cost of Physicians' Services in Ontario" (2001) 92 Can. J. Public Health 437.

[14]   WHO, *WHO Report on the Global Tobacco Epidemic, 2008* (Geneva: WHO, 2008), online: <http://www.who.int/tobacco/mpower/mpower_report_full_2008.pdf> at 14.

[15]   WHO, *The World Health Report 2003* (Geneva: WHO, 2003) at 91.

[16]   See *e.g.*, Rob Cunningham, *Smoke & Mirrors: The Canadian Tobacco War* (Ottawa: International Development Research Centre, 1996) at 32; Michael Grossman & Philip Price, *Tobacco Smoking and the Law in Canada* (Toronto: Butterworths, 1992) at 1-6.

[17]   *RJR-MacDonald Inc. v. Canada (Attorney General)*, [1995] S.C.J. No. 68, [1995] 3 S.C.R. 199 at para. 48 (S.C.C.), *per* La Forest J.

Comprehensive tobacco control policies pursue a number of intermediate goals with the ultimate aim of reducing the human and economic cost of tobacco consumption. They attempt to minimize the number of people who consume tobacco products. Because of the addictive properties of tobacco, those who begin smoking are likely to continue and eventually suffer from tobacco-related disease. These efforts, in particular those that aim to prevent people from taking up smoking, are crucial. One aspect of this is known as "demand reduction", and includes restrictions on marketing and price increases through taxation. The other entails restricting the supply of tobacco products, particularly to young people ("supply reduction"). Another major goal of tobacco control is to minimize the harm to individuals from SHS and, for those who smoke, from their own consumption ("harm reduction"). Finally, judicial and other measures can be used to impose accountability for the harm caused by tobacco consumption, with the aim of deterring harmful conduct and shifting the costs of ameliorating the harm done by tobacco products.

This chapter reviews examples of all of these types of measures. Although it is useful to define and distinguish them, it will become apparent that there are important and complex relationships between the various approaches. For example, efforts to restrict supply will obviously have an impact on demand, and measures to reduce exposure to SHS have been shown to have an impact on smokers' behaviour, contributing to reduced consumption and cessation. Accountability mechanisms, especially damage awards, costs and settlements in litigation, can have an impact on the price of tobacco products, which influences demand. In particular, various types of measures contribute to the specific objective of reducing tobacco use among young people.

Not all of the measures that make up a comprehensive tobacco control strategy are legal measures; education and public information campaigns, for example, are crucial parts of any such effort. This chapter focuses on the role that law has to play in tobacco control — that is, the use of legislation and judicial mechanisms as part of tobacco control strategies — and on the legal issues that may arise when various control measures are implemented.

II.   THE LEGAL FRAMEWORK

The law relating to tobacco control encompasses a wide range of areas of law at local, provincial, national and international levels. This section briefly outlines the international and domestic legal framework that is relevant to the specific measures discussed in the remainder of the chapter. An understanding of the legal framework is essential to appreciate the responsibilities, capacities and limitations of the various levels of government involved in tobacco control.

(a) International Law

At the international level, the World Health Organization ("WHO") has primary responsibility for health issues, and under its former Director-General, Gro Harlem Bruntland, took up a leading role in tobacco control. Other UN agencies are involved in specific aspects of tobacco control, such as the Food and Agriculture Organization (tobacco production), UNICEF (tobacco use by young people), and the International Labour Organization (smoking in the workplace). In 1998, the UN established an Ad Hoc Interagency Task Force on Tobacco Control to co-ordinate the relevant activities of UN agencies. The World Bank has also taken an interest in tobacco control, focusing on the economic impact of tobacco use and tobacco control in developing countries.

The most significant recent development in the international legal framework relevant to tobacco control is the conclusion of the *WHO Framework Convention on Tobacco Control* ("FCTC"). The FCTC was negotiated under the auspices of the WHO and was adopted by the World Health Assembly on 21 May 2003.[18] The Convention came into force on 27 February 2005, and as of January 2008, 168 states had signed the treaty and 158 were parties (*i.e.*, had signed and ratified or acceded).[19] Canada signed the FCTC on 15 July 2003 and ratified it on 26 November 2004.

The FCTC recognizes and commits state parties to a comprehensive range of tobacco control measures. State parties are permitted and indeed encouraged to adopt measures more stringent than those required by the Convention (Article 2(1)). Its provisions require states to adopt and implement measures to:

- provide "protection from exposure to tobacco smoke in indoor workplaces, public transport, indoor public places, and, as appropriate, other public places" (Article 8);

- provide for testing, measurement, and regulation of the contents of tobacco products (Article 9);

- require the disclosure to "governmental authorities [of] information about the contents and emissions of tobacco products", and public

---

[18] *WHO Framework Convention on Tobacco Control*, 21 May 2003, 2302 U.N.T.S. 166.

[19] WHO, "Full List of Signatories and Parties to the WHO Framework Convention on Tobacco Control" (2008), online: <http://www.who.int/fctc/signatories_parties/en/index.html>.

disclosure of the toxic contents of tobacco products and their emissions (Article 10);

- ensure that "packaging and labelling do not promote a tobacco product by any means that are false, misleading, deceptive or likely to create an erroneous impression", including a false impression that the product is less harmful than others; that packaging and labelling include approved health warnings meeting certain criteria, and information about the product's contents and emissions (Article 11);

- promote public awareness of tobacco control issues, including public access to information about the health risks and addictive characteristics of tobacco (Article 12);

- ensure that packaging is marked with information that will assist in combating illicit trade in tobacco products, including marking of the permitted final destination of the product (Article 15);

- prohibit sales of tobacco products to persons under 18 or the age set by national law (and related measures designed to discourage sales to minors) (Article 16); and

- promote economically viable alternatives to tobacco for workers, growers and sellers (Article 17).

Although most of the Convention's provisions are expressed in mandatory language, several articles allow more flexibility to states. The provision on price and tax measures affirms their importance in reducing tobacco consumption. It urges states to adopt tax and price policies that would contribute to this goal and to prohibit or restrict duty-free sales of tobacco products (Article 6), but allows states a fairly wide discretion in setting tax and price levels. According to Article 13, states are also required to "undertake a comprehensive ban of all tobacco advertising, promotion and sponsorship" or, if their constitutional principles do not permit a comprehensive ban, to "apply restrictions" to advertising, promotion and sponsorship. Specific marketing restrictions are set out in Article 13(4), but again, measures are to be taken "in accordance with [the state's] constitution or constitutional principles". This dilution of the requirement of a comprehensive ban weakens the treaty's stance on tobacco marketing, and is troubling in light of evidence that only a comprehensive ban appears likely to be effective in reducing demand. Arguably, though, the compromise was necessary to obtain the agreement of states such as the United States which took the position that a comprehensive ban would violate constitutionally protected freedom of expression.[20] On the question of liability, Article 19 urges states to "consider taking legislative action or promoting their existing laws, where necessary, to deal with criminal and civil liability, including compensation where appropriate" and to co-operate in exchanging information and providing mutual legal assistance in relevant proceedings.

Finally, Part VII of the FCTC contains articles providing for international co-operation and sharing of information. It has been suggested that these provisions "though mild-sounding to some, could be the key to the treaty's success", since their implementation would "assure that nearly all countries around the globe have active, well-informed, and reasonably well-funded tobacco control experts" who would have the benefit of international contacts, that successful strategies could be quickly shared, and that weaknesses in states' policies would not escape attention.[21] The WHO has been actively working to monitor global tobacco control efforts and assist member states, especially developing countries, to build capacity and implement the FCTC.[22]

Other obligations in several areas of international law are also relevant to tobacco control. International human rights law contains the right to the "highest attainable standard of physical and mental health", which arguably requires states to implement effective measures to reduce the health impact of tobacco use.[23] The *Convention on the Rights of the Child* requires states to protect the health and well-being of children and to ensure education and access to information that promote children's development and health.[24] The right to freedom of expression, which has been raised in connection with marketing restrictions (as will be discussed below), is protected in the *International Covenant on Civil and Political*

---

[20]   See *e.g.*, Gregory F. Jacob, "Without Reservation" (2004) 5 Chicago J. Int'l L. 287, Christine P. Bump, "Close but No Cigar: The WHO Framework Convention on Tobacco Control's Futile Ban on Tobacco Advertising" (2003) 17 Emory Int'l L. Rev. 1251.

[21]   Stephen D. Sugarman, "International Aspects of Tobacco Control and the Proposed WHO Treaty" in Robert L. Rabin & Stephen Sugarman, eds., *Regulating Tobacco* (Oxford: Oxford University Press, 2001) 245 at 271. Sugarman was writing before the adoption of the FCTC but his comments remain valid in light of the final provisions.

[22]   WHO, *WHO Report on the Global Tobacco Epidemic, 2008* (Geneva: WHO, 2008), online: <http://www.who.int/tobacco/mpower/mpower_report_full_2008.pdf>;   WHO,   *Building Blocks for Tobacco Control: A Handbook* (Geneva: WHO, 2004), online: <http:// www.who.int/tobacco/resources/publications/tobaccocontrol_handbook/en/index.html>.

[23]   *International Covenant on Economic, Social and Cultural Rights*, 16 December 1966, 993 U.N.T.S. 3, art. 12.

[24]   *Convention on the Rights of the Child*, 20 November 1989, 1577 U.N.T.S. 3, Articles 17, 24, and 29. Article 24 (right to health) specifically mentions protection from environmental pollution.

Rights, but is subject to restrictions provided by law that are necessary, *inter alia*, for the protection of public health.[25]

International trade law is also relevant because of the restrictions it may place on governments adopting tobacco control measures.[26] Briefly, the issue is that efforts to restrict marketing or sales of tobacco products, regulate product contents, or use taxes to manipulate the price of tobacco products may potentially act as barriers to trade and conflict with states' trade law obligations. Article XX(b) of the *General Agreement on Tariffs and Trade* ("GATT") does contain an exception for measures that are "necessary to protect human ... life or health".[27] The effect of these agreements, then, will depend on the interpretation both of the obligations and the health exception. A dispute regarding Thailand's tobacco legislation, decided under the GATT in the late 1980s, gives some indication of how these issues might be dealt with. In this case (known as the *Thai Cigarettes* case) the United States challenged Thailand's policy prohibiting the import of cigarettes without a licence (which Thailand admitted amounted to a virtual prohibition on imports), while allowing the sale of domestic cigarettes through a state-owned enterprise, and imposing higher internal taxes on imported cigarettes.[28] Thailand unsuccessfully argued that these measures were permitted by the Article XX(b) exception because they were part of Thailand's policy to protect health by reducing tobacco consumption. The GATT panel ruled that although this was a valid objective, the impugned measures could not be considered "necessary" to protect human health because other less trade-restrictive measures could be used to pursue the objective. It did, however, recognize that other measures to reduce the supply and consumption of tobacco products might be consistent with GATT obligations. This and other cases

---

[25]   *International Covenant on Civil and Political Rights*, 16 December 1966, 999 U.N.T.S. 171, art. 19.

[26]   See *e.g.*, Cynthia Callard *et al.*, "An introduction to International Trade Agreements and their impact on Public Measures to Reduce Tobacco Use" (2001), online: Physicians for a Smoke-Free Canada <http://www.smoke-free.ca/pdf_1/Trade&Tobacco-April%202000. pdf>.

[27]   *General Agreement on Tariffs and Trade* ("GATT"), 30 October 1947, 58 U.N.T.S. 187. Other relevant agreements contain similar exceptions: see *e.g.*, *General Agreement on Trade in Services* ("GATS"), Annex 1B to the *Marrakesh Agreement Establishing the World Trade Organization*, 15 April 1994, 1867 U.N.T.S. 3 (entered into force 1 January 1995), Article XIV(b); *North American Free Trade Agreement Between the Government of Canada, the Government of Mexico and the Government of the United States*, 17 December 1992, Can. T.S. 1994 No. 2, 32 I.L.M. 289 (entered into force 1 January 1994), Art. 2101.

[28]   GATT, *Thailand — Restrictions on Importation of and Internal Taxes on Cigarettes*, 7 November 1990, 37th Supp. B.I.S.D. (1990) 200.

suggest that governments have significant, but not unlimited, scope under the WTO agreements for designing tobacco control measures.[29]

Issues have also recently arisen under the North American Free Trade Agreement regarding the potential for tobacco policy to result in an alleged expropriation of investment. Grand River Enterprises Six Nations, Ltd., a corporation owned by members of the Six Nations (Iroquois Confederacy) in Ontario, has filed a claim under Chapter 11 of the North American Free Trade Agreement ("NAFTA") alleging that the implementation of the Master Settlement Agreement between the tobacco industry and the American state governments violates U.S. obligations with respect to investment, including non-discrimination, minimum standards of treatment and compensation for expropriation.[30] Some of these claims were time barred, however the remaining claims will proceed to arbitration.[31]

(b) Canadian Law

A number of different areas of law are potentially relevant to tobacco control measures, including tort law, consumer protection, occupational health and safety, and taxation. The body of relevant legislation includes tobacco-specific enactments at the federal, provincial and municipal levels, as well as a range of other legislation that may have implications for tobacco control. Many of these will be discussed in later sections of the chapter.

As in many areas of public health, Canadian tobacco control policy must take account of the division of powers between the provincial and federal governments. Both levels of government have enacted legislation that is designed to pursue one or more of the tobacco control policy goals outlined above. The main federal statute is the *Tobacco Act*, enacted in 1997 and amended in 1998.[32] The *Tobacco Act* covers product standards and information, access, labelling, and restrictions on advertising and

---

[29]   On the relationship between trade and health, see *e.g.*, M. Gregg Bloche, "WTO Deference To National Health Policy: Toward an Interpretive Principle" (2002) 5 J. Int'l Econ. L. 825; WHO & WTO, "WTO Agreements and Public Health: A Joint Study by the WHO and the WTO Secretariat" (Geneva: WTO/WHO, 2002).

[30]   *Grand River Enterprises Six Nations, Ltd. v. United States of America* (NAFTA/UNCITRAL Arbitration) (Particularized Statement of Claim, 30 June 2005).

[31]   *Grand River Enterprises Six Nations, Ltd. v. United States of America* (NAFTA/UNCITRAL Arbitration) (Decision on Objections to Jurisdiction, 20 July 2006).

[32]   *Tobacco Act*, S.C. 1997, c. 13; *Act to Amend the Tobacco Act*, S.C. 1998, c. 38. Earlier statutes have included the *Tobacco Restraint Act*, R.S.C. 1985, c. T-12 (first enacted in 1908); the *Tobacco Products Control Act*, R.S.C. 1985, c. 14 (4th Supp.); and the *Tobacco Sales to Young Persons Act*, S.C. 1993, c. 5; all of these have now been repealed.

promotion. In addition, the federal *Non-Smokers' Health Act* bans smoking in federally regulated workplaces[33] and the *Excise Act, 2001* deals with licensing and taxation.[34] Provincial governments have enacted a range of statutes dealing with marketing, sales to minors, bans on smoking in workplaces and public places, and other matters.

Clearly, there are areas of overlap between federal and provincial enactments. Their respective jurisdictions as set out in ss. 91 and 92 of the *Constitution Act, 1867*[35] determine what measures each level of government is permitted to take, and in the event of a conflict between valid federal and provincial laws, the doctrine of paramountcy will apply. In addition, extraterritorial application of laws may render them invalid on constitutional grounds. The tobacco companies have on several occasions raised such issues in challenging federal and provincial legislation as *ultra vires*.

In *RJR-MacDonald Inc. v. Canada (Attorney General),*[36] the federal *Tobacco Products Control Act* (the predecessor to the present *Tobacco Act*) was challenged as *ultra vires* Parliament and a violation of the *Charter.*[37] The federal government argued that the legislation was validly enacted pursuant to its jurisdiction over criminal law or under the peace, order and good government clause. The majority of the Supreme Court of Canada held that the legislation was a valid exercise of the criminal law power. The law created prohibitions (against advertising and promotion of tobacco products, and against sale of products without the prescribed warnings) accompanied by penal sanctions, and had an underlying purpose that was aimed at preventing injury to the public. The protection of health had traditionally been one of the purposes of criminal law, and the mere fact that tobacco consumption and promotion had not been criminalized in the past did not prevent the prohibitions at issue from being criminal law. The government had prohibited advertising and promotion rather than tobacco consumption itself because a prohibition on sale and consumption of tobacco was "not a practical policy option at this time".[38] Prohibitions on advertising and the requirement for health warnings on products had the same purpose of "protecting Canadians from harmful and dangerous products" and this was a valid criminal law

---

[33] *Non-Smokers' Health Act*, R.S.C. 1985, c. 15 (4th Supp.). It also amended the *Hazardous Products Act*, R.S.C. 1985, c. H-3 in relation to cigarette advertising.

[34] *Excise Act, 2001*, S.C. 2002, c. 22.

[35] *Constitution Act, 1867* (U.K.), 30 & 31 Vict., c. 3, reprinted in R.S.C. 1985, App. II, No. 5.

[36] [1995] S.C.J. No. 68 (S.C.C.).

[37] Part I of the *Constitution Act, 1982*, being Schedule B to the *Canada Act 1982* (U.K.), 1982, c. 11.

[38] *RJR-MacDonald Inc. v. Canada (Attorney General)*, [1995] S.C.J. No. 68 at para. 34 (S.C.C.).

purpose.[39] The argument that the legislation could not properly be considered criminal law because it prohibited only ancillary acts such as promotion was rejected, as was an argument that the legislation should be considered regulatory rather than criminal law because it contained exemptions to its prohibitions. Having found the legislation to be a valid exercise of the criminal law power, the Court declined to determine whether or not it also fell within the peace, order and good government power. As will be discussed below, the legislation was ultimately found to violate the *Charter*, and was subsequently replaced by the current *Tobacco Act*.

The courts have also addressed potential conflicts between the federal *Tobacco Act* and provincial legislation which covers essentially the same subject matter. In *Rothmans, Benson & Hedges Inc. v. Saskatchewan*, a challenge was brought against the retail display prohibition in Saskatchewan on the grounds that it was inoperative because of the doctrine of federal legislative paramountcy. The Saskatchewan *Tobacco Control Act* prohibits the advertisement, promotion or display of tobacco products in premises where minors are permitted, including retail displays (the so-called "shower curtain law").[40] The Supreme Court of Canada, reversing a decision of the Saskatchewan Court of Appeal,[41] upheld the provincial legislation, noting that a retailer could comply with both federal and provincial provisions, and the federal provisions did not create an *entitlement* to display tobacco products, but merely defined the scope of its promotion prohibition.[42] Both the federal and provincial statutes have the same purposes, so there is no inconsistency between their provisions merely because one is stricter.[43]

The question of extra-territorial application of tobacco legislation has been raised as a further constitutional issue in recent cases. In *J.T.I. Macdonald Corp. v. Canada (Attorney General)*, several tobacco companies challenged the new federal *Tobacco Act* on several grounds, including the alleged extra-territorial effect of a section of the Act that prohibits tobacco promotion in Canada by means of a publication, broadcast or other communication that originates outside Canada.[44] The decision of the Superior Court of Québec acknowledged the extra-territorial reach of the provision but denied that this made it *ultra vires* the

---

[39]   *Ibid.*, at para. 43. See also paras. 41-42 regarding health warnings.

[40]   *Tobacco Control Act*, S.S. 2001, c. T-14.1, s. 6.

[41]   *Rothmans, Benson & Hedges Inc. v. Saskatchewan*, [2003] S.J. No. 606 (Sask. C.A.), rev'd [2005] S.C.J. No. 1 (S.C.C.).

[42]   *Rothmans, Benson & Hedges Inc. v. Saskatchewan*, [2005] S.C.J. No. 1, 2005 SCC 13 at para. 17-18 (S.C.C.).

[43]   *Ibid.*, at para. 25-26.

[44]   *Tobacco Act*, S.C. 1997, c. 13, s. 31(3).

federal Parliament, which "has the legislative authority to give extra-territorial effect to its laws".[45]

However, provincial legislation which is extra-territorial in its purpose and effects may be constitutionally invalid, if this extra-territorial effect is its pith and substance rather than being incidental to the exercise of provincial jurisdiction. The British Columbia *Tobacco Damages and Health Care Costs Recovery Act* (which will be further discussed below in Section VII (c) of this chapter) was challenged on this basis. The Act creates an action by the provincial government "against a [tobacco] manufacturer to recover the cost of health care benefits caused or contributed to by a tobacco related wrong".[46] It also defines a "tobacco related wrong" and provides for recovery on an aggregate basis and for certain presumptions to be made in the context of tobacco litigation. These provisions were challenged as being *ultra vires*, in part because of their extra-territorial effects. The Supreme Court of Canada rejected this argument, and upheld the legislation.[47]

Tobacco control legislation has also been challenged under the *Charter*, most notably as infringing freedom of expression (in the case of advertising bans). The first major case was *RJR-MacDonald*, in which the previous federal legislation was found to be a valid exercise of federal jurisdiction but an unjustified infringement of s. 2(*b*) of the *Charter*. The prohibition on advertising and promotion was conceded to infringe freedom of expression under s. 2(*b*); a majority of the Supreme Court of Canada also held that provisions requiring unattributed health warnings on tobacco packages and limiting the other information that could be displayed on packages infringed freedom of expression.[48] The Court was split (five to four) on the question of justification, with the majority holding that the provisions could not be justified under s. 1 because they impaired rights more than necessary. In the opinion of the majority,

[45]   *JTI Macdonald Corp. v. Canada (Attorney General)*, [2002] Q.J. No. 5550 at para. 441 (Qué. S.C.). This issue was not raised on appeal: *J.T.I. Macdonald Corp. v. Canada (Attorney General)*, [2005] Q.J. No. 10915 (Qué. C.A.), var'd *Canada (Attorney General) v. JTI-Macdonald Corp.*, [2007] S.C.J. No. 30, 2007 SCC 30 (S.C.C.).

[46]   *Tobacco Damages and Health Care Costs Recovery Act*, S.B.C. 2000, c. 30, s. 2(1). This statute is an amended and renamed version of the *Tobacco Damages Recovery Act*, S.B.C. 1997, c. 41, which was found to be unconstitutional on the ground of extraterritoriality in *JTI-Macdonald Corp. v. British Columbia (Attorney General)*, [2000] B.C.J. No. 349, 184 D.L.R. (4th) 335 (B.C.S.C.).

[47]   *British Columbia v. Imperial Tobacco Canada Ltd.*, [2005] S.C.J. No. 50, 2005 SCC 49 (S.C.C.).

[48]   *RJR-MacDonald Inc. v. Canada (Attorney General)*, [1995] S.C.J. No. 68 at para. 124 (S.C.C.), *per* McLachlin J. Justice La Forest (dissenting) doubted that the labelling provisions constituted an infringement, but was of the opinion that they would be "fully justifiable under s. 1" in any case (at para. 116).

measures less intrusive than a comprehensive advertising ban could achieve the same objective, and the government had failed to show why warning labels must be unattributed and why placing other information on packages would defeat the legislative objective.[49] The provision banning the use of tobacco trade marks on non-tobacco articles was also thought to fail the rational connection test because the majority doubted that this practice would increase tobacco consumption.[50] As a result, the impugned provisions were struck down, as were two other sections which could not be adequately severed.

The more recent *Tobacco Act* was enacted following this decision and clearly represents the federal government's attempt to tailor provisions in accordance with the Court's ruling. The subsequent challenge to this legislation was dealt with by the Québec courts and, ultimately, the Supreme Court of Canada in *Canada (Attorney General) v. JTI-Macdonald Corp.*[51] The Superior Court of Québec upheld the legislation, rejecting challenges under s. 2(*b*) as well as s. 7 (regarding alleged vagueness and overbreadth) and s. 8 (regarding powers of inspection and seizure, and reporting requirements),[52] but was reversed in part by the Québec Court of Appeal.[53]

On appeal and cross appeal to the Supreme Court of Canada, six aspects of the legislation were considered. First, the impact of ss. 18 and 19 of the Act was argued by the manufacturers to preclude the publication of industry-sponsored research favourable to the tobacco industry, since the exception in s. 18(2) to the general ban on promotion in s. 19 covers "literary, dramatic, musical, cinematographic, scientific, educational or artistic" works only where no consideration is given for the use or depiction of tobacco products. The Court, however, held that "promotion" in this context should be read to mean only "commercial promotion directly or indirectly targeted at consumers", and therefore scientific research publications would fall outside its scope.[54] The manufacturers also argued that three provisions of the Act were vague and overbroad, and therefore unjustifiable infringements: the prohibition in s. 20 of promotion that is "likely to create an erroneous impression" about tobacco

---

[49]   *Ibid.*, at para. 174, McLachlin J.

[50]   *Ibid.*, at para. 159, McLachlin J.

[51]   *Canada (Attorney General) v. JTI-Macdonald Corp.*, [2007] S.C.J. No. 30, 2007 SCC 30 (S.C.C.).

[52]   *JTI Macdonald Corp. v. Canada (Attorney General)*, [2002] Q.J. No. 5550 (Qué. S.C.), var'd [2005] Q.J. No. 10915 (Qué. C.A.), var'd [2007] S.C.J. No. 30 (S.C.C.).

[53]   *JTI Macdonald Corp. v. Canada (Attorney General)*, [2005] Q.J. No. 10915 (Qué. C.A.), var'd [2007] S.C.J. No. 30 (S.C.C.).

[54]   *Canada (Attorney General) v. JTI-Macdonald Corp.*, [2007] S.C.J. No. 30, 2007 SCC 30 at paras. 56-57 (S.C.C.).

products, in addition to "false, misleading or deceptive promotion"; the prohibition in s. 22(3) on advertising that "could be construed on reasonable grounds to be appealing to young persons"; and the prohibition on "lifestyle" advertising in s. 22(3). However, in all three cases the Supreme Court held that, provided they were properly interpreted, the provisions could be upheld as justifiable under s. 1 of the *Charter*. The fifth argument raised by the manufacturers was that the prohibitions on sponsorship promotion (ss. 24-25) were unconstitutional infringements of their freedom of expression, but the Court disagreed and upheld the provisions, including the ban on using corporate names in sponsorship promotion or on sports or cultural facilities. Finally, the manufacturers challenged regulations under the Act (the *Tobacco Product Information Regulations*) that increased the size of mandatory warning labels from 33 to 50 per cent of the principal display surface of tobacco product packaging.[55] The Court held that the requirement did infringe s. 2(*b*) of the *Charter*, but that the infringement was justified.

In the result, all of the challenged provisions of the Act and regulations were upheld as constitutional. The decision represents an interesting example of the "dialogue" between the courts and Parliament with respect to the validity of legislation under the *Charter*. Both the Court's approach to the analysis and the government's approach to justifying its choices are noticeably different as compared to the earlier *RJR-MacDonald* case, and both appear to have affected the outcome. The Court's conclusions on the constitutionality of several provisions, however, were conditional on those provisions being interpreted a certain way, which may in some respects be narrower than what had been intended. Also notable is the fact that in its analysis on several points, the Court referred to the FCTC as relevant to determining whether Parliament's choices could be justified.[56]

Finally, tobacco control legislation must take account of constitutionally protected Aboriginal rights, in view of the tradition of tobacco use in certain cultural and spiritual practices of First Nations peoples in Canada. Several statutes provide explicit exemptions for these traditional uses of tobacco by Aboriginal peoples.[57] In addition, there are

---

[55]   *Tobacco Product Information Regulations*, S.O.R./2000-272.

[56]   *Canada (Attorney General) v. JTI-Macdonald Corp.*, [2007] S.C.J. No. 30, 2007 SCC 30 at paras. 66-67, 138 (S.C.C.).

[57]   See *Smoke-Free Ontario Act*, S.O. 1994, c. 10, s. 13; *Non-Smokers Health Protection Act*, C.C.S.M. c. S125, s. 7(2)(b); *Tobacco Control Act*, S.S. 2001, c. T-14.1, s. 4(5). These exempt gifts of tobacco for cultural or spiritual use from the prohibition on furnishing tobacco to young persons. The Ontario provision and recent amendments to the Manitoba Act (*Non-Smokers Health Protection Act*, S.M. 2004, c. 17, s. 3, adding s. 5.1 to the Act) also contains an exemption from the prohibition on smoking in designated places and

issues regarding exemptions from taxation on tobacco purchases by Aboriginal purchasers.[58] In keeping with its jurisdiction over Aboriginal affairs, the federal government has undertaken to develop specific tobacco control programs for First Nations and Inuit communities.[59]

III. DEMAND REDUCTION

It is by now well-established that not only are tobacco products harmful, they are also addictive.[60] Studies suggest that the substantial majority of smokers would like to quit, but few are successful in doing so.[61] With this in mind, a key public health aim must be to prevent as many people as possible from beginning to smoke, in addition to reducing the consumption of those who have already begun.[62] Reducing the demand for tobacco products pits public health authorities against the marketing efforts of the tobacco industry, which obviously has the contrary aim of increasing demand and consumption. Demand reduction measures therefore include restrictions on tobacco marketing (advertising, promotion and sponsorship) and the dissemination of contrary messages to discourage consumption, known as "counter-marketing". They also include measures to increase the price of tobacco products, with the expectation that this will decrease demand. Reducing demand among children and young people is particularly important given that smoking initiation in the vast majority of cases occurs before the age of 18.[63]

---

provides for a separate area in a health facility, home or institution for traditional use of tobacco.

[58] See e.g., Howard L. Morry, "Aboriginal Peoples and the Law: Taxation of Aboriginals in Canada" (1992) 21 Man. L. J. 426 at paras. 137-39.

[59] Steering Committee of the National Strategy to Reduce Tobacco Use in Canada, *New Directions for Tobacco Control in Canada: A National Strategy* (Ottawa: Minister of Public Works and Government Services, 1999) at 9, 16.

[60] Evidence suggests that most smokers are dependent on nicotine according to the medical definition of substance dependence: *Reducing Tobacco Use: A Report of the Surgeon General* (Georgia: U.S. Department of Health and Human Services, Centers for Disease Control and Prevention, National Center for Chronic Disease Prevention and Health Promotion, Office on Smoking and Health, 2000) at 129, online: <http://www.cdc.gov/tobacco/data_statistics/sgr/sgr_2000/>.

[61] *Ibid.*, at 97.

[62] Demand reduction measures will ideally decrease the consumption of current smokers as well as discouraging smoking initiation; however, specific efforts to encourage reduction and cessation among smokers will be discussed below under harm reduction.

[63] *Reducing Tobacco Use: A Report of the Surgeon General* (Georgia: U.S. Department of Health and Human Services, Centers for Disease Control and Prevention, National Center for Chronic Disease Prevention and Health Promotion, Office on Smoking and Health, 2000) at 162, online: <http://www.cdc.gov/tobacco/data_statistics/sgr/sgr_2000/>; K.E. Warner *et al.*, "Innovative approaches to youth tobacco control: introduction and overview" (2003) 12

This section will discuss three main types of measures to reduce the demand for tobacco products: taxation and price, restrictions on marketing, and packaging and labelling requirements.

(a) Taxation and Price

The taxation of tobacco products has a long history, but was not until relatively recently motivated by public health concerns.[64] Rather, the primary concern was to raise revenue, and in fact, tobacco was targeted as a source of revenue largely due to the assumption that price would not significantly affect demand for tobacco (that is, because of the nature of the product, in particular its addictive properties, demand for it would be relatively stable regardless of price).[65] More recently, governments have used taxation as a way of increasing the price of tobacco products, in the hope that this will reduce demand. Whether or not demand reduction is the stated objective of taxation, the imposition of substantial taxes on tobacco products, and the resulting increases in price, is an important part of comprehensive tobacco control policies.[66] There is evidence to suggest that price does in fact have a significant influence on demand.[67] In particular, the evidence suggests that young people are disproportionately influenced by price increases; as a result, "[m]ost students of tobacco control policy believe that raising prices — typically accomplished through

---

[64]   (Suppl. 1) Tobacco Control 1 at 4; J. E. Henningfield *et al.*, "Regulatory strategies to reduce tobacco addiction in youth" (2003) 12 (Suppl. 1) Tobacco Control 14 at 14.

[65]   Frank J. Chaloupka, Melanie Wakefield & Christina Czart, "Taxing Tobacco: The Impact of Tobacco Taxes on Cigarette Smoking and Other Tobacco Use" in Robert L. Rabin & Stephen Sugarman, eds., *Regulating Tobacco* (Oxford: Oxford University Press, 2001) 39 at 39-40. But see *e.g.*, Rob Cunningham, *Smoke & Mirrors: The Canadian Tobacco War* (Ottawa: International Development Research Centre, 1996) at 33, describing early attempts to control the sale of cigarettes through high licence fees.

[66]   Chaloupka, Wakefield & Czart, *ibid.*, at 39.

[67]   The objective of taxation is still relevant, however, because it determines the optimal level of taxation and the use of revenues.

        See *e.g.*, *Reducing Tobacco Use: A Report of the Surgeon General* (Georgia: U.S. Department of Health and Human Services, Centers for Disease Control and Prevention, National Center for Chronic Disease Prevention and Health Promotion, Office on Smoking and Health, 2000) at 195-96, online: <http://www.cdc.gov/tobacco/data_statistics/sgr/sgr_2000/> at 337. This report, after a comprehensive review of available evidence, estimated that a 10 per cent increase in price could be predicted to reduce consumption by 3 to 5 per cent. Frank J. Chaloupka, Melanie Wakefield & Christina Czart, "Taxing Tobacco: The Impact of Tobacco Taxes on Cigarette Smoking and Other Tobacco Use" in Robert L. Rabin & Stephen Sugarman, eds., *Regulating Tobacco* (Oxford: Oxford University Press, 2001) at 57 cite research suggesting that this effect could be even higher for large tax increases.

tax increases — is the single most effective means of reducing youth smoking quickly and substantially".[68]

Increasing taxation for the purpose of deterring consumption, in co-operation with the provinces, is part of the federal government's tobacco control strategy.[69] Taxes on tobacco products manufactured in or imported into Canada are imposed by the federal and provincial governments. The federal *Excise Act, 2001* imposes duty on tobacco at the rates set out in schedules to the Act, subject to certain exemptions.[70] Provincial legislation (typically in the form of specific tobacco tax statutes) imposes additional taxes.[71] Whereas the federal duty is payable by the manufacturer or importer, the provincial taxes are payable at the point of sale and collected and remitted by the seller; if consumers bring tobacco products into the province they are liable to pay the same tax as if they had been bought in that province. The provincial taxes are, for the most part, fixed amounts per unit.[72] This type of tax structure is easier to administer than *ad valorem* taxes, which are based on a percentage of price, but fixed rates are vulnerable to erosion due to inflation.[73] In some provinces, dealers are specifically prohibited from advertising or otherwise stating that they will

---

[68]   K.E. Warner *et al.*, "Innovative approaches to youth tobacco control: introduction and overview" (2003) 12 (Suppl 1) Tobacco Control 1 at 1. See also Chaloupka, Wakefield & Czart, *ibid.*; *Reducing Tobacco Use, ibid.*, at 337.

[69]   Steering Committee of the National Strategy to Reduce Tobacco Use in Canada, *New Directions for Tobacco Control in Canada: A National Strategy* (Ottawa: Minister of Public Works and Government Services, 1999) at 15.

[70]   *Excise Act, 2001*, S.C. 2002, c. 22, ss. 42 (duty on tobacco), 43 (additional duty on cigars); ss. 45-48 (duty relieved in certain cases); Schedule 1 (Rates of Duty on Tobacco Products), Schedule 2 (Additional Duty on Cigars).

[71]   See *e.g.*, *Tobacco Tax Act*, R.S.O. 1990, c. T.10; *Tobacco Tax Act*, R.S.A. 2000, c. T-4; *Tobacco Tax Act*, R.S.B.C. 1996, c. 452; *Tobacco Tax Act, 1998*, S.S. 1998, c. T-15.001; *Tobacco Tax Act*, C.C.S.M. c. T80; *Tobacco Tax Act*, R.S.Q. c. I-2; *Tobacco Tax Act*, R.S.N.B. 1973, c. T-7; *Tobacco Tax Act*, R.S.Y. 2002, c. 219; *Tobacco Tax Act*, R.S.N.L. 1990, c. T-5; *Health Tax Act*, R.S.P.E.I. 1988, c. H-3; *Tobacco Tax Act*, R.S.N.W.T. 1988, c. T-5; *Tobacco Tax Act (Nunavut)*, R.S.N.W.T. 1988, c. T-5; *Tobacco Tax Act*, S.P.E.I. 2007, c. 19 (awaiting proclamation). In Nova Scotia, the tobacco tax provisions are contained in Part III of the *Revenue Act*, S.N.S. 1995-96, c. 17.

[72]   The Northwest Territories and Nunavut legislation takes a different approach and sets the tax rate at 90 per cent of the taxable price, regardless of the actual price paid (or 12.2 cents where no taxable price has been prescribed): *ibid.*, s. 2. Separate taxes are imposed on cigars in all of the statutes (typically as a percentage of the retail price).

[73]   Frank J. Chaloupka, Melanie Wakefield & Christina Czart, "Taxing Tobacco: The Impact of Tobacco Taxes on Cigarette Smoking and Other Tobacco Use" in Robert L. Rabin & Stephen Sugarman, eds., *Regulating Tobacco* (Oxford: Oxford University Press, 2001) at 45-46. *Ad valorem* taxes, on the other hand, are vulnerable to price manipulation by industry and retailers (*ibid.*), although this can be avoided by fixing prices or minimum prices for tax valuation purposes.

absorb or refund the tax payable, to prevent retailers from nullifying or minimizing the price increase.[74]

Various objections to increased taxation on tobacco products have been raised. The most important of these is the concern that when taxes are high and vary between jurisdictions, smuggling is likely to become more prevalent. In the mid-1990s, taxes were lowered in response to concerns about smuggling, a move which was criticized as harmful and unnecessary by tobacco control advocates.[75] The alternative, of course, is to tackle the problem of smuggling directly; efforts to suppress tobacco smuggling will be discussed below in Section IV (b) of this chapter. Another way of imposing an additional tax burden on tobacco production is through income taxes; the *Income Tax Act* provides for a surtax on the profits of tobacco manufacturers.[76]

(b) Marketing Restrictions

Cigarettes and other tobacco products are consumer goods; however, unlike most other consumer goods, they are addictive and their use is hazardous to the health of consumers and the public. Therefore, while most consumer goods are permitted to be marketed and advertised — subject to certain restrictions, such as that the advertisement not be misleading — governments have sought to restrict the advertising and other forms of marketing that are designed to induce people to consume tobacco products. The tobacco industry resists many of these restrictions, arguing that their marketing activities are designed primarily to increase their market share and promote brand loyalty, not increase overall consumption.[77] Branding is, indeed, "an essential part of tobacco product

---

[74] See *e.g.*, *Tobacco Tax Act*, R.S.B.C. 1996, c. 452, s. 4; *Tobacco Tax Act*, R.S.O. 1990, c. T.10, s. 15; *Tobacco Tax Act*, R.S.Y. 2002, c. 219, s. 4; *Health Tax Act*, R.S.P.E.I. 1988, c. H-3, s. 6.

[75] Canadian Cancer Society *et al.*, *Surveying the Damage: Cut-Rate Tobacco Products and Public Health in the 1990s* (Ottawa: Canadian Cancer Society *et al.*, 1999). For further discussion, see Rob Cunningham, *Smoke & Mirrors: The Canadian Tobacco War* (Ottawa: International Development Research Centre, 1996) at 122-35.

[76] *Income Tax Act*, R.S.C. 1985, c. 1 (5th Supp.), ss. 182-83.

[77] U.S. Department of Health and Human Services, *Reducing Tobacco Use: A Report of the Surgeon General* (Georgia: U.S. Department of Health and Human Services, Centers for Disease Control and Prevention, National Center for Chronic Disease Prevention and Health Promotion, Office on Smoking and Health, 2000) at 162, online: <http://www.cdc. gov/tobacco/data_statistics/sgr/sgr_2000/>. See *e.g.*, Imperial Tobacco Canada, "Our Position: Facts About Imperial Tobacco Canada" (2006), online: <http://www.imperialtobacco canada.com/onewebca/sites/IMP_5TUJVZ.nsf/vwPagesWebLive/EBA51B60505FE0F3C1 256E6E00643304?opendocument&SID=&DTC=>. In this document the company states that the purpose of its marketing efforts is to "encourage adult smokers to choose our brands over competitor brands" (at 2).

marketing".[78] However, governments and tobacco control advocates also believe that marketing increases consumption and encourages smoking initiation, and in fact logically must be directed at these objectives, otherwise consumption — and profits — would inexorably decline as existing smokers quit or die: the industry needs "replacement smokers".[79] Consequently, restricting the marketing of tobacco has become a public health priority. As in other areas, the prevention of youth smoking, here through the suppression of marketing directed at or likely to influence youth, is a key objective.

There are several different kinds of marketing that tobacco control measures have targeted. The first and most obvious is advertising, including broadcast, print, outdoor (billboard and sign), and point of sale (retail) advertising. Other marketing activities include sponsorship of events, promotions such as free gifts and contests, distribution of free samples, direct mail marketing, and package design.[80] The tobacco industry spends large sums of money on marketing: tobacco is the second most heavily advertised product in the United States (after automobiles) and the industry spends billions of dollars annually on marketing there, and an estimated $20 million annually in Canada.[81] These expenditures have persisted, albeit with some fluctuations, despite attempts to restrict marketing, reinforcing suspicions that the industry is adept at finding ways of circumventing restrictions and finding new marketing techniques to replace those that are prohibited.[82]

Several different strategies have been designed to minimize and counteract the impact of tobacco marketing. One strategy is counter-marketing: the dissemination of information, particularly about the health

[78]   John Slade, "Marketing Policies" in Robert L. Rabin & Stephen Sugarman, eds., *Regulating Tobacco* (Oxford: Oxford University Press, 2001) 72 at 80.

[79]   U.S. Department of Health and Human Services, *Reducing Tobacco Use: A Report of the Surgeon General* (Georgia: U.S. Department of Health and Human Services, Centers for Disease Control and Prevention, National Center for Chronic Disease Prevention and Health Promotion, Office on Smoking and Health, 2000) at 162, online: <http://www.cdc.gov/tobacco/data_statistics/sgr/sgr_2000/>.

[80]   For an overview of various marketing efforts, see John Slade, "Marketing Policies" in Robert L. Rabin & Stephen Sugarman, eds., *Regulating Tobacco* (Oxford: Oxford University Press, 2001) at 88-95.

[81]   U.S. Department of Health and Human Services, *Reducing Tobacco Use: A Report of the Surgeon General* (Georgia: U.S. Department of Health and Human Services, Centers for Disease Control and Prevention, National Center for Chronic Disease Prevention and Health Promotion, Office on Smoking and Health, 2000) at 161-62, online: <http://www.cdc.gov/tobacco/data_statistics/sgr/sgr_2000/>; Physicians for a Smoke-Free Canada, "Tobacco Industry Advertising Expenditures in Canada 1987-2000", online: <http://www.smoke-free.ca/factsheets/pdf/AdvertExpend2000.PDF>.

[82]   John Slade, "Marketing Policies" in Robert L. Rabin & Stephen Sugarman, eds., *Regulating Tobacco* (Oxford: Oxford University Press, 2001) at 95-97.

effects of smoking, designed to discourage people from consuming tobacco. This includes media and education campaigns, but also mandatory labelling and warning requirements, which will be discussed in the section immediately following. This section reviews examples of the most direct approach, which is to prohibit or restrict the various types of marketing activities.

Part IV of the federal *Tobacco Act*[83] sets out restrictions on promotion. "Promotion" is broadly defined to include any direct or indirect "representation about a product or service by any means, ... including any communication of information about a product or service and its price or distribution, that is likely to influence and shape attitudes, beliefs and behaviours about the product or service".[84] Section 19 prohibits the promotion of tobacco products or related brand elements except as authorized by the Act and regulations, and s. 31(1) prohibits the publication, broadcasting, or other dissemination of prohibited promotions. Certain forms of promotion are specifically prohibited: promotion by any means that are "false, misleading or deceptive or that are likely to create a false impression about the characteristics, health effects or health hazards of the tobacco product or its emissions" (s. 20), promotion by means of testimonial or endorsement (s. 21), "lifestyle advertising", and advertising "that could be construed on reasonable grounds to be appealing to young persons".[85] Information and brand-preference advertising of tobacco products is permitted in direct mail to adults or adult magazines, and in places where young persons are not permitted (s. 22(2)). Other provisions restrict the sale and promotion of non-tobacco products displaying a tobacco brand element (ss. 26-28), prohibit the use of brand elements and manufacturers' names in sponsorship or on sporting or cultural facilities (ss. 24-25), and prohibit sales promotions such as gifts with purchase, cash rebates, games and contests, and the distribution of free tobacco products or accessories (s. 29).[86] Subject to regulations, retail signs and displays of products and accessories are permitted (s. 30).

---

[83]   *Tobacco Act*, S.C. 1997, c. 13.

[84]   *Ibid.*, s. 18(1). Section 18(2) exempts certain activities from the operation of Part IV, such as literary, artistic or scientific works or reports, commentaries or opinions depicting or referring to tobacco products or brands, provided that no consideration is given by a tobacco retailer or manufacturer for these works.

[85]   *Ibid.*, s. 22(3); lifestyle advertising is defined in s. 22(4).

[86]   *Ibid.* On the interpretation of s. 29, see *Larny Holdings Ltd. v. Canada (Minister of Health)*, [2002] F.C.J. No. 1026, [2003] 1 F.C. 541 (F.C.T.D.); and *Falls Management Co. v. Canada (Minister of Health)*, [2005] F.C.J. No. 1157, 2005 FC 924 (F.C.T.D.), rev'd [2006] F.C.J. No. 236 (F.C.A.).

These provisions represent the federal government's attempt to tailor marketing restrictions in a way that would avoid unjustifiable infringements of the right to freedom of expression as interpreted by the Supreme Court of Canada in the 1995 decision of *RJR-MacDonald*.[87] As discussed above, the Supreme Court of Canada upheld the provisions that were challenged by the industry, finding them to be justified under s. 1 of the *Charter*, provided they were properly interpreted and applied.[88]

A number of provincial and territorial statutes also have restrictions on marketing of tobacco products. Some restrictions duplicate the federal *Tobacco Act* provisions, such as prohibiting sponsorship and endorsements,[89] or misleading and deceptive advertising.[90] However, in some cases provincial restrictions may be more stringent than the federal provisions. For example, most jurisdictions now prohibit or significantly restrict retail displays of tobacco products,[91] although retail display is permitted by the federal legislation.[92] Though these provisions seem to be contradictory, the Supreme Court of Canada held in *Rothmans, Benson & Hedges Inc. v. Saskatchewan* that the doctrine of federal legislative paramountcy does not preclude the operation of stricter provincial legislation unless they are actually inconsistent in the sense that it is impossible to comply with both statutes or one frustrates the purpose of the other, which is not the case here.[93]

British Columbia's legislation contains a broad prohibition on any promotion or advertisement of tobacco use except in accordance with the Act and regulations, and in particular prohibits advertising and promotion that may interfere with government initiatives "to prevent injury to the health of a consumer or purchaser of tobacco or to restrain the use and consumption of tobacco".[94] A few statutes prohibit the sale of products, including confectionary, in the form of a cigarette or other tobacco

---

[87] *RJR-MacDonald v. Canada (Attorney General)*, [1995] S.C.J. No. 68, [1995] 3 S.C.R. 199 (S.C.C.).

[88] *Canada (Attorney General) v. JTI-Macdonald Corp.*, [2007] S.C.J. No. 30, 2007 SCC 30 (S.C.C.).

[89] *Tobacco Act*, R.S.Q. c. T-0.01, ss. 22, 24(4).

[90] *Ibid.*, s. 24(2); *Tobacco Control Act*, R.S.B.C. 1996, c. 451, s. 2(1)(b).

[91] See *e.g.*, *Tobacco Reduction Act*, S.A. 2005, c. T-3.8, s. 7.1; *The Tobacco Control Act*, S.S. 2001, c. T-14.1, s. 6; The *Non-Smokers Health Protection Act*, C.C.S.M. c. N92, ss. 7.2, 7.3; *Smoke-Free Ontario Act*, S.O. 1994, c. 10, s. 3.1; *Tobacco Sales Act*, S.N.B. 1993, c. T-6.1, s. 6.21; *Tobacco Access Act*, S.N.S. 1993, c. 14, s. 9A; *Tobacco Act*, R.S.Q. c. T-0.01, s. 20.2; *Tobacco Control Act*, S.Nu. 2003, c. 13, s. 8; *Smoke-Free Places Act*, S.Y. 2008, c. 8, s. 8 (this section will come into force on 15 May 2009: see s. 10).

[92] *Tobacco Act*, S.C. 1997, c. 13, s. 30.

[93] *Rothmans, Benson & Hedges Inc. v. Saskatchewan*, [2005] S.C.J. No. 1, 2005 SCC 13 (S.C.C.).

[94] *Tobacco Control Act*, R.S.B.C. 1996, c. 451, s. 2(1)(c).

product,[95] a prohibition which targets candy cigarettes and other similar products appealing to children. Federal and provincial legislation sets the minimum size of cigarette packages (usually at 20 cigarettes);[96] the primary aim of this requirement is to prevent the sale of smaller packages that appeal particularly to young people.[97]

One specific concern has been the marketing of certain brands of cigarettes as "light" or "mild". Studies have shown that many consumers believe light and mild cigarettes to be less harmful to their health, but it is now recognized that the evidence does not support this belief.[98] The concern, therefore, is that individuals may choose to consume these products rather than quitting smoking, in the mistaken belief that they are reducing their risk. As a result, many advocates have called for a ban on using these terms, which are arguably misleading to consumers. The federal government in 2001 called upon the tobacco industry to voluntarily stop using these terms to describe their products, with no apparent effect.[99] It could be argued that even in the absence of specific prohibition, marketing using these descriptors already violate the more general prohibitions on misleading or deceptive advertising in tobacco legislation (as mentioned above) or trade practices legislation.[100] A group of Canadian physicians applied to the Competition Commissioner in 2003 for an inquiry, alleging that the use of these descriptors constitutes false and misleading representations under the *Competition Act*.[101] In 2006– 2007, the Commissioner reached agreements with a number of cigarette manufacturers (including the three largest in Canada) under which they

---

[95]   *Tobacco Access Act*, S.N.S. 1993, c. 14, s. 8; *Tobacco Control Act*, S.Nu. 2003, c. 13, s. 4.

[96]   *Tobacco Act*, S.C. 1997, c. 13, s. 10; *Tobacco Control Regulation*, B.C. Reg. 232/2007, s. 4; *Tobacco Sales Act*, S.N.B. 1993, c. T-6.1, s. 4; *Tobacco Tax Act*, R.S.N.L. 1990, c. T-5, s. 6(4); *Tobacco Access Act*, S.N.S. 1993, c. 14, s. 7(a); *Tobacco Control Act*, S.Nu. 2003, c. 13, s. 10; *Smoke-Free Ontario Act*, S.O. 1994, c. 10, s. 5(2); *Tobacco Act*, R.S.Q. c. T-0.01, s. 19; *Tobacco Control Act*, S.S. 2001, c. T-14.1, s. 5. British Columbia and Nova Scotia also prohibit the sale of loose cigarettes, for the same reason: *Tobacco Control Act*, R.S.B.C. 1996, c. 451, s. 2(3); *Tobacco Access Act*, S.N.S. 1993, c. 14, s. 7(b).

[97]   Nancy A. Rigotti, "Reducing the Supply of Tobacco to Youths" in Robert L. Rabin & Stephen Sugarman, eds., *Regulating Tobacco* (Oxford: Oxford University Press, 2001) 143 at 148.

[98]   M.J. Ashley, J. Cohen & R. Ferrence, "'Light' and 'Mild' Cigarettes: Who Smokes Them? Are They Being Misled?" (2001) 92 Can. J. Public Health 407.

[99]   Physicians for a Smoke-Free Canada, "Whatever Happened to the Ban on 'Light' and 'Mild'?" (Spring 2004) Report to Members at 3, online: <http://www.smoke-free.ca/pdf_1/spring2004.pdf>.

[100] Class actions recently filed in Canada have focused on light and mild cigarettes, alleging misleading and deceptive marketing practices: see the discussion below in Section VII (b).

[101] *Ashley v. Canada (Commissioner of Competition)*, [2006] F.C.J. No. 568, 2006 FC 459 (F.C.T.D.) (unsuccessful application to the Federal Court to order the Commissioner to complete this inquiry).

would voluntarily cease using these descriptors on their packaging.[102] In 2007, the federal government published proposed regulations banning the use of "light" and "mild" as descriptors on tobacco and related products.[103]

(c) Packaging, Labelling and Warnings

In addition to placing restrictions on marketing by the tobacco industry and retailers, comprehensive tobacco control policies attempt to counteract these efforts by disseminating information about the health risks of tobacco use. Education and counter-marketing campaigns are important parts of these strategies, and there have been recent initiatives to make these more effective by applying the same marketing principles used by tobacco companies to get the anti-smoking message across to the public and young people in particular.[104]

Legislative measures here include restrictions on packaging, mandatory warnings (on packages, at retail outlets and on advertisements), and mandatory disclosure of contents. Packages are required by the federal *Tobacco Act* to display warnings with a form and content prescribed by the *Tobacco Products Information Regulation*.[105] The prescribed warnings contain short statements in bold lettering about the health effects of tobacco products and full-colour graphic images, and must cover at least 50 per cent of the principal display surfaces of the package.[106] These warnings, when adopted in 2000, were the strongest in the world, and have since become the "gold standard" for warning labels.[107] The regulations also require prescribed health information to be printed on leaflet inserts or on another part of the package, covering 60 per cent to 70 per cent of the surface area in each case,[108] and the amounts

---

[102] Competition Bureau, News Release, "Competition Bureau Reaches Further Agreements with Six Cigarette Companies to Stop Using 'Light' and 'Mild' on Cigarette Packages" (31 July 2007), online: <http://www.competitionbureau.gc.ca/epic/site/cb-bc.nsf/en/02383e.html>.

[103] *Promotion of Tobacco Products and Accessories Regulations (Prohibited Terms)*, C. Gaz. 2007.I.2239.

[104] See M.C. Farrelly *et al.*, "Youth tobacco prevention mass media campaigns: past, present, and future directions" (2003) 12 Tobacco Control 35.

[105] *Tobacco Act*, S.C. 1997, c. 13, s. 15(1); *Tobacco Products Information Regulation*, S.O.R./2000-272.

[106] *Tobacco Products Information Regulation, ibid.*, s. 5(2). The prescribed warnings can be viewed online at Health Canada, <http://www.hc-sc.gc.ca/hl-vs/tobac-tabac/legislation/label-etiquette/graph/index_e.html>.

[107] See *e.g.*, *WHO Framework Convention on Tobacco Control*, 21 May 2003, 2302 U.N.T.S. 166, Art. 11.

[108] *Tobacco Products Information Regulation*, S.O.R./2000-272, s. 7. The prescribed notices can be viewed online at Health Canada, <http://www.hc-sc.gc.ca/hl-vs/tobac-tabac/legislation/label-etiquette/message/index_e.html>.

of toxic emissions or constituents to be displayed on the package.[109] Some provincial statutes also enable regulations prescribing warnings to be carried on tobacco packages.[110]

In addition to warnings carried on tobacco product packages, federal and provincial legislation require the display of signs warning of the health effects of tobacco in locations where these products are sold.[111] Finally, Québec requires any tobacco advertising, where permitted, to contain health warnings attributed to the Minister.[112]

IV. SUPPLY REDUCTION

Another obvious way of reducing the consumption of tobacco products and its harmful effects is to restrict the availability of those products. Although an outright ban on tobacco was an early objective of tobacco control in Canada and elsewhere and is occasionally proposed,[113] it is generally accepted that "a prohibition upon the sale or consumption of tobacco is not a practical policy option at this time" given the prevalence of smoking and the addictive properties of tobacco.[114] However, there are other specific measures designed to reduce the supply of tobacco products and in particular to keep them out of the hands of children and young people. In some jurisdictions, sales of tobacco products are prohibited in certain specified locations, such as schools, child care and health care

---

[109]   *Ibid.*, ss. 9, 10. An amendment proposed in May 2008 would remove this requirement: *Regulations Amending the Tobacco Products Information Regulation*, C. Gaz. 2008.I.1717.

[110]   *Smoke-Free Ontario Act*, S.O. 1994, c. 10, ss. 5(1), 19(1)(*d*); *Tobacco Act*, R.S.Q. c. T-0.01, s. 28; *The Non-Smokers Health Protection Act*, C.C.S.M. c. N92, s. 9(1)(e); *Tobacco Control Act*, R.S.B.C. 1996, c. 451, s. 11(2)(a). To date those regulations which have been enacted require packages to carry the warnings prescribed by federal legislation: *General*, O. Reg. 613/94, s. 3.

[111]   *Tobacco Act*, S.C. 1997, c. 13, s. 9; *Tobacco Control Regulation*, B.C. Reg. 232/2007, s. 5(1)(a); *Tobacco Sales Act*, S.N.B. 1993, c. T-6.1, s. 3; *General Regulation — Tobacco Sales Act*, N.B. Reg. 94-57, s. 4(2); *Tobacco Control Act*, S.N.L. 1993, c. T-4.1, s. 5; *Tobacco Access Act*, S.N.S. 1993, c. 14, s. 9; *Tobacco Access Regulations*, N.S. Reg. 9/96, s. 3, Schedules A-E; *Tobacco Control Act*, S.Nu. 2003, c. 13, s. 11; *Smoke-Free Ontario Act*, S.O. 1994, c. 10, s. 6; *Tobacco Act*, R.S.Q. c. T-0.01, s. 20.4; *Tobacco Control Act*, S.S. 2001, c. T-14.1, s. 7. Saskatchewan's provision also prohibits the display of any such sign that is *not* supplied or approved by the department or authorized under the federal *Tobacco Act*.

[112]   *Tobacco Act*, R.S.Q. c. T-0.01, s. 24.

[113]   See Rob Cunningham, *Smoke & Mirrors: The Canadian Tobacco War* (Ottawa: International Development Research Centre, 1996) at 32, describing early support for total prohibition in parts of Canada and the proposal or adoption of prohibition laws in many U.S. states. For an example of a recent proposal to ban tobacco, see "How Do You Sleep at Night, Mr. Blair?", Editorial (2003) 362 Lancet 1865.

[114]   *RJR-MacDonald Inc. v. Canada (Attorney General)*, [1995] S.C.J. No. 68 at para. 34 (S.C.C.), *per* La Forest J.

facilities, and pharmacies.[115] The prohibition on sale of tobacco to minors, the best established of all tobacco control measures, will be discussed in the following section. The suppression of illicit trade, in particular through anti-smuggling measures, which will be discussed briefly below, is also an important part of supply reduction.

(a)   Restrictions on Supply to Young People

The sale of tobacco products to minors has been prohibited in Canada and most of the United States since the late 19th century.[116] Traditionally, legislation has focused on prohibiting sales as a way of cutting off the commercial supply of tobacco to young people, but more recently, some attempts have been made to restrict non-commercial or "social" sources. These non-commercial sources include friends and family members who give or sell cigarettes to minors, and are an increasingly important source of supply to young people, particularly those who are just starting to smoke.[117]

The federal legislation and legislation in almost all provinces and territories prohibits the supply of tobacco products to persons under a prescribed age (either 18 or 19);[118] some also prohibit the act of purchasing tobacco on behalf of or for the purpose of resale to a minor.[119] These provisions attempt to catch non-commercial as well as commercial sources. Some jurisdictions also explicitly prohibit sales to persons who

[115]   *Tobacco Sales Act*, S.N.B. 1993, c. T-6.1, s. 6.1; *Tobacco Control Act*, S.N.L. 1993, c. T-4.1, s. 4.1; *Tobacco Access Act*, S.N.S. 1993, c. 14, s. 9B; *Tobacco Control Act*, S.Nu. 2003, c. 13 s. 9; *Smoke-Free Ontario Act*, S.O. 1994, c. 10, s. 4; *Tobacco Act*, R.S.Q. c. T-0.01 ss. 17, 17.1, 18; *Tobacco Control Act*, S.S. 2001, c. T-14.1 s. 8.

[116]   Rob Cunningham, *Smoke & Mirrors: The Canadian Tobacco War* (Ottawa: International Development Research Centre, 1996) at 32-33; Michael Grossman & Philip Price, *Tobacco Smoking and the Law in Canada* (Toronto: Butterworths, 1992) at 3-48–3-51.

[117]   Nancy A. Rigotti, "Reducing the Supply of Tobacco to Youths" in Robert L. Rabin & Stephen Sugarman, eds., *Regulating Tobacco* (Oxford: Oxford University Press, 2001) 143 at 146-47; J. Forster *et al.*, "Social Exchange of Cigarettes by Youth" (2003) 12 Tobacco Control 148.

[118]   *Tobacco Act*, S.C. 1997, c. 13, s. 8(1); *Tobacco Control* Act, R.S.B.C. 1996, c. 451, s. 2(2); *Non-Smokers Health Protection Act*, C.C.S.M. c. S125, s. 7(1); *Tobacco Control Act*, S.N.L. 1993, c. T-4.1, s. 4(1); *Tobacco Control Act*, S.Nu. 2003, c. 13, s. 3(1); *Smoke-Free Ontario Act*, S.O. 1994, c. 10, s. 3(1); *Tobacco Control Act*, S.S. 2001, c. T-14.1, s. 4; *Tobacco Control Act*, S.N.W.T. 2006, c. 9, s. 3(1); *Tobacco Sales Act*, S.N.B. 1993, c. T-6.1, s. 5(1); *Tobacco Access Act*, S.N.S. 1993, c. 14, s. 5(1); *Tobacco Sales and Access Act*, R.S.P.E.I. 1988, c. T-3.1, s. 4(1); *Tobacco Act*, R.S.Q. c. T-0.01, s. 13.

[119]   *Tobacco Sales Act*, S.N.B. 1993, c. T-6.1, s. 6; *Tobacco Access Act*, S.N.S. 1993, c. 14, s. 5(2); *Tobacco Sales and Access Act*, R.S.P.E.I. 1988, c. T-3.1, s. 4(2). The *Tobacco Act*, R.S.Q. c. T-0.01, s. 14.3, prohibits sale to a person known to be purchasing tobacco for a minor.

appear to be under the prescribed age, unless the seller knows or is shown proof that the buyer is of age.[120] The mere fact that a minor appeared to be over the prescribed age will not be a defence.[121] However, a defence will exist where the supplier is shown proof of age, has no reasonable grounds to believe that the documentation produced is not legitimate, and therefore believes on reasonable grounds that the individual is of age.[122] Retailers are required by federal and provincial legislation to post signs with the prescribed form and content stating that it is prohibited to sell tobacco products to minors.[123] The *Tobacco Control Act* in Nunavut requires retailers to have policies, practices and procedures, and training and monitoring programs to prevent sales to minors (s. 5).

The difficulties in enforcing prohibitions on social supply to minors are recognized in some of the legislation which provides that parents and guardians who supply tobacco to minors in private places are exempt from the prohibition.[124] The federal *Tobacco Act* provision only covers the supply of tobacco to a young person in a public place.[125] The Newfoundland and Labrador *Tobacco Control Act*, s. 4(4), provides an exception for the supply of tobacco to a minor who is living in an adult correctional facility. Finally, as noted above, several jurisdictions also

---

[120] *Smoke-Free Ontario Act*, S.O. 1994, c. 10, s. 3(2) [prohibits sale to person appearing to be under 25 years unless proof that person is at least 19 years]; *Tobacco Control Act*, S.S. 2001, c. T-14.1, s. 4; *Tobacco Control Act*, S.N.W.T. 2006, c. 9, s. 3(2); *Tobacco Sales and Access Act*, R.S.P.E.I. 1988, c. T-3.1, s. 4(4); *Tobacco Control Act*, S.Nu. 2003, c. 13, s. 3(2).

[121] *Tobacco Control Act*, S.N.L. 1993, c. T-4.1, s. 4(2); *Tobacco Access Act*, S.N.S. 1993, c. 14, s. 5(3); *Tobacco Sales and Access Act*, R.S.P.E.I. 1988, c. T-3.1, s. 4(2).

[122] Most of the relevant statutes have some provision to this effect, although they are worded differently; see *Tobacco Act*, S.C. 1997, c. 13, s. 8(2); *Tobacco Control Act*, R.S.B.C. 1996, c. 451, s. 2(2.1); *Non-Smokers Health Protection Act*, C.C.S.M. c. S125, s. 7(3); *Smoke-Free Ontario Act*, S.O. 1994, c. 10, s. 3(3); *Tobacco Act*, R.S.Q. c. T-0.01, s. 14; *Tobacco Control Act*, S.S. 2001, c. T-14.1, s. 4(2), (3). The Atlantic provinces take a slightly different approach and provide that where a purchaser appears to be under-age, proof of age in a prescribed form must be provided before the product can be sold: *Tobacco Sales Act*, S.N.B. 1993, c. T-6.1, s. 5(2); *Tobacco Control Act*, S.N.L. 1993, c. T-4.1, s. 4(3); *Tobacco Access Act*, S.N.S. 1993, c. 14, s. 5(4); *Tobacco Sales and Access Act*, R.S.P.E.I. 1988, c. T-3.1, s. 4(4).

[123] *Tobacco Act*, S.C. 1997, c. 13, s. 9; *Tobacco (Access) Regulations*, S.O.R./99-93, s. 4; *Tobacco Sales Act*, S.N.B. 1993, c. T-6.1, s. 3; *General Regulation — Tobacco Sales Act*, N.B. Reg. 94-57, s. 4(1); *Tobacco Access Act*, S.N.S. 1993, c. 14, s. 9; *Tobacco Access Regulations*, N.S. Reg. 9/96, s. 3, Schedules A-C; *Smoke-Free Ontario Act*, S.O. 1994, c. 10, s. 6; *General*, O. Reg. 48/06, s. 11; *Tobacco Sales and Access Act*, R.S.P.E.I. 1988, c. T-3.1, s. 6; *General Regulations*, P.E.I. Reg. EC22/92, s. 2; *Tobacco Control Act*, S.S. 2001, c. T-14.1, s. 7.

[124] *Non-Smokers Health Protection Act*, C.C.S.M. c. S125, s. 7(2); *Tobacco Control Act*, S.S. 2001, c. T-14.1, s. 4(4); *Tobacco Control Act*, S.N.W.T. 2006, c. 9, s. 3(6)(a).

[125] *Tobacco Act*, S.C. 1997, c. 13, s. 8(1).

provide for exceptions where tobacco is supplied to a young person for use in traditional Aboriginal ceremonies or practices.[126]

Enforcement and compliance are crucial to the success of these laws in reducing youth access to tobacco products. Studies have shown that unless compliance rates are high (80-90 per cent or higher), prohibitions on sales to minors will have little perceptible effect on access.[127] Under federal and provincial legislation, providing tobacco to a minor is an offence punishable in most cases by a fine, the amount of which increases with each subsequent offence.[128] A number of statutes also provide for suspension of licences or temporary bans on selling tobacco products where vendors have been convicted of these offences, and require signs to be posted on the premises informing consumers of the conviction and suspension.[129] Inspectors or enforcement officers may be appointed under these statutes, and have various powers, including the power to enter premises where tobacco products are sold, make inquiries, investigate complaints of alleged violations, and conduct or arrange for test purchases to determine whether retailers are complying with statutory requirements.[130]

Another way of preventing access to tobacco by minors is prohibiting or restricting sales by means that make it difficult or impossible to verify age, such as vending machines and mail order sales. Vending machines may either be prohibited altogether[131] or restricted to

---

[126] See *Smoke-Free Ontario Act*, S.O. 1994, c. 10, s. 13(2); *Non-Smokers Health Protection Act*, C.C.S.M. c. S125, s. 7(2)(b); *Tobacco Control Act*, S.S. 2001, c. T-14.1, s. 4(5); *Tobacco Control Act*, S.N.W.T. 2006, c. 9, s. 3(6)(b). These exempt gifts of tobacco for cultural or spiritual use from the prohibition on furnishing tobacco to young persons.

[127] Canadian Cancer Society, "A Critical Analysis of Youth Access Laws" (2002), online: Canadian Cancer Society <http://www.cancer.ca/vgn/images/portal/cit_776/48/38/69664397cw_criticalanalysisyouthaccesslaws_en.pdf> at 20.

[128] *Tobacco Act*, S.C. 1997, c. 13, s. 45; *Non-Smokers Health Protection Act*, C.C.S.M. c. S125, s. 8(1); *Tobacco Control Act*, S.N.L. 1993, c. T-4.1, s. 7; *Tobacco Access Act*, S.N.S. 1993, c. 14, s. 12(1); *Smoke-Free Ontario Act*, S.O. 1994, c. 10, s. 15; *Tobacco Sales and Access Act*, R.S.P.E.I. 1988, c. T-3.1, s. 8; *Tobacco Control Act*, S.S. 2001, c. T-14.1, s. 20. British Columbia's legislation allows for a term of imprisonment in addition to or instead of a fine: *Tobacco Control Act*, R.S.B.C. 1996, c. 451, s. 12(1).

[129] *Tobacco Act*, S.C. 1997, c. 13, s. 59 (these orders are optional); *Tobacco Control Act*, S.N.L. 1993, c. T-4.1, s. 7; *Tobacco Access Act*, S.N.S. 1993, c. 14, s. 12(2); *Smoke-Free Ontario Act*, S.O. 1994, c. 10, ss. 16, 18; *Tobacco Control Act*, S.S. 2001, c. T-14.1, s. 23 (temporary ban upon second or subsequent conviction).

[130] *Tobacco Act*, S.C. 1997, c. 13, s. 35; *Tobacco Sales Act*, S.N.B. 1993, c. T-6.1, s. 7(3); *Tobacco Control Act*, S.N.L. 1993, c. T-4.1, s. 3(2); *Tobacco Access Act*, S.N.S. 1993, c. 14, s. 10; *Tobacco Access Regulations*, N.S. Reg. 9/96, s. 4; *Tobacco Act*, R.S.Q. c. T-0.01, s. 34(11); *Tobacco Control Act*, S.S. 2001, c. T-14.1, s. 17.

[131] *Tobacco Control Act*, S.Nu. 2003, c. 13, s. 12; *Smoke-Free Ontario Act*, S.O. 1994, c. 10, s. 7; *Tobacco Sales and Access Act*, R.S.P.E.I. 1988, c. T-3.1, s. 5; *Tobacco Act*, R.S.Q. c. T-0.01, s. 16.

certain locations.[132] The federal *Tobacco Act* (s. 13) prohibits the sale of tobacco products by mail, and Québec's *Tobacco Act* (s. 20) requires sales to be made in the physical presence of the vendor and purchaser (except for vending machines as permitted in the Act). Finally, the federal *Tobacco Act* (s. 11), New Brunswick *Tobacco Sales Act* (s. 6.2), Nunavut *Tobacco Control Act* (s. 7) and Québec *Tobacco Act* (s. 15) also prohibit retail displays that allow persons to handle the tobacco before paying for it, a measure designed to prevent shoplifting, especially by young people. Internet sales represent the newest challenge to youth access laws. The volume of Internet sales has grown rapidly in recent years, and studies suggest that most sites do not have adequate age verification procedures and rates of compliance with youth access laws are very low.[133]

Alberta remains the only Canadian province without legislation prohibiting the sale of tobacco products to minors (though the federal prohibition would still apply); rather, it prohibits the possession and consumption of tobacco by minors (under 18 years).[134] Contravention of the relevant provision is an offence punishable by a fine of not more than $100; the police are empowered to seize any tobacco products believed to be related to an offence and upon conviction these items are destroyed or disposed of.[135] Nova Scotia, in addition to prohibiting supply to minors, also prohibits possession of tobacco by anyone under the age of 19; a police officer may search a suspected person and confiscate any tobacco found, but possession is not an offence.[136] The *Tobacco Control Act* in the Northwest Territories prohibits young persons from purchasing or attempting to purchase tobacco or tobacco accessories.[137]

This type of law, known as a "possession, use and purchase" ("PUP") law, is an alternative (or complement) to prohibitions on sales to

---

[132] *Tobacco Act*, S.C. 1997, c. 13, s. 12 (permitted in private places and bars, taverns and beverage rooms); *Tobacco Sales Act*, S.N.B. 1993, c. T-6.1, s. 6.3 (prohibited in retail stores); *Tobacco Access Act*, S.N.S. 1993, c. 14, s. 6 (prohibited in any place accessible to the public); *Tobacco Control Act*, S.S. 2001, c. T-14.1, s. 9 (permitted in private places or public places that minors are not allowed to enter).

[133] See *e.g.*, Kurt M. Ribisl *et al.*, "Internet sales of cigarettes to minors" (2003) 290 JAMA 1356 (finding that approximately 90 per cent of attempts by minors to buy cigarettes online without providing age verification were successful); J.A. Bryant *et al.*, "Online Sales: Profit without Question" (2002) 11 Tobacco Control 226 (approximately 70 per cent of orders by minors were filled without age verification).

[134] *Prevention of Youth Tobacco Use Act*, R.S.A. 2000, c. P-22, s. 2. The Yukon also appears not to have legislation in place covering this issue; again, though, the federal *Tobacco Act* provisions would apply.

[135] *Ibid.*, s. 4.

[136] *Smoke-free Places Act*, S.N.S. 2002, c. 12, s. 11.

[137] *Tobacco Control Act*, S.N.W.T. 2006, c. 9, s. 3(4.1).

minors, and has become increasingly common in the United States.[138] Nevertheless, such laws have been controversial. According to those who favour this approach, fairness requires that if retailers can be punished for selling cigarettes to young people, then young people should also be subject to penalties for buying or consuming them. In addition they hope that prohibiting the use or possession of tobacco will send a message to youths that smoking is unacceptable, deter young people from smoking and give them a reason to resist peer pressure to smoke. However, others are concerned that it is unfair to shift the responsibility for preventing youth smoking to minors themselves, given that they are presumed to be unable to make responsible decisions about smoking due to their age. This is seen to be contradictory to the rationale for preventing sales to minors, and to implicitly accept the tobacco industry's argument that smokers rather than the industry are responsible for smoking and its consequences.[139] In addition, concerns have been raised about the effectiveness of these laws and their potential to undermine the role of parents and schools in discipline.[140] The current state of Canadian legislation suggests that many remain unconvinced of the benefits of PUP laws, but it remains to be seen whether they become more widespread.

(b) Illicit Trade

Tobacco smuggling is considered to be a public health issue because it undermines taxation and price strategies to reduce demand and often has the effect of flooding the market with cheap tobacco products. A substantial proportion of tobacco products are thought to be smuggled (an estimated 5 per cent of all cigarettes sold worldwide, 30 per cent of market in Canada in 1993 at the height of the smuggling problem and 20 per cent currently in the U.K.).[141] The tobacco industry often cites the risk of smuggling and other contraband (such as stolen and counterfeit products) as an argument for lower taxes.[142] Given the importance of

---

[138] Nancy A. Rigotti, "Reducing the Supply of Tobacco to Youths" in Robert L. Rabin & Stephen Sugarman, eds., *Regulating Tobacco* (Oxford: Oxford University Press, 2001) at 166-67; M. Wakefield & G. Giovino, "Teen Penalties for Tobacco Possession, Use and Purchase: Evidence and Issues" (2003) 12 Tobacco Control 6.

[139] Rigotti, *ibid.*, at 167-68; Wakefield & Giovino, *ibid.*

[140] Wakefield & Giovino, *ibid.*

[141] Stephen D. Sugarman, "International Aspects of Tobacco Control and the Proposed WHO Treaty" in Robert L. Rabin & Stephen Sugarman, eds., *Regulating Tobacco* (Oxford: Oxford University Press, 2001) at 253.

[142] See *e.g.*, Rob Cunningham, *Smoke & Mirrors: the Canadian Tobacco War* (Ottawa: International Development Research Centre, 1996) at 125; Michelle Leverett *et al.*, "Tobacco Use: The Impact of Prices" (2002) 30 J.L. Med. & Ethics 88 at 92; Imperial Tobacco Canada, News Release, "Another Tobacco Theft Further Proof that High Taxation

maintaining high prices through taxation to a comprehensive tobacco control regime, the preferred option from a public health perspective is to combat illicit trade rather than cut taxes.[143]

Article 15 of the FCTC deals with elimination of illicit trade in tobacco products, including smuggling, illicit manufacturing and counterfeiting. It commits each party to "adopt and implement effective legislative, executive, administrative or other measures to ensure that" tobacco products are marked in order to allow determination of their origin, monitoring and control of their movement and legal status, and determination of whether they are legally for sale in a particular domestic market (para. 2). Parties are also required to take other measures to eliminate illicit trade, such as collecting and sharing information on cross-border trade and providing for penalties and confiscation of proceeds (para. 4). International, regional and subregional co-operation is called for (para. 6). The 2007 Conference of the Parties to the FCTC agreed to begin negotiating a protocol on illicit trade in tobacco products.[144]

Some measures to combat smuggling have been implemented in Canada. For example, the federal *Excise Act, 2001* requires all manufacturers of tobacco products to be licensed (s. 25). Licensed manufacturers or importers must stamp the product and package it in a package printed with prescribed information before it is released into the

---

is Resulting in Increased Crime, Says Canadian Tobacco Manufacturer" (10 August 2004) (regarding theft and counterfeit imports).

[143]   See *e.g.*, U.S. Department of Health and Human Services, *Reducing Tobacco Use: A Report of the Surgeon General* (Georgia: U.S. Department of Health and Human Services, Centers for Disease Control and Prevention, National Center for Chronic Disease Prevention and Health Promotion, Office on Smoking and Health, 2000) at 337, online: <http://www. cdc.gov/tobacco/data_statistics/sgr/sgr_2000/>; Frank J. Chaloupka, Melanie Wakefield & Christina Czart, "Taxing Tobacco: The Impact of Tobacco Taxes on Cigarette Smoking and Other Tobacco Use" in Robert L. Rabin & Stephen Sugarman, eds., Regulating Tobacoo (Oxford: Oxford University Press, 2001) at 57; K.E. Warner *et al.*, "Innovative Approaches to Youth Tobacco Control: Introduction and Overview" (2003) 12 (Suppl. 1) Tobacco Control 1 at 1. The Canadian government did lower taxes in the mid-1990s because of concerns about smuggling, but has been criticized for this: Canadian Cancer Society *et al.*, *Surveying the Damage: Cut-Rate Tobacco Products and Public Health in the 1990s* (Ottawa: Canadian Cancer Society *et al.*, 1999). Rob Cunningham, *Smoke & Mirrors: The Canadian Tobacco War* (Ottawa: International Development Research Centre, 1996) at 122-35. It is also worth noting that smuggling does not occur only in response to differential taxation and may occur even when taxes are low: Neil Boister & Richard Burchill, "Stopping the Smugglers: Proposals for an Additional Protocol to the World Health Organization's *Framework Convention on Tobacco Control*" (2002) 3 Melbourne J. I. L. 33 at 37.

[144]   WHO, "New Guidelines Adopted on Smoke-Free Environments: Parties to Tobacco Control Treaty Agree to Negotiate Protocol on Illicit Tobacco Trade" (News Release, 6 July 2007), online: <http://www.who.int/mediacentre/news/releases/2007/pr38/en/index.html>. For a discussion of proposals for a protocol, see Boister & Burchill, *ibid.*, at 47-51.

market (ss. 34, 35).[145] The sale, purchase or possession of unstamped or unpackaged tobacco (with certain exceptions) is prohibited (ss. 30, 32), as is purchase or receipt for sale of tobacco from an unlicensed manufacturer or of unstamped or fraudulently stamped tobacco (s. 29). Tobacco products must be sold and distributed in their original packages (s. 33). Stamping of tobacco products indicates that duty has been paid (and the absence of stamping is notice that duty has not been paid: s. 36). Provincial legislation also provides for registration of manufacturers, importers, exporters and transporters, permits for wholesalers and dealers, and the marking and stamping of tobacco products to indicate whether duty has been paid and the province in which the products are to be sold.[146]

One way of preventing smuggling into Canada is to target exports of tobacco products which will subsequently be smuggled back into the country. At the height of the smuggling problem in the early 1990s, there was a dramatic increase in exports to the United States; a large proportion of these found their way back onto the Canadian market as contraband.[147] In order to discourage this and increase the price of contraband tobacco, an export tax was introduced (briefly in 1992 and again in 1994).[148] Currently, the *Excise Act, 2001* imposes a special duty on all Canadian-manufactured tobacco exports, with some exceptions.[149]

The tobacco industry has little incentive to reduce smuggling, as it provides another outlet for sales of its products, often at a low price that makes them even more attractive to consumers. In recent years, tobacco companies have been accused of complicity with smuggling in civil and criminal actions in a number of countries.[150] In 1999, the Canadian government filed a suit against RJR-Macdonald and related companies in U.S. Federal Court in New York state, alleging that the defendants had fraudulently deprived the government of revenue and profited illicitly from their participation in smuggling cigarettes from the United States

---

[145] The prescriptions regarding packaging and information required to be printed are contained in the *Stamping and Marking of Tobacco Products Regulations*, S.O.R./2003-288.

[146] See *e.g.*, *Tobacco Tax Act*, R.S.O. 1990, c. T.10; *General*, R.R.O. 1990, Reg. 1034; *Tobacco Tax Act*, R.S.B.C. 1996, c. 452; *Tobacco Tax Act Regulation*, B.C. Reg. 66/2002.

[147] Rob Cunningham, *Smoke & Mirrors: The Canadian Tobacco War* (Ottawa: International Development Research Centre, 1996) at 125.

[148] *Ibid.*, at 127, 132.

[149] *Excise Act, 2001*, S.C. 2002, ss. 56-58, Sched. 3.

[150] For accounts of some of these cases in the U.S., the U.K. and Europe, see Neil Boister & Richard Burchill, "Stopping the Smugglers: Proposals for an Additional Protocol to the World Health Organization's *Framework Convention on Tobacco Control*" (2002) 3 Melbourne J. I. L. at 38-40; Elizabeth J. Farnam, "Racketeering, RICO and the Revenue Rule in Attorney General of Canada v. R.J. Reynolds: Civil RICO Claims for Foreign Tax Law Violations" (2002) 77 Wash. L. Rev. 843.

into Canada.[151] The action was dismissed on the grounds of a rule that the U.S. courts could not be used to enforce another country's revenue laws, and this dismissal was upheld on appeal.[152] Subsequently, civil and criminal proceedings have been initiated in Canadian courts against several companies and individuals in relation to these alleged activities.[153] The government of Québec obtained a judgment under its tax legislation claiming almost $1.4 billion in unpaid taxes, penalties and interest from JTI-Macdonald Corp., said to be owed because of the company's evasion of taxes through involvement in smuggling.[154] In July 2008, Imperial Tobacco and Rothmans Benson & Hedges pleaded guilty to charges in relation to their alleged role in aiding contraband tobacco sales. The two companies agreed to pay fines and a civil settlement amounting to a total of approximately $1.15 billion.[155]

V. HARM REDUCTION

Harm reduction refers to a broad range of measures that attempt to reduce the detrimental health effects of tobacco use. Helping people to quit smoking, or to reduce their consumption and the health impact of smoking, is part of a comprehensive tobacco control strategy. This is probably the most controversial area of tobacco control policy; harm reduction for smokers is controversial even among tobacco control advocates.[156]

---

[151]   *Attorney General of Canada v. R.J. Reynolds Tobacco Holdings Inc.*, 103 F.Supp. 2d 134 (N.D.N.Y. 2000).

[152]   *Attorney General of Canada v. R.J. Reynolds Tobacco Holdings Inc.*, 103 F.Supp. 2d 134 (N.D.N.Y. 2000), aff'd 268 F. 3d 103 (2d Cir. 2001), cert. denied 123 S. Ct. 513 (2002). For discussion of this case (and criticism of the decision to dismiss), see Elizabeth J. Farnam, "Racketeering, RICO and the Revenue Rule in Attorney General of Canada v. R.J. Reynolds: Civil RICO Claims for Foreign Tax Law Violations" (2002) 77 Wash. L. Rev. 843.

[153]   See *e.g.*, *R. v. JTI-Macdonald Corp.*, [2006] O.J. No. 2710 (Ont. S.C.J.); *R. v. JTI-Macdonald Corp.*, [2005] O.J. No. 5179 (Ont. S.C.J.) (both dealing with pre-trial issues). Former vice-president of sales of RJR-MacDonald (now JTI-Macdonald) pleaded guilty and provided information about the company's role in smuggling operations: "Senior Tobacco Exec Won't Go to Jail in Massive Fraud Case" *CBC News* (4 May 2006), online: <http://www.cbc.ca/canada/story/2006/05/04/cigarette-fraud.html>.

[154]   *Québec (Sous-ministre du Revenu) v. JTI-Macdonald Corp.*, [2004] J.Q. no 8978 (Qué S.C.). The company filed for protection from creditors shortly afterwards based on concerns about its "continued viability" pending the legal proceedings: *Re JTI-Macdonald Corp.*, [2004] O.J. No. 3671 (Ont. S.C.J.).

[155]   "Tobacco Giants to Pay up to $1.15B over contraband sales", online: CBC News <http://www.cbc.ca/canada/story/2008/07/31/tobacco-settlement.html>.

[156]   See *e.g.*, S. Chapman, "Harm Reduction" (2003) 12 Tobacco Control 341; L.T. Kozlowski, "First, Tell the Truth: A Dialogue on Human Rights, Deception, and the Use of Smokeless Tobacco as a Substitute for Cigarettes" (2003) 12 Tobacco Control 34.

This section will discuss cessation and alternative harm reduction strategies, as well as testing and disclosure requirements for tobacco products.

(a) Support for Smoking Cessation and Reduction

Encouraging smoking cessation is a key part of a comprehensive public health strategy for tobacco control. Education and public information have important roles here,[157] and marketing restrictions and smoke-free laws, discussed elsewhere in this chapter, indirectly encourage cessation. There are also several issues relating specifically to the legal and policy framework for cessation initiatives. First, there is the question of health care providers' duties with respect to patients who smoke. It has been suggested that a physician's duty of care to her patient includes a duty to advise a patient of the dangers of smoking and offer assistance with cessation.[158] There is arguably also a duty to advise patients who smoke of the health risks to third parties who may be exposed to their smoke.[159] Other health professionals such as nurses and pharmacists also have an important role in supporting cessation, and fulfilment of this role is recognized as part of good clinical practice.[160]

Inclusion of cessation counselling in health professionals' education and provision of funding for cessation-related services are important factors enabling these activities. A related issue concerns the availability

---

[157]   See *e.g.*, Steering Committee of the National Strategy to Reduce Tobacco Use in Canada, *New Directions for Tobacco Control in Canada: A National Strategy* (Ottawa: Minister of Public Works and Government Services, 1999) at 19-21 for an overview of activities, including media campaigns, brochures and other information, and quitlines (telephone information and counselling services).

[158]   For discussion, see Penny A. Washington, "Scope of a Physician's Duty When Counselling Patients on Smoking Cessation" (Legal opinion prepared by Bull, Housser & Tupper for Physicians for a Smoke-Free Canada, 1999), online: Physicians for a Smoke-Free Canada <http://www.smoke-free.ca/pdf_1/bht-opinion-cessation.PDF>. This opinion suggests that "Canadian courts would likely find that a physician who does not routinely counsel smoking patients on cessation is not meeting the requisite standard of care. Whether such a finding would result in a successful claim for damages would depend on whether the individual plaintiff could overcome ... significant causation hurdles" (*ibid.*, at 25).

[159]   *Ibid.*; Penny A. Washington, "Potential Liability of Physicians When Counselling Patients Regarding Exposure to Environmental Tobacco Smoke" (Legal opinion prepared by Bull, Housser & Tupper for Physicians for a Smoke-Free Canada, 1999), online: Physicians for a Smoke-Free Canada <http://www.smoke-free.ca/pdf_1/bht-opinion-second-hand-smoke.pdf>. This could be argued, for example, by analogy with *Pittman Estate v. Bain*, [1994] O.J. No. 463, 112 D.L.R. (4th) 257 (Ont. Gen. Div.).

[160]   See *e.g.*, Canadian Medical Association, "Tobacco: The Role of Health Professionals in Smoking Cessation" (Joint Statement, 2001), online: <http://policybase.cma.ca/dbtw-wpd/PolicyPDF/PD01-05.pdf>.

of cessation aids such as nicotine replacement therapy ("NRT"). In Canada, nicotine patches and gum (the most widely used forms of NRT) are available without a prescription; buproprion (an antidepressant which may help with nicotine withdrawal) requires a prescription.[161] Some provincial cessation programs include subsidies for these products for participants, and in other cases these products are covered by provincial drug insurance plans.[162] Concerns about the price of NRT products in Canada have been dealt with by the Patented Medicines Review Board.[163]

Given the effects of tobacco on foetuses and infants, smoking cessation programs for pregnant and postpartum women are an important priority area.[164] The issue of smoking by pregnant women also raises important and difficult questions about the type and degree of control that can properly be exercised over women's behaviour during pregnancy.[165]

(b) Product Information Disclosure

Information about tobacco product ingredients and characteristics is needed to assess the risks of such products, communicate these to consumers, and determine whether content should be regulated or

---

[161]   Health Canada, "Quit Smoking Aids" (2008), online: <http://www.hc-sc.gc.ca/hl-vs/tobac-tabac/body-corps/aid_e.html>.

[162]   See e.g., Tobacco Steering Committee of the National Strategy to Reduce Tobacco Use in Canada, New Directions for Tobacco Control in Canada: A National Strategy (Ottawa: Minister of Public Works and Government Services, 1999) at 19; Michele Tremblay et al., "Physicians Taking Action Against Smoking: An Intervention Program to Optimize Smoking Cessation Counselling by Montreal General Practitioners" (2001) 165 C.M.A.J. 601 at 606.

[163]   Mark C. Taylor, "Public Policy and Smoking Cessation: Beyond Pharmacological Solutions" (Paper presented at the Public Forum: Nicotine Issue — New Approaches to Cessation, 31 May 1999), online: Physicians for a Smoke-Free Canada <http://www.smoke-free.ca/pdf_1/CessationMay99.PDF> at 8.

[164]   For a review and assessment of some such programs, see Karen M. Devries & Lorraine J. Greaves, "Smoking Cessation for Pregnant Women" (2004) 95 Can. J. Public Health 278. For a review of the evidence with respect to harms during pregnancy, see U.S. Department of Health and Human Services, The Health Consequences of Smoking: A Report of the Surgeon General (Georgia: U.S. Department of Health and Human Services, Centers for Disease Control and Prevention, National Center for Chronic Disease Prevention and Health Promotion, Office on Smoking and Health, 2004) c. 5, online: CDC <http://www.cdc.gov/tobacco/data_statistics/sgr/sgr_2004/index.htm>.

[165]   A discussion of these issues is beyond the scope of this chapter. See e.g., Barry M. Lester et al., "Substance Use During Pregnancy: Time for Policy to Catch Up with Research" (2004) 1 Harm Reduction J., online: Harm Reduction Journal <http://www.harmreductionjournal.com/home>; Laury Oaks, Smoking and Pregnancy: The Politics of Fetal Protection (New Brunswick, N.J.: Rutgers University Press, 2001) (especially c. 7: "Cigarette Smoking as Fetal Abuse"); Sandra Rodgers, "The Legal Regulation of Women's Reproductive Capacity in Canada" in Jocelyn Downie, Timothy Caulfield & Colleen Flood, eds., Canadian Health Law and Policy, 2d ed. (Markham, Ont.: Butterworths, 2002) at 331.

modified to reduce harm. Mandatory disclosure of tobacco product information is surprisingly rare (in comparison with requirements for other hazardous products or consumer goods), but may become more common when the FCTC comes into force; Article 10 provides for states to implement measures for disclosure to government and the public of the constituents and emissions of tobacco products.

The federal *Tobacco Reporting Regulations* require manufacturers (defined in s. 1 to include importers) to submit periodic reports containing information about ingredients (including additives), data on listed constituents (such as nicotine) and emissions, and information about research activities, sales and marketing.[166] The regulations prescribe methods of collecting the constituent and emissions data. Legislation elsewhere provides for reporting regulations but these have not yet been adopted.[167]

The industry has opposed these requirements on a number of grounds. The federal regulations were unsuccessfully challenged in the Québec courts as *ultra vires* and an infringement of s. 8 of the *Charter* (unreasonable search or seizure).[168] Another concern is that the reporting requirements compel tobacco companies to disclose trade secrets. A more general concern relates to the reliability of information obtained through product testing. This can be addressed to some extent by prescribing testing methods. However, further research is required to determine the extent to which laboratory test results provide an accurate indicator of the smoke that is actually inhaled and its effects.

(c) Regulation of Tobacco Products and Alternatives

The most difficult and controversial area of harm reduction is the development and promotion of "harm-reducing products": tobacco products that may minimize harm to consumers or alternative nicotine delivery system ("ANDS") products. It might seem that reducing the harm caused by tobacco products must be a good thing, but in fact the matter is not so clear. Since tobacco products have multiple toxic constituents and harmful effects, designing a product that reduces the overall health impact significantly is likely to be difficult. Observers are justifiably sceptical of

---

[166] S.O.R./2000-273.

[167] *Tobacco Act*, R.S.Q. c. T-0.01, s. 30. British Columbia's *Tobacco Testing and Disclosure Regulation*, B.C. Reg. 282/98 has been repealed: B.C. Reg. 393/2007.

[168] *JTI Macdonald Corp. v. Canada (Attorney General)*, [2002] Q.J. No. 5550 at paras. 492 & ff (Qué. S.C.); *JTI Macdonald Corp. v. Canada (Attorney General)*, [2005] Q.J. No. 10915 at paras. 166-92 (Qué. C.A.). This issue was not raised on appeal to the Supreme Court of Canada: *Canada (Attorney General) v. JTI-Macdonald Corp.*, [2007] S.C.J. No. 30, 2007 SCC 30 (S.C.C.).

industry claims that a new product is less harmful, given the long history of such claims that have proven to be false.[169]

Even if a genuinely harm-reducing product could be developed, experts fear that reducing the harm of tobacco consumption could undermine the ultimate goal of decreasing its prevalence.[170] Evidence suggests that the availability of cigarettes that are — or are perceived to be — less harmful is likely to discourage smokers from quitting and may encourage some people to smoke who otherwise might not.[171] As a result, there are serious questions about whether making cigarettes less harmful would actually result in reduced harm for individuals or a net public health benefit.[172] At the same time, although cessation is obviously the preferred outcome, the statistics suggest that relatively few smokers manage to quit successfully.[173] In addition, some forcefully argue that it is ethically wrong to deprive individuals of opportunities to reduce their risk just because we are concerned about the net impact of harm reducing products or we would prefer that they abstain from tobacco use altogether.[174] Therefore, additional measures to reduce harm are required, but they need to be carefully designed.[175]

One option is eliminating or limiting nicotine or additives so that products are less addictive or attractive to consumers, thereby decreasing overall consumption. Reducing nicotine, however, may lead smokers who

---

[169] Physicians for a Smoke-Free Canada, "The Tobacco Industry is Trolling for Big Fish: 10 Lessons from Canada on Tobacco Product Regulations" (October 2006), online: <http://www.smoke-free.ca/pdf_1/lessonsfromcanada-final.pdf>.

[170] See e.g., Kenneth E. Warner, "Reducing Harm to Smokers: Methods, Their Effectiveness, and the Role of Policy" in Robert L. Rabin & Stephen Sugarman, eds., Regulating Tobacco (Oxford: Oxford University Press, 2001) 111 at 114.

[171] See e.g., S. Shiffman et al., "Smoker and Ex-Smoker Reactions to Cigarettes Claiming Reduced Risk" (2004) 13 Tobacco Control 78.

[172] For an example of a recent debate, see N. Gray & P. Boyle, "The Case of the Disappearing Nitrosamines: a Potentially Global Phenomenon" (2004) 13 Tobacco Control 13, and the responding editorial: W.A. Farone, "Accepting Premature Deaths from Smoking: Could Partial Reduction of Some Toxic Components in Cigarettes Lead to Reductions in Premature Deaths From Smoking?" (2004) 13 Tobacco Control 1.

[173] Kenneth E. Warner, "Reducing Harm to Smokers: Methods, Their Effectiveness, and the Role of Policy" in Robert L. Rabin & Stephen Sugarman, eds., Regulating Tobacco (Oxford: Oxford University Press, 2001) at 111, states that although the vast majority of smokers want to quit, only about 3 per cent actually manage to quit each year.

[174] See e.g., L.T. Kozlowski, "First, Tell the Truth: A Dialogue on Human Rights, Deception, and the Use of Smokeless Tobacco as a Substitute for Cigarettes" (2003) 12 Tobacco Control 34; C. Bates et al., "European Union Policy on Smokeless Tobacco: A Statement in Favour of Evidence Based Regulation for Public Health" (2003) 12 Tobacco Control 360.

[175] Kenneth E. Warner, "Reducing Harm to Smokers: Methods, Their Effectiveness, and the Role of Policy" in Robert L. Rabin & Stephen Sugarman, eds., Regulating Tobacco (Oxford: Oxford University Press, 2001) at 132-33.

are already addicted to compensate by smoking more — which would ultimately be counterproductive as far as their own health is concerned.[176] Imposing standards that limit the toxic constituents of tobacco smoke could directly reduce the harm caused by consuming tobacco products. The introduction of "low tar" or "light" cigarettes was purportedly intended to achieve this. Although it is now accepted that these products are in fact no less harmful, there is evidence to suggest that some people have continued to smoke or taken up smoking because of the reassurance these products provided.[177] This experience has served as a caution to those proposing harm-reducing tobacco products. A range of other options have been cautiously explored, such as modifying filters and reducing harmful additives.[178] However, mistrust of industry claims and the difficulty of obtaining and evaluating reliable evidence in order to compare risks make this a challenging area to regulate.

Were consensus to develop that regulating cigarette content should be pursued, this could be done in much the same way as other types of consumer goods are regulated. Canadian legislation allows for tobacco product standards to be set.[179] The federal government has adopted regulations on the ignition propensity of cigarettes to prevent fires caused by cigarettes,[180] but standards have yet to be adopted with respect to content or emissions. Some have also argued that nicotine should be regulated as a drug, leading to a much more comprehensive regulatory framework for tobacco products (as well as other nicotine delivery devices).[181] Debate about the feasibility and merits of this approach has been ongoing internationally, recently centred around renewed proposals for regulation by the U.S. Food and Drug Administration.[182]

---

[176] On this debate, see *e.g.*, Jack E. Henningfield *et al.*, "Reducing the Addictiveness of Cigarettes" (1998) 7 Tobacco Control 281, and the responses to this article: Letters to the editor (1999) 8 Tobacco Control 106.

[177] See John R. Hughes, "Do 'Light' Cigarettes Undermine Cessation?" (2001) 10 Tobacco Control 41, for a summary and discussion of some studies.

[178] WHO, "Advancing Knowledge on Regulating Tobacco Products" (2000), online: <http://www.who.int/entity/tobacco/media/en/OsloMonograph.pdf> at 32-36, 41-42; L.T. Kozlowski *et al.*, "Maximum Yields Might Improve Public Health: If Filter Vents Were Banned: A Lesson from the History of Vented Filters" (2006) 15 Tobacco Control 262; Michael Rabinoff *et al.*, "Pharmacological and Chemical Effects of Cigarette Additives" (2007) 97 Am. J. Public Health 1981.

[179] *Tobacco Act*, R.S.Q. c. T-0.01, s. 30; *Tobacco Act*, S.C. 1997, c. 13, ss. 5, 7.

[180] *Cigarette Ignition Propensity Regulations*, S.O.R./2005-178.

[181] See *e.g.*, N. Gray *et al.*, "Toward a Comprehensive Long-term Nicotine Policy" (2005) 14 Tobacco Control 161; N. Gray, "The Need for Tobacco Regulation" (2006) 15 Tobacco Control 145; Jacques Le Houezec, Albert Hirsch & Yves Martinet, "Time for a Nicotine and Tobacco Regulatory Authority in France" (2006) 15 Tobacco Control 343.

[182] Michael Givel, "Philip Morris' FDA Gambit: Good for Public Health?" (2005) 26 J. Public Health Pol'y 450; Richard A. Daynard, "Public Health vs. Philip Morris: Is it a Zero-Sum

Other possibilities include the promotion of smokeless tobacco products and non-tobacco ANDS (such as inhalers or other means of ingesting nicotine) as alternatives to smoking. These products may allow people who are addicted to nicotine to obtain it through means that are less harmful than smoking tobacco. Again, there is an important debate in progress about whether these alternatives will result in a net benefit and whether they should be pursued as a matter of policy. There is evidence that smokeless tobacco products pose significantly less health risks as compared to smoking, but they are still not risk-free.[183] In addition, some are concerned that the use of smokeless tobacco might actually *increase* smoking rates by serving as a "gateway" to tobacco use, although the available evidence seems to suggest that this is not true and that smokeless tobacco may provide a less harmful alternative for nicotine-addicted smokers and ex-smokers.[184] The controversy surrounding a European Union ban on certain smokeless tobacco products has illustrated these opposing views.[185] Non-tobacco ANDS are also being explored as potential harm reducing products, but raise similar issues. Questions arise as to how ANDS should be regulated and whether their marketing should be restricted. This is another evolving area in which little consensus has been reached. However, pressure for reform has come from critics pointing out that the most dangerous products (cigarettes) remain the least regulated and most available, while alternatives are subject to stricter regulation or even prohibitions in some cases.[186]

VI. PROTECTION FROM SECOND-HAND SMOKE

Given that smoking continues to be prevalent in Canadian society, one of the crucial goals of tobacco control policy is protecting non-

---

Game?" (2005) 26 J. Public Health Pol'y 469; P.A. McDaniel & R.E. Malone, "Understanding Philip Morris's Pursuit of US Government Regulation of Tobacco" (2005) 14 Tobacco Control 193; Michael Givel, "FDA Legislation: Time to Shift US Federal Anti-tobacco Advocacy Tactics" (2007) 16 Tobacco Control 217; Matthew Myers, "FDA Legislation: A Strong Bill that Represents a Major Step Forward" (2007) 16 Tobacco Control 289.

[183] See *e.g.*, J. Foulds *et al.*, "Effect of smokeless tobacco (snus) on smoking and public health in Sweden" (2003) 12 Tobacco Control 349; Ritesh Gupta *et al.*, "Smokeless Tobacco and Cardiovascular Risk" (2004) 164 Arch. Int. Med. 1845. The health effects of smokeless tobacco products (in particular the risk of oral cancer) seems to vary significantly between various forms of these products: Foulds *et al.*, *ibid.*

[184] Foulds *et al.*, *ibid.*; C. Bates *et al.*, "European Union Policy on Smokeless Tobacco: A Statement in Favour of Evidence Based Regulation for Public Health" (2003) 12 Tobacco Control 360.

[185] Bates *et al.*, *ibid.* See also Coral E. Gartner & Wayne D. Hall, "Should Australia Lift its Ban on Low Nitrosamine Smokeless Tobacco Products?" (2008) 188 Med. J. Australia 44.

[186] Gartner & Hall, *ibid.*

smokers from second-hand smoke (SHS, also referred to as "environmental tobacco smoke", "involuntary smoking" or "passive smoking").[187] The smoking-attributable deaths in Canada in 2002 included over 800 deaths from SHS.[188] A recent report of the U.S. Surgeon General concluded that there is no "safe level" of exposure to second-hand smoke.[189] The primary goal of restrictions on smoking is to protect people from unwanted exposure to the toxins contained in SHS and their health effects, but they also contribute to demand reduction and play a role in encouraging people to reduce or quit smoking. Although public awareness of the health risks of SHS is relatively low,[190] there is a significant and growing (though variable) level of support for smoking bans in Canada.[191]

There are restrictions on smoking across Canada at the federal, provincial and municipal levels, though they vary in scope.[192] In Canada and other jurisdictions, a common pattern has been noted in the development of smoking bans: the earliest examples were specific bans on smoking in certain public places such as schools, public transport and government buildings, followed by restrictions in private workplaces, and finally, increasingly comprehensive bans covering public places.[193]

---

[187] On the controversial question of terminology, see S. Chapman, "Other People's Smoke: What's in a Name? Opinions Differ Over What Term Should Be Used To Describe 'Other People's Smoke'" (2003) 12 Tobacco Control 113.

[188] Dolly Baliunas et al., "Smoking-attributable Mortality and Expected Years of Life Lost in Canada 2002: Conclusions for Prevention and Policy" (2007) 27 Chronic Diseases in Canada 154 at 157.

[189] U.S. Department of Health and Human Services, The Health Consequences of Involuntary Exposure to Tobacco Smoke: A Report of the Surgeon General (Georgia: U.S. Department of Health and Human Services, Centers for Disease Control and Prevention, Coordinating Center for Health Promotion, National Center for Chronic Disease Prevention and Health Promotion, Office on Smoking and Health, 2006) at 11.

[190] See e.g., Mary Jane Ashley et al., "Knowledge About Tobacco and Attitudes Toward Tobacco Control: How Different are Smokers and Non-smokers?" (2000) 91 Can. J. Public Health 376.

[191] Ashley et al., ibid.; Nicole A. Guia et al., "Support for Tobacco Control Policies" (2003) 94 Can. J. Public Health 36; Health Canada, "Canadian Tobacco Use Monitoring Survey ('CTUMS'): Summary of Results for the First Half of 2007 (February-June)", online. <http://www.hc-sc.gc.ca/hl-vs/tobac-tabac/research-recherche/stat/_ctums-esutc_2007/wave-phase-1_summary-sommaire_e.html>.

[192] For a useful overview of Canadian laws in this area see Non-Smokers' Rights Association, "Provincial and Territorial Smoke-free Legislation/Regulations/Policies" (January 2007), online: <http://www.nsra-adnf.ca/cms/File/pdf/prov_smokefree_leg_reg_policies_January_2007.pdf>.

[193] Peter D. Jacobson & Lisa M. Zapawa, "Clean Indoor Air Restrictions: Progress and Promise" in Robert L. Rabin & Stephen Sugarman, eds., Regulating Tobacco (Oxford: Oxford University Press, 2001) 207 at 221; Rob Cunningham, Smoke & Mirrors: The Canadian Tobacco War (Ottawa: International Development Research Centre, 1996) c. 10.

(a)   Smoke-Free Public Places and Workplaces

Restrictions on smoking in public places exist in provincial/ territorial and municipal legislation. The scope of these restrictions varies across the country, but there is a clear trend toward more comprehensive smoking bans, responding to evidence suggesting that restricting smoking to designated areas does not effectively minimize the harms from SHS exposure.[194] As a result, there have been significant legislative changes over the last few years. Most Canadian jurisdictions now have laws banning smoking in all enclosed public places.[195] British Columbia's ban will come into force on 31 March 2008.[196] Prince Edward Island has a public smoking ban but allows smoking in designated enclosed areas.[197] Comprehensive bans covering most public places including bars and restaurants now apply in many municipalities, whether or not such a ban also exists in provincial legislation.[198] Some provincial statutes explicitly provide that where there are overlapping provincial and municipals laws, the stricter of these laws will prevail.[199]

While even comprehensive bans have typically only covered indoor or enclosed public places,[200] some legislation includes at least some outdoor spaces such as restaurant patios; sporting facilities; school grounds; or areas near doors, windows and air intakes of public

[194]   See *e.g.*, T. Cains *et al.*, "Designated 'No Smoking' Areas Provide from Partial to No Protection from Environmental Tobacco Smoke" (2004) 13 Tobacco Control 17; M. Pion & M.S. Givel, "Airport Smoking Rooms Don't Work" (2004) 13 Tobacco Control 37.

[195]   *Tobacco Reduction Act*, S.A. 2005, c. T-3.8, s. 3(a); *The Tobacco Control Act*, S.S. 2001, c. T-14.1, s. 11; *The Non-Smokers Health Protection Act*, C.C.S.M. c. N92, s. 2(1)(a); *Smoke-Free Ontario Act*, S.O. 1994, c. 10, s. 9(1); *Tobacco Act*, R.S.Q. c. T-0.01, s. 2; *Smoke-free Places Act*, S.N.B. 2004, c. S-9.5, s. 3(a); *Smoke-free Places Act*, S.N.S. 2002, c. 12, s. 5(1); *Smoke-Free Environment Act, 2005*, S.N.L. 2005, c. S-16.2, s. 4(1); *Tobacco Control Act*, S.N.W.T. 2006, c. 9, s. 8(1); *Tobacco Control Act*, S.Nu. 2003, c. 13, s. 14; *Smoke-Free Places Act*, S.Y. 2008, c. 8, s. 4. The Québec, Nova Scotia, Newfoundland and Labrador, and Yukon provisions set out lists of places in which smoking is not permitted rather than prohibiting it in public places generally, but the lists are sufficiently comprehensive to be considered full bans.

[196]   *Tobacco Sales (Banning Tobacco and Smoking in Public Places) Amendment Act, 2007*, S.B.C. 2007, c. 12, s. 3 (which will add s. 2.3 to the *Tobacco Control Act*, R.S.B.C. 1996, c. 451).

[197]   *Smoke-free Places Act*, R.S.P.E.I. 1988, c. S-4.2, ss. 4, 8-9.

[198]   See Non-Smokers' Rights Association, "Compendium of Smoke-free Workplace and Public Place By-laws" (March 2008), online: <http://www.nsra-adnf.ca/cms/file/pdf/ Compendium_March_2008.pdf>.

[199]   See *e.g.*, *The Non-Smokers Health Protection Act*, C.C.S.M. c. N92, s. 6; *Smoke-Free Ontario Act*, S.O. 1994, c. 10, s. 12; *Tobacco Control Act*, S.Nu. 2003, c. 13, s. 15.

[200]   *E.g.*, *Tobacco Control Act*, S.S. 2001, c. T-14.1, s. 11; *Non-Smokers Health Protection Act*, C.C.S.M. c. N92, s. 2.

buildings.[201] Even the most comprehensive smoking bans still provide for some exemptions, though increasingly only in designated areas that are limited in size, enclosed and have separate ventilation. Common exemptions include residential care facilities and hotels or other lodgings.[202]

There is growing public awareness of the effects of SHS on employees and concerns about the limits of employees' ability to control their own exposure. Protecting employees from SHS is an important objective of smoking bans, and some of these bans have been explicitly formulated as occupational health and safety laws. For example, the federal *Non-smokers' Health Act* restricts smoking in workplaces within the jurisdiction of the federal government, which include government offices and federally regulated industries.[203] Prohibitions or restrictions on smoking in private sector workplaces are included in the statutes of most Canadian jurisdictions.[204] It is also arguable that even in the absence of explicit legislative provisions, occupational health and safety law would require employers to ban or restrict smoking in order to protect workers' health.[205] Some statutes provide protection for "whistleblowers" (employees who report violations or otherwise seek to have the legislation enforced).[206] Workers' exposure to SHS has also been the subject of litigation and claims for compensation (see Section VII (b) below).

(b) Issues and Challenges

Smoking restrictions have been opposed and challenged by the tobacco industry and others, in particular industry associations (often with

---

[201]   *E.g., Tobacco Reduction Act*, S.A. 2005, c. T-3.8, s. 3(d); *Smoke-Free Ontario Act*, S.O. 1994, c. 10, s. 9(2), (6); *Tobacco Act*, R.S.Q. c. T-0.01, ss. 2.1, 2.2; *Smoke-free Places Act*, S.N.B. 2004, c. S-9.5, s. 3(f); *Smoke-free Places Act*, S.N.S. 2002, c. 12, s. 5(2)-(4).

[202]   *E.g., Tobacco Reduction Act*, S.A. 2005, c. T-3.8, s. 5; *Tobacco Control Act*, S.S. 2001, c. T-14.1, s. 11(3)(a); *The Non-Smokers Health Protection Act*, C.C.S.M. c. N92, s. 3; *Tobacco Control Act*, S.N.W.T. 2006, c. 9, s. 8(2).

[203]   *Non-smokers' Health Act*, R.S.C. 1985, c. 15 (4th Supp.).

[204]   *Tobacco Reduction Act*, S.A. 2005, c. T-3.8, s. 3(b); *The Non-Smokers Health Protection Act*, C.C.S.M. c. N92, s. 2(1)(b); *Smoke-Free Ontario Act*, S.O. 1994, c. 10, s. 9(1); *Tobacco Act*, R.S.Q. c. T-0.01, s. 2(9); *Smoke-free Places Act*, S.N.B. 2004, c. S-9.5, s. 3(b); *Smoke-free Places Act*, S.N.S. 2002, c. 12, s. 7; *Smoke-Free Environment Act, 2005*, S.N.L. 2005, c. S-16.1, s. 4(1)(a); *Smoke-free Places Act*, R.S.P.E.I. 1988, c. S-4.2, s. 4 (except in designated enclosed areas: ss. 8-9); *Tobacco Control Act*, S.Nu. 2003, c. 13, s. 13.

[205]   For discussion, see Wendy Hyman, "Environmental Tobacco Smoke in the Workplace: The Legal Impact of Federal and Ontario Occupational Health and Safety Legislation" (1996) 4 Health L. J. 221.

[206]   See *e.g., Tobacco Control Act*, S.Nu. 2003, c. 13, s. 13(6); *Smoke-Free Ontario Act*, S.O. 1994, c. 10, s. 9(4). Workplace smoking and employers' treatment of smokers and non-smokers also raise a number of employment law issues which will not be dealt with here.

the support of the tobacco industry).[207] Some argue that decisions about whether to ban smoking in public places, especially food and beverage establishments, should be left to the market; others oppose such bans because of fears of lost business, though the evidence supporting such claims is at best equivocal.[208] Legal challenges to smoking restrictions have been attempted in some cases, arguing for example that restrictions are arbitrary, discriminatory, or beyond the powers of the authority adopting them.[209]

Several statutes exempt traditional uses of tobacco by aboriginal peoples from smoking bans.[210] The Manitoba *Non-Smokers Health Protection Act* also excludes its application to reserve lands.[211] This exemption was recently challenged by the owner of a tavern outside a reserve who argued that the differential application of the ban on- and off-reserve was discriminatory. Mr. Jenkinson and his company ("Creekside Hideaway Motel Ltd.") appealed convictions for multiple breaches of the Act on the basis that they violated the *Charter*.[212] Justice Clearwater, in a somewhat problematic judgment, found that s. 15 had indeed been violated and that the infringement could not be saved by s. 1, therefore striking down the exemption (s. 9.4) and directing an acquittal.[213] This

---

[207] See *e.g.*, J. Drope & S. Glantz, "British Columbia Capital Regional District 100% Smokefree Bylaw: A Successful Public Health Campaign Despite Industry Opposition" (2003) 12 Tobacco Control 264; J.V. Dearlove *et al.*, "Tobacco Industry Manipulation of the Hospitality Industry to Maintain Smoking in Public Places" (2002) 11 Tobacco Control 94.

[208] M. Scollo *et al.*, "Review of the Quality of Studies on the Economic Effects of Smoke-Free Policies on the Hospitality Industry" (2003) 12 Tobacco Control 13; Rita Luk, Roberta Ferrence & Gerhard Gmel, "The Economic Impact of a Smoke-Free Bylaw on Restaurant and Bar Sales in Ottawa, Canada" (2006) 101 Addiction 738.

[209] See *e.g.*, *Restaurant and Food Services Assn. of British Columbia v. Vancouver (City)*, [1998] B.C.J. No. 53 (B.C.C.A.); *Albertos Restaurant v. Saskatoon (City)*, [2000] S.J. No. 725, 2000 SKCA 135 (Sask. C.A.); *Pub and Bar Coalition of Ontario v. Ottawa (City)*, [2002] O.J. No. 2240 (Ont. C.A.); *Filos Restaurant Ltd. v. Calgary (City)*, [2007] A.J. No. 159, 2007 ABQB 97 (Alta. Q.B.).

[210] See *e.g.*, *Smoke-Free Ontario Act*, S.O. 1994, c. 10, s. 13(3), (4); *The Non-Smokers Health Protection Act*, C.C.S.M. c. N92, s. 5.1; *Tobacco Control Act*, S.S. 2001, c. T-14.1, s. 11(3)(c); *Smoke-free Places Act*, S.N.B. 2004, c. S-9.5, s. 2(2).

[211] *The Non-Smokers Health Protection Act*, C.C.S.M. c. N92, s. 9.4, which provides that the Act does not apply to "penitentiaries, federally regulated airports, Canadian Forces bases or to any other place or premises occupied by a federal work, undertaking or business, or on lands reserved for Indians". The New Brunswick legislation has a similar provision except that it does not mention reserve lands: *Smoke-free Places Act*, S.N.B. 2004, c. S-9.5, s. 2(3).

[212] *R. v. Jenkinson*, [2006] M.J. No. 250, 2006 MBQB 185 (Man. Q.B.), rev'd [2008] M.J. No. 78 (Man. C.A.). In the Provincial Court they had also argued that the provisions were *ultra vires* the province, but this point was not pursued on appeal to the Court of Queen's Bench.

[213] *R. v. Jenkinson*, [2006] M.J. No. 250, 2006 MBQB 185 at para. 25 (Man. Q.B.), rev'd [2008] M.J. No. 78 (Man. C.A.). The provision struck down was not the provision under

decision is under appeal to the Manitoba Court of Appeal,[214] but the Manitoba government has stated that in the meantime it will apply the smoking ban to reserves.[215]

With smoking restrictions becoming increasingly comprehensive, there are few places left that are unregulated. However, preventing exposure to SHS in private places and residences raises difficult issues. Exposure to SHS in the home is a serious health problem,[216] especially for children,[217] but banning smoking in private residences would be considered by many to be an unacceptable interference with privacy, in addition to being very difficult to enforce. The problem of SHS risks in the home can be dealt with in a limited way through family law (for example as a factor potentially affecting custody determinations) and child protection (in exceptional cases where the life of a child, for example one with severe asthma, may be at risk).[218] Bans on smoking in private vehicles when children are present have been advocated in Canada, following examples from the United States.[219] In December 2007, Nova Scotia became the first Canadian province to ban smoking in cars

---

which the appellants had been convicted but Clearwater J. held that they should not be convicted of charges "laid in the face of the discriminatory exemption section".

[214]   *R. v. Jenkinson*, [2007] M.J. No. 39, 2007 MBCA 19 (Man. C.A.) (preliminary ruling on intervenor status).

[215]   Government of Manitoba, News Release, "Province to Extend Smoking Ban to First Nations" (13 September 2006), online: <http://www.gov.mb.ca/chc/press/top/2006/09/2006-09-13-04.html>.

[216]   A recent study estimated that over 1,000 deaths occurred in 1998 from SHS exposure in the home: Eva M. Makomaski Illing & Murray J. Kaiserman, "Mortality Attributable to Tobacco Use in Canada and its Regions, 1998" (2004) 95 Can. J. Public Health 38 at 43.

[217]   See *e.g.*, U.S. Department of Health and Human Services, *Reducing Tobacco Use: A Report of the Surgeon General* (Georgia: U.S. Department of Health and Human Services, Centers for Disease Control and Prevention, National Center for Chronic Disease Prevention and Health Promotion, Office on Smoking and Health, 2000) at 195-96, online: <http://www.cdc.gov/tobacco/data_statistics/sgr/sgr_2000/> (health effects on children from SHS including bronchitis, pneumonia, ear diseases, asthma and possibly sudden infant death syndrome). Of the smoking-attributable deaths in Canada in 2002, almost 100 deaths were among children less than one year old: Dolly Baliunas *et al.*, "Smoking-attributable Mortality and Expected Years of Life Lost in Canada 2002: Conclusions for Prevention and Policy" (2007) 27 Chronic Diseases in Canada 154 at 157.

[218]   See *e.g.*, Physicians for a Smoke-Free Canada, "Second Hand Smoke and Children's Health: Custody and Access" (August 2002), online: <http://www.smoke-free.ca/pdf_1/custody%20and%20access.pdf>; Ontario Medical Association, "Exposure to Second-Hand Smoke: Are We Protecting Our Kids?" (Position Paper by the Ontario Medical Association) (2004), online: <http://www.oma.org/Health/tobacco/smoke2004.pdf>.

[219]   See *e.g.*, Ontario Medical Association, *ibid.*; Ontario Medical Association, News Release, "Ontario's Doctors Applaud Sault MPP for Taking Action to Protect Children's Health" (6 December 2007), online: <http://www.oma.org/Media/news/pr071206.asp>.

when minors are present.[220] In the first half of 2008, the Yukon and Ontario followed suit.[221] Another issue that is gaining increasing attention is SHS in multi-unit dwellings, which is typically dealt with as a matter of landlord-and-tenant law.[222]

Residential facilities such as long-term care facilities need to balance protection from SHS with accommodation of residents who may be addicted smokers; they are typically included within legislative provisions as "public places" but permitted to allow smoking in designated areas.[223] Smoking in correctional facilities raises even more difficult issues. The prevalence of smoking in correctional facilities is much higher than in the general population (according to some studies, as high as 80 per cent), which results in resistance to and difficulties in implementing smoking restrictions.[224] It also means, though, that the risk of SHS-related harm is unusually high, and this in a context where individuals are held involuntarily. Workers in correctional facilities are also affected. As a result, there have been complaints and legal action both from inmates opposing smoking restrictions[225] and from inmates and employees wanting protection from SHS.[226] These competing interests may be balanced by

---

[220]   Bill 6, *An Act to Amend Chapter 12 of the Acts of 2002, the Smoke-Free Places Act*, 2nd Sess., 60th Gen. Assembly, Nova Scotia, 2007 (assented to 13 December 2007).

[221]   *Smoke-Free Places Act*, S.Y. 2008, c. 8, s. 4(1)(q) (in force 15 May 2008); *Smoke-Free Ontario Amendment Act, 2008*, S.O. 2008, c. 12 (assented to 18 June 2008).

[222]   Non-Smokers' Rights Association, "A Review of Decisions Made by Adjudicators of Landlord and Tenant Boards" (December 2007), online: <http://www.nsra-adnf.ca/cms/file/pdf/Board_decisions_Dec2007.pdf>.

[223]   See *supra*, note 202 and accompanying text.

[224]   Matthew J. Carpenter *et al.*, "Smoking in correctional facilities: a survey of employees" (2001) 10 Tobacco Control 38.

[225]   *Regina Correctional Centre Inmate Committee v. Saskatchewan (Department of Justice)*, [1995] S.J. No. 350, 133 Sask. R. 61 (Sask. Q.B.); *McNeill v. Ontario (Ministry of the Solicitor General & Correctional Services)*, [1998] O.J. No. 2288, 126 C.C.C. (3d) 466 (Ont. Gen. Div.); *Saskatoon Correctional Centre Inmate Committee v. Government of Saskatchewan*, [2000] S.J. No. 307, 193 Sask. R. 248 (Sask. Q.B.); *Inmate Welfare Committee of William Head Institution v. William Head Institution*, [2003] F.C.J. No. 411, 2003 FCT 288 (F.C.T.D.); *Vaughn v. Ontario*, [2003] O.J. No. 5304 (Ont. S.C.J.). Most of these have been unsuccessful, but in *McCann v. Fraser Regional Correctional Centre*, [2000] B.C.J. No. 559 (B.C.S.C.), the court held that implementing a smoking ban on five days' notice violated prisoners' security of the person and constituted cruel and unusual punishment, primarily because the short time frame did not allow adequate measures to be put in place to assist smokers in adjusting to the ban.

[226]   *Re Ontario Public Service Employees' Union*, [1996] O.O.H.S.A.D. No. 18 (Office of Adjudication); *Galarneau c. Canada (Procureur general)*, [2004] F.C.J. No. 886, 2004 FC 718 (F.C.), aff'd [2005] F.C.J. No. 42, 2005 FC 39 (F.C.); "Prisoner sues Ottawa over smoking cellmate" CBC News (17 June 2002), online: <http://www.cbc.ca/canada/story/2002/06/17/prison_smoke020617.html>. In the U.S., the Supreme Court has held that failure to protect a prisoner from exposure to SHS may violate the right to freedom from cruel or unusual punishment: *Helling v. McKinney*, 113 S. Ct. 2475 (1993).

allowing smoking only in designated areas or outdoors, but there has been a movement toward full bans on the grounds of health protection and more effective enforcement.[227]

VII.   LITIGATION

Litigation is an increasingly important way of using the law to address the impact of tobacco use. Civil litigation has dominated attempts to assign accountability, although criminal proceedings and public inquiries offer possibilities as well.[228] A full discussion of tobacco litigation is beyond the scope of this chapter, but this section aims to give an overview of the potential benefits and difficulties of using litigation as part of tobacco control efforts, and of some important recent developments in the Canadian context.

(a) Litigation as a Tobacco Control Strategy

There are differing views of the utility and legitimacy of litigation as part of a comprehensive tobacco control strategy.[229] Proponents of litigation as a public health strategy point to several ways in which tobacco lawsuits contribute to tobacco control efforts.[230] Lawsuits increase

[227] See e.g., Physicians for a Smoke-Free Canada, News Release, "Smoking Ban in Federal Prisons a Healthy Step Forward" (27 June 2007), online: <http://www.smoke-free.ca/eng_home/news_press_2007-06-25b.htm>. However, Québec recently backtracked from implementing a full ban following protests: "Québec prison inmates step outdoors for a smoke" CBC News (8 February 2008), online: <http://www.cbc.ca/canada/ottawa/story/2008/02/08/qc-smokingban-prison0208.html?ref=rss>.

[228] On criminal proceedings, see U.S. Department of Health and Human Services, Reducing Tobacco Use: A Report of the Surgeon General (Georgia: U.S. Department of Health and Human Services, Centers for Disease Control and Prevention, National Center for Chronic Disease Prevention and Health Promotion, Office on Smoking and Health, 2000) at 256-59, online: <http://www.cdc.gov/tobacco/data_statistics/sgr/sgr_2000/>; on public inquiries, see D. Douglas Blanke, Towards Health with Justice: Litigation and Public Inquiries as Tools for Tobacco Control (Geneva: World Health Organization, 2002) at 47-50.

[229] See e.g., Benedickt Fischer & Jurgen Rehm, "Some Reflections on the Relationship of Risk, Harm and Responsibility in Recent Tobacco Lawsuits, and Implications for Public Health" (2001) 92 Can. J. Public Health 7, and the response by Roberta Ferrence et al., "Tobacco Industry Litigation and the Role of Government: A Public Health Perspective" (2001) 92 Can. J. Public Health 89. For discussion of the debate, see Peter D. Jacobson & Soheil Soliman, "Litigation as Public Health Policy: Theory or Reality?" (2002) 30 J.L. Med. & Ethics 224.

[230] Jacobson & Soliman, ibid., at 225-26; Ferrence et al., ibid., at 39; R. Daynard, "Why Tobacco Litigation? Just How Important is Litigation in Achieving the Goals of the Tobacco Control Community?" (2003) 12 Tobacco Control 1; Robert L. Rabin, "The Third Wave of Tobacco Tort Litigation" in Robert L. Rabin & Stephen Sugarman, eds., Regulating Tobacco (Oxford: Oxford University Press, 2001) 176 at 198-203.

public awareness of the damage caused by tobacco products and of tobacco industry behaviour that has undermined public health goals. The resulting awareness and "denormalization" of tobacco supports other efforts to decrease tobacco consumption. Related to this is the disclosure of documents during litigation, which has made available internal documents revealing the strategies and knowledge of tobacco companies. Without tobacco litigation, it has been suggested, "the full story of conscious industry disregard for the health effects of its profit-making activity might never have become a part of the public record".[231] Next, it is hoped that litigation will exert a deterrent effect on manufacturers, encouraging them to act more responsibly. Furthermore, it is hoped that large damage awards against the industry might lead to price increases for tobacco products and thereby reduce demand in much the same way as taxation. Finally, in some cases, remedies awarded or settlements made as a result of such litigation have provided funds for research or tobacco control efforts, or put in place control measures beyond those already provided for by legislation.

Although many agree that litigation strategies have value for these reasons, there are also significant difficulties. As a public health strategy, litigation is unpredictable and uncertain; in practice litigation is "an exceedingly blunt weapon" and according to one authority, "deterrence considerations operate so haphazardly as to lose virtually all meaning".[232] It is also limited in the range of issues it can address and the types of remedies it can provide, meaning that at best it is a partial solution and at worst it may distort or distract from comprehensive public health efforts.[233] Moreover, litigation is typically extremely costly and time-consuming: most cases will involve tobacco companies as defendants, and these companies are notorious for a "scorched earth" strategy that aims to use the industry's massive financial resources to make "every case, regardless of the amount at stake, a never-ending quagmire of expense for the plaintiff and the plaintiff's attorneys".[234] It is not unusual for cases — even those which seem to have good prospects for success — to be abandoned at various stages because of lack of funds to continue the proceedings. Taking into account these difficulties but also the value litigation may contribute, tobacco lawsuits have the potential to be an important part of tobacco control, but only as a complement to legislative and other measures.

---

[231] Rabin, *ibid.*, at 202-203.

[232] Rabin, *ibid.*, at 200, 199. See also Peter D. Jacobson & Soheil Soliman, "Litigation as Public Health Policy: Theory or Reality?" (2002) 30 J.L. Med. & Ethics 224 at 227.

[233] Jacobson & Soliman, *ibid.*

[234] D. Douglas Blanke, *Towards Health with Justice: Litigation and Public Inquiries as Tools for Tobacco Control* (Geneva: World Health Organization, 2002) at 18.

By far the largest body of cases in this area have been litigated in the United States, although tobacco litigation in various forms has more recently spread to many countries.[235] In the United States, there have been three "waves" of tobacco litigation.[236] In the first wave, beginning in 1954, individual plaintiffs sued for damages, alleging negligence, misrepresentation and breach of warranty; all of these suits were defeated by tobacco companies' arguments that they were not aware of potential harms and that causation had not been proved. The second wave of cases in the 1980s and 1990s were based on product liability and failure to warn, but these again were unsuccessful. The defendants argued that consumers were aware of the risks of smoking. However, in part through some of this litigation, greater access was gained to internal industry documents, on the basis of which it became possible to argue that the defendants knew of the health risks and addictive nature of their products, and that they had deliberately concealed this information. This opened up new possibilities for the third wave of cases, and in particular new legal theories, better prospects for success and the possibility of punitive damages for intentionally harmful or deceptive conduct. Since the mid-1990s, the third wave of litigation has encompassed a large number of diverse cases, involving a variety of plaintiffs, causes of action and remedies. These have included individual and class actions by smokers and by persons affected by SHS on a number of grounds, and actions by governments or other third parties for recovery of health care costs attributable to tobacco consumption. Although tobacco litigation is a relatively recent phenomenon in Canada, there have been some examples of each of these in the Canadian context.

(b)   Individual and Class Actions

Individuals who have suffered tobacco-related harms have brought actions against tobacco companies on a number of grounds. The range of possible claims includes negligence (failure to warn and/or negligent product design), misrepresentation, fraud, product liability, express or implied warranty, unjust enrichment or deceptive advertising (under consumer protection or advertising statutes).[237] Plaintiffs may claim compensatory damages (e.g., for financial losses, cost of medical care),

---

[235] For overviews, see Blanke, *ibid.*, at 33-43; Richard A. Daynard *et al.*, "Tobacco Litigation Worldwide" (2000) 320 BMJ 111.

[236] These are summarized in Blanke, *ibid.*, at 16-32; Robert L. Rabin, "The Third Wave of Tobacco Tort Litigation" in Robert L. Rabin & Stephen Sugarman, eds., *Regulating Tobacco* (Oxford: Oxford University Press, 2001) 176 at 198-203; Stephen D. Sugarman, "Mixed Results from Recent United States Tobacco Litigation" (2002) 10 Tort L. Rev. 94 at 95 & ff.

[237] For a review of possible causes of action, see Blanke, *ibid.*, at 55-56.

exemplary (punitive) damages, equitable remedies (*e.g.*, disgorgement of profits), declarations or injunctions (*e.g.*, to refrain from certain practices, for public disclosure of information).[238] Cases in the United States have showed the difficulties of successfully maintaining these actions, but have produced a few positive results for plaintiffs.[239] In Canada, the first individual case was brought in 1988 but was dismissed for failing to meet the limitation period,[240] and another claim for damages based on misrepresentation and failure to warn has so far been unsuccessful.[241] Another action, brought by an individual plaintiff, Mirjana Spasic, and continued (after her death from lung cancer) by her estate, has been ongoing since 1997, with numerous procedural motions in the Ontario courts.[242] This action is of particular significance because it alleges, in addition to negligence and misrepresentation, the tort of spoliation of evidence in relation to the destruction of documents.[243] The lengthy proceedings and number of motions and appeals in this case have led several commentators to characterize it as an example of the tobacco industry litigation strategy described in the previous section.[244]

The aggregation of claims into class actions offers the potential to "level the playing field" in tobacco litigation by taking advantage of

---

[238] *Ibid.*, at 57-58.

[239] See Stephen Sugarman, "Mixed Results from Recent United States Tobacco Litigation" (2002) 10 Tort L. Rev. 94 at 99-103 (plaintiff victories) and 103-105 (defence victories).

[240] *Perron v. R.J.R. MacDonald Inc.*, [1996] B.C.J. No. 2093 (B.C.C.A.) (plaintiff knew of all the facts required to commence his action by 1983; limitation period had expired by 1988).

[241] *Battaglia v. Imperial Tobacco*, [2001] O.J. No. 5541 (Ont. S.C.J.) (dismissing the claim, stating that the "plaintiff is the only one who has control" over his smoking, and that the misrepresentations "were relied on but not to the detriment of the Plaintiff'; at paras. 82-83); [2002] O.J. No. 5074 (Ont. S.C.J.) (setting aside a motion dismissing the appeal); [2003] O.J. No. 4360 (Ont. Div. Ct.) (dismissing an application to admit fresh evidence on the pending appeal).

[242] *Spasic Estate v. Imperial Tobacco Ltd.*, [2003] O.J. No. 1797 (Ont. Div. Ct.); [2003] O.J. No. 824 (Ont. S.C.J.); [2002] O.J. No. 2152 (Ont. S.C.J.); [2001] O.J. No. 4985 (Ont. S.C.J.); [2000] O.J. No. 2690, 188 D.L.R. (4th) 577 (Ont. C.A.); [1998] O.J. No. 4906 (Ont. Gen. Div.); [1998] O.J. 6529 (Ont. Gen. Div.); [1998] O.J. No. 125 (Ont. Gen. Div.), application for leave to appeal dismissed with costs [2000] S.C.C.A. No. 547 (S.C.C.).

[243] The defendants have attempted, unsuccessfully, to have this novel claim struck from the statement of claim: see the decisions cited above, *ibid.*

[244] Stephen E. Smith, "'Counterblastes' to Tobacco: Five Decades of North American Tobacco Litigation" (2002) 14 Windsor Rev. Legal & Social Issues 1 at 28; Jeff Berryman, "Canadian Reflections on the Tobacco Wars: Some Unintended Consequences of Mass Tort Litigation" (2004) 53 Int'l & Comp. L. Q. 579 at 590. See D. Douglas Blanke, *Towards Health with Justice: Litigation and Public Inquiries as Tools for Tobacco Control* (Geneva: World Health Organization, 2002) at 18.

"economy of scale in trial preparation".[245] Many such actions have been attempted in the United States, although few have been successful.[246] One hurdle which must be overcome in class proceedings is the certification of the class, which may pose difficulties in tobacco litigation due to the potential size and diversity of the class of individuals involved.[247] In February 2004, an Ontario court refused to certify a class in what would have been the first major class action in Canada (filed in 1995).[248] The class would have included "all residents of Ontario, whether living or deceased, who have ever smoked cigarette products manufactured, marketed, or sold by the defendants [and] ... all persons having derivative claims" under family law legislation, and would have included several million claimants.[249] Although the court held that certification should be denied in this case because there was not sufficient commonality between the claimants, and the proceeding as framed would not be the preferable procedure for dealing with these claims, it was "not intend[ed] that these reasons should stand for the proposition that no class proceeding relating to tobacco use can ever be certified".[250] Following the denial of certification, the defendants sought costs both against the plaintiffs and personally against their counsel, but the court refused to award costs, primarily due to the public interest nature of the litigation.[251] An action was also brought in Ontario against Imperial Tobacco Canada for negligence and products liability in relation to a fire caused by one of its cigarettes, but certification of the class in this case was refused in 2005.[252]

---

[245]   Robert L. Rabin, "The Third Wave of Tobacco Tort Litigation" in Robert L. Rabin & Stephen Sugarman, eds., *Regulating Tobacco* (Oxford: Oxford University Press, 2001) at 181-82.

[246]   See *e.g.*, Stephen D. Sugarman, "Mixed Results from Recent United States Tobacco Litigation" (2002) 10 Tort L. Rev. 94 at 105-10.

[247]   *Ibid.*, at 106. Jeff Berryman, "Canadian Reflections on the Tobacco Wars: Some Unintended Consequences of Mass Tort Litigation" (2004) 53 Int'l & Comp. L. Q. 579 at 589 suggests that Canadian courts tend to be more liberal than their U.S. counterparts in this respect (although this was written before the decision in *Caputo*, discussed below). See D. Douglas Blanke, *Towards Health with Justice: Litigation and Public Inquiries as Tools for Tobacco Control* (Geneva: World Health Organization, 2002) at 18.

[248]   *Caputo v. Imperial Tobacco Ltd.*, [2004] O.J. No. 299, 236 D.L.R. (4th) 348 (Ont. S.C.J.) (refusing certification); [2005] O.J. No. 842, 250 D.L.R. (4th) 756 (Ont. S.C.J.) (additional reasons); [2006] O.J. No. 537 (Ont. S.C.J.) (seeking discontinuance).

[249]   *Caputo v. Imperial Tobacco Ltd.*, [2004] O.J. No. 299, 236 D.L.R. (4th) 348 at para. 1 (Ont. S.C.J.).

[250]   *Ibid.*, at para. 86.

[251]   *Caputo v. Imperial Tobacco Ltd.*, [2005] O.J. No. 842, 250 D.L.R. (4th) 756 (Ont. S.C.J.). For a critical comment, see David Collins, "Recent Tobacco Class Action Litigation in the Ontario Superior Court" (2006) 39 U.B.C. L. Rev. 389.

[252]   *Ragoonanan v. Imperial Tobacco Canada Ltd.*, [2000] O.J. No. 4597 (Ont. S.C.J.) (dismissing defendant's application to strike out the plaintiff's pleadings); [2005] O.J. No. 867 (Ont. S.C.J.) (dismissing defendant's application for summary judgment); [2005] O.J.

In Québec, however, class proceedings have been ongoing since 1998, and two classes were certified in 2005.[253]

Class proceedings have also targeted the marketing of "light" and "mild" cigarettes as false and misleading promotion contrary to consumer protection legislation. A class action against Imperial Tobacco was commenced in British Columbia in 2003 and certified in 2005.[254] An appeal challenging the certification was allowed in part, allowing the action to proceed but limiting the class to those whose claims arose in May 1997 or later due to limitations issues.[255] The defendant had added the Canadian government as a third party in this action, because of its role in regulating tobacco products, and specifically the alleged activities and representations of Health Canada and Agriculture Canada in relation to "light" and "mild" cigarettes.[256] However, the third party notice was struck by a 2007 decision of the British Columbia Supreme Court, which found that even if the alleged facts were proved, Canada could not be liable to the plaintiffs or defendant on the grounds argued.[257] Proceedings regarding "light" and "mild" cigarettes were also commenced in Newfoundland in 2004 and the application for certification was heard in late 2007.[258] A similar application in Québec was refused in 2006 on the grounds that the

---

No. 4697 (Ont. S.C.J.) (refusing certification of class for class action), aff'd [2008] O.J. No. 1644 (Ont. Div. Ct.) (appeal and cross-appeal dismissed). For a scathing critique of the decision dismissing the application for summary judgment in this case, see David Collins, "Recent Tobacco Class Action Litigation in the Ontario Superior Court" (2006) 39 U.B.C. L. Rev. 389.

[253] *Conseil québécois sur le tabac et la santé v. JTI-MacDonald Corp.*, [2005] J.Q. no 4161 (Qué. S.C.). One class is to be represented by the Conseil (para. 128) and the second by Cécilia Létourneau (para. 138). Motion to dismiss the class action dismissed: *Conseil québécois sur le tabac et la santé v. JTI-MacDonald Corp.*, [2007] J.Q. no 1143, 2007 QCCS 645 (Qué. S.C.). Motion for leave to appeal dismissed: *Imperial Tobacco Canada Ltd. v. Conseil québécois sur le tabac et la santé*, [2007] J.Q. no 4415, 2007 QCCA 694 (Qué. C.A.); *JTI-MacDonald Corp. v. Létourneau*, [2007] J.Q. no 4412, 2007 QCCA 695 (Qué. C.A.); *Rothmans, Benson & Hedges v. Létourneau*, [2007] J.Q. no 4402, 2007 QCCA 690 (Qué. C.A.); *Rothmans, Benson & Hedges v. Conseil québécois sur le tabac et la santé*, [2007] J.Q. no 4403, 2007 QCCA 691 (Qué. C.A.). Several other procedural matters were dealt with in 2008: *Conseil québécois sur le tabac et la santé v. JTI-MacDonald Corp.*, [2008] J.Q. no 5270, 2008 QCCS 2481 (Qué. S.C.); *Létourneau v. JTI-Macdonald Corp.*, [2008] J.Q. no 4553, 2008 QCCS 2188 (Qué. S.C.); *Conseil québécois sur le tabac et la santé v. JTI-MacDonald Corp.*, [2008] J.Q. no 950, 2008 QCCS 500 (Qué. S.C.).

[254] *Knight v. Imperial Tobacco Canada Ltd.* [2005] B.C.J. No. 216, 250 D.L.R. (4th) 347 (B.C.S.C.), var'd [2006] B.C.J. No. 1056 (B.C.C.A.).

[255] *Knight v. Imperial Tobacco Canada Ltd.*, [2006] B.C.J. No. 1056, 2006 BCCA 235 (B.C.C.A.).

[256] *Knight v. Imperial Tobacco Canada Ltd.*, [2007] B.C.J. No. 1461, 2007 BCSC 964 at para. 9 (B.C.S.C.) (quoting allegations summarized by Imperial Tobacco in its submissions).

[257] *Ibid.*

[258] *Sparkes v. Imperial Tobacco Canada Limited*: see Ches Crombie Barristers, "Light Cigarettes", online: <http://www.chescrosbie.com/library/light-cigarettes.cfm>.

claims overlapped substantially with those in the class proceedings already certified in 2005, and should therefore have been dealt with as part of those proceedings rather than by way of a separate action.[259]

Litigation has also been used as a way of addressing harms caused by SHS. This has included not only individual and class actions against tobacco companies, but also actions against employers or service providers who fail to provide a smoke-free environment, and claims for workers' compensation and disability benefits by employees harmed by SHS in the workplace.[260] In the United States, the first tobacco class action suit was on behalf of flight attendants who had been exposed to SHS in airline cabins.[261] To date, no such cases have yet been reported in Canada; they present significant difficulties for plaintiffs in terms of establishing causation and linking particular manufacturers to the harm suffered.[262] Compensation has been awarded where tobacco-related disease has resulted from exposure to SHS in the workplace, notably in the case of well-known anti-tobacco advocate Heather Crowe, a non-smoker with lung cancer caused by decades of working in a smoke-filled environment.[263]

(c) Actions by Government

As discussed earlier, the federal and some provincial governments in Canada have pursued civil and criminal proceedings against tobacco companies for their alleged participation in cigarette smuggling.[264] A number of other countries and the European Union have filed similar suits in U.S. courts. In 1999 the United States government filed proceedings against tobacco companies under the *Racketeer Influenced and Corrupt Organizations Act* ("RICO").[265] In August 2006, a federal district court found that the companies knowingly deceived the public about the risks

---

[259]   *Gagnon c. Imperial Tobacco Ltée.*, [2006] J.Q. no 7350 (Qué. S.C.), referring to the class actions certified in *Conseil québécois sur le tabac et la santé v. JTI-MacDonald Corp.*, [2005] J.Q. no 4161 (Qué. S.C.).

[260]   E.L. Sweda, "Lawsuits and Secondhand Smoke" (2004) 13 Tobacco Control 61.

[261]   *Broin v. Philip Morris Companies, Inc.*, 641 So.2d 888 (Fla. App. 1994), review denied, 654 So.2d 919 (Fla. 1995). This action, commenced in 1991, was certified and went to trial but was settled before completion of the trial: Robert L. Rabin, "The Third Wave of Tobacco Tort Litigation" in Robert L. Rabin & Stephen Sugarman, eds., *Regulating Tobacco* (Oxford: Oxford University Press, 2001) at 194.

[262]   Stephen D. Sugarman, "Mixed Results from Recent United States Tobacco Litigation" (2002) 10 Tort L. Rev. 94 at 115-16.

[263]   See Physicians for a Smoke-Free Canada, "The Heather Crowe Campaign", online: <http://www.smoke-free.ca/heathercrowe>.

[264]   See above in Section IV (b) of this chapter.

[265]   18 U.S.C. §1961-1968.

and addictiveness of smoking, and ordered them to publish corrective statements and to stop using terms such as "light" and "low tar" because they mislead consumers.[266]

The most important developments in the Canadian context, besides the smuggling cases, involve recovery of health care costs by provincial governments. These follow the attempts of state governments and private insurers in the U.S., with mixed results: many claims have been dismissed, but the state actions were settled in a series of large, very important settlements in the late 1990s.[267] In Canada, Ontario attempted to recover health care costs from tobacco companies, through litigation in U.S. federal court, but this action was dismissed.[268] Several provinces have legislation providing for recovery of health care costs caused by a third party's negligence, which could be used as the basis of this type of action.[269] They may, however, face several barriers (e.g., on questions of causation), leading several jurisdictions to explore the possibility of specific legislation to address the issue.

In 1997, British Columbia enacted the *Tobacco Damages Recovery Act*, subsequently amended and renamed the *Tobacco Damages and Health Care Costs Recovery Act*.[270] The legislation establishes, in s. 2, a direct action by the government "against a [tobacco] manufacturer to recover the cost of health care benefits caused or contributed to by a tobacco related wrong". Recovery may be on an individual or aggregate basis; the right of recovery exists regardless of any recovery by the individual or another person and does not require the government to establish the identities, costs or causes of tobacco related diseases in particular individuals. A "tobacco related wrong" is defined for the

---

[266]   *United States et al. v. Philip Morris USA Inc. et al.*, 449 F. Supp. 2d 1 (2006). Motion to stay this judgment and order denied: *United States et al. v. Philip Morris USA Inc. et al.*, 449 F. Supp. 2d 988 (2006); motion for clarification of order granted in part: *United States et al. v. Philip Morris USA Inc. et al.*, 477 F. Supp. 2d 191.

[267]   Robert L. Rabin, "The Third Wave of Tobacco Tort Litigation" in Robert L. Rabin & Stephen Sugarman, eds., *Regulating Tobacco* (Oxford: Oxford University Press, 2001) 176 at 190-93; *SG Report 2000* U.S. Department of Health and Human Services, *Reducing Tobacco Use: A Report of the Surgeon General* (Georgia: U.S. Department of Health and Human Services, Centers for Disease Control and Prevention, National Center for Chronic Disease Prevention and Health Promotion, Office on Smoking and Health, 2000), online: <http://www.cdc.gov/tobacco/data_statistics/sgr/sgr_2000/> at 238-42.

[268]   D. Douglas Blanke, *Towards Health with Justice: Litigation and Public Inquiries as Tools for Tobacco Control* (Geneva: World Health Organization, 2002) at 53, note 84; Stephen E. Smith, "'Counterblastes' to Tobacco: Five Decades of North American Tobacco Litigation" (2002) 14 Windsor Rev. Legal & Social Issues 1 at 29-30.

[269]   *Health Insurance Act*, R.S.O. 1990, c. H.6, s. 36.0.1; *Hospitals Act*, R.S.A. 2000, c. H-12, Part 5. Regarding the Ontario provision, see Smith, *ibid.*, at 30. These provisions are in addition to a right of subrogation in respect of injuries to covered persons.

[270]   S.B.C. 2000, c. 30.

purpose of this action as "a breach of a common law, equitable or statutory duty or obligation owed by a manufacturer to persons in British Columbia who have been exposed or might become exposed to a tobacco product" (s. 1(1)). For recovery on an aggregate basis, the government must prove such a breach, that exposure to the product can cause or contribute to disease, and that the defendant's product was offered for sale in British Columbia during the period of the breach (s. 3(1)). Subsection 3(2) requires a court to presume that the relevant population would not have been exposed to the product but for the breach, and that exposure caused or contributed to disease in a portion of that population. If these provisions apply, subsections 3(3) and 3(4) provide for determination of the proportion of liability of each defendant, on the basis of market share unless a defendant can prove that its breach did not cause or contribute to exposure or disease.[271] Statistical and other population-based evidence can be used to establish causation and to quantify costs (s. 5).[272] Section 4 provides for joint and several liability of two or more defendants for the cost of health care benefits where one of the defendants has breached a relevant duty and been held liable, and the defendants have conspired or acted in concert, or acted in a principal and agent relationship with respect to the breach, or they would be jointly or vicariously liable for damages under the common law, equity or legislation.

Pursuant to these provisions, the British Columbia government has filed a statement of claim against a group of Canadian and related foreign companies and the Canadian Tobacco Manufacturers' Council.[273] The statement of claim alleges a number of different breaches by manufacturers, including provision of a defective and hazardous product, failure to warn, inducing minors to smoke, and misrepresentation (in breach of common law and statutory duties). As discussed above (in Section II (b)), this legislation was challenged by tobacco manufacturers, arguing that several of its provisions have extraterritorial application, and that the provisions on presumptions and retroactive application undermine judicial independence and the rule of law. However, the Supreme Court of Canada in 2005 rejected these arguments and upheld the legislation.[274] The British

---

[271] Sections 7 and 8 also provide for apportionment of liability (s. 7 on the basis of risk contribution in proceedings other than aggregate actions).

[272] This provision applies to actions by or on behalf of individuals and in class proceedings as well as in actions by the government.

[273] This statement of claim is available online: British Columbia Ministry of Health Services <http://www.health.gov.bc.ca/tobacco/pdf/agbc22.pdf>; and a summary at <http://www.health.gov.bc.ca/tobacco/writ.html>.

[274] *British Columbia v. Imperial Tobacco Canada Ltd.*, [2005] S.C.J. No. 50, 2005 SCC 49 (S.C.C.).

Columbia claim has proceeded following this decision,[275] and several other provinces have now enacted similar legislation.[276]

VIII. CONCLUSION

Tobacco control is an area of public health law that is of crucial importance, given the massive human and economic cost of tobacco-related disease and the range of legal issues that it raises. Canada has been one of the world's leaders in developing comprehensive, effective tobacco control policy. This complex and dynamic area of the law continues to evolve, as witnessed by recent developments in smoke-free legislation and litigation by both public and private actors. In the last few years, the Supreme Court of Canada has upheld three important pieces of tobacco control legislation,[277] addressing a variety of constitutional issues and solidifying the legal basis for tobacco control measures. Yet, as the tobacco epidemic continues to claim lives in Canada and around the world, advocates and governments are challenged to build on existing efforts and develop new approaches.[278]

---

[275]   See *British Columbia v. Imperial Tobacco Canada Ltd.*, [2006] B.C.J. No. 2080, 2006 BCCA 398 (B.C.C.A.) [rejecting a further challenge by foreign defendants on the basis of extraterritoriality]; leave to appeal refused [2006] S.C.C.A. No. 443 (S.C.C.). A third party claim against the federal government in this case was recently dismissed: *British Columbia v. Imperial Tobacco Canada Ltd.*, [2008] B.C.J. No. 609, 2008 BCSC 419 (B.C.S.C.).

[276]   *Tobacco Health Care Costs Recovery Act*, S.N.L. 2001, c. T-4.2 (not yet proclaimed); *Tobacco Damages and Health Care Costs Recovery Act*, S.S. 2007, c. T-14.2 (not yet proclaimed); *Tobacco Damages and Health Care Costs Recovery Act*, S.M. 2006, c. 18 (not yet proclaimed); *Tobacco Damages and Health-care Costs Recovery Act*, S.N.S. 2005, c. 46 (not yet proclaimed); *Tobacco Damages and Health Care Costs Recovery Act*, S.N.B. 2006, c. T-7.5.

[277]   *Rothmans, Benson & Hedges Inc. v. Saskatchewan*, [2005] S.C.J. No. 1, 2005 SCC 13 (S.C.C.) (*Tobacco Control Act*, S.S. 2001, c. T-14.1); *British Columbia v. Imperial Tobacco Canada Ltd.*, [2005] S.C.J. No. 50, 2005 SCC 49 (S.C.C.) (*Tobacco Damages and Health Care Costs Recovery Act*, S.B.C. 2000, c. 30); *Canada (Attorney General) v. JTI-Macdonald Corp.*, [2007] S.C.J. No. 30, 2007 SCC 30 (S.C.C.) (*Tobacco Act*, S.C. 1997, c. 13).

[278]   For examples of some more radical proposals, see N. Gray *et al.*, "Toward a Comprehensive Long-term Nicotine Policy" (2005) 14 Tobacco Control 161; C. Callard, D. Thompson & N. Collishaw, "Transforming the Tobacco Market: Why the Supply of Cigarettes Should Be Transferred from For-Profit Corporations to Non-Profit Enterprises with a Public Health Mandate" (2005) 14 Tobacco Control 278; R. Borland, "A Strategy for Controlling the Marketing of Tobacco Products: A Regulated Market Model" (2003) 12 Tobacco Control 374; Ron Borland, "Why Not Seek Clever Regulation? A Reply to Liberman" (2006) 15 Tobacco Control 339.

8

INJURIES: SOCIETY'S NEGLECTED EPIDEMIC

Tracey M. Bailey, Louis Hugo Francescutti and Trevor L. Strome[*]

I. OVERVIEW

When the public is asked what diseases it fears the most, the answers typically range from cancer and heart disease to emerging and infectious diseases such as Avian Influenza (H5N1) Virus, Severe Acute Respiratory Syndrome ("SARS"), Acquired Immune Deficiency Syndrome ("AIDS"), West Nile Virus, and Bovine Spongiform Encephalitis ("BSE" — "Mad Cow Disease"). The public's opinions, however, are based in part on unbalanced media coverage, a skewed estimate of the risk associated with contracting such illnesses, and fear of the unknown. The disease that should be of most concern, especially to individuals under the age of 45, happens to be a disease about which most people know very few facts — injury. Injuries kill more people under 45 years of age, and cause more years of potential life lost, than any other disease.[1] Despite this, injuries are considered to be little more than "accidents" or an "unfortunate fact of life". (Would anyone consider cancer to be an "accident"?) Yet unlike many other deadly diseases, experts know a good deal about what causes injuries and under what conditions; in theory, we know exactly how to prevent them.

The goal of this chapter is to introduce the concept of injury control and research as an endeavour necessary to reduce the medical and financial toll of injury on society. In doing so, this chapter will unveil the magnitude of the

[*] The authors would like to thank Elizabeth Robertson, Gergely Hegedus and Colin Ouellette for their research assistance.
[1] S.P. Baker et al., The Injury Fact Book (Oxford: Oxford University Press, 1992).

injury problem, identify strategies and interventions proven to help prevent injury, and investigate the implications and impact of public policy on injury occurrence. After reading this chapter, the reader will better understand the scope of the injury problem and will be armed with the information necessary to navigate the entangled web of public policy and injury control.

II. INJURY — THE NEGLECTED EPIDEMIC

Injuries seem to be viewed by society as random occurrences over which we have no control — as "accidents". As the saying goes, "when your time is up, it's up" — but this rather fatalistic view of the world perpetuates needless suffering and cost due to injury. Many times the term "freak accident" appears in a news headline even though it is clear the event being described occurred as a result of a bad choice rather than bad luck. If "accidents" are the result of bad choices, then it stands to reason that if different (or better) choices are made, injuries can be prevented.

The word "injury" has its roots in the Latin *injuria* — "*in*" meaning "not" and "*jus*" meaning "right". Basically, injuries are "not right". The word injury, unfortunately, is often associated with the word "accident". The "classic" definition of injury is any specific and identifiable bodily impairment or damage that usually results from an acute exposure to either thermal, mechanical, electrical or chemical energy.[2] Injury can also occur in the absence of an essential of life such as heat or oxygen. "Trauma" is a severe injury that threatens life or limb. Someone fracturing a wrist after falling while roller-blading is an example of an injury being caused by an acute exposure (the fall) to mechanical energy (hitting the ground). Similarly, a scald caused by exceedingly hot bath water is an example of an acute exposure to thermal energy.

In the study of the injury epidemic, injury researchers utilize an epidemiological model that examines the three major components of an injury event: the *agent*, *host*, and *vector* or *environment*.[3] Applying the epidemiological model to West Nile Virus ("WNV"), the agent is the virus itself, and the vector is the mosquito that carries the virus. The mosquito then subsequently bites, and infects, the host (the human). Applying the epidemiological model to a burn injury, the agent is heat energy, the vector is exposure to scalding water, applied to an individual (the host). See Table 1 to compare the agent host and vector for these two scenarios. In the study of injuries, it is essential to understand how the agent, vector, and host interact to

---

[2]   J.J. Gibson, "The Contribution of Experimental Psychology to the Formulation of the Problem of Safety — A Brief for Basic Research" in *Behavioural Approaches to Accident Research* (New York: Association for the Aid of Crippled Children, 1961) at 77-89.

[3]   Leon S. Robertson, *Injury Epidemiology* (New York: Oxford University Press, 1992) at 147-67.

determine how to prevent injuries from occurring — much the same way the study of these factors is necessary to arrest the spread of infectious disease.

Table 1: West Nile Virus versus Burn Injury

	Agent	Vector	Host
West Nile Virus	*Flavivirus*	Mosquito (*i.e.*, *Culex pipiens*)	Human
Burn Injury	Heat energy	Exposure to scalding water	Human

Injuries are usually classified as being either intentional or unintentional. Intentional injuries typically result from a violent act directed at oneself or at another. Intentional injuries directed at oneself include a suicide, attempted suicide or para-suicide (an act that mimics a suicide attempt). They can be indicative of an underlying mental state that puts people at risk for such behaviour and require special medical attention. Intentional interpersonal injury is an act of violence towards another person. Types of interpersonal injury include sexual abuse/assault, physical abuse/assault, elder abuse, child abuse, family violence and homicide. In many cases, acts of intentional interpersonal injury are indicators of problems in the social environment (family, community or otherwise) of the individuals involved.

Unintentional injuries are usually what come to mind when the word "injury" is mentioned. It is important to realize, however, that "unintentional" does NOT imply "accidental" or "unpredictable". Unlike acts of intentional injury described above, nobody intends to be injured in a motor vehicle crash, while playing their favourite sport, or during work at a construction site. Of the types of unintentional injuries, those categorized as transportation-related comprise the largest percentage of occurrences.[4] Types of transportation-related injuries include motor vehicle collisions, pedestrian injuries, motorcycle injuries, and injuries while using sports and recreation-type vehicles (snowmobiles, bicycles, all-terrain vehicles, *etc.*). Other major categories of unintentional injuries include falls, poisonings, burns, and injuries caused by medical procedures.

III. BURDEN OF INJURY

The three most common measures to compare the absolute and relative impacts of health conditions are the number of deaths (mortality),

---

[4] Injury and Child Maltreatment Section, *Health Canada Analysis of Statistics Canada Data* (Ottawa, 2003).

the number of disabilities (morbidity), and potential-years-of-life-lost
("PYLL"). PYLL is an aggregate measure commonly used in injury
research that illustrates the loss to society as a result of premature deaths
due to injury and is "the sum, over all persons dying from that cause, of
the years that these persons would have lived had they experienced
normal life expectation".[5] For example, a young person dying at age 18
from an injury would result in 57 potential years of life lost given an
individual life expectancy of 75.

The scope of the injury problem in terms of mortality, morbidity and
potential-years-of-life lost is staggering. In Canada, there were 13,906
deaths[6] in 2003 and 226,436 hospitalizations due to unintentional injury
between April 2002 and March 2003.[7] More telling, however, is that
unintentional injury is the *leading cause of death* for people between the
ages of 1 and 44, and the fourth leading cause of death for all Canadians.[8]
Overall, injuries continue to be the second leading cause of premature
mortality (after cancer), measured by potential years of life lost.[9]

The leading causes of deaths due to unintentional injury in Canada
(2004) were motor vehicle collisions (29.3 per cent), falls (24.8 per cent),
and poisoning (10.6 per cent).[10] The leading causes of hospitalizations due
to injury in Canada are falls, motor vehicle incidents, and self-inflicted
injuries[11] (see additional detail in table below).

Table 2: Leading Causes of Hospitalizations due to Injury, Canada 2004

Cause	Percent of Injury Hospitalizations
Falls	49.1
Motor vehicle collisions	8.7
Self inflicted	8.3
Struck by/against	4.0
Assault	3.8
Poisonings	3.2

[5]   J.M. Last, *A Dictionary of Epidemiology*, 3d ed. (Oxford: Oxford University Press, 1995).
[6]   See Public Health Agency of Canada, online: <http://www.phac-aspc.gc.ca/injury-bles/facts-eng.php>.
[7]   See Public Health Agency of Canada, online: <http://www.phac-aspc.gc.ca/injury-bles/facts-eng.php>.
[8]   See Public Health Agency of Canada, online: <http://www.phac-aspc.gc.ca/injury-bles/facts-eng.php>.
[9]   National Scientific Advisory Committee, *Listening for Direction on Injury* (2004).
[10]   See Public Health Agency of Canada, online: <http://dsol-smed.phac-aspc.gc.ca/dsol-smed/is-sb/c_mort_matrix_e.html>.
[11]   See Public Health Agency of Canada, online: <http://dsol-smed.phac-aspc.gc.ca/dsol-smed/is-sb/c_hosp_matrix_e.html>.

Injury comes at an alarming cost to society. It is difficult, however, to pin an "exact" number on the financial cost. This is because the Canadian health care system is not primarily financially oriented and because of the myriad ways serious injury can impact one's life and society in general. One investigation into the cost of injury, conducted by Health Canada, estimates in 1998, $12.7 billion or 8 per cent of the total economic burden of illness in Canada could be ascribed to injury.[12] Some have even questioned these figures as being underestimates of the true burden. Needless to say, the figures speak for themselves. As the health care system struggles to meet current demand we can no longer afford to waste dollars treating a preventable disease.

Figure 1: Total Costs of Diseases/Disorders, Canada 1998

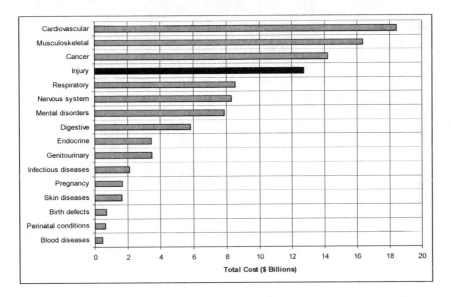

Source: Public Health Agency of Canada, *Economic Burden of Illness in Canada, 1998* (Ottawa: Health Canada, 2002).

The costs associated with injury can be broken down into *direct* and *indirect* costs. Direct costs are a result of the injury event itself, including medical transportation and treatment costs, and property damage repair or replacement. Indirect costs associated with an injury are longer-term,

---

[12]   Public Health Agency of Canada, *Economic Burden of Illness in Canada, 1998* (Ottawa: Health Canada, 2002).

including lost productivity and other costs to society. According to another investigation into the cost of injury by the SmartRisk Foundation, unintentional injuries accounted for over $4.2 billion in direct costs per year; although approximately six per cent of injury patients ended up in hospital, hospitalization costs accounted for 23 per cent of total direct costs.[13] The indirect cost of injuries was estimated at $4.5 billion.[14] Permanent disability accounted for $2.7 billion (60 per cent) whereas injuries causing death accounted for $1.8 billion.[15]

IV. INJURY PREVENTION

The best way to reduce the impact of injuries on society is prevention. Research has shown that injuries are inherently preventable through some combination of individual choice, societal value, and intervening barrier between the person and the source of injury. Injury researchers study the myriad types of injury and determine which events, circumstances, environmental factors, and other variables are most highly correlated with the occurrence of injury.   In addition, researchers investigate and evaluate the various interventions available to determine which ones are most effective at preventing injury. The presence and/or absence of effective interventions or injury risk factors can be used to *predict* the occurrence of injuries. Knowing when injuries are likely to occur and deliberately applying the most effective interventions in known high-injury-risk situations can lead to the *prevention* of injuries.

One would expect that a disease such as injury with such enormous direct and indirect monetary and non-monetary impact would be a high funding priority for health research agencies. Unfortunately, this appears not to be the case. In terms of research expenditure as a percentage of total economic burden, injury ranks next to last in comparison to all other diagnostic categories. Surprisingly, for every dollar that is spent on treating injuries, less than one cent is spent on injury prevention.[16] Compare this to cancer, where for every dollar spent on cancer treatment nine cents is spent on cancer research.[17]

Funding directed to injury prediction and prevention research and on control measures is well spent due to the tremendous return on investment. Everyone has heard the phrase "An ounce of prevention is

---

[13]   SmartRisk Foundation, *The Economic Burdon of Unintentional Injury in Canada* (Ottawa, 1998).

[14]   *Ibid.*

[15]   *Ibid.*

[16]   Centers for Disease Control and Prevention, *Working to Prevent and Control Injury in the United States: Fact Book for the Year 2000* (Atlanta, 2000).

[17]   *Ibid.*

worth a pound of cure". Given that there are 16 ounces in a pound, many interventions are worth even *more* than a pound of cure by a factor of two or more. Every dollar that is spent on a bicycle helmet saves $30 in direct and indirect costs of injury. For each dollar spent on a child car seat, the result is up to $32 savings in direct and indirect costs. A dollar that is spent on a smoke detector can save the healthcare system and society $65. Even every dollar that is spent on traffic check-stops saves $8.[18] A traffic safety initiative in the State of Victoria, Australia, was able to demonstrate a return of 22 dollars for every dollar invested in the initiative.

Figure 2: Research Funding as Percentage of Total Economic Burden, by Disease/Disorder, Canada 1998

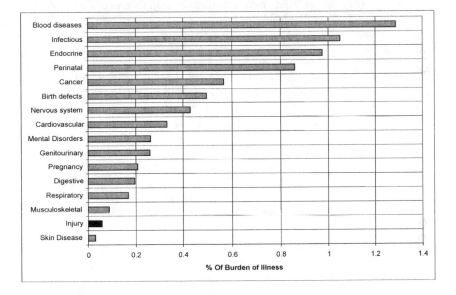

Source: Public Health Agency of Canada, *Economic Burden of Illness in Canada, 1998* (Ottawa: Health Canada, 2002).

There are actually three forms of prevention, each taking aim at different timeframes along the injury event continuum. Preventing injuries from occurring in the first place is known as *primary prevention*. An example of this would be preventing an alcohol-related collision with an on-board ignition interlock system, or preventing a workplace injury by wearing the proper safety gear and being trained for the job. Once an injury has occurred, *secondary prevention* is the process of reducing the

---

[18]   *Ibid.*

impact of that injury on the individual through efficient and effective treatment. Effective secondary prevention requires efficient and effective Emergency Medical Services and hospital facilities to be rapidly available. For example, helicopter medevac services can help airlift trauma victims to an appropriate medical facility to receive necessary medical care as soon as possible after the occurrence of the injury. Finally, *tertiary prevention* involves returning the injured individual as closely as possible to the pre-injury state, and involves the utilization of various therapeutic resources such as physical and occupational therapy. This would include, for example, the various therapies necessary over an extended period to re-integrate a brain injury survivor back into society. It is clear from these examples that as one progresses from primary through to tertiary prevention, the interventions become more costly, time-consuming and generally involve more recovery effort on the part of the injury survivor and his or her friends and family.

Primary, secondary and tertiary prevention together form the framework of the Injury Control Model. Injury control involves the integration and co-ordination of professionals and systems whose focus is injury research, prediction, and prevention; emergency medical services; acute care; and rehabilitation services (see Figure 3 for the conceptual injury control model).

Figure 3: Injury Control Model

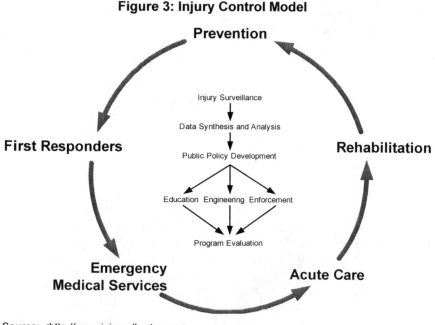

Source: <http://www.injuryalberta.com>.

Primary, secondary and tertiary prevention efforts cannot be effective without a strong base. This strong base requires data, research and action. Effective prevention efforts require data that help answer the questions "who", "what" and "when". (These basic data points include *who* was injuried, *what* type of injury occurred, *when* did the injury occur, *what* was the cause of the injury, *who* provided treatment, *what* treatment was provided, and *what* was the outcome.) The best data to help answer these questions comes from sources such as injury surveillance systems and medical records.

Once data about the basic questions has been collected, researchers study it to improve our understanding of how and why injuries occur. Areas that researchers investigate include the patterns in the occurrence of injuries, how various factors contributed to those occurrences, which interventions were the most effective in preventing (or reducing the impact of) injuries, and which treatments were the most effective in helping return the patient to the pre-injury state. Studying how and why injuries occur increases our ability to better predict and prevent injuries. Outcomes research (understanding which treatments worked the best), on the other hand, helps determine how to provide the very best medical care for survivors of injury to return them as closely as possible to their pre-injury state.

Once research has been conducted, risk factors identified and interventions proposed, it is important for the resulting knowledge from research to be disseminated back to prevention practitioners so they can take action to help reduce the number of injuries. It is relatively easy to conceptualize how to enable secondary prevention (such as through the provisioning of Emergency Medical Services) or tertiary prevention (such as ensuring rehabilitation services are available and properly funded). The ultimate goal, however, should be to prevent injuries from occurring in the first place (primary prevention).

Although the outright prevention of injuries has the potential to reduce individual and societal hardship as well as to save society the most money in direct and indirect costs, the enabling factors of primary prevention may not be as easy to enumerate. There are, in fact, four major categories of injury countermeasures that have proven effective to combat the occurrence of injury. *Education*, *Enforcement*, *Environment Modification* and *Economic Incentives* (the "Four E's") utilize different, yet often interconnected, strategies to reduce the occurrence of injuries.[19]

---

[19]   Lawrence R. Berger & Dinesh Mohan, *Injury Control: A Global View* (New York: Oxford University Press, 1996).

The goals of injury-related education are generally to change individuals' attitudes toward injuries and injury prevention and, more specifically, to inform the population of an injury risk and how to avoid it. By increasing awareness and changing attitudes, education campaigns aim to change people's behaviours from risk-taking to risk-reducing. Education campaigns vary in size and complexity from safety posters in the workplace to expensive national media campaigns. Although probably the most visible and frequently undertaken of the countermeasures, education is considered the least effective when *implemented in isolation*.[20] Educational interventions have varying success because they rely on an individual to change his or her behaviour over the long term. This is akin to overcoming a bad habit (or adopting a good habit) on the basis of knowledge and awareness alone. Just as smokers who are aware of the cancer risk posed by cigarettes often continue to smoke in the absence of other types of intervention (such as a nicotine patch), people who know that alcohol greatly reduces the ability to drive safely sometimes continue to drive while impaired. If an education campaign is able to result in a real and long-lasting change in behaviour, it is most powerful when used in concert with other intervention efforts. Even so, the education of the population about injuries, their societal impact, and their prevention is a crucial step in reducing the overall occurrence of injury.

Environmental modifications can be categorized into two sub-classes. The *physical* environment is comprised of the physical surroundings of an individual. The *social* environment includes the set of attitudes and beliefs towards injury and the value placed on preventing them. Modifications to the physical environment are sometimes referred to as "engineering" interventions. Important work by injury prevention pioneers recognized that the effectiveness of injury prevention efforts could be magnified by making a physical change in the environment that removes a person from harm's way, or reduces exposure to an injury-causing agent, without requiring active human intervention.[21] (For example, building an overpass walkway over a busy road eliminates a pedestrian's exposure to heavy traffic and greatly reduces the risk of a traffic-related injury.) Changes to the physical environment are considered to be *passive* measures because they typically represent some sort of physical barrier between the individual and the source of injury, or the removal or reduction of the injury source altogether.

---

[20]   T. Christoffel & S. Gallagher, *Injury Prevention and Public Health* (Gaithersberg, MD: Aspen Publishers, 1999).

[21]   William Haddon, Jr., "Advances in the Epidemiology of Injuries as a Basis for Public Policy" (Sep.-Oct. 1980) 95(5) Public Health Rep. 411-21.

Research has shown that the social environment consists of attitudes, norms, beliefs, and fashions, and plays a very strong part in shaping the behaviour of an individual[22] (depending, of course, on the individual's susceptibility to such influences). Changes to the social environment are somewhat less tangible and more challenging to implement than changes to the physical environment. Possible changes to the social environment include shaping prevailing attitudes and beliefs to accept and promote risk-reducing behaviour, or when that is not possible, to provide a buffer to individuals from the negative (risk-promoting) attitudes prevalent in society. For example, as society's acceptance of drinking and driving has generally decreased, so has the overall occurrence of impaired driving. This is because an individual might be more greatly deterred from driving under the influence if the individual's social circle views driving under the influence as unacceptable, in addition to the individual knowing that this is risky behaviour.

Economic incentives (or disincentives) promote risk-reducing behaviour through financial means. Economic strategies serve to financially reward or punish individuals on the basis of their demonstrated previous and current behaviour; in this case, as it relates to their decisions to engage in activities that are at high-risk for injuring themselves or others. A very high-profile (and often controversial) example of economic strategies to "promote" risk-reducing activity is the increase of insurance premiums for individuals who have been involved in motor vehicle collisions (and the corresponding "decrease" for individuals not involved in motor vehicle collisions). Another (positive) example of an economic incentive is the practice that many bicycle retailers have of offering discounts on bicycle helmets with the purchase of a new bicycle. In many ways, economic incentives (and sanctions) go hand-in-hand with enforcement efforts.

Enforcement, which can tie in closely to economic incentives, refers to the necessity of adhering to the significant (and growing) body of legislation and policy that is designed to reduce the occurrence, risk and effect of injuries. Enforcement typically addresses one or more of the injury strategies to target high-priority injury problems based on seriousness, expense, or both. Enforcement typically mandates (or prohibits) specific behaviours and activities. While such legislation or policy may exist, enforcement, or the lack of it, will often be key to whether or not a particular intervention will be successful.

---

[22]   Leon S. Robertson, *Injury Epidemiology* (New York: Oxford Press, 1992) at 101-21.

V. STRATEGIES FOR SUCCESS

Armed with the tools to identify how and why injuries occur, effective strategies are necessary to enact the changes that can result in significant reductions in the number and impact of injuries. One of the pioneers of injury research, William Haddon, Jr., identified ten countermeasures that illustrate how the environment can be modified by removing an injury hazard, modifying the injury hazard, protecting and modifying those at risk from the hazard, and ensuring that systems are in place to treat those suffering exposure to the hazard. The ten countermeasures identified by Haddon (with some examples) are:[23]

Table 3: Haddon's Injury Countermeasures

	Strategy	Example(s)
1	Prevent the creation of the hazard.	Prohibit toys that are unsafe for children (*i.e.*, baby walkers).
2	Reduce the amount of the hazard.	Package medications in smaller bottles. Reduce speed limits.
3	Prevent release of a pre-existing hazard.	Ensure proper storage and lock-up of dangerous household products (*i.e.*, cleaning products).
4	Modify the spatial distribution of the hazard.	Install airbags in cars. Ensure areas around playground equipment are sufficiently padded with sand or other soft material.
5	Separate (in time or space) the hazard from the person.	Build overpass pedestrian walkways. Schedule road construction for night-time.
6	Separate (by a material barrier) the hazard from the person.	Build concrete medians between oncoming lanes of traffic. Install safety-gates at stairwells in homes with small children.
7	Modify the basic qualities of the hazard.	Build cribs with slats too narrow to entrap and/or strangle a child.
8	Make people more resistant to injury.	Promote good health and physical fitness practices in the population.
9	Counter damage already done by the hazard.	Train people to conduct first aid. Ensure the availability of highly trained emergency medical services.
10	Stabilize, repair and rehabilitate the injured person.	Ensure the availability of acute care services as well as physical and occupational therapy programs.

---

[23] William Haddon, Jr., "Advances in the Epidemiology of Injuries as a Basis for Public Policy" (Sept.-Oct. 1980) 95(5) Health Rep. 411-21.

To achieve real change in an individual's attitudes and behaviours towards injury requires the overcoming of (at times) significant resistance (for example, "I'm not going to wear a bicycle helmet ... they look stupid"). To be sure, adopting an injury-aware mindset requires a departure from old (perhaps fatalistic or even naïve) ways of thinking and *actively* changing one's behaviours until a risk-aware mindset *is* the way of thinking. The earlier in life that one incorporates injury control ideals into their way of thinking, the easier it is to accomplish change. This is one reason why so many injury prevention efforts are aimed at children and young adults. When people are introduced to the available better choices during a time when they are most responsive to such messages, there is a greater chance they will adopt behaviours and attitudes that will last a lifetime. (For example, children who grow up wearing helmets while riding their bicycles often do not even consider the other "unsafe" alternative, even as they grow into adulthood.)

As with almost every large scale societal "movement", the prevention of injuries ultimately begins with the individual. It is the individual who ultimately decides to reduce his or her likelihood of personal injury by knowing the options and making proactive and risk-avoiding (or at least risk-reducing) choices. In addition to refraining from risky behaviour, there are many other strategies people can use "in their own space" to identify potential sources of injury and take measures to address them. Things as simple as planning fire escape routes from their homes, ensuring that vehicles (automobiles and bicycles) are in proper repair, and clearing sidewalks of ice and snow in the winter help to reduce the occurrence and severity of injury. People can also engage in activities and training that help reduce the risk of injury to others, or help reduce the effect of an injury that has occurred. For example, people trained in emergency first aid are often the first responders on the scene of an injury, and can play a major role in preventing further injury to an injured person until the arrival of professionally trained emergency services personnel.

While an individual's attitude affects one's own behaviour, it is the social environment (*i.e.*, the community) that has a great impact upon one's attitudes. As behaviours and attitudes congruent with the principles of injury control increase in prevalence in society, they can begin to influence the behaviours and choices of individuals within a peer group. In other words, as more people begin making better choices and changing their attitudes, the overall makeup of the social environment in which they live begins to change. A growing awareness of injuries and their prevention within a community can result in the community becoming more proactive towards preventing injuries. This overall change in societal attitudes can result in the decreased acceptance of behaviour that puts people in harm's way. Increased importance and support then begins to be placed on enforcement, economic and environmental injury countermeasures. Ultimately, the community becomes willing to spend time and money on changes to reduce the occurrence and risk of injury. For example, playgrounds can be made more injury resistant by adding more sand around tall structures, and dangerous intersections can be made safer by placing a crosswalk or traffic lights. "Community Watch" or "Block Parent" programs help elevate the general feeling of safety and security in a neighbourhood by providing safe-houses and by warning troublemakers that they are being watched. School and extracurricular activities become more injury-conscious when coaches, players and parents are less willing to accept unsafe and un-sportsmanlike conduct during matches. As the receptiveness of the community towards injury control increases, education interventions are no longer working in isolation and there is therefore a reduced chance that such interventions will "wear off".

This willingness to accept changes such as those just suggested also lends itself to an increased amenability towards a growing body of legislation and legal measures aimed in large part at the reduction of injury. Not all are without controversy[24] but as public awareness of these issues grows and the effectiveness of such measures is established, the population slowly becomes more accepting of greater governmental regulation in this area. The next section of this chapter will examine the breadth of legislative activity in the field of injury prevention and in managing injury when it occurs. All three levels of government (federal, provincial and municipal) have been active in various ways, according to the authority they have to regulate in this area.

VI. LAW'S ROLE IN PREVENTING INJURY

There are many things that governments can do to prevent and control injuries. Many of these are non-legislative in nature, such as education of the public and the funding of research programs. However, it is arguable that governments can exert the greatest influence through their ability to make laws and to enforce those laws. It has been asserted that "law is the primary tool of government".[25]

---

[24]   Recent examples include the debate over the amended *Firearms Act*, S.C. 1995, c. 39 and the recent political wrangling about the suggested implementation of an Alberta province-wide smoking ban. For media coverage of the *Firearms Act*, see online: <http://www.ctv.ca/servlet/ArticleNews/mini/CTVNews/1087336336712_22?s_name=election2004&no_ads=>; <http://www.cbc.ca/news/background/guncontrol>. For media coverage of the Alberta smoking ban, see: <http://www.cbc.ca/canada/calgary/story/2006/10/18/calgary-smoke ban.html>; <http://www.canada.com/edmonton/edmontonjournal/news/story.html?id=cd90d 46b-3f27-412a-8d88-27c9bab04fa9>.

[25]   Tom Christoffel & Stephen P. Teret, *Protecting the Public: Legal Issues in Injury Prevention* (Oxford: Oxford University Press, 1993) at 7.

Laws may be aimed at a number of goals: not only at the attempted modification of the behaviour of individuals (to make safer choices, for example), but towards the alteration of products or environments to create safer devices or surroundings for individuals. Economic incentives or disincentives can be created, in addition to other forms of punitive consequences, for unwanted actions, such as the imposition of fines for drunk driving (in addition to or rather than jail time),[26] or a fine under occupational health and safety legislation (which can impose severe financial penalties on businesses for failure to comply with safety standards in the workplace). Laws can also require the education or training of individuals.

Lawrence Gostin has enunciated seven models for government intervention in public health.[27] Of these seven models, the first five of them relate, at least in part, to various ways the government can use its law making authority: to tax and spend; to alter the informational environment; to alter the built environment; to alter the socio-economic environment; and to directly regulate persons, professionals and businesses.[28] His sixth model, indirect regulation through the tort system,[29] may include legal actions involving governments; they obviously relate to the law making ability of the judiciary and the role they can play in this area. Finally, his seventh model, deregulation,[30] is an important reminder of the need to evaluate laws that are already in place. Legislation that was thought to be of assistance in achieving certain goals at one point in time may have proven to be counter productive.

Specifically, what can the law set out to do? Laws may either mandate or prohibit certain actions. For example, a given law may require one to wear a seatbelt, while another will prohibit an individual from speeding or from riding in the back (payload area) of a pickup truck.

The aim of the legislation will also vary. It may be directed at either people, places (environments), or things.[31] An individual may be required to wear a motorcycle helmet, refrain from assaulting others, or report unsafe conditions on their work site (aimed at the person). The barriers on a roadway may need to meet certain standards of safety when constructed,

---

[26]   *Criminal Code*, R.S.C. 1985, c. C-46, s. 255(1)(*a*)(ii).

[27]   All seven of these are referenced in his Foreword to this book and set out an extremely useful framework for contemplating the role of government.

[28]   Lawrence O. Gostin, "Health of the People: The Highest Law?" (2004) 32:3 J.L. Med. & Ethics 511-513; Lawrence O. Gostin, "Law and Ethics in Population Health" (2004) 28:1 Australian & New Zealand Journal of Public Health 8-9.

[29]   Gostin, "Health of the People", *ibid.*, at 513; Gostin, "Law and Ethics", *ibid.*, at 10.

[30]   *Ibid.*

[31]   Tom Christoffel & Stephen P. Teret, *Protecting the Public: Legal Issues in Injury Prevention* (Oxford: Oxford University Press, 1993) at 11-12.

or a work site may need to be maintained in a certain condition (aimed at the environment or place). Finally, a vehicle may need to be manufactured to include certain safety features such as airbags, or sleepwear may be directed to be fire-retardant (aimed at the thing).

Legislation may also be targeted to the places in which individuals find themselves at various points in their day. Some is aimed at the home (offence or safe products legislation, for example); the workplace (occupational health and safety and workers' compensation legislation); in transport (highway traffic and motor vehicle, railway, aeronautics or marine legislation); or at play.[32]

Laws may also be directed at different types or causes of injuries. For example, we have already discussed the distinction between intentional and unintentional injuries. However, often injuries are categorized by their cause and one may find it helpful to look at legislation in those terms. Major etiological categories include assault, homicide, suicide, transportation-related, falls, poisonings, burns, injuries as a result of a medical intervention, asphyxiation or firearms.

Regardless of how we choose to organize our thoughts around legislation in this area, in all cases, the laws in question are responding to socially unacceptable levels of injury from varying sources; their aim is to prevent injury or reduce levels of harm when injury occurs. Much has been done but, clearly, there are many types of injuries which may be further reduced through legislation, among other things.

Commentary on the history of injury law in the United States has discussed the gradual shift in direction over the last few decades from a focus on individual responsibility based on the belief that most "accidents" were due to the choices made by individuals, to focus on actions (and laws) which deal with modifying the environment to make it safer.[33] Eventually, however, experts in the field came to the realization that various approaches have a significant role to play and solutions are often multi-dimensional. "In recent years ... this intellectual tension [between behavioural intervention and environmental intervention] has

[32]   See, for example, *Athletics Control Act*, R.S.O. 1990, c. A.34, *An Act respecting Safety in Sports*, R.S.Q. c. S-3.1.

[33]   Health Canada, Injury Prevention Centre, "Building Toward Breakthroughs in Injury Control: A Legislative Perspective on the Prevention of Unintentional Injuries Among Children and Youth in Canada" (Ottawa: Minister of Public Works and Government Services Canada, 1996), online: Public Health Agency of Canada <http://www.phac-aspc.gc.ca/dca-dea/publications/break_e.html>.

receded and behavioural perspectives are now increasingly viewed as complementary rather than antagonistic to environmental perspectives."[34]

VII. GOVERNMENTAL POWERS TO ENACT INJURY CONTROL LEGISLATION (JURISDICTION)

As is the case with many areas of Canadian law, legislation around injury control does not fit neatly within the jurisdiction of any one level of government. Rather, all levels of government are involved to varying degrees depending on the focus of regulation.

Section 92 of the *Constitution Act, 1867* is understood to give extensive jurisdiction over health issues to the provinces. This includes authority over hospitals[35] (except marine hospitals), and the delivery of health care (through "property and civil rights"[36] and "matters of a local or private nature").[37] The authority over property and civil rights also gives provincial governments jurisdiction over most private sector activities, and as a result over areas such as industrial activity, occupational safety, workers compensation and so on. Many other activities relating to injury, such as the regulation of health professionals, could be enumerated under this. The regulation of public highways comes within matters of a local or private nature. Provincial governments also have jurisdiction over local works and undertakings (with federal exceptions such as railways and shipping), municipal institutions, provincial prisons, and the imposition and punishment by fine, penalty or imprisonment for enforcing any law of the province, among other things.

Municipal governments have the powers delegated to them by provincial governments through municipal legislation. These powers include many important responsibilities pertaining to local health and public safety, including water, sanitation and sewage, and police services. Moreover, provinces are often content to leave some of the more controversial public health issues, such as restrictions on smoking in public places, to municipal councils.[38]

---

[34]   Richard J. Bonnie & Bernard Guyer, "Injury as a Field of Public Health: Achievements and Controversies" (2002) 30:2 J.L. Med. & Ethics 274.

[35]   *Constitution Act, 1867* (U.K.), 30 & 31 Vict., c. 3, s. 92(7), reprinted in R.S.C. 1985, App. II, No. 5.

[36]   *Ibid.*, s. 92(13).

[37]   *Ibid.*, s. 92(16).

[38]   In Alberta, for example, smoking in public areas was, until very recently, regulated for the most part by municipalities and not the provincial government. However, the provincial government recently passed amendments to its *Tobacco Reduction Act*, S.A. 2005, c. T-3.8 in November 2007, which now prohibit smoking in public and work places across the province. For more information, see Chapter 7, "Tobacco Control and the Law in Canada".

The powers accorded to the federal government in s. 91 of the *Constitution Act, 1867* include several areas significant to public health and safety such as criminal law, quarantine and the establishment and maintenance of marine hospitals, navigation and shipping, trade and commerce, Aboriginals (or as s. 91 of the *Constitution Act, 1867* sets out: "Indians"), the military, and penitentiaries. As well, the introductory paragraph to s. 91 gives Parliament jurisdiction over the "peace, order and good government" of Canada. Understood originally as a residual clause giving Parliament authority over subject matters not specifically enumerated in ss. 91 or 92, POGG has come to be interpreted as giving Parliament legislative authority: (1) of a plenary nature, in circumstances of national emergency; and (2) over distinct matters not clearly within provincial jurisdiction that attain a "national dimension". The latter has been the basis for judicial recognition of federal authority over such diverse matters as aeronautics, standard product labelling, narcotics control measures, and marine pollution.[39] In spite of the fact that health (and, thus the health related aspects of injury) mainly falls under the jurisdiction of provincial governments, Parliament has been able to exert a great deal of influence over the area through the use of its taxation powers.[40] While the Constitution divides legislative responsibilities between the federal and provincial governments, our courts have recognized the principle that either government may *spend* the taxes it raises on any matter it chooses, whether or not the matter is within its jurisdiction.[41] The federal government has used its greater taxing power to induce the provinces to enter into standard-setting agreements as a condition of receiving federal monies — thus the *Canada Health Act*.

To co-ordinate many of its activities in the health field, Parliament established the Department of Health. The *Department of Health Act*[42] sets out several specific duties for the Department and the Minister of Health, including[43] "the protection of the people of Canada against risks to health", and "the establishment and control of safety standards and safety information requirements for consumer products and of safety information requirements for products intended for use in the workplace". The federal government funds extensive health research programs, including several going to injury prevention. The establishment of the Canadian Institutes of Health Research, Institute of Population and Public Health, which

---

[39]   *Constitution Act, 1867* (U.K.), 30 & 31 Vict., c. 3, s. 91, reprinted in R.S.C. 1985, App. II, No. 5.

[40]   See *Canada Health Act*, R.S.C. 1985, c. C-6 and the *Federal-Provincial Fiscal Arrangements Act*, R.S.C. 1985, c. F-8.

[41]   *Winterhaven Stables Ltd. v. Canada (Attorney General)*, [1988] A.J. No. 924, 53 D.L.R. (4th) 413 (Alta. C.A.).

[42]   *Department of Health Act*, S.C. 1996, c. 8.

[43]   *Ibid.*, s. 4(2)(*b*), (*d*).

supports research into injury prevention, and workplace and occupational health (among other things), is one example. Another example is the development of model codes for construction and fire safety.[44] Policy development accompanied by funds or other resources can be effective even if there is no jurisdiction to legislate.

The following section lists certain legislative and regulatory measures which govern injury control in Canada. A comprehensive list is beyond the confines of this chapter. Given the lack of literature in this area, the aim is to reference and at least discuss briefly some major pieces and areas of legislation pertaining to injury in Canada.

VIII.   AREAS OF LEGISLATIVE ACTIVITY

An attempt to categorize legislation could be according to types of injury (for example, falls, burns, asphyxiation, poisoning, *etc.*). It could also be done according to the level of government which enacted it. Here, the attempt has been to group legislation according to broad areas of control. There are no clear lines, however, between these areas and as will become evident, there is overlap between a number of them.

(a) Violence

When one thinks of legislation enacted to deal with violence and the "intentional injuries" that result, the first thing to spring to mind is the *Criminal Code*.[45] An analysis of the interaction between the criminal law and public health is covered in Chapter 13, "Criminal Justice and Public Health",[46] so this will not be discussed here. Provincial legislation dealing with the protection of vulnerable adults[47] or minors[48] is also an obvious example (and this is also covered in Chapter 13). However, other examples of legislation need to be mentioned, if at least briefly, to set the

---

[44]   Canadian Commission on Building and Fire Codes ("CCBFC") has developed six model codes for construction and fire. This Commission was established by the National Research Council of Canada. The codes as created are not within federal jurisdiction, yet have been adopted by provinces. Part of the possible rationale for provinces and territories to buy into this is their ability to consult with this national commission and provide input into the content of the model codes. Canadian Commission on Building and Fire Codes, online: National Research Council <http://www.nationalcodes.ca/ccbfc/index_e.shtml>.

[45]   *Criminal Code*, R.S.C. 1985, c. C-46.

[46]   See Chapter 13 for a discussion of areas such as family violence, mental illness and drug offences, and whether the criminal law has a deterrent effect, among other related issues.

[47]   For example, the *Protection for Persons in Care Act*, R.S.A. 2000, c. P-29; *Protection for Persons in Care Act*, C.C.S.M. c. P144; *Protection for Persons in Care Act*, S.N.S. 2004, c. 33.

[48]   See the *Child, Youth and Family Enhancement Act*, R.S.A. 2000, c. C-12; *Child and Family Services Act,* R.S.O. 1990, c. C.11; *Family Services Act,* S.N.B. 1980, c. F-2.2.

scene. These include provincial mental health legislation under which a person can be certified and essentially held against their will in an institution if they meet the applicable criteria, such as "suffering from mental disorder [and] in a condition presenting or likely to present a danger to the person or others".[49] There are also provincial Acts addressing compensation for victims of violence generally,[50] and even victims of domestic violence specifically.[51] This latter type of law addresses issues such as removing the respondent from the home, and providing for restraining orders. It also provides the authority to order a respondent to pay monetary compensation to the victim and any children.

One issue, however, that has been the subject of much debate in government, academic circles and the public (and media) that relates to violence and injury is the federal firearms legislation. Parliament has always legislated in this area. However, the *Firearms Act*, which came into force on December 5, 1995, created a furore. The new statute extended regulation from automatic weapons and handguns to "ordinary" guns, such as shot guns. This was controversial as it affected individuals such as hunters and farmers who had not been subject to the prior legislation.

The object of the Act and its regulations is to "help reduce firearms-related death, injury and crime and to promote public safety through universal licensing of firearms owners" and the registration of firearms in Canada.[52] The legislation, in addition to regulating the manufacture and import of firearms, addresses two key things. First is the requirement that the owner of firearms be licensed. In determining whether or not an applicant should receive a licence to own or possess firearms, a criminal record indicating violence or a history of mental illness may result in an applicant being denied.[53] An applicant also has to pass a safety course

---

[49]   *Mental Health Act*, R.S.A. 2000, c. M-13, s. 2(*a*), (*b*). The *Mental Health Amendment Act*, 2007, S.A. 2007, c. 35 (awaiting proclamation) will change the second part of this criteria to "likely to cause harm to the person or others or to suffer substantial mental or physical deterioration or serious physical impairment ...".

[50]   For example, *Victims Restitution and Compensation Payment Act*, S.A. 2001, c. V-3.5; *Compensation for Victims of Crime Act*, R.S.O. 1990, c. C.24.

[51]   Such as *Protection Against Family Violence Act*, R.S.A. 2000, c. P-27; The *Victims of Domestic Violence Act*, S.S. 1994, c. V-6.02; *Victims of Family Violence Act*, R.S.P.E.I. 1988, c. V-3.2; *Family Violence Protection Act*, S.N.L. 2005, c. F-3.1.

[52]   Canada Firearms Program, *About Us*, online: <http://www.cfc-cafc.gc.ca>.

[53]   *Firearms Act*, S.C. 1995, c. 39, s. 5(1): "A person is not eligible to hold a licence if it is desirable, in the interests of the safety of that or any other person, that the person not possess a firearm, a cross-bow, a prohibited weapon, a restricted weapon, a prohibited device, ammunition or prohibited ammunition"; s. 5(2): depends on whether (a) the person "has been convicted" of certain offences, (b) whether they have "been treated for a mental illness ... [if] associated with violence or threatened or attempted violence on the part of the person against any person", or (c) whether the person "has a history of behaviour that

covering safe firearms use and so on prior to obtaining a licence.[54] Secondly, each firearm must be registered. An individual cannot receive a registration certificate for a firearm unless he or she has a licence which allows him or her to possess that type of firearm.[55]

Another section of the Act prohibits the transfer of a firearm to anyone unless the person with the firearm has "no reason to believe that the individual (*a*) has a mental illness that makes it desirable, in the interests of safety of that individual or any other person, that the individual not possess a firearm; or (*b*) is impaired by alcohol or a drug".[56] There are other specific conditions under the Act that deal directly with the lending of a firearm.[57] A number of offences are set out and include, for example, a prohibition on knowingly making a false statement regarding an application for a licence, registration certificate or authorization.[58]

The constitutionality of this legislation was challenged in *Reference re: Firearms Act (Can.)*.[59] Dale Gibson noted how charged this issue had become: "If words were bullets, many victims would by now have been claimed by the incessant word-slinging between proponents and opponents of gun control ever since the Government of Canada first announced its intention to introduce the legislation that became the Firearms Act of 1995 ... So far, the chief consequence of the duelling among politicians, lobbyists, journalists, cocktail analysts, lawyers, and judges has been to slow the full implementation of the Act; and the only casualties have been those persons unlucky enough to get in the way of firearms discharges that the operation of effective gun control laws might

---

includes violence or threatened or attempted violence on the part of the person against any person".

[34] For case law dealing with refusals to grant a licence, see *R. v. Pagnotta*, [2001] B.C.J. No. 2260, 2001 BCSC 444 (B.C.S.C.); *Scouten v. Kinloch*, [2004] B.C.J. No. 1750, 2004 BCPC 301 (B.C. Prov. Ct.) (appeal of refusal of licence); *British Columbia (Chief Firearms Officer) v. Fahlman*, [2004] B.C.J. No. 1246, 2004 BCCA 343 (B.C.C.A.) (nature of a review by the Provincial Court of the denial of a licence); *Pogson v. Alberta (Chief Firearms Officer)*, [2004] A.J. No. 248, 358 A.R. 210, 2004 ABPC 41 (Alta. Prov. Ct.) (court overturned the applicant's rejection for a licence despite evidence she was an alcoholic, *etc.*), rev'd [2005] A.J. No. 281, 2005 ABQB 179 (Alta. Q.B.) (decision also set standard of review in Alberta); *Beattie v. Ottawa (City) Police Service*, [2004] O.J. No. 4454 (Ont. S.C.J.) (raises privacy issues involved in application); *Alberta (Chief Firearms Officer) v. Rolls*, [2004] A.J. No. 912, 2004 ABQB 582 (Alta. Q.B.) (recent Alberta case re nature of review of refusal to grant licence).

[55] *Firearms Act*, S.C. 1995, c. 39, s. 13.

[56] *Ibid.*, s. 22.

[57] *Ibid.*, s. 33.

[58] *Ibid.*, s. 106(1).

[59] [2000] S.C.J. No. 31, [2000] 1 S.C.R. 783, 2000 SCC 31 (S.C.C.).

have prevented."[60] In 1998, a unanimous bench of the Supreme Court upheld the legislation as constitutionally valid and within the jurisdiction of the federal government. As part of its discussion, the Court considered the purpose for which Parliament had enacted this legislation: "viewed from its purpose and effects, the *Firearms Act* is in 'pith and substance' directed to public safety".[61] The Court also noted that "given the general acceptance of the gun control legislation that has existed for the past hundred years, the constitutional validity of which has always been predicated on Parliament's concern for public safety, it is difficult now to impute a different purpose to Parliament".[62]

If Canadians think the debate here was heated, we need not look very far to find even stronger views on this issue. It is part of a continuing debate in the U.S. as well where the powerful gun lobby has been active in attempts to keep this area as free from regulation as possible. There have been a number of laws introduced in this area and constitutional challenges to the legislation are fairly plentiful.[63] The force of the pro-firearm camp is so strong that it has even affected research in the area of firearms and injury. As Bonnie and Guyer have noted, "[w]hen the Republican Party took control of the House of Representatives after the mid-term elections in 1994, the continued existence of the CDC injury centre was in doubt. In the end, Congress forbade the use of CDC funds to support gun control".[64]

A related issue which has become a subject for debate across Canada is whether governments should require reporting of gunshot wounds and other injuries by health care professionals and/or health services institutions. Four provinces in Canada to date have enacted such legislation. Ontario's *Mandatory Gunshot Wound Reporting Act, 2005* requires facilities that treat persons for gunshot wounds to disclose that person's name and location to police.[65] The preamble states that "gunfire poses serious risks to public safety and that mandatory reporting of

---

[60]   Dale Gibson,"The Firearms Reference in the Alberta Court of Appeal" (1999) 37 Alta. L. Rev. 1071.

[61]   *Reference re: Firearms Act (Can.)*, [2000] S.C.J. No. 31, [2000] 1 S.C.R. 783 at 801 (S.C.C.)

[62]   *Ibid.* at 800 (S.C.C.)

[63]   See Jon S. Vernick & Stephen P. Teret, "New Courtroom Strategies Regarding Firearms: Tort Litigation Against Firearm Manufacturers and Constitutional Challenges to Gun Laws" (1999) 36 Hous. L. Rev. 1713 (for a discussion of constitutional challenges to gun legislation in the U.S.); see also "Tort Law – Civil Immunity – Congress Passes Prohibition of Qualified Civil Claims Against Gun Manufacturers and Distributors" (2005-2006) 119 Harv. L. Rev. 1939.

[64]   Richard J. Bonnie & Bernard Guyer, "Injury as a Field of Public Health: Achievements and Controversies" (2002) 30:2 J.L. Med. & Ethics 267 at 269.

[65]   S.O. 2005, c. 9, s. 2(1).

gunshot wounds will enable police to take immediate steps to prevent further violence, injury or death". Thus, the enunciated purpose relates to public safety and the prevention of injury. Saskatchewan's and Manitoba's recently enacted *The Gunshot and Stab Wounds Mandatory Reporting Act* are similar to the Ontario legislation, though as the titles make clear, they apply to stab wounds as well as gunshot wounds.[66] Nova Scotia's *Gunshot Wounds Mandatory Reporting Act* is in keeping with the Ontario legislation.[67] Alberta has taken a different course in amending its *Health Information Act* to provide discretion to custodians of health information to disclose certain information to police if he or she "reasonably believes (a) that the information relates to the possible commission of an offence under a statute or regulation of Alberta or Canada, and (b) that the disclosure will protect the health and safety of Albertans".[68] However, whether or not legislation such as this actually prevents injury and does not merely serve to assist police in the discovery or investigation of offences is unclear and raises a number of issues. This type of enactment blurs the roles between a health care professional's duty to provide health services and generally protect the confidentiality of those they serve, and that of the police whose role it is to investigate crime.[69] There is not much research to suggest that mandatory reporting of gunshot wounds decreases further immediate violence or injury. However, the argument has been made on the basis of studies in other areas that this may be effective and needs to be scrutinized further.[70] The issue, however, has recently created a controversy in medical circles around the role of physicians in reporting crime, and of ensuring patient confidentiality.[71] It

---

[66] S.S. 2007, c. G-9.1 (came into force 1 September 2007); S.M. 2008, c. 21 (assented to 12 June 2008 but at the time of writing had not yet been proclaimed).

[67] S.N.S. 2006, c. 30 (came into effect on 1 June 2008).

[68] R.S.A. 2000, c. H-5, s. 37.3.

[69] See Wayne Renke, "The Constitutionality of Mandatory Reporting of Gunshot Wounds Legislation" (2005) 14:1 Health Law Review 3 and Traccy M. Bailey & Steven Penney, "Healing, not Squealing: Recent Amendments to Alberta's Health Information Act" (2006) 15:2 Health Law Review 3 regarding this point, as well as discussion about the constitutionality of such legislation.

[70] Jonnathan P. Shepherd, "Emergency Medicine and Police Collaboration to Prevent Community Violence" (2001) 38:4 Annals of Emergency Medicine 430.

[71] Howard Ovens, "Why Mandatory Reporting of Gunshot Wounds is Necessary: A Response from the OMA's Executive of the Section on Emergency Medicine" (2004) 170:8 C.M.A.J. 1040, online: <http://www.cmaj.ca/cgi/content/full/170/8/1256>; H. Ovens & H. Morrison, "The Case for Mandatory Reporting of Gunshot Wounds in the Emergency Department" in *OMA Section on Emergency Medicine Position Paper* (November 2003), online: Ontario Medical Association <http://www.oma.org/pcomm/omr/nov/03maintoc.htm>; Merril A. Pauls & Jocelyn Downie, "Shooting Ourselves in the Foot: Why Mandatory Reporting of Gunshot Wounds is a Bad Idea" (2004) 170:8 C.M.A.J. 1255, online: <http://www. cmaj.ca/cgi/content/full/170/8/1255>; A. Frampton, "Reporting of Gunshot Wounds by Doctors in Emergency Departments: A Duty or a Right Some Legal & Ethics Issues Surrounding Breaking Patient Confidentially" (2005) 22 Emerg. Med. J. 84-86.

has been argued that the obligation to report gunshot wounds may only serve to deter those with such injuries from seeking out treatment. However, limited studies to date purport that this is not the case.[72] This is definitely an area which calls out for further examination and study.[73]

(b) Product Safety

The word "product" can encompass a vast array of items, devices and substances. Governments have not attempted to oversee the regulation of all products through direct legislation. There are no statutes governing, for example, manufacturing standards for each and every product that is on the market today. However, with respect to products that have been deemed to be particularly hazardous (either because of a flaw in their construction or in their very nature), legislative steps have been taken to impose rules on certain persons. Most of the focus in terms of the force of law is not on consumers of products, but on those who would import, manufacture or sell these products. Consumers have mainly been the focus of educational campaigns, or labelling and/or instructions that accompany the products they purchase.

The federal government has enacted a huge array of legislation dealing with product safety. This includes laws dealing with consumer products, products for use in the workplace (discussed later in this chapter), pharmaceuticals, natural health products, medical devices, cosmetics, radiation emitting devices and pesticides. Even a cursory review of all of the federal legislation in the area is beyond the scope of the chapter. However, this section will attempt to mention some of the key pieces of legislation, define the scope of that legislation, and in certain instances, discuss some key issues in the area at present.[74]

---

[72]   J.P. May, D. Hemenway & A. Hall, "Do Criminals Go to the Hospital When They Are Shot?" (2002) 8 Injury Prevention 236.

[73]   Hence the call for surveillance. See L.J. Paulozzi et al., "CDC's National Violent Death Reporting System: Background and Methodology" (2004) 10 Injury Prevention 47.

[74]   As an obvious starting point for further research into this area, see Health Canada's website at <http://www.hc-sc.gc.ca>. Other legislation in the area of product safety covers a broad array of issues such as: (1) the regulation of radiation emitting devices, including those used in radiology departments across the country. See Radiation Emitting Devices Act, R.S.C. 1985, c. R-1. The Consumer and Clinical Radiation Protection Bureau of Health Canada's mandate is to assist in reducing health and safety risks that may occur as a result of the use of radiation through such devices as x-rays, ultrasound, and lasers. They work in relation to this Act, but also the Canada Labour Code, R.S.C. 1985, c. L-2, the Food and Drugs Act, R.S.C. 1985, c. F-27 and the Medical Devices Regulations, S.O.R./98-282. In addition to the legislation, there are safety codes that have been developed with respect to medical devices and other sources of radiation such as baggage x-ray inspection systems; (2) acceptable levels of radiation for workers employed at nuclear facilities. See s. 3(a) of the Nuclear Safety and Control Act, S.C. 1997, c. 9 which states that "[t]he purpose of this Act

(i) Hazardous Products Act

A key statute currently governing this area is the federal *Hazardous Products Act*.[75] Although it has been labelled as "antiquated",[76] its stated aim is "... to prohibit the advertising, sale and importation of hazardous products".[77] Certain items such as drugs, medical devices, explosives, tobacco, radioactive nuclear substances and pest control products are specifically excluded as they are dealt with under other federal legislation.[78]

The term "hazardous product" is defined in the legislation to include "prohibited", "restricted" or "controlled" products. The Act itself is divided into three sections to deal with these different categories. Prohibited products are dealt with in Part I of the Act and Part I of Schedule I under the Act. Part I of the Act and Part II of Schedule I deal with restricted products. Controlled products are discussed under Part II of the Act and Schedule II. These controlled products will be discussed later in this chapter in the section on Health and Safety in the Workplace.

Both prohibited and restricted products are essentially consumer goods. If the product has been included in the prohibited list, it cannot be advertised, sold or imported. However, if it is in the restricted category, conditions may be set under the regulations with respect to these products.

What can be included in Schedule I as a prohibited or restricted product is set out in s. 6(1) of the Act as follows:

> (a) any product, material or substance that is or contains a poisonous, toxic, flammable, explosive, corrosive, infectious, oxidizing or reactive product, material or substance or other product, material or substance of a similar nature that ... is or is likely to be a danger to the health or safety of the public; or

is to provide for (a) the limitation, to a reasonable level and in a manner that is consistent with ... the health and safety of persons and the environment that are associated with the development, production and use of nuclear energy, and the production, possession and use of nuclear substances, prescribed equipment and prescribed information". Regulations can, among other things, set limits for amounts of radiation various classes of persons may be exposed to. Regulations govern nuclear facilities (which more appropriately fits under occupational health and safety), but also things such as radiation devices (product safety); (3) the control of pesticides (discussed in Chapter 11, "Public Health and Environmental Protection in Canada"); and (4) explosives (*Explosives Act*, R.S.C. 1985, c. E-17).

[75] *Hazardous Products Act*, R.S.C. 1985, c. H-3.
[76] Kathleen Cooper, "Lead Poisoning in Children", Letter to the Editor (2004) 171:5 C.M.A.J. 429.
[77] *Hazardous Products Act*, R.S.C. 1985, c. H-3.
[78] *Ibid.*, s. 3. The *Explosives Act*, R.S.C. 1985, c. E-17, *Food and Drugs Act*, R.S.C. 1985, c. F-27 and the *Nuclear Safety and Control Act*, S.C. 1997, c. 9 are all dealt with briefly later in this section. The *Tobacco Act*, S.C. 1997, c. 13 is discussed in Chapter 7 of this book. *Pest Control Products Act*, S.C. 2002, c. 28.

(*b*) any product designed for household, garden or personal use, for use
in sports or recreational activities, as life-saving equipment or as a
toy, plaything or equipment for use by children that … is or is likely
to be a danger to the health and safety of the public by reason of its
design, construction or contents.

A reading of Schedule I reveals the types of products which have to
date been included within the scope of this legislation. Examples of
prohibited products are children's sleepwear (if it has not met certain
standards for flammability), face protectors for hockey or lacrosse players
(which do not meet the standards), furniture or other children's items
coated with substances containing excessive lead levels,[79] baby walkers
(notorious for the injuries they caused before they were banned),[80] and
non-safety glass shower doors or enclosures. Examples of restricted
products include many types of toys (dolls with stuffing in them are just
one illustration of the numerous toys which fall into this category), glazed
ceramics and glasswear, cribs and playpens, car seats for children, ice
hockey helmets, and tents. There is a long set of regulations dealing with
specific items listed in this part. For example, the *Cribs and Cradles
Regulations*[81] is several pages long and deals with labelling that must be
permanently affixed to cribs (including specified warnings), and the
testing that must be undertaken to ensure a particular type of crib meets
the safety standards which are set out. One of the requirements in relation
to cribs which has been the subject of public education endeavours is that
the slats of the crib must be no more than a maximum distance apart.
Not only does this regulation describe what the standard is, but it sets out
just how the testing must be conducted to ensure the slats meet the
specifications.

---

[79] Although some of the debate around regulation under the *Hazardous Products Act* has
focused on whether the standards are stringent enough to ensure safety, and whether they
are up to date. For example, the levels of lead acceptable in certain products have been
criticized in the past as completely outdated. See Kathleen Cooper, "Lead Poisoning in
Children", Letter to the Editor (2004) 171:5 C.M.A.J. 429 (where Kathleen Cooper reported
that "as of March 2004 Canada had yet to pass regulations, proposed in 2003, that would
see the adoption of the standard that the United States put in place over 25 years ago"
regarding acceptable lead levels in paint). However, since then, the *Surface Coating
Materials Regulations*, S.O.R./2005-109 have been brought into force, as well as new
standards regarding children's furniture, toys and other items (amendments in 2005 to Part
I, Schedule I of the *Hazardous Products Act*, items 2, 9 and 42). On the topic of lead and
children, Health Canada issues warnings to Canadians about children's products and lead.
A recent example: Health Canada, Advisory 2007-114, "Health Canada Advises Canadians
About Children's Potential Exposure to Lead" (6 September 2007), online: <http://www.
hc-sc.gc.ca/ahc-asc/media/advisories-avis/_2007/2007_114-eng.php>.

[80] Health Canada, Consumer Product Safety, "Regulatory Review and Recommendation regarding
Baby Walkers Pursuant to the Hazardous Products Act", online: <http://www.hc-sc.gc.ca/
cps-spc/pubs/cons/walker-review-marchette/index-eng.php>.

[81] *Cribs and Cradles Regulations*, S.O.R./86-962.

Before the inclusion of a product on either list, voluntary measures may be requested from industry. Inclusion may only occur if voluntary compliance is found not to be effective, or if the cost in terms of injury subject to voluntary measures is deemed to be too great. One example of a product which ultimately made the prohibited list is the recent ban on baby walkers. Testing had been conducted on their safety, and voluntary standards had been in place since 1989 which resulted in these being removed from a large part of the Canadian market. However, for various reasons, including the continued availability of walkers through garage sales, through some retail outlets, and through the Internet, the inclusion into the prohibited category was proposed by Health Canada.[82] They were ultimately banned on April 7, 2004, with then Minister of Health, Pierre Pettigrew, stating that: "It is the safety of our children that is of the most vital importance and today I am pleased to announce that Canada is the first country in the world to ban the sale of these products."

To make a comparison with an item initially proposed for the restricted list, the issue of lead in children's jewellery is an illustrative one. According to the Regulatory Impact Analysis Statement published in the Canada Gazette as of November 19, 2003, there were no current standards in Canada "for migratable lead limits in consumer products" at that time.[83] The Statement discusses the recent history of this issue. Following up on a complaint by a parent whose child had elevated levels of lead in her blood as a result of sucking on a pendant, Health Canada made a request to industry in April 1999 asking them to seek information from their suppliers about whether lead had been added to products intended for children under the age of 15 years, or to test those products so that the lead content did not exceed a specified limit. With respect to jewellery intended for those over 15 years, they asked that such products be labelled to warn consumers that there are risks associated with mouthing jewellery containing lead and that it should not be used by children. However, in this case it does not appear that this voluntary request had much effect on industry, particularly compared with the baby walker example. When Health Canada surveyed the market over a year later, 94 per cent of the jewellery contained lead in excess of the recommended levels and only one warning label was observed in the entire sample. A further letter was then sent to industry, and a consumer advisory was issued in an attempt to warn Canadians of this danger (albeit approximately six months after the survey was completed). As is usual in

---

[82]   Health Canada, Consumer Product Safety, "Regulatory Review and Recommendation regarding Baby Walkers Pursuant to the Hazardous Products Act", online: <http://www.hc-sc.gc.ca/cps-spc/pubs/cons/walker-review-marchette/index-eng.php>.

[83]   Children's Jewellery Regulations: Regulatory Impact Analysis Statement, C. Gaz. 2003, I.137: 47 (*Hazardous Products Act*), online: <http://canadagazette.gc.ca/partI/2003/20031122/html/regle8-e.html>.

Regulatory Impact Analysis Statements, a number of options were laid out and assessed. However, the proposal was to make children's jewellery containing excess amounts of lead illegal. The *Children's Jewellery Regulations* came into force on June 1, 2005.[84] They established maximum amounts of total and migratable lead. Subsequently, a further Regulatory Impact Analysis Statement was published. This lead to the repeal of the *Children's Jewellery Regulations* but the addition of these standards to Part I of Schedule I, thus moving this to the prohibited list.[85]

In a move to overhaul the outdated legislation in this area, the Minister of Health, Tony Clement, introduced Bill C-52, *An Act respecting the safety of consumer products*, on April 8, 2008.[86] If this is enacted, it will repeal and replace Part I of the *Hazardous Products Act*.[87] Its stated purpose it to "protect the public by addressing or preventing dangers to human health or safety that are posed by consumer products in Canada, including those that circulate within Canada and those that are imported".[88] There are a number of significant changes to the current regime which this Bill has introduced. Some of the most notable provisions include the ability of the Minister to order manufacturers or importers to conduct tests and provide information to confirm compliance with the law;[89] new provisions regarding the reporting of dangerous incidents involving products;[90] the power to issue recall orders to manufacturers, importers or vendors[91] (currently, Health Canada can advise a recall but it has no authority to require it); and increased fines and penalties (both in terms of offences and administrative violations) for contravention of the Act or of orders issued under it.[92]

---

[84]   S.O.R./2005-132. These were added to Part II of Schedule I of the *Hazardous Products Act*.

[85]   Item 42 of Schedule I, Part I, *Hazardous Products Act*. As discussed previously, Health Canada will issue warnings such as the one posted on 9 July 2004, to throw away children's jewellery purchased from a vending machine. This warning also contained the general advice that consumers should question retailers about whether there is lead in jewellery before purchasing it. It is questionable as to whether the information contained in a warning such as this actually reaches the majority of Canadians who will subsequently purchase jewellery for children; see online: <http://www.hc-sc.gc.ca/cps-spc/pubs/cons/jewellery-bijoux-eng.php>.

[86]   Bill C-52, *An Act respecting the safety of consumer products*, 2nd Sess., 39th Parl., 2008. At the time of writing, the Bill had also passed Second Reading and was with the Standing Committee on Health.

[87]   *Hazardous Products Act*, R.S.C. 1985, c. H-3.

[88]   Bill C-52, *An Act respecting the safety of consumer products*, 2nd Sess., 39th Parl., 2008, cl. 3.

[89]   *Ibid.*, cl. 12.

[90]   *Ibid.*, cl. 14.

[91]   *Ibid.*, cl. 32.

[92]   *Ibid.*, cl. 40-70.

(ii)   Food and Drugs Act

The *Food and Drugs* Act regulates food, drugs, cosmetics and therapeutic devices which are all defined under the legislation.[93] A number of issues are dealt with, including the importing, manufacturing or processing, labelling, packaging, advertisement, and sale of these products. They are aimed, as is the *Hazardous Products Act*, at ensuring the safety of Canadians in the use of food, pharmaceuticals, natural health products, cosmetics and devices used in the health care setting. In the Act itself, specific prohibitions are set out in respect of each of these categories. For example, in the case of devices, the legislation states that "[n]o person shall sell any device that, when used according to directions or under such conditions as are customary or usual, may cause injury to the health of the purchaser or user thereof".[94] One prohibition that is common to all items regulated under the Act states that they cannot be advertised or sold as a "treatment, preventative or cure for any of the diseases, disorders or abnormal physical states referred to in Schedule A". Examples of diseases in Schedule A include alcoholism, cancer and kidney disease. This is to prevent false claims with respect to products offered for sale, *etc*. It is an attempt to control, in part, the claims of unscrupulous vendors or healers of cures for these diseases. Much of the detail, however, is found in the applicable regulations.[95] Advisories and warnings are also issued by Health Canada in this area as well. For example, the recent warning about certain COX-2 inhibitors such as Celebrex was posted on the Therapeutic Products Directorate's web page[96] (and was also widely reported in the media).

---

[93]   "Drug" is defined in part as "any substance ... for use in the diagnosis, treatment, mitigation or prevention of a disease, disorder or abnormal physical state, or its symptoms, in human beings ...". "Cosmetic" is described as "any substance ... for use in cleansing, improving or altering the complexion, skin, hair or teeth, and includes deodorants and perfumes". "Device" is defined as "any article, instrument, apparatus or contrivance ... for use in (a) the diagnosis, treatment, mitigation or prevention of a disease, disorder or abnormal physical state, or its symptoms, in human beings ... (b) restoring, correcting, or modifying a body function or the body structure of human beings ... (c) the diagnosis of pregnancy in human beings ... or (d) the care of human beings... during pregnancy and at and after birth of the offspring, including care of the offspring, and includes a contraceptive device but does not include a drug": *Food and Drugs Act*, R.S.C. 1985, c. F-27, s. 2. "Food" is not mentioned as it is discussed in Chapter 12, "Foodborne Illness and Public Health".

[94]   *Food and Drugs Act, ibid.*, s. 19.

[95]   *Cosmetic Regulations*, C.R.C. c. 869; *Food and Drug Regulations*, C.R.C. c. 870; *Marihuana Exemption (Food and Drugs Act) Regulations*, S.O.R./2003-261; *Medical Devices Regulations*, S.O.R./98-282; *Natural Health Products Regulations*, S.O.R./2003-196; and *Processing and Distribution of Semen for Assisted Conception Regulations*, S.O.R./96-254.

[96]   The mission of the Therapeutic Products Directorate is to "contribute to the health of Canadians and to the effectiveness of the health care system by regulating pharmaceuticals

In terms of prevention of specific injuries, specific facets of this legislation have led to a reduction in injury, or the seriousness of injury in numerous areas. One illustration of this is the regulation of child resistant packaging of certain pharmaceuticals. Under Part C of the *Food and Drugs Regulations*, for example, the regulation requires that "no person shall sell a [specified] drug ... unless (i) where the drug is recommended solely for children, it is packaged in a child resistant package ...".[97]

Legislative renewal of this area has been under consideration for the last decade. Health Canada's health protection legislative renewal initiative,[98] which began in 1998, was aimed in part at the revamping of the *Food and Drugs Act*.[99] Other pieces of legislation that were intended to be part of the comprehensive process were the *Quarantine Act*,[100] the *Hazardous Products Act*[101] and the *Radiation Emitting Devices Act*.[102] Though one new comprehensive piece of legislation was contemplated, much of the renewal work has been carried out in a piecemeal fashion once again. Bill C-51, *An Act to amend the Food and Drugs Act and to make consequential amendments to other Acts*[103] is a recent development. Introduced on April 8, 2008, with Bill C-52,[104] discussed in the last section, it proposes substantial changes to the current legislative scheme.

Some new terminology is used in the Bill; one example is "therapeutic product", defined as including drugs and devices, as well as cells, tissues or organs in certain circumstances.[105] Some key changes that have also been proposed include changes to the licensing of therapeutic products;[106] increased powers for inspectors;[107] powers to compel changes in labelling;[108] power to order a recall of a therapeutic product or

---

and medical devices and by providing Canadians with access to information to make informed choices". See Health Canada, Therapeutic Products Directorate Strategic Plan 2006–2009, "The Way Forward", online: <http://www.hc-sc.gc.ca/dhp-mps/pubs/drug-medic/tpd_stratplan_dpt_planstrat_2006-eng.php#1>.

[97] *Food and Drug Regulations*, C.R.C. c. 870, Part C, C.01.031(1).

[98] Health Canada, *Shared Responsibilities, Shared Vision: Renewing the Federal Health Protection Legislation (A Discussion Paper)* (Ottawa: Health Canada, 1998), online: <http://www.hc-sc.gc.ca/ahc-asc/alt_formats/hpfb-dgpsa/pdf/pubs/shared-respon-partag-eng.pdf>.

[99] *Food and Drugs Act*, R.S.C. 1985, c. F-27.

[100] *Quarantine Act*, S.C. 2005, c. 20.

[101] *Hazardous Products Act*, R.S.C. 1985, c. H-3.

[102] *Radiation Emitting Devices Act*, R.S.C. 1985, c. R-1.

[103] Bill C-51, *An Act to amend the Food and Drugs Act and to make consequential amendments to other Acts*, 2nd Sess., 39th Parl., 2008.

[104] Bill C-52, *An Act respecting the safety of consumer products*, 2nd Sess., 39th Parl., 2008.

[105] Bill C-51, *An Act to amend the Food and Drugs Act and to make consequential amendments to other Acts*, 2nd Sess., 39th Parl., 2008, cl. 3(6).

[106] *Ibid.*, cl. 18.1 - 20.3.

[107] *Ibid.*, cl. 22 - 23.9.

[108] *Ibid.*, cl. 20.1.

cosmetic;[109] and substantially increased penalties for contravention of the Act.[110]

One interesting change of note is the repeal of s. 3 of the Act,[111] as well as Schedule A. This is particularly interesting as new regulations relating to this have recently come into force.[112] On the face of the suggested repeal, those with concerns about legislative gaps on this front may be somewhat comforted by the inclusion of new sections in Bill C-51 such as s. 12 (prohibiting advertising, selling or importing for sale therapeutic products without the necessary requirements) or s. 14 (prohibiting deceptive labelling, advertising, etc.).[113] However, the gap or lack thereof may well depend upon interpretation of these sections by Health Canada.

(iii) Controlled Drugs and Substances Act[114]

Certain injuries are caused directly by the abuse of drugs or indirectly through crime fuelled by the use of drugs. This federal Act deals specifically with narcotics and other "controlled substances". Schedules in the Act itself set out which drugs are designated. Examples include morphine, cocaine, methadone, amphetamines, anabolic steroids, cannabis and ephedrine. The specifics of regulation are dependant upon which schedule the drug is listed under. Generally, the legislation regulates the importing and exporting, production, distribution and possession of these specified drugs. More specifically, it prohibits persons from possessing certain substances (unless authorized) or from seeking or obtaining certain substances from a medical practitioner unless they disclose certain information (for example, whether or not they have acquired that particular substance from others in the preceding 30 days). It also prohibits trafficking in these drugs that are otherwise legal if an individual is not authorized to be in possession of them. As a result, it may be an offence to be in possession of a quantity of codeine. The rationale behind sentencing for an offence is clearly laid out in s. 10(1) which states that: "Without restricting the generality of the *Criminal Code*, the

---

[109]   *Ibid.*, cl. 24.

[110]   *Ibid.*, cl. 31.

[111]   *Food and Drugs Act*, R.S.C. 1985, c. F-27.

[112]   The *Regulations Amending Certain Regulations Made under the Food and Drugs Act (Project 1539)* were registered on 13 December 2007, and came into force on 1 June 2008. They revised the list in Schedule A and exempted natural health products and some drugs from the prohibition against making preventative claims for the diseases or conditions listed.

[113]   Bill C-51, *An Act to amend the Food and Drugs Act and to make consequential amendments to other Acts*, 2nd Sess., 39th Parl., 2008, cl. 12, 14.

[114]   S.C. 1996, c. 19.

fundamental purpose of any sentence for an offence under this Part is to contribute to the respect for the law and the maintenance of a just, peaceful and safe society while encouraging rehabilitation, and treatment in appropriate circumstances, of offenders and acknowledging the harm done to victims and to the community."[115]

(c) Transportation

Transportation of persons and goods is another area where the legislative scheme is a meshing of regulation by all three levels of government. While the most common rules of the road which Canadians are generally most familiar with are governed by provincial acts[116] such as Alberta's *Traffic Safety Act*, there are many pieces of legislation which have been enacted with safety and the prevention or reduction of injury as one of the main focuses. This section will take a cursory look at the main pieces of legislation in the Canadian context, and then briefly focus on some of the prime areas of public discourse in the area of transportation and injury prevention.

The legislation that exists in this area covers a wide range of sub-areas. It begins with federal legislation which essentially deals with product safety in this area. The *Motor Vehicle Safety Act* sets out in its preamble that it is "[a]n Act to regulate the manufacture and importation of motor vehicles and motor vehicle equipment to reduce the risk of death, injury and damage to property and the environment". Under this Act, authorized companies may apply national safety marks on motor vehicles, restraints for children and the disabled, and tires. However, they cannot do so unless standards under the legislation have been met.[117] The regulations set out the details of the standards of manufacture and other requirements. Warnings that must be included or affixed are also the subject of the details of the regulations.[118] Inspectors have powers to see if standards are being met, including those to search premises, inspect vehicles, and seize property. Offences for violations under the Act are set out as well.[119]

---

[115]   *Ibid.*, s. 10(1).

[116]   *Traffic Safety Act*, R.S.A. 2000, c. T-6; *Motor Vehicle Act*, R.S.B.C. 1996, c. 318; *Highway Traffic Act*, C.C.S.M. c. H60; *Motor Vehicle Act*, R.S.N.B. 1973, c. M-17; *Highway Traffic Act*, R.S.N.L. 1990, c. H-3; *Motor Vehicle Act*, R.S.N.S. 1989, c. 293; *Highway Traffic Act*, R.S.O. 1990, c. H.8; *Highway Traffic Act*, R.S.P.E.I. 1988, c. H-5; *Highway Safety Code*, R.S.Q. c. C-24.2; *Traffic Safety Act*, S.S. 2004, c. T-18.1.

[117]   *Motor Vehicle Safety Act*, S.C. 1993, c. 16, s. 3.

[118]   For example, s. 7(f)(i) of the *Motor Vehicle Restraint Systems and Booster Cushions Safety Regulations* S.O.R./98-159 sets out that the manufacturer must warn that a particular type of child seat is forward facing only.

[119]   *Motor Vehicle Safety Act*, S.C. 1993, c. 16, ss. 17-18.

Other areas of federal regulation include air, rail and marine transportation,[120] and inter-provincial transport. The federal *Aeronautics Act*, for example, grants the Minister responsible the authority, among other things, to investigate matters of safety.[121] Some of the provisions of the *Canada Marine Act* relate to safety, including one of its stated objects. It also contains some traffic control provisions[122] (there to provide for safe navigation among other things), and the requirement that a port authority take measures to maintain order and safety in the port.[123]

The *Railway Safety Act* (which works in conjunction with the federal *Canada Transportation Act*[124] and with provincial laws), which covers the construction of railways, the operation and maintenance of railways and equipment, and the inspection of railways, has a number of clear statements related directly to safety. Its objectives are to: "(*a*) promote and provide for the safety of the public and personnel, and the protection of property and the environment, in the operation of railways; (*b*) encourage the collaboration and participation of interested parties in improving railway safety; (*c*) recognize the responsibility of railway companies in ensuring the safety of their operations; and (*d*) facilitate a modern, flexible and efficient regulatory scheme that will ensure the continuing enhancement of railway safety".[125] Inspectors under the Act are able to order that something not be used (or place conditions on its use) if they are of the opinion that it is unsafe, and this applies not only to those operating railways, but to operators of motor vehicles using a crossing as well.[126] It also includes provisions to ensure that those in certain safety sensitive positions be required to undergo regular medical examinations. There is an obligation on those individuals to advise the physician or optometrist that they hold a position which is "critical to safe railway operations".[127] The physician or optometrist must notify a designated physician or optometrist of the railway company if they believe on reasonable grounds that the patient "has a condition that is likely to pose a threat to safe railway operations". As well, in addition to setting out offences for breach of the Act, the legislation requires a railway to

---

[120] The federal *Marine Liability Act*, S.C. 2001, c. 6 governs liability and lawsuits relating to causes of action relating to shipping, including claims related to injured or deceased persons.

[121] *Aeronautics Act*, R.S.C. 1985, c. A-2, s. 4.2(*n*).

[122] *Canada Marine Act*, S.C. 1998, c. 10, s. 58.

[123] *Ibid.*, s. 61.

[124] *Canada Transportation Act*, S.C. 1996, c. 10.

[125] *Railway Safety Act*, R.S.C. 1985, c. 32 (4th Supp.), s. 3.

[126] *Ibid.*, s. 31.

[127] *Ibid.*, s. 35.

establish a safety management system and to maintain records to assess its safety performance (including accident rates).[128]

The federal *Canadian Transportation Accident Investigation and Safety Board Act* applies to aviation, marine and railway "occurrences", including accidents (and certain occurrences regarding pipelines) and establishes a board which can investigate "transportation occurrences", "make findings as to their causes", identify "safety deficiencies", "[make] recommendations ... to eliminate or reduce ... safety deficiencies" and make public reports in respect of its findings.[129]

The *Motor Vehicle Transport Act, 1987* regulates motor vehicle transport by inter-provincial undertakings. For example, it would govern the safety of bus and truck transport between provinces. This is obviously an area which needs to be co-ordinated with provincial laws and regulations that may only be made under this Act after consulting the provincial governments of the provinces who will be affected. It deals with the issuing of licences. While a commercial driver may already have a provincial licence, a licence under this Act will likely be required if he or she crosses provincial borders.[130]

The final piece of federal legislation that will be briefly reviewed is the *Canada Transportation Act* which sets out a national transportation policy. While its focus is mainly economic considerations, safety is part of the legislated mandate. Section 5 says in part that "a safe, economic, efficient ... network of ... transportation services ... is essential to serve the transportation needs of shippers and travellers, ... and that those objectives are most likely to be achieved when ... (*a*) the national transportation system meets the highest practicable safety standards ...". This Act also establishes the Canadian Transportation Agency which is given authority under other federal legislation. The agency can hold inquiries and issue orders, and has powers of a superior court in terms of compelling witnesses, the production of documents, the enforcement of its orders, and so on.[131]

Provincial Acts govern a variety of other matters including general rules regarding safe use of roads (for example, speed limits, traffic control devices, use of booster seats[132] and prohibitions on driving while speaking

---

[128] *Ibid.*, s. 37.

[129] *Canadian Transportation Accident Investigation and Safety Board Act*, S.C. 1989, c. 3, s. 7.

[130] *Motor Vehicle Transport Act, 1987*, R.S.C. 1985, c. 29 (3rd Supp.), s. 8.

[131] *Canada Transporation Act*, S.C. 1996, c. 10, ss. 5, 7.

[132] While legislation mandating the use of car seats for infants and young children is in effect in every province and territory in Canada, legislation requiring booster seats for older children is relatively new and not yet implemented across the country. To date, seven provinces have enacted such legislation, with three provinces bringing this into effect in

on a cell phone[133]); licensing and permits (dealing with items such as general and commercial licences, permits, driver training and examination, and the new trend toward more detailed graduated licencing);[134] vehicle inspections (general and commercial); dangerous goods transportation[135] and the transportation of goods in general; road restrictions and bans; buses and trucks; off-highway vehicles;[136] and in some cases, rail and air traffic. It is beyond the scope of this chapter to

---

2008: *Motor Vehicle Act Regulations*, B.C. Reg. 218/2007; *Seat Belt Regulation — Motor Vehicle Act*, N.B. Reg. 83/163; and *Highway Traffic Act*, R.S.N.L. 1990, c. H-3, s. 178.1.

[133]   To date, three provinces have banned the use of hand-held devices while driving: *Highway Traffic Act*, R.S.N.L. 1990, c. H-3, s. 176.1 (the first such legislation to be enacted, it came into effect 1 April 2003); *Highway Safety Code*, R.S.Q. c. C-24.2, s. 439.1; *Motor Vehicle Act*, R.S.N.S. 1989, c. 293, s. 100D. Bill 204, *Traffic Safety (Hand-Held Communication Devices) Amendment Act, 2008*, 1st Sess., 27th Leg., Alberta, 2008 had passed first reading and was referred to the Standing Committee on the Economy during second reading at the time of writing.

[134]   According to Ontario's *Highway Traffic Act*, R.S.O. 1990, c. H.8, Part IV, s. 31(b): "[t]he purpose of this Part is to protect the public by ensuring that ... driving privileges are granted to novice and probationary drivers only after they acquire experience and develop or improve safe driving skills in controlled conditions". See also *Operator Licensing and Vehicle Control Regulation*, Alta. Reg. 320/2002, s. 33; *Graduated Driver Licensing Regulations*, P.E.I. Reg. EC225/07.

[135]   The federal *Transportation of Dangerous Goods Act, 1992*, S.C. 1992, c. 34 also applies to federal matters (*i.e.*, dangerous goods on a ship outside of Canada, or on aircraft registered in Canada). Its preamble states it is "[a]n Act to promote public safety in the transportation of dangerous goods". Under s. 4(1)(a), agreements can be made with the provinces regarding the administration of this Act. It prohibits transport or import of dangerous goods unless safety requirements have been met (s. 5(a)). There is also a duty to report accidental release of dangerous goods under certain circumstances (s. 18(1)), and also to take "reasonable emergency measures to reduce or eliminate any danger to public safety that results or may reasonably be expected to result from the release" (s. 18(2)).

[136]   Newfoundland's *Motorized Snow Vehicles and All-Terrain Vehicles Act*, R.S.N.L. 1990, c. M-20 and Ontario's *Motorized Snow Vehicles Act*, R.S.O. 1990, c. M.44 are examples of stand alone legislation in this area. Other provinces have dealt with this in more comprehensive legislation: for example, Alberta's *Off-Highway Vehicle Regulation*, Alta. Reg. 319/2002 under its *Traffic Safety Act*, R.S.A. 2000, c. T-6, ss. 117-22. Calls for further regulation of this area, and in particular legislation aimed at the use of ATVs and minors, has grown. The lack of regulation regarding children is startling. Though all provinces and territories except the Yukon have enacted provisions relating to the use of ATVs, their use by children is largely unrestricted. In many jurisdictions, children are free to drive ATVs if on private land, sometimes on public land, with the only requirement in some instances being the presence of an adult. In most instances, no training is required, and in Alberta and British Columbia, not even a helmet is necessary. See: *Off-Highway Vehicle Regulation*, Alta. Reg. 319/2002 under its *Traffic Safety Act*, R.S.A. 2000, c. T-6, ss. 117-22; *Motor Vehicle (All Terrain) Act*, R.S.B.C. 1996, c. 319; *The Off-Road Vehicles Act*, S.M. 1987 88, c. 64; *Off-Road Vehicle Act*, S.N.B. 1985, c. O-1.5; *Motorized Snow Vehicles and All-Terrain Vehicles Act*, R.S.N. 1990, c. M-20; *All-Terrain Vehicles Act*, R.S.N.W.T. 1988, c. A-3; *Off-highway Vehicles Act*, R.S.N.S. 1989, c. 323, s. 10; *All-Terrain Vehicles Act*, R.S.N.W.T. 1988, c. A 3; *Off Road Vehicles Act*, R.S.O. 1990, c. O.4; *An Act respecting off-highway vehicles*, R.S.Q. V-1.2; *The All Terrain Vehicles Act*, S.S. 1988-89, c. A-18.02.

look at all of these areas. It will turn instead to a discussion of some of the key areas that have been the subject of court cases and public debate.

Legislation has been enacted mandating the wearing of motorcycle helmets (and moving away, then, from using education only to attempt to convince drivers that this is a sound and safe practice). These statutory provisions have been challenged on numerous grounds. In *R. v. Fisher*,[137] two accused (one the driver, the other the passenger on a motorcycle) admitted that they had been in contravention of s. 172.3(1) of Manitoba's *Highway Traffic Act*. However, they argued that this provision violated their s. 7 *Charter* rights as a person was more likely to be involved in an accident on a motorcycle if wearing a helmet than if not. They attributed the increased likelihood to heat build-up in the helmet, loss of peripheral vision and the loss or decrease in ability to hear with a helmet on. Both sides presented expert evidence. Justice Gyles found that there was likely no breach of the accused's security of the person, but that if there was "compulsory helmet legislation is a reasonable limit which can be demonstrably justified in a free and democratic society, in view of the evidence establishing head injury reduction".[138] On appeal, Scollin J. said there was no *Charter* breach to deal with. He declared that "[the] provision requiring the wearing of a helmet is an integral part of a broad legislative scheme to promote highway safety and to minimize the overall human and economic cost of accidents. On an unselfish, moderate and practical understanding of the right to security of the person, such provisions create duties to others which in no way affect *Charter* rights".[139]

The accused in *R. v. Sluis*[140] also attempted the argument that the requirement to wear a motorcycle helmet in the relevant B.C. legislation violated his s. 7 *Charter* rights as it increased the danger of using a motorcycle (at least for some) and restricted his freedom unreasonably. Justice Esson said there was not "sufficient substance to warrant granting leave to appeal. The complaint of Mr. Sluis is ... one which should be directed towards the legislature and government which has jurisdiction in the matter".[141]

One case did set limits on the ability to mandate the use of motorcycle helmets but this was in the context of human rights legislation and the protected ground of religion. In *Dhillon v. British Columbia*

---

[137]   [1984] M.J. No. 32, 42 C.R. (3d) 291, 29 M.V.R. 137 (Man. Prov. Ct.), aff'd [1985] M.J. No. 454, 37 Man. R. (2d) 81 (Man. Q.B.).

[138]   *Ibid.*, at para. 38 (Prov. Ct.).

[139]   *Ibid.*, at para. 12 (Q.B.).

[140]   [1988] B.C.J. No. 1197 (B.C.C.A.) (In Chambers).

[141]   *Ibid.*

(Ministry of Transportation and Highways, Motor Vehicle Branch),[142] the complainant tried to take a road test on a motorcycle and was refused as he would not wear a helmet. Mr. Dhillon was a devout Sikh and, as such, had a religious obligation to wear a turban. His complaint stated that he was denied a service customarily available to the public and that this was contrary to the *Human Rights Act* of British Columbia. The human rights tribunal found that the duty to wear a turban was a *bona fide* religious obligation, and that the respondent had failed to accommodate him to the point of undue hardship as required by the legislation. The tribunal considered the magnitude of the risk and who would bear the risk of failing to wear a helmet. Although the evidence showed that an already high-risk activity would become even riskier without a helmet, the marginal risk was minimal and would be borne mainly by the unhelmeted rider. While there would be increased costs due to those injured, they were not so great that they would be an undue hardship. As a result, the relevant section was declared discriminatory and the respondent was to refrain from proceeding as it had in the future.

However, the recently released decision of *R. v. Badesha*[143] fails to follow the *Dhillon* judgment.[144] Judge Blacklock noted he was not bound to follow that case[145] and set out extensive reasons for upholding the Ontario legislation mandating the wearing of helmets as constitutional and in line with the provincial human rights legislation, even where the religious beliefs of the Sikh applicant in question were infringed. The judge found that the applicant's refusal to wear a helmet, either instead of or over his turban, was based on sincerely held religious beliefs. He acknowledged a breach of s. 2(*a*) of the *Charter*[146] but went on to hold that the breach was justifiable under s. 1. In finding in this way, he took into account "the relatively limited nature of the intrusion on the Applicant's freedom of religion ... the benefits to his *own* personal safety, the interest of his own family, *other users* of the road and *the public* in general ...".[147] He went on to find that there had been no breach of s. 15 of the *Charter*[148]

---

142 [1999] B.C.H.R.T.D. No. 25.

143 *R. v. Badesha*, [2008] O.J. No. 854, 2008 ONCJ 94 (Ont. C.J.).

144 [1999] B.C.H.R.T.D. No. 25.

145 Indeed, Judge Blacklock noted the following: "I do not think to be frank that the analysis of reasonable accommodation as employed in that case fits comfortably with the way in which the Supreme Court of Canada has developed that concept in the other cases that have been put before me during this argument. It should also be noted that some of those cases were only decided at a point in time subsequent to the argument of or final decision in Dhillon" (*R. v. Badesha*, [2008] O.J. No. 854 at para. 70, 2008 ONCJ 94 (Ont. C.J.)).

146 *Canadian Charter of Rights and Freedoms*, ss. 1, 2(*a*), Part I of the *Constitution Act, 1982*, being Schedule B to the *Canada Act 1982* (U.K.), 1982, c. 11.

147 *R. v. Badesha*, [2008] O.J. No. 854 at para. 74, 2008 ONCJ 94 (Ont. C.J.).

148 *Canadian Charter of Rights and Freedoms*, s. 15, Part I of the *Constitution Act, 1982*, being Schedule B to the *Canada Act 1982* (U.K.), 1982, c. 11.

as neither the purpose or effect of the legislation was in conflict with the protection afforded by this section. Finally, he addressed the human rights arguments that had been advanced. While he found the human rights legislation to be applicable, he said that to require Ontario to accommodate the applicant and others in his situation would constitute an undue hardship on the province as "it would compel the Province to abandon a reasonable safety standard".[149] This was also a case where an accommodation would not be possible and so the application was dismissed. It was noted that this decision would not preclude provinces from legislating exceptions to their own helmet requirements, but where there were no such exceptions, the legislation should stand.[150]

As with a number of injury prevention strategies, an approach which utilizes a number of methods is usually the most successful. The work done to increase the use of bicycle helmets is no different.[151] While educational and public awareness campaigns are important,[152] helmet use increases once mandatory legislation is introduced.[153] Australia and New Zealand have mandatory bicycle helmet laws which apply to all ages[154]

---

[149]   *R. v. Badesha*, [2008] O.J. No. 854 at para. 97, 2008 ONCJ 94 (Ont. C.J.).

[150]   *Ibid.*, at para. 71: "The fact that other jurisdictions have opted for statutory exceptions regarding observant Sikhs is also not controlling". At para. 99: "I want to emphasize again, that the outcome of this case turned on what I determined was or was not required as a matter of constitutional law and *The Ontario Human Rights Code*. What the Province may choose to do in this area, as a matter of policy now, or in the future, of course remains a matter for the Legislature". Justice Blacklock was referring to the helmet exemption laws for Sikhs in Manitoba and British Columbia: *Safety Helmets Standards and Exemptions Regulation*, Man. Reg. 167/2000, *Motorcycle Safety Helmet Exemption Regulation*, B.C. Reg. 237/99.

[151]   The Canadian Association of Road Safety Professionals, "Support for the Mandatory Use of Bicycle Helmets for All Ages" (Position Paper), online: <http://www.carsp.ca/index.php?0=page_content&1=98&2=196>.

[152]   Possibly for political reasons as legislation mandating the use of bicycle helmets was not introduced in British Columbia, Australia or New Zealand until the voluntary use of helmets had increased: U.K., Elizabeth Towner *et al.*, Department of Transport, "Bicycle helmets: review of effectiveness (No. 30)" (November 2002), online: <http://www.dft.gov.uk/pgr/roadsafety/research/rsrr/themel/bicyclehelmetsreviewofeffect4726>.

[153]   A. Macpherson & A. Spinks, "Bicycle helmet legislation for the uptake of helmet use and prevention of head injuries" (2007) Cochrane Database of Systematic Reviews, Issue 2, Art. No. CD005401; Robert D. Foss & Douglas J. Beirness, "Bicycle Helmet Use in British Columbia: Effects of the Helmet Use Law" (Chapel Hill, NC: University of North Carolina Highway Safety Research Centre & Traffic Injury Research Foundation, 2000); G.B. Rodgers, "Effects of State Helmet Laws on Bicycle Helmet Use by Children and Adolescents" (2002) 8 Injury Prevention 42.

[154]   Delia Hendrie, Matthew Legge & Diana Rosman, "An Economic Evaluation of the Mandatory Bicycle Helmet Legislation in Western Australia" (Department of Public Health) online: <http://www.officeofroadsafety.wa.gov.au/documents/AneconomicevaluationofbicyclehelmetlegislationinWA-1999_Deliasconferencepaper.pdf>; United Kingdom, Department of Transport "Bicycle helmets: review of effectiveness (No. 30)" (November 2002), online: <http://www.dft.gov.uk/pgr/roadsafety/research/rsrr/theme1/bicyclehelmetsreviewofeffect4726?page=7>.

and studies done there have shown the implementation of laws to correlate with an increase in use.[155] In the United States, California was the first state to implement such legislation which came into effect in 1987.[156] In Canada, five provinces to date have such laws.[157] The application of those laws vary as some apply to all riders, while others only apply to minors, or in one instance to infants in a carrier. In Ontario, where the law originally applied to everyone, it was amended to apply only to minors after a change in the political party holding power in government.

Bicycle helmet laws have faced challenges in the courts. In *R. v. Warman*,[158] an appeal of a conviction for failure to wear a bicycle helmet was dismissed. Mr. Warman had argued that the law violated his right of free choice and discriminated against him as certain individuals were exempted from the legislation (due to religious considerations) and he was not. Justice Blair said that "while acknowledging the importance of freedom of choice, I conclude that society in the public interest must occasionally place constraints on this freedom ... [A]lthough British Columbia's bicycle helmet law infringes on Mr. Warman's free choice, the infringement is of an insubstantial nature in light of society's need to promote the welfare and well being of its citizens, particularly those operating bicycles on the province's highways".[159] He further held that it had not been shown that the law discriminated against the religious or other rights of Mr. Warman. The exemption for others from the legislation did not lead to the finding that those who do not fall within the exemption face discrimination.[160] A fairly recent challenge was also made to Nova Scotia's legislation. It was upheld as constitutional despite arguments that it violated the accused's rights to liberty and freedom of expression.[161]

---

[155] M.H. Cameron, S. Gantzer & S.V. Newstead, "Bicyclists Head Injuries in Victoria Three Years After the Introduction of Mandatory Helmet Use", Report No. 75 (Victoria: Monash University Accident Research Centre, 1994); J. Marshall & M. White, "Compulsory Helmet Wearing Legislation for Bicyclists in South Australia", Report No. 8/94 (Walkerville, South Australia: Office of Road Safety, 1994).

[156] Bicycle Helmet Safety Institute, "Helmet Laws for Bicycle Riders", online: <http://www.helmets.org/mandator.htm>.

[157] *Traffic Safety Act*, R.S.A. 2000, c. T-6, *Vehicle Equipment Regulation*, Alta. Reg. 322/2002, s. 97(1) (under 18); *Motor Vehicle Act*, R.S.B.C. 1996, c. 318, s. 184 (under 16); *The Highway Traffic Act*, C.C.S.M. c. H60 s. 147(2) (child passengers); *Motor Vehicle Act*, R.S.N.B. 1973, c. M-17, s. 177 (minors); *Motor Vehicle Act*, R.S.N.S. 1989, c. 293, s. 170 (all persons); *Highway Traffic Act*, R.S.O. 1990, c. H.8, s. 104 (all persons riding on highway and under 16 any time); *Highway Traffic Act*, R.S.P.E.I. 1988, c. H-5, s. 194(2)(a.1) (all persons).

[158] [2001] B.C.J. No. 2733, 2001 BCSC 1771 (B.C.S.C.).

[159] *Ibid.*, at paras. 5-6.

[160] *Ibid.*, at para. 8.

[161] "Judge tosses out challenge to N.S. bike helmet law" *CBC News* (1 March 2005), online: <http://www.cbc.ca/news/story/2004/03/01/nshelmet040301.html>.

Seatbelt legislation has also been the subject of *Charter* challenges. The laws mandating the wearing of seatbelts have been upheld in decisions across the country. One of the first was *R. v. Leger*.[162] This was followed by a number of other decisions. In *R. v. Thompson*,[163] following upon a conviction under the provincial legislation, the argument was made that the applicable section violated the freedom of religion of the applicant. He set out a set of personal beliefs, including the belief in free will, and said that the *Charter* guaranteed his right to believe in what he chose to, and the right to act in ways which supported those beliefs. Justice Anderson stated that even if he were to accept that the beliefs as set out constituted a religion (which he did not), freedom of religion is not an unbounded freedom but one which is subject to provincial laws with the aim of public safety. He held that the alleged breach of freedom of religion was so insubstantial that it did not even amount to a breach of s. 2.

In *R. v. Nikkel*,[164] a similar argument was made before a county court judge in British Columbia, only this time based on s. 7 of the *Charter*. The judge quoted from *R. v. Thompson* and said that the same reasoning applied to this challenge, namely that "the liberty here espoused by the appellant is subject to the laws of the Province relating to public safety and that the alleged infringement is so insubstantial as not to be considered as a breach of Section 7 of the *Charter*".[165] The later decision of the B.C. Court of Appeal in *R. v. Kennedy*[166] confirmed previous decisions finding the legislation constitutionally valid.

The Nova Scotia Court of Appeal dealt with this issue as well in *R. v. Doucette*[167] in which the individual convicted for failure to wear his seatbelt attempted to argue that the provincial legislation infringed his right under s. 7 of the *Charter*, as well as s. 15. The argument as to the right to life, liberty and security of the person suggested that these were threatened as seatbelts could actually cause injury as opposed to preventing it. The argument with respect to s. 15 asserted that as classes of persons were exempt from the application of the legislation, this violated Mr. Doucette's right to equality under the law. In response to the argument regarding equality, the court found it to be without merit. They stated that "[t]here are obviously valid reasons for exempting certain classes of persons from the requirement to use seat belts and, in doing so,

---

[162]   [1985] Q.J. No. 38, 39 M.V.R. 60 (Qué. S.C. (Crim. Div.)).
[163]   [1986] B.C.J. No. 388, 28 C.C.C. (3d) 575, 41 M.V.R. 158 (B.C.C.A.), aff'd [1986] B.C.J. No. 850 (B.C.C.A.).
[164]   [1986] B.C.J. No. 2876 (B.C. Co. Ct.).
[165]   *Ibid.*, at para. 4.
[166]   [1987] B.C.J. No. 2028, 18 B.C.L.R. (2d) 321, 3 M.V.R. (2d) 88 (B.C.C.A.).
[167]   [1987] N.S.J. No. 113, 77 N.S.R. (2d) 279 (N.S.C.A.).

the government has not discriminated against the appellant ...".[168] In terms of the alleged breach of s. 7, the court held that there was no *prima facie* breach of s. 7 rights, but that if a breach was to be alleged, it fell on the person making the allegation to adduce evidence to establish this. In this case, no evidence as to the dangerousness of seatbelts had been introduced and so the appellant failed on this argument as well.

In the Alberta case of *R. v. Maier*,[169] the accused was convicted at trial and was not successful in arguing that the law violated his s. 7 rights. Unlike in *R. v. Doucette*, expert evidence had been introduced on both sides as to whether or not seatbelts caused or ameliorated injury. The trial judge found no breach of s. 7 as he found that based on the evidence that had been introduced, seat belts and other restraint devices had the effect of reducing death and injury. There was a temporary reprieve for Mr. Maier as the Court of Queen's Bench Justice appealed to found that based on the evidence, seat belts do cause injury and this violated s. 7. He further found the legislation was not upheld by s. 1. The Court of Appeal, however, reversed that decision and reinstated the conviction. They found that it was improper for the appeal judge to reverse findings of fact made by the trial judge. Indeed, they stated that: "it is not shown that the seat-belt increases the wearer's risk of injury or death by whatever small amount. Indeed, the contrary is shown. The risk of injury or death is decreased when a seat-belt is worn; moreover, failure to wear a seat-belt puts other persons, both in the vehicle and outside it, at increased risk ... Mr. Maier has not shown that the legislation infringes his rights under the ... *Charter* ...".[170]

The public health campaign against drinking and driving has in general been an interesting one to follow. As with numerous public health goals, a number of methods have been employed in the quest to reduce impaired driving. More severe legal penalties have been one part of that. Penalties for impaired driving have increased in the last several years as a result of growing public awareness of the seriousness of impaired driving and the devastating consequences as a result of publicized incidents. Under Alberta's *Traffic Safety Act*, for example, if an accused is found guilty of impaired driving or failing to provide a breath sample under s. 253 or s. 254 of the *Criminal Code*, they automatically have their licence suspended for one year.[171] This increases to three years if convicted twice in ten years, and to five years if convicted three times in that period.[172] However, there is at least some evidence that if penalties are

[168] *Ibid.*, at para. 21.
[169] [1989] A.J. No. 65 (Alta. Q.B.).
[170] [1989] A.J. No. 1169, 101 A.R. 126 at 29 (Q.L.) (Alta. C.A.).
[171] *Traffic Safety Act*, R.S.A. 2000, c. T-6, s. 83(1).
[172] *Ibid.*, s. 83(2), (3).

too severe, the beneficial effects may be short-lived. At least according to one study, the more successful approach is less severe penalties accompanied by regular enforcement.[173] Thus, the use of check stops to catch impaired drivers, hopefully before injury is suffered, has been shown to be an important factor. Alberta Transportation has stated that the goal of check stops is not only to catch and convict those who are driving under the influence; it is also aimed at changing the attitude of the public (and is meant to be educational as well).

Check stops, however, have been the subject of legal challenges. In *R. v. Dedman*,[174] the accused was stopped at a check stop by police. After initiating conversation with him, the smell of alcohol was detected on his breath. He tried but failed to provide a breath sample at the road side and was thus charged with failing, without reasonable excuse, to comply with a demand to provide a sample under the *Criminal Code*.[175] A key issue was whether police had authority to require the accused to stop his vehicle at the check stop. The majority of the Supreme Court of Canada agreed that his acquittal at trial should be set aside. They found that police did have authority at common law to randomly stop vehicles at a check stop (though they said at that time it was not authorized by statute). They held that one of the duties of a police officer is to protect life, and from that duty arises a duty to control traffic. Justice Le Dain, in writing for the majority, stated that:

> ... the right to circulate in a motor vehicle on the public highway [i]s a "liberty" ... however ... the right is not a fundamental liberty like the ordinary right of movement of the individual, but a licensed activity that is subject to regulation and control for the protection of life and property.[176]

> Because of the seriousness of the problem of impaired driving, there can be no doubt about the importance and necessity of a program to improve the deterrence of it. The right to circulate on the highway free from unreasonable interference is an important one, but it is, as I have said, a licensed activity subject to regulation and control in the interest of safety. ... I would accordingly hold that there was common law authority for the random vehicle stop for the purpose contemplated by the R.I.D.E. program.[177]

---

[173]   Lawrence R. Berger & Dinesh Mohan, *Injury Control: A Global View* (Oxford: Oxford University Press, 1996) at 219-20.

[174]   [1985] S.C.J. No. 45, [1985] 2 S.C.R. 2 (S.C.C.).

[175]   *Criminal Code*, R.S.C. 1985, c. C-46, s. 234.1(2).

[176]   *R. v. Dedman*, [1985] S.C.J. No. 45, [1985] 2 S.C.R. 2 at para. 68 (S.C.C.).

[177]   *Ibid.*, at para. 69.

Thus, in this case, restrictions on individual liberty were justified in the name of safety and in furtherance of the aim to prevent injury.[178]

(d) Health and Safety in the Workplace

The regulation in this area is abundant. The federal government and all provinces and territories have passed laws dealing with occupational health and safety, product safety in the workplace and workers compensation in the event of an injury or death. This chapter is not intended to cover all of the legislation, regulations, codes and case law that cover this area; for that several books would be required. It is intended only as an introduction to the general legislative lay of the land with references for further inquiry.[179]

(i) Occupational Health and Safety Legislation

While occupational health and safety legislation does vary somewhat across the jurisdictions, there are many similarities.[180] Generally, there are provisions setting out responsibilities of workers,[181] supervisors, and employers[182] (and others)[183] to establish and maintain safe

---

[178] Subsequently, certain provinces passed legislation giving police statutory authority to stop vehicles. The Supreme Court of Canada said that while this breached s. 9 of the *Charter*, it was upheld by s. 1, see *R. v. Hufsky*, [1988] S.C.J. No. 30, [1988] 1 S.C.R. 621 at 633 (S.C.C.); *R. v. Ladouceur*, [1990] S.C.J. No. 53, [1990] 1 S.C.R. 1257 (S.C.C.).

[179] For a good starting point in this area in Canada, updated annually, see Norman A. Keith, *Canadian Health and Safety Law: A Comprehensive Guide to the Statutes, Policies and Case Law*, looseleaf (Aurora, Ont.: Canada Law Book, 1997). For an overview of the law in Ontario, see Michael Grossman, *The Law of Occupational Health and Safety in Ontario*, 2nd ed. (Markham, Ont.: Butterworths, 1994). See also "Lancaster's Bi-Weekly Health & Safety/Workers' Compensation Law E-Bulletin" (Toronto: Lancaster House, 2003); Cheryl A. Edwards, *OH&S Due Diligence In Ontario: A Practical Guide*, 2nd ed. (Toronto: Thomson Carswell, 2006); and Alberta, "Occupational Health and Safety Code 2006: Explanation Guide" (Edmonton: Alberta Human Resources and Employment, 2006).

[180] For a summary of legislation in Canada, as well as other information regarding the legislation, see the Canadian Centre for Occupational Health and Safety's website where specific similarities are succinctly set out: <http://www.ccohs.ca/oshanswers/legisl/responsi.html>.

[181] The *Canada Labour Code*, R.S.C. 1985, c. L-2, s. 126 sets out, for example, that employees must use safety equipment; follow prescribed procedures; and report anything hazardous, as well as all accidents and all contraventions of the Act. Section 2 of Alberta's *Occupational Health and Safety Act*, R.S.A. 2000, c. O-2 places a duty on workers to take reasonable care to protect the health and safety of themselves and others.

[182] One example is s. 124 of the *Canada Labour Code*, *ibid.*, which states that: "Every employer shall ensure that the health and safety at work of every person employed by the employer is protected." A number of specific duties are then outlined in s. 125 and s. 125.1 (for example, an employer must ensure buildings meet standards, install guard-rails according to standards, and "investigate, record and report ... all accidents, occupational

working environments. There are also sections dealing with the rights of workers to refuse to work if there are grounds to believe that there is a danger to themselves or others working at the site.[184] Another key issue which has been established is the duty to report accidents, injuries or other types of specified occurrences.[185]

The main piece of federal legislation regulating occupational health and safety is Part II of the *Canada Labour Code*.[186] Section 122.1 sets out that "[t]he purpose of this Part is to prevent accidents and injury to health arising out of, linked with or occurring in the course of employment to which this Part applies".[187] Given the limited jurisdiction of the federal government to regulate this area, it generally applies only to employment "… in connection with the operation of any federal work, undertaking or business" or by a federal corporation or the "public service of Canada".[188] A number of regulations dealing with specific areas of federal jurisdiction have also been enacted.[189]

While the role of the federal government in establishing laws in this area in Canada is limited, it has sought to play a part in co-ordinating efforts amongst all levels of government through its *Canadian Centre for Occupational Health and Safety Act*.[190] The legislation establishes a centre

---

diseases and other hazardous occurrences known to the employer"). These are just a few of the many obligations which are listed.

[183] *Occupational Health and Safety Act*, R.S.A. 2000, c. O-2, s. 2(3), (4), (5). Duties also imposed on suppliers to ensure as far as reasonably practicable to do so that tools, equipment, *etc.* are safe; that tools, equipment and hazardous materials comply with the Act; and that every contractor ensures, as far as it is reasonably practicable to do so, that the employer complies with the Act, among other things.

[184] One example is found in s. 35 of Alberta's *Occupational Health and Safety Act, ibid.*, dealing with "imminent danger" on the work site. It states that where there are "reasonable and probable grounds" to believe there is an imminent danger on the work site, a worker shall not work and shall notify his or her employer. The employer is prohibited from taking disciplinary action or dismissing a worker because they have complied with the Act in this regard (s. 36).

[185] Legislation also sets out obligations to report accidents and other incidents. For example, s. 18 of Alberta's *Occupational Health and Safety Act, ibid.*, states that if a serious injury or accident occurs, a report must be made and an investigation must be conducted (sometimes even if no injury has occurred, *e.g.*, the upset of a crane). A report in this case is excluded from evidence in a trial, fatality inquiry, and certain other proceedings under s. 18(5).

[186] R.S.C. 1985, c. L-2.

[187] *Ibid.*, s. 122.1.

[188] *Ibid.*, s. 123.

[189] *Aviation Occupational Health and Safety Regulations*, S.O.R./87-182; *Canada Occupational Health and Safety Regulations*, S.O.R./86-304; *Coal Mining Occupational Health and Safety Regulations*, S.O.R./90-97; *Marine Occupational Safety and Health Regulations*, S.O.R./87-183; *Oil and Gas Occupational Safety and Health Regulations*, S.O.R./87-612; and *On Board Trains Occupational Safety and Health Regulations*, S.O.R./87-184.

[190] *Canadian Centre for Occupational Health and Safety Act*, R.S.C. 1985, c. C-13. See the Centre's website at <http://www.ccohs.ca>.

to: "promote the fundamental right of Canadians to a healthy and safe working environment by creating a national institute concerned with the study, encouragement and cooperative advancement of occupational health and safety, in whose governing body the interests and concerns of workers, trade unions, employers, federal, provincial and territorial authorities, professional and scientific communities and the general public will be represented".[191] Objects of the Centre include the facilitation of "consultation and cooperation among federal, provincial and territorial jurisdictions, and participation by labour and management in the establishment and maintenance of high standards of occupational health and safety appropriate to the Canadian situation; ... assist[ance] in the development and maintenance of policies and programs aimed at the reduction or elimination of occupational hazards; and to serve as a national center for statistics and other information in relation to occupational health and safety".[192] It also gives the Centre powers to create systems to collect and analyze information.[193] Some provinces have taken measures to incorporate co-operation under this Act into their provincial legislation.[194]

However, the federal government has made an impact in this area with recent amendments to the *Criminal Code* brought into force on March 31, 2004. Those amendments created new legal duties in this area that affect everyone, regardless of whether a workplace falls under federal or provincial jurisdiction. These changes saw the imposition of a new federal criminal law duty on persons directing the work of others. Section 217.1 states that: "Every one who undertakes, or has authority, to direct how another person does work or performs a task is under a legal duty to take reasonable steps to prevent bodily harm to that person, or any other person, arising from that work or task."[195] This section came about as a result of the Westray mining disaster in Nova Scotia where 26 coal miners were killed in an explosion despite repeated reports of unsafe working conditions.[196] Neither the company nor senior managers were successfully convicted under the *Criminal Code* for their failure to take steps to rectify the danger. This new duty as outlined in the *Criminal Code*, in conjunction with related sections dealing with corporate criminal

---

[191]   *Ibid.*, s. 2.
[192]   *Ibid.*, s. 5(*b*), (*c*) and (*d*).
[193]   *Ibid.*, s. 6.
[194]   *Occupational Health and Safety Act*, R.S.A. 2000, c. O-2, s. 26: the Minister can enter into agreements with other persons or governments to conduct research, establish training programs, or set up educational programs.
[195]   *Criminal Code*, R.S.C. 1985, c. C-46, s. 217.1.
[196]   See "Bill C-45 Overview" online: <http://www.ccohs.ca/oshanswers/legisl/billc45.html>.

liability,[197] creates novel and severe penalties for those who fail in their duty.

All provinces and territories have established occupational health and safety legislation. They all have stand-alone Acts with the exception of British Columbia which has incorporated these provisions into its *Workers Compensation Act*.[198] The laws cover most workplaces, with some specified exceptions.[199] In addition to the general aims of this type of legislation discussed above, the Acts set out the ability to inspect work sites (including the authority to examine documents, seize items or samples, conduct tests, and obtain statements from individuals).[200] Orders can be made to cease work or to take measures to rectify an unsafe situation.[201] Offences are set out in the Acts and penalties can theoretically be quite severe.[202]

(ii)   Controlled Products Legislation

The handling of "controlled products" at work sites is also the subject of both federal and provincial legislation.[203] Under the federal

---

[197]   See, in particular, *Criminal Code, R.S.C.* 1985, c. C-46, ss. 22.1-22.2, which radically altered corporate liability under the *Criminal Code* in several ways. One significant item of note: liability for omissions is expanded — this encompasses the failure of supervisors, for example, to take steps to ensure safe working conditions. For an insightful discussion of the amendments to these two sections, see Eric Colvin & Sanjeev Anand, *Principles of Criminal Law*, 3rd ed. (Toronto: Thomson Carswell, 2007) at 122-30.

[198]   *Workers Compensation Act*, R.S.B.C. 1996, c. 492; *Occupational Health and Safety Act*, R.S.A. 2000, c. O-2; *Workplace Safety and Health Act*, C.C.S.M. c. W210; *Occupational Health and Safety Act*, S.N.B. 1983, c. O-0.2; *Occupational Health and Safety Act*, R.S.N.L. 1990, c. O-3; *Safety Act*, R.S.N.W.T. 1998, c. S-1 and *Mine Health and Safety Act*, S.N.W.T. 1994, c. 25; *Occupational Health and Safety Act*, S.N.S. 1996, c. 7; *Safety Act*, R.S.N.W.T. 1988, c. S-1, as amended by s. 76.05 of *Nunavut Act*, S.Nu 2003, c. 25 and *Mine Health and Safety Act (Nunavut)*, S.N.W.T. 1994, c. 25; *Occupational Health and Safety Act*, R.S.O. 1990, c. O.1; *Occupational Health and Safety Act*, R.S.P.E.I. 1988, c. O-1.01; *An Act respecting occupational health and safety*, R.S.Q. c. S-2.1; *Occupational Health and Safety Act*, S.S. 1993, c. O-1.1; *Occupational Health and Safety Act*, R.S.Y. 2002, c. 159.

[199]   See for example: *Farming and Ranching Exemption Regulation*, Alta. Reg. 27/1995, which exempts farming and ranching from the operation of the Act.

[200]   *Occupational Health and Safety Act*, R.S.A. 2000, c. O-2, s. 8.

[201]   *Ibid.*, s. 9 (Officer can order work to stop or measures to be taken if work site unsafe).

[202]   *Ibid.*, s. 41 (for contravention of the Act, regulations or Code: for a first offence a fine of up to $500,000 with additional fines of up to $30,000 per day for continuing offences, plus up to six months in jail; for a second offence a fine of up to $1 million with additional fines of up to $60,000 per day for continuing offences, plus up to 12 months imprisonment. There is a separate offence for providing false information during an inspection or investigation to an officer designated under the Act, or to a peace officer).

[203]   Part II of the federal *Hazardous Products Act*, R.S.C. 1985, c. H-3; provincial occupational health and safety legislation, for example, s. 30 of the *Occupational Health and Safety Act*, R.S.A. 2000, c. O-2.

legislation (Part II of the *Hazardous Products Act*, as well as Schedule II),[204] the sale or import of "controlled products"[205] "intended for use in a work place in Canada" is regulated. Products cannot be sold or imported unless they meet certain requirements, and offences are set out to deal with contraventions of the Act.[206] As a result of provincial legislation, controlled products under the federal scheme are integrated into the provincial regulations.[207]

In addition, the *Hazardous Products Act* requires the exchange of certain information with respect to controlled products. The obligation on a supplier to provide the chemical identity of a controlled product is an example of an exchange of information which should take place under this system.[208] This is a type of right to know legislation about the products that are being supplied to and used at work sites and is important in the event that a worker is exposed to a controlled product and requires emergency medical treatment. This body of law is tied as well to the federal *Hazardous Materials Information Review Act*[209] which establishes a commission with powers to deal with trade secret issues regarding the ingredients in products. As a result of the co-ordination of federal and provincial laws, however, all workplaces in Canada where controlled products are used are subject to the same rules. The commission

---

[204] As well as the *Controlled Products Regulations*, S.O.R./88-66.

[205] This covers items such as compressed gas, poisonous materials and corrosive materials. Products that are regulated under the federal: *Explosives Act*, R.S.C. 1985, c. E-17; the *Food and Drugs Act*, R.S.C. 1985, c. F-27; *Pest Control Products Act*, R.S.C. 1985, c. P-9; *Nuclear Safety and Control Act*, S.C. 1997, c. 9; and *Tobacco Act*, S.C. 1997, c. 13 are excluded from the application of the *Hazardous Products Act*. Hazardous waste, and the consumer products regulated in Part II of Schedule I, wood or wood products and manufactured articles are also excluded from the application of this section of the *Hazardous Products Act*.

[206] *Hazardous Products Act*, R.S.C. 1985, c. H-3, s. 28(1) provides penalties for contravention of the Act or regulations. Summary conviction offences are liable to a fine of up to $100,000 or imprisonment of up to six months or both. Indictable offences are liable to a fine of up to $1 million or imprisonment up to two years or both.

[207] The *Occupational Health and Safety Regulation*, Alta. Reg. 62/2003 of Alberta, for example, incorporates federal regulations into the Act. According to s. 2: "For the purposes of section 1(c) of the Act, a product, material or substance specified by the *Controlled Products Regulations* made pursuant to paragraph 15(1)(a) of the *Hazardous Products Act* (Canada) to be included in any of the classes listed in Schedule II to the *Hazardous Products Act* (Canada) is designated as a controlled product."

[208] See the *Controlled Products Regulation*, S.O.R./88-66 under the *Hazardous Products Act*, R.S.C. 1985, c. H-3 and the following website: <http://www.ccohs.ca/oshanswers/legisl/msdss.html> for information such as "What is a Material Safety Data Sheet?". Essentially, it is a document that contains information about chemical products, how to work safely with them and the potential effects on health of these products. These sheets are the documents which are required for designated products as a result of the above legislation.

[209] *Hazardous Materials Information Review Act*, R.S.C. 1985, c. 24 (3rd Supp.). See also the *Hazardous Materials Information Review Regulations*, S.O.R./88-456.

established under the federal Act also has powers as may be conferred on it by any province under their own occupational health and safety legislation, so that there is one system in place (and not 14) to deal with issues that arise. This integrated system is referred to as the Workplace Hazardous Materials Information System ("WHMIS").[210]

(e) Safe Buildings

In Canada, as with a number of areas already discussed, the federal, provincial and municipal levels of government all play a role in developing the regulations that are ultimately in place to regulate buildings and their systems. The aspects covered are diverse and include rules regarding design, manufacture, construction, installation, operation, and the maintenance of buildings and various systems (for example, fire, electrical, gas and plumbing).

On the federal scene, the Canadian Commission on Building and Fire Codes ("CCBFC") has developed six model codes for construction and fire, including the National Building Code of Canada.[211] Members are appointed by the National Research Council. They "receive policy advice from the Provincial/Territorial Policy Advisory Committee on Codes ("PTPACC") which is made up of representatives from the provincial and territorial ministries responsible for building, plumbing and fire safety regulation".[212] This gives the provinces and territories the ability to provide input into the model codes. "The National Research Council of Canada established the Associate Committee on the National Building Code in the 1940s and the Associate Committee on the National Fire Code in 1956 to encourage uniformity of building and fire regulations throughout Canada. These two committees were replaced by the Canadian Commission on Building and Fire Codes in 1991." Legislation is in the realm of the provinces.[213] However, the legislation and codes are often enforced in part by municipalities.

What is particularly interesting from a public health perspective is the power that can be wielded in the name of injury prevention, not through building codes and legislation specifically, but through public health statutes. For example, in Alberta's *Public Health Act*,[214] Executive Officers can become involved with enforcing safe standards regarding buildings — even where the premises were constructed according to the

---

[210]   See "WHMIS – General", online: <http://www.ccohs.ca/oshanswers/legisl/intro_whmis.html>.

[211]   See online: <http://www.nationalcodes.ca/ncd_home_e.shtml> for background information on the development of the Codes.

[212]   See online: <http://www.nationalcodes.ca/ccbfc/index_e.shtml>.

[213]   See, for example, Alberta's *Safety Codes Act*, R.S.A. 2000, c. S-1.

[214]   *Public Health Act*, R.S.A. 2000, c. P-37.

codes that existed at the time. This is done pursuant to s. 62 whereby orders may be issued if there are "reasonable and probable grounds to believe that a nuisance exists" on either public or private property.[215] Orders that may be made under this section are vast and include a number of different powers, including the power to require work done. "Nuisance" is defined broadly as "a condition that is or that might become injurious or dangerous to the public health ...".[216] "Public health" is not defined and thus need not be interpreted narrowly. As set out in a recent decision of the Public Health Appeal Board, Boardwalk Equities Inc. had been ordered by an Executive Officer under s. 62 to alter the balusters of the guards around stairs and dining areas so that the spacing between them was narrower. A complaint had been made about the railings and the safety concerns included the possibility that a child could slip his or her head through the spaces and be injured by this. The Officer ordered that this be rectified even though at the time that the building was constructed the railings met code. The decision of the Officer was upheld on appeal to the Public Health Appeal Board,[217] and their decision was also upheld on judicial review.[218] A subsequent application for a declaration that particular sections of the *Housing Regulation*[219] and the *Minimum Housing and Health Standards*,[220] both created pursuant to the *Public Health Act*,[221] were *ultra vires* the power of the Lieutenant Governor in Council under the legislation was dismissed,[222] and this was also upheld on appeal.[223]

IX. TORT LITIGATION AND INJURY CONTROL

Much of this chapter has focused on the measures taken by governments to control injury through legislation. However, statutory and regulatory measures are not the only legal mechanisms which can be used as tools to control injury. As discussed in Professor Renke's chapter in

---

[215] *Ibid.*, s. 62(1).
[216] *Ibid.*, s. 1(ee).
[217] In the matter of an appeal to the Public Health Appeal Board by Boardwalk Equities Inc. from the Executive Officer's Order Issued by the Capital Health Authority on June 17, 2003, Appeal No.: 07/2003, Hearing dates: February 9 and 10, and April 21, 2004.
[218] *Boardwalk Equities Inc. v. Capital Health Authority*, [2005] A.J. No. 41, 378 A.R. 117, 2005 ABQB 34 (Alta. Q.B.).
[219] *Housing Regulation*, Alta. Reg. 173/99.
[220] *Minumum Housing and Health Standards* created pursuant to s. 4 of the *Housing Regulation*, Alta. Reg. 173/99.
[221] *Public Health Act*, R.S.A. 2000, c. P-37.
[222] *BPCL Holdings Inc. v. Alberta*, [2006] A.J. No. 1287, 2006 ABQB 757 (Alta. Q.B.), aff'd [2008] A.J. No. 451 (Alta. C.A.). It had been argued, in part, by the applicants that the provisions in question (housing standards) lacked a connection to public health. Justice Slatter disagreed.
[223] *BPCL Holdings Inc. v. Alberta*, [2008] A.J. No. 451, 429 A.R. 311, 2008 ABCA 153 (Alta. C.A.).

this book, "Criminal Justice and Public Health" (Chapter 13), criminal law sets out to prevent injury and promote health, and may be effective as one weapon in the arsenal against injury. Civil litigation in the courts is another, and it sometimes provides the means to effect changes in the behaviour of individuals or businesses to prevent injury. In particular, tort actions have served as key to redress injuries that have been suffered, with the additional aim of deterring future conduct which could perpetrate further harm.

What is a tort? Justice Cory of the Supreme Court of Canada defined it in the following way:

> It provides a means whereby compensation, usually in the form of damages, may be paid for injuries suffered by a party as a result of the wrongful conduct of others. It may encompass damages for personal injury suffered, for example, in a motor vehicle accident or as a result of falling in dangerous premises ... A primary object of the law of tort is to provide compensation to persons who are injured as a result of the actions of others.[224]

If tort law is to compensate an already injured party, how does it prevent injury? A look at the aims of tort law can be helpful in recognizing its potential application in this regard. Some of the purposes have been set out by Professor Lewis Klar as follows:[225] (1) to compensate those injured through the fault of others; (2) to provide justice (to hold accountable those whose actions have injured another); (3) to deter others from acting in a certain injurious manner (the prospect of having to pay substantial compensation for undesirable conduct such as drinking, driving and injuring others as a result has been argued to have a deterrent effect); (4) to educate (a particular judgment can let society, or a specific segment of it, know that certain conduct is no longer deemed acceptable);[226] and (5) as an ombudsman: "[tort law] can be used to apply pressure upon those who wield political, economic or intellectual power".[227] In addition to these, the goal of tort law has been expressly described as the "reduction of the occurrence, and severity, of injury-

---

[224]   *Hall v. Hebert*, [1993] S.C.J. No. 51, [1993] 2 S.C.R. 159, 15 C.C.L.T (2d) 93 at 118 (S.C.C.).

[225]   Lewis Klar, *Tort Law*, 3d ed. (Toronto: Thomson Carswell, 2003) at 9-18.

[226]   An example is liability of commercial hosts. With respect to commercial host liability, see: *Menow v. Jordan House Ltd.*, [1973] S.C.J. No. 80, [1974] S.C.R. 239 (S.C.C.) and *Stewart v. Pettie*, [1995] S.C.J. No. 3, [1995] 1 S.C.R. 131 (S.C.C.). Two recent examples of liability being imposed on a commercial host are: *Holton v. MacKinnon*, [2005] B.C.J. No. 57 (B.C.S.C.) and *Laface v. McWilliams*, [2005] B.C.J. No. 470, 2005 BCSC 291 (B.C.S.C.), aff'd *Laface v. Boknows Hotels Inc. and McWilliams*, [2006] B.C.J. No. 1111, 2006 BCCA 227 (B.C.C.A.).

[227]   Allen M. Linden, *Canadian Tort Law*, 7th ed. (Markham, Ont.: Butterworths, 2001) at 22.

causing events".[228] How effective tort litigation has been in this regard is a matter of controversy[229] and the degree to which it is seen as an effective instrument to this end varies. However, there is little doubt that in certain instances, at least, court decisions have led the way to improved safety conditions.[230]

Although there are a number of tort actions one can commence depending on the circumstances, the tort action that is used in the majority of cases involving injury is the negligence action.[231] In such a case, the onus is on the plaintiff to prove four elements on a balance of probabilities: (1) that the defendant owed her a duty of care; (2) that he breached the standard of care expected of him; (3) that the plaintiff has sustained injuries; and (4) that these injuries are as a result of the conduct of the defendant.[232] There are also a number of defences which may be used on behalf of defendants to eliminate or reduce their liability, even where the plaintiff is able to establish the listed elements. The key defence is that of contributory negligence (where the plaintiff is partially liable due to their actions).[233]

There are, of course, a number of limitations to tort actions. To begin with, it is often very difficult for the plaintiff to establish the element of causation, particularly in certain types of tort actions.[234] Tort litigation is also expensive and costs to the parties can be an enormous

---

[228] "Towards a Jurisprudence of Injury: The Continuing Creation of a System of Substantive Justice in American Tort Law, 1984" (by Special Committee on the Tort Liability System in its report to the American Bar Association).

[229] There have been a number of critiques of tort law and a fault-based compensation system. See, for example, Sugarman, "Doing Away with Tort Law" (1985) 73 Calif. L. Rev. 555.

[230] See N. Weber, *Product Liability: The Corporate Response* (1987), The Conference Board Report No. 893 at 21, cited in Lewis Klar, *Tort Law*, 3d ed. (Toronto: Thomson Carswell, 2003) at 15.

[231] For a discussion of the complex area of tort law, and of other types of tort actions, L. Klar, *Tort Law*, 3d ed. (Toronto: Carswell, 2003) and Allen M. Linden, *Canadian Tort Law*, 7th ed. (Markham, Ont.: Butterworths, 2001).

[232] This is an oversimplification of what must be established in a negligence action. For a detailed discussion of these elements, as well as other types of tort actions, see Klar, *Tort Law, ibid.*; Linden, *Canadian Tort Law, ibid.*

[233] For example, even where a plaintiff has established that the defendant driver is liable for the motor vehicle collision which has caused her injuries, she may be found partially liable due to her failure to wear a seatbelt where this has likely contributed to her injuries: *Galaske v. O'Donnell*, [1994] S.C.J. No. 28, 112 D.L.R. (4th) 109 (S.C.C.).

[234] See the discussion of mass exposure or toxic tort litigation in Lawrence O. Gostin, *Public Health Law: Power, Duty, Restraint* (Berkeley and Los Angeles, CA; London, U.K.: University of California Press, 2000) at 282-88. See also Ellen I. Picard & Gerald B. Robertson, *Legal Liability of Doctors and Hospitals in Canada*, 4th ed. (Toronto: Thomson Carswell, 2007) at 270: "Often it is extremely difficult for the patient to prove... the actual cause of the injury." See also Gerald B. Robertson, "Informed Consent Ten Years Later: The impact of Reibl v. Hughes" (1991) 70 Can. Bar Rev. 423 at 447.

drawback, especially for those without the resources to pursue (or defend) their claims. This type of legal action is also reactive rather than proactive. Someone has already been harmed and although there may be a deterrent effect as already mentioned which may prevent future injury, it is too late for the injured plaintiff in the case at hand.[235]

Most injuries occur at home, on the road or at work. These venues have largely been covered in the overview of legislation. In considering tort actions, and negligence actions specifically, some key areas are worthy of brief mention as they are key sources of common law in this area.

(a) Product Safety Litigation

Product safety, or the lack thereof, has been a huge source of tort litigation in the area of injury. In the United States, these types of cases are decided on the basis of strict liability.[236] However, this is not the case in Canada where these issues are still considered on the basis of negligence.[237] As Justice Linden has put it in his *Canadian Tort Law*, "the protection afforded a Canadian consumer by Canadian courts is less than that accorded to an American consumer by United States civil courts".[238] In Canada, in a tort action related to product liability, there are three main duties owed to purchasers of products (as well as other reasonably foreseeable users): those related to (1) design,[239] (2) manufacture, and (3) marketing.[240] Tort law has been a means to prod manufacturers to create

---

[235] For a discussion of other drawbacks, see Gostin's *Public Health Law, ibid.*, at 303-305.

[236] For a general discussion of strict liability in the context of tort law, see Lewis Klar, *Tort Law*, 3d ed. (Toronto: Thomson Carswell, 2003) at 553-97.

[237] See Jamie Cassels & Craig E. Jones, *The Law of Large-Scale Claims: Product Liability, Mass Torts, and Complex Litigation in Canada* (Toronto: Irwin Law, 2005). See also Lara Khoury, "Causation and Health in Medical, Environmental and Product Liability" (2007) 25 Windsor Y.B. Access Just. 135 (for a discussion of causation in the area).

[238] Allen M. Linden, *Canadian Tort Law*, 7th ed. (Markham, Ont.: Butterworths, 2001) at 569.

[239] For example, the design of defective car brakes led to liability in *Phillips v. Ford Motor Co.*, [1970] O.J. No. 1484, [1970] 2 O.R. 714 (Ont. H.C.J.), rev'd [1971] O.J. No. 1564, [1971] 2 O.R. 637 (Ont. C.A.).

[240] See Lewis Klar, *Tort Law*, 3d ed. (Toronto: Thomson Carswell, 2003) at 331-43; See particularly *Hollis v. Dow Corning Corp.*, [1995] S.C.J. No. 104, [1995] 4 S.C.R. 634 (S.C.C.) in which breast implants ruptured, injuring the plaintiff. She sued both the manufacturer and the physicians. At trial, the judge found that the implants had been negligently manufactured. This was overturned at the B.C. Court of Appeal. However, they upheld the portion of the trial decision which found the manufacturer liable for a failure to warn of the inherent risks. This was despite the fact that the "learned intermediary", the physician, had also failed to warn the patient of the risks. As the manufacturer had not passed on the information to the physician, they could not rely on this principle to avoid liability.

safer products where direct regulation by government has failed to do so. As aptly put by Vernick *et al.*:

> Product liability continues to be an important tool for the prevention of injuries. Although it is sometimes difficult to attribute specific changes to specific cases, the weight of the anecdotal and empirical evidence suggests that litigation has made some products safer. Prevention occurs through the imposition of monetary damages, media attention, information gathering, and litigation's ability to foster subsequent legislative or regulatory change.[241]

(b) Occupiers' Liability

For those injured as a result of dangers on premises (such as icy sidewalks), the negligence action is again a source of compensation for injuries suffered, but also an incentive to property owners and occupiers to maintain their property in a manner that is safe for those coming onto it. It is important in part "given the large number of injuries and deaths caused by accidents occurring on private premises ...".[242] Generally, whether by way of the common law or a statute, a duty has been found to be owed by occupiers to those coming onto their property (the duty varying with the role of the person entering; *i.e.*, visitor versus trespasser). While the common law has developed a number of rules dealing with this area of the law, in many provinces in Canada, occupiers' liability legislation has become extremely important as it has supplanted a number of the precedents found in past decisions of the courts. For example, Alberta's *Occupiers' Liability Act* sets out a statutory duty on occupiers to visitors to "take such care as in all the circumstances of the case is reasonable to see that the visitor will be reasonably safe in using the premises for the purposes for which the visitor is invited or permitted by the occupier to be there or is permitted by law to be there".[243] While a discussion of this area is beyond the abilities of this chapter, it is important to raise awareness of the significance of this area for injury and tort litigation.[244]

(c) Motor Vehicle Collisions

Negligence actions as a result of injuries sustained in motor vehicle collisions have resulted in an enormous body of reported legal decisions.

---

[241] "Role of Litigation in Preventing Product-related Injuries" in Jon Vernick *et al.*, *Epidemiologic Reviews*, vol. 25 (2003) at 90-98.

[242] Lewis Klar, *Tort Law*, 3d ed. (Toronto: Thomson Carswell, 2003) at 525.

[243] *Occupiers' Liability Act*, R.S.A. 2000, c. O-4, s. 5.

[244] For an analysis of the law in this area, see Lewis Klar, *Tort Law*, 3d ed. (Toronto: Thomson Carswell, 2003) at c. 15; A.M. Linden, L. Klar & B. Feldthusen, *Canadian Tort Law: Cases, Notes & Materials*, 12th ed. (Markham, Ont.: LexisNexis Butterworths, 2004) at c. 14.

In addition to the potential of facing criminal charges for certain driving behaviour and the prospect of an increase in insurance premiums for being at-fault for a collision, the real possibility, and even likelihood, that a civil claim will be launched in the event of injuries occurring can arguably serve as one more reason for people to drive cautiously and within certain reasonable limits. In most cases, the lawsuit is commenced against the driver and owner of the vehicle. However, in certain situations, other defendants may be included. For example, the potential for liability as a result of injuries caused because of drinking and driving has been extended beyond the driver and owner (and the passenger who fails to wear his seatbelt) to those who have served the driver the alcohol consumed.[245]

However, it is important to note that in this massive area of tort and motor vehicle collisions, there has been significant movement by certain jurisdictions away from a scheme which compensates injured parties on the basis of fault. In Alberta, for example, while negligence actions are alive and well, certain limited no-fault benefits are available and typically cover limited medical expenses and loss of income. However, in certain other provinces, such as Ontario, Québec and Manitoba, tort actions have been severely restricted or done away with altogether for those injured in automobile collisions.[246]

(d)   Workers Compensation Legislation

In the past, tort actions could be launched against employers or co-workers as a result of an employee being injured or killed at the workplace. This has been changed across Canada with the introduction of workers compensation legislation. All of the provinces and territories now have this type of statutory arrangement. Essentially, it provides a scheme whereby employers are required to pay into this system,[247] which in turn provides payment to workers or their families who are injured or killed at work.[248] In return for the requirement to financially support this system, employers (and others) are immune from tort litigation launched by

---

[245]   *Jordan House Ltd. v. Menow*, [1973] S.C.J. No. 80, 38 D.L.R. (3d) 105 (S.C.C.); *Stewart v. Pettie*, [1995] S.C.J. No. 3, 121 D.L.R. (4th) 222 (S.C.C.).

[246]   For an explanation of the variations, see A.M. Linden, L. Klar & B. Feldthusen, *Canadian Tort Law: Cases, Notes & Materials*, 12th ed. (Markham, Ont.: LexisNexis Butterworths, 2004) at 779-91.

[247]   *Workers Compensation Act*, R.S.A. 2000, c. W-15, s. 94: employers that fall under the Act must pay premiums.

[248]   *Ibid.*, s. 14: the Act applies to all workers and employers in all industries in Alberta unless they have been deemed exempt.

workers or their families for damages.[249] The Acts establish processes for assessing injury or disability, and whether in a given situation an employee is entitled to compensation and expenses. The Acts also set out how assessments on employers will be made. The assessment may include an amount to "enable the Board to carry out its obligations under ... the Occupational Health and Safety Act".[250] Practically speaking, if employers fail to provide safe workplaces, their WCB costs will increase.

(e)   Patient Safety and Medical Malpractice Actions

Awareness is increasing that the health care system itself, the system designed to ameliorate harm and injury, can in fact be a source of injury to the patients it serves. While it is outside the scope of this chapter to survey this area, it is important to mention it briefly as a field of study in the area of injury control. The subject came under closer scrutiny with the publication of the Institute of Medicine's report, *To Err is Human: Building a Safer Health System*[251] which garnered the attention of the media and many others and drew attention to the fact that medical error was widespread (perhaps more so than previously acknowledged or realized) and greater attention needed to be paid to the reduction of such error. Largely as a result of that report, research has been burgeoning to assess the magnitude of this problem. In the Canadian context, *The Canadian Adverse Events Study: The Incidence of Adverse Events Among Hospital Patients in Canada* was published in 2004, setting out that "an estimated 7.5% of patients admitted to acute care hospitals in Canada in the fiscal year 2000 experienced 1 or more [adverse events]" and that "36.9% of these patients were judged to have highly preventable [adverse events]".[252] Other related research undertakings are underway funded by a variety of sources, one of the most noteworthy being the Canadian Patient Safety Institute, created and funded by Health Canada to work on initiatives in the area.[253]

---

[249]   *Ibid.*, s. 21: "no action lies for the recovery of compensation under this Act and all claims for compensation shall be determined by the Board". Neither the worker, his or her legal representative nor his or her dependants can sue the employer; s. 23. if an accident occurs, and this Act applies, the worker is entitled to compensation under this Act but they cannot sue the employer or any other worker (whether injured or dead).

[250]   *Ibid.*, s. 99 is used as an example though all provinces and territories have a similar scheme it is believed.

[251]   Committee on Quality of Health Care in America, Institute of Medicine (Washington: National Academy Press, 1999).

[252]   G. Ross Baker *et al.*, "The Canadian Adverse Events Study: The Incidence of Adverse Events Among Hospital Patients in Canada" (2004) 170:11 C.M.A.J. 1678 at 1683; see also Canadian Institute of Health Information Fifth Annual Report, "Health Care in Canada 2004" (9 June 2004).

[253]   Canadian Patient Safety Institute, online: <http://www.cpsi-icsp.ca>.

The tort system has been the traditional means, in large measure, for individuals to seek compensation for injuries they have suffered as a result of conduct on the part of health professionals and the institutions they work in. Medical malpractice actions have been one of the main tools for addressing these types of injuries.[254] Other means have included hearings and disciplinary proceedings conducted by the self-regulating bodies governing particular health care professionals (physicians, for example). Tort reform has been examined in the past in Canada[255] and, indeed, is part of the focus of a recently completed report for Health Canada.[256] However, as that report states, little reform is likely due to a lack of will on the part of either the public or politicians.[257] Given the likelihood that injuries will continue to be compensated for via the tort system, some of the most important legal issues that are the subject of much recent attention include the duty to disclose adverse events to patients,[258] growing obligations to

---

[254] See Ellen I. Picard & Gerald B. Robertson, *Legal liability of doctors and hospitals in Canada*, 4th ed. (Toronto: Thomson Carswell, 2007) for an excellent analysis of medical malpractice litigation in Canada.

[255] For an early example, see J.R.S. Pritchard, "Liability and Compensation in Health Care" (A Report to the Conference of Deputy Ministers of Health of the Federal/Provincial/ Territorial Review on Liability and Compensation Issues in Health Care) (Toronto: University of Toronto Press, 1990).

[256] Joan M. Gilmour, *Patient Safety, Medical Error and Tort Law: An International Comparison* (Toronto: York University, 2006).

[257] *Ibid.*, at 75.

[258] Regarding legal obligations to disclose, see Gerald Robertson, "When Things Go Wrong: The Duty to Disclose Medical Error" (2002) 28 Queens L. J. 353 at 362; Philip C. Hebert, Alex V. Levin & Gerald Robertson, "Bioethics for Clinicians: Disclosure of Medical Error" (2001) 164:4 C.M.A.J. 509; Gerald B. Robertson for the Commission of Inquiry on Hormone Receptor Testing, "The Legal Duty of Physicians to Disclose Medical Errors" (2008); and Tracey M. Bailey & Nola M. Ries, "Legal Issues in Patient Safety: The Example of Nosocomial Infection" (2005) 8 Healthcare Quarterly Special Issue on Patient Safety 140-45. Regarding ethical duties, see Canadian Medical Association, *Revised Code of Ethics*, s. 14; David Spurgeon, "Quebec Doctors Must Tell Patients About Medical 'Accidents'" (2002) 325 BMJ 1192. For examples of guidelines of regulatory bodies for physicians in Canada: College of Physicians and Surgeons of Saskatchewan recently made it explicit that physicians are expected to disclose errors made to patients; Colleges in Québec, Manitoba and Ontario also have policies regarding duty to disclose harm. See also College of Physicians and Surgeons of Saskatchewan, "Policy: Physician Disclosure of Adverse Events and Errors that Occur in the Course of Patient Care" (April 2002); College of Physicians and Surgeons of Ontario, "Disclosure of Harm – #1-03" (February 2003), online: <http://www.cpso.on.ca/Policies/disclosure.htm>; College of Physicians and Surgeons of Manitoba, "Physician Disclosure of Harm that Occurs in the Course of Patient Care – 169", online: <http://www.cpsm.mb.ca/statements/169.php>; Québec, *Code of Ethics of Physicians*, s. 56, online: <http://www.cmq.org/DocumentLibrary/UploadedContents/CmsDocuments/ cmqcodedeontoan.pdf>. For other disclosure guidelines recently developed, see: Health Quality Council of Alberta, "Disclosure of Harm to Patients and Families" (2006), online: <www.hqca.ca>; Canadian Patient Safety Institute, "Canadian Disclosure Guidelines" (2008), online: <http://www.patientsafetyinstitute.ca/uploadedFiles/Resources/cpsi_english._april28.pdf>; The Canadian Medical Protective Association, "Communicating with your patient about harm: Disclosure of Adverse Events" (2008).

report such events to third parties,[259] and the legal effect of apologies provided after an adverse event.[260]

X.   EVALUATING THE EFFECTIVENESS OF LAW AND OTHER MEASURES

Governments can pass laws, and they and others can educate and work to create safer products and environments. However, how does one assess whether these efforts are working and if there are more effective means, or more cost-effective ways of dealing with the burden of injury? One of the key things that must be done is the gathering of information to study injury. Surveillance systems for infectious diseases have existed for decades, monitoring the progression of diseases and aiding the development of prevention programs for populations at risk. Although injuries are a major burden on the health care system, surveillance systems to monitor and control the occurrence of injuries are only in their infancy. As awareness of the predictable and preventable nature of injuries continues to grow, and as injuries are viewed less as "accidents" and "acts of God", efforts to develop injury surveillance systems and injury prevention and control programs are increasing in number and sophistication.

Accurate, timely and readily available information is the cornerstone for effective injury control efforts. Many of the injuries that require medical attention, however, are never uploaded into any comprehensive database for use in injury surveillance systems. Estimates suggest that up to 25 per cent of all injuries are treated by either a clinic or a physician[261] and never reach an ED (although potentially this percentage could be much higher). Although many injured patients present to their family physician or primary care clinic, the relevant injury data is either not entered into an electronic system, or if it is, this data is never uploaded to any surveillance database. Even medical record systems installed at many hospitals may not be accessible to regular surveillance efforts. This failure to record and/or access such a potential wealth of surveillance data in a standardized and accessible format impedes assessment of a community's

---

[259]   Saskatchewan was the first province to enact legislation requiring mandatory reporting of medical errors to the Department of Health of the province: *Regional Health Services Act*, S.S. 2002, c. R-8.2, s. 58; see also *An Act respecting health services and social services* R.S.Q. c. S-4.2, s. 8.

[260]   For a discussion of recent legislative initiatives in Canada, see Tracey M. Bailey, Elizabeth C. Robertson & Gergely Hegedus, "Erecting Legal Barriers: New Apology Laws in Canada and the Patient Safety Movement: Useful Legislation or a Misguided Approach?" (2007) 28:2 Health Law in Canada 33.

[261]   J.M. Williams *et al.*, "The Emergency Department Log as a Simple Injury-Surveillance Tool" (1995) 25 Ann. Emerg. Med. 686 at 691.

health care needs and "limits the ability to scientifically assess the effectiveness of interventions".[262] Most injury data are still composed of mortality and hospitalization statistics, although such statistics represent only the "tip of the iceberg". For every childhood injury resulting in death, there are 45 hospitalizations and 1,300 Emergency Department ("ED") visits.[263] Furthermore, the impact of an injury spreads beyond the injured person to family, employers, the health care system and the community.[264] Because the vast majority of injuries do not result in death, injury surveillance based on mortality statistics alone is clearly inadequate. It has been shown that the patterns of occurrence and the associated risk factors are different for fatal and nonfatal injuries,[265] and injury surveillance systems must be made sensitive to that fact. Williams *et al.* state: "although one goal of injury control and prevention research is capture of the underlying cause of injury and the existence of co-morbid factors associated with various injury events, this type of information is the most difficult and costly to collect".[266]

There are several Canadian injury surveillance systems in operation today. For example, the Health Surveillance and Epidemiology Division of the Public Health Agency of Canada hosts a web site called "Injury Surveillance Online" from which injury researchers and other stakeholders can obtain the most recently available nationwide injury statistics. Data on "Injury Surveillance Online" is collected from a variety of sources, including:

- Statistics Canada (mortality)
- Canadian Institute for Health for Health Information (hospitalization), and
- Injury and Child Maltreatment Section of the Public Health Agency (emergency department visits).

Although a very good source of the most recently available data, there is usually a two- to three-year time lag for analyzed data to be posted

---

[262] H.G. Garrison, C.W. Runyan, J.E. Tintinalli *et al.*, "Emergency Department Surveillance: An Examination of Issues and a Proposal for a National Strategy" (1994) 24 Ann. Emerg. Med. 849.

[263] S.S. Gallagher *et al.*, "The Incidence of Injuries Amongst 87,000 Massachusetts Children and Adolescents: Results of the 1980-81 Statewide Childhood Injury Prevention Program Surveillance System" (1984) 74 American Journal of Public Health 1340 at 1347.

[264] L.H. Francescutti, "Injury Control: Are You Accountable?" (1997) Canadian Journal of CME 109 at 119.

[265] C.W. Runyan & J.M. Bowling, "Emergency Department Record Keeping and the Potential for Injury Surveillance" (1992) 32 J Trauma 187 at 189.

[266] J.M. Williams *et al.*, "Development of an Emergency Department-Based Injury Surveillance System" (1996) 27 Ann. Emerg. Med. 59 at 65.

due to the complexities of collecting, analyzing and synthesizing data from the provinces and territories.

The Canadian Hospitals Injury Reporting and Prevention Program ("CHIRPP") was initiated in 1990 to investigate the rates, etiology and outcomes of injuries to children and is a computerized information system that collects and analyzes data on injuries and poisonings from the emergency departments of 16 hospitals across Canada. The primary focus of the program is on children and youth 19 years of age and younger.

The Canadian Agricultural Injury Surveillance Program ("CAISP"), established in 1995, is a national program funded by the Canadian Agriculture Safety Program ("CASP"). The purpose of CAISP is to collect and interpret information on agricultural injuries from across Canada. CAISP has worked towards ensuring that agricultural injury data is collected, coded and disseminated in a standard manner across Canada. The collaborative approach adopted by CAISP results in a more efficient use of surveillance resources and more effective information dissemination.

As injury data collection continues to benefit from growing adoption of electronic reporting tools and standardized reporting formats, the timeliness and ease of access to injury data will continue to improve. These technological changes will enable even more meaningful research to be conducted to evaluate and determine the most effective injury control methodologies.

XI. BARRIERS TO SUCCESS

It is clearly established that injuries have a major health and financial impact on society, yet there is no concerted and high-profile urgency attached to injury control as there is to other diseases such as diabetes and breast cancer. This is especially surprising since injuries are the major killers of people under age 44. Although Canada has seen a slight decline in injury rates over the past several years, significant reductions in injuries are not occurring as they are in countries such as Sweden.[267]

Despite all the data pointing to injuries as a very high-priority health concern, there is little evidence of serious concerted commitment and action to address the issue. There seem to be several barriers to the success of injury control measures. Perhaps one of the biggest barriers to success is the continued lack of awareness of the true nature of injuries.

---

[267] Barbara Sibbald, "Canada Ranks in Middle in Child-Injury Mortality Rate, Report Indicates" (2001) 164:10 C.M.A.J. 1483.

Despite media campaign after media campaign, the pervasive attitude is that injuries are "accidents" — that there is not much we can do to prevent them. If injuries are (incorrectly) deemed to be unpredictable (and therefore unpreventable) events, people may be unwilling to endure the "inconvenience" of making better choices to reduce their risk of injury. Moreover, people tend to think that "injuries won't happen to them", and that they somehow are invincible. This may be due in part to the very mixed messages people receive from society and through the media. Invariably, risky behaviour is portrayed as exciting and attractive in the media, whereas safety-oriented behaviour most often is spotlighted in the opposite fashion. The sobering message of anti-drinking-and-driving commercials somehow seems to be lost in the noise of the beer commercials.

Another potential barrier is our social, political and legal devotion to the autonomy of the individual. Invariably, legal measures taken to control injury restrict personal freedoms. This raises legal and ethical issues regarding when such restrictions are appropriate and whether less-restrictive means can be used as effectively with less impact on the ability of the individual to make personal choices. As has been seen with past legislative measures (seatbelt legislation, for example), the public has been reluctant to embrace such measures — at least until the effectiveness of them has been established.[268] A common argument that has been made is that one of the "costs" that should always be considered when assessing a measure is the loss to the individual of their personal freedom.[269] Injury prevention strategies are often trying to protect people from their own behaviour, however, and this is seen as paternalistic. There are several counter-arguments to this which have been used, including[270] the lack of information or awareness individuals may or may not have before deciding on whether or not to take a risk; the exposure of society to harm, at least indirectly (by costs to the health system and elsewhere); lost productivity to society when someone is injured; and cases where the benefits to society outweigh the costs.

Picking up on one of those counter-arguments, another barrier to the success of injury prevention is the fact that regulation costs money. A cost

---

[268]   "Opposition to mandatory seatbelt laws virtually evaporated in the face of unequivocal evidence that the safety gains (lives saved and disability avoided) far outweighed the costs of enforcement and the slight reduction in freedom", Richard J. Bonnie & Bernard Guyer, "Injury as a Field of Public Health: Achievements and Controversies" (2002) 30:2 J.L. Med. & Ethics 274 at 276.

[269]   R.J. Bonnie, "The Efficacy of Law as a Paternalistic Instrument" in G. Melton, ed., *Nebraska Symposium on Human Motivation, 1985: Law as a Behavioral Instrument* (Lincoln: University of Nebraska Press, 1986) at 131-211.

[270]   Richard J. Bonnie & Bernard Guyer, "Injury as a Field of Public Health: Achievements and Controversies" (2002) 30:2 J.L. Med. & Ethics 274 at 275-76.

benefit analysis should be made with respect to measures taken by governments (and this is often attempted). However, the assessment may not always be accurate due to a lack of information. As well, other measures may be seen as more cost-effective. Education is often less expensive than legal regulation; however, it is often not as effective.

There are many injury prevention programs, ranging from school-based playground safety slogans to workplace occupational injury reduction efforts. Yet unlike cardiovascular disease or diabetes, there is no national co-ordinating centre to help orchestrate and provide resources for ongoing injury prevention and control research and programs. All the groups and organizations working in isolation or in small clusters to reduce injuries are up against an immense barrage of influences that promote (or at least condone) behaviour that puts people at risk of injury. Injury control lacks a large lobby group and suffers from a lack of leadership and co-ordination that only a national injury organization can provide. It is easy to know who to call in order to make a donation to diabetes or cancer research, but who should one call to make a donation to injury research?

Injuries need the same attention that has been afforded to diseases such as cancer, diabetes, and heart attack and stroke. The challenge before Canada today is to immediately develop a well-funded and implemented national injury control strategy; a strategy that would actively engage the provinces and territories at the local/municipal level. We need a strategy that will adapt the best elements from countries that have demonstrated previous success in reducing their burden of injury. Without such a strategy and commitment, injuries will continue to be the leading cause of death for Canadians under the age of 45.

XII. CONCLUSION

This chapter provides the reader with an introduction to the intricacies of public health law as it relates to the issues of injuries and their prevention. The debate will likely never cease as to where the right to personal choice and freedom ends and the law begins. One thing that is clear, however, is that legislators, like all injury stakeholders, should have but one goal in mind: to reduce the occurrence (and therefore cost) of injury in society. Public health law is a powerful tool when used in combination with the other intervention types; in fact, the law impacts upon all means of intervention to some degree or another. Legislators and other injury stakeholders must work together to ensure that the most effective legislation is introduced so as to have the greatest impact upon the reduction of injuries while ensuring the rights and freedoms of individuals to live, work and play in a safe, risk-reducing environment.

9

OBESITY AND THE LAW

Nola M. Ries and Barbara von Tigerstrom[*]

I.   INTRODUCTION

We live in an obesogenic era, where numerous factors conspire to promote unhealthy weight gain among significant portions of the population. Food is abundant and immense willpower is needed to resist ubiquitous temptation to over-consume. Work and recreation are largely sedentary for many who spend hours in front of computers to earn income and more hours in front of television screens in passive entertainment. The outcome of this typical, modern life of overeating and under-exercising is an epidemic of weight gain; there is a fundamental mismatch[1] between our physical needs and our "hostile food environment".[2]

Rising numbers of overweight and obese individuals, particularly among children, are a growing public health problem. Being overweight or obese is linked with numerous diseases, including type 2 diabetes, heart disease, hypertension and certain cancers. "[G]lobally, being either overweight or obese has been estimated to be the seventh most significant risk factor for mortality and the eighth most significant risk factor for

[*]   Portions of this chapter are reprinted from Nola M. Ries, "Piling on the Laws, Shedding the Pounds? The Use of Legal Tools to Address Obesity" (2008) Health L.J. (Suppl.) 101. The authors acknowledge funding support from the Canadian Institutes of Health Research, Grant # MOP81162.
[1]   We borrow the term "mismatch" from Peter Gluckman & Mark Hanson, *Mismatch: Why Our World No Longer Fits Our Bodies* (Oxford: Oxford University Press, 2006). See esp. pp. 158-77 for their discussion of obesity and metabolic mismatch.
[2]   We borrow this phrase from the testimony of Bruce Silverglade, Director of Legal Affairs, Center for Science in the Public Interest, before the U.S. House of Representatives, Committee on Government Reform, *Hearings of the Role of the Government in Combating Obesity* (3 June 2004) at 2, online: <http://www.cspinet.org/new/pdf/GovReftsy.pdf>.

disease."[3] Obesity may, in fact, increase morbidity more than poverty or smoking in some populations.[4]

Almost 60 per cent of Canadian adults are overweight or obese,[5] and obesity rates have increased dramatically among children in Canada.[6] An estimated 60 per cent of obese children aged 5 to 10 have at least one risk factor for cardiovascular disease, such as high cholesterol or blood pressure.[7] Children and adolescents who are overweight or obese today are likely to become obese adults and drive up rates of preventable conditions like coronary heart disease and associated health care costs and deaths.[8]

Obesity and related conditions have major economic impacts: they drive up public health care expenditures and have indirect economic costs

---

[3]   Nuffield Council on Bioethics, *Public Health: Ethical Issues* (London: Nuffield Council on Bioethics, 2007) at 82, citing A.D. Lopez *et al.*, "Global and Regional Burden of Disease and Risk Factors, 2001: Systematic Analysis of Population Health Data" (2006) 367 Lancet 1747. For a comprehensive overview of health concerns associated with obesity, see Tommy L.S. Visscher & Jacob C. Seidell, "The Public Health Impact of Obesity" (2001) 22 Annual Review of Public Health 355.

[4]   R. Sturm & K.B. Wells, "Does Obesity Contribute as much to Morbidity as Poverty or Smoking?" (2001) 115 Public Health 229. The authors conclude (at 234): "The association of obesity with chronic conditions and poorer quality of life is at least as high, if not higher, than the association of poverty, smoking, or drinking with chronic conditions and poorer quality of life. Moreover, the prevalence of obesity is higher than that of poverty, daily smoking, or heavy drinking."

[5]   Michael Tjepkema, "Measured Obesity: Adult Obesity in Canada", *Nutrition: Findings from the Canadian Community Health Survey*, Issue No. 1 (2005), online: Statistics Canada <http://www.statcan.ca/english/research/82-620-MIE/2005001/pdf/aobesity.pdf>.
Overweight refers to body mass index ("BMI") between 25 and 29.9, and obese refers to BMI above 30. Levels of morbid obesity in Canada (BMI above 40) increased 225 per cent between 1985 and 2003: P.T.Katzmarzyk & C. Mason, "Prevalence of Class I, II and III Obesity in Canada" (2006) 174:2 Canadian Medical Association Journal 156.

[6]   M.S. Tremblay *et al.*, "Temporal Trends in Overweight and Obesity in Canada, 1981–1996" (2002) 26:4 International Journal of Obesity 538. In childhood obesity, Canada ranks fifth out of 34 countries that are members of the Organisation for Economic Cooperation and Development (OECD). See Canada, House of Commons, Standing Committee on Health, *Healthy Weights for Healthy Kids*, 39th Parl., 1st Sess. (March 2007) (Chair: Rob Merrifield) at 1; online: <http://www.ccfn.ca/pdfs/HealthyWeightsForHealthyKids.pdf>.

[7]   Institute of Medicine, *Preventing Childhood Obesity: Health in the Balance* (Washington, D.C.: National Academies Press, 2004).

[8]   Kirsten Bibbins-Domingo *et al.*, "Adolescent Overweight and Future Adult Coronary Heart Disease" (2007) 357 New Eng. J. Med. 2371. The authors attribute over 100,000 excess deaths from coronary heart disease by 2036 to current rates of overweight adolescents. A retrospective study published in the same issue of this journal confirmed a positive association between overweight adolescents and a higher risk of coronary heart disease as adults: Jennifer L. Baker, Lina W. Olsen & Thorkild I.A. Sorensen, "Childhood Body-Mass Index and the Risk of Coronary Heart Disease in Adulthood" (2007) 357 New Eng. J. of Med. 2329.

in terms of lost productivity, disability and premature death.[9] Some fear that "[s]kyrocketing obesity levels may portend an epidemic of chronic diseases and related treatment costs that threaten to overwhelm the public and private sectors".[10] Annual total costs of obesity in Canada and the United States have been calculated respectively at $4.3 billion[11] and $139 billion.[12] It has been estimated in the United States that "[l]ower obesity rates alone could produce productivity gains of $254 billion and avoid $60 billion in treatment expenditures per year".[13]

Many factors interact in complex ways to affect body weight, including individual biological factors (genetic predisposition, age, sex); social, economic and cultural factors (income, education, cultural norms regarding food); lifestyle, behavioural and health factors (eating patterns, activity levels); and environmental factors (food availability and cost; community environment; industry behaviour, such as food marketing and labelling, menu items and serving sizes).[14] Considering the enormous costs associated with obesity, many levels of government — from municipalities to national departments of health — are turning much attention to regulatory and policy interventions that may be implemented to address some of these factors in an attempt to control this public health epidemic. Indeed, obesity has been termed the "new frontier of public health law".[15]

This chapter examines the use of legal tools to address rising rates of overweight and obesity. It begins with an overview of the role of regulation in public health and discusses justifications for legislative intervention to address health risks and problems. Arguments about the appropriate role of the state in regulating an area — food choices and body weight — that some consider a matter of personal responsibility are briefly considered. Discussion of regulatory interventions in this chapter

---

[9]   C.L. Birmingham et al., "The Cost of Obesity in Canada" (1999) 160:4 Canadian Medical Association Journal 483 and E. Finkelstein et al., "The Costs of Obesity Among Full-time Employees" (2005) American Journal of Health Promotion (September-October) 45.

[10]   Milken Institute, An Unhealthy America: The Economic Burden of Chronic Disease — Charting a New Course to Save Lives and Increase Productivity and Economic Growth (Santa Monica, CA: Milken Institute, 2007) at 3.

[11]   P.T. Katzmarzyk & I. Janssen, "The Economic Costs Associated with Physical Inactivity and Obesity in Canada: An Update" (2004) 29:1 Canadian Journal of Applied Physiology 90.

[12]   E. Finkelstein et al., "Economic Causes and Consequences of Obesity" (2005) 26 Annual Review of Public Health 239.

[13]   Milken Institute, An Unhealthy America: The Economic Burden of Chronic Disease — Charting a New Course to Save Lives and Increase Productivity and Economic Growth (Santa Monica, CA: Milken Institute, 2007) at 2.

[14]   Kim D. Raine, Overweight and Obesity in Canada: A Population Health Perspective (Ottawa: Canadian Institute for Health Information, 2004).

[15]   Michelle M. Mello, David M. Studdert & Troyen A. Brennan, "Obesity — The New Frontier of Public Health Law" (2006) 352 New Eng. J. Med. 2601.

focuses on those aimed at the food environment. Humans need food to survive but, increasingly, an overabundance of food, especially food that is calorie-dense and nutrient-poor, is contributing to conditions that have a negative impact on health and may even contribute to declining life expectancy.[16] Legislators in many jurisdictions are enacting laws to influence or control consumer food choices and food industry practices. These include rules and restrictions on food labelling, advertising, ingredients and access. Other regulatory interventions focus on physical activity (*e.g.*, mandating a specific number of daily minutes of physical activity in schools) and the built environment (*e.g.*, using zoning by-laws and urban planning measures to mandate bicycle and walking paths, parks and playgrounds and to restrict the location and/or number of fast-food outlets). This chapter does not focus on these latter interventions, but they have been addressed elsewhere.[17] Law as a tool to address obesity also includes litigation by private or public plaintiffs against food manufacturers or others who are alleged to engage in legally actionable conduct that promotes obesity. The chapter comments briefly on litigation as a public health strategy.

II.   THE ROLE OF REGULATION IN PUBLIC HEALTH

Governments engage in many activities to protect and promote the public's health, ranging from educational campaigns to raise awareness of factors that increase or decrease health risks to legal interventions that regulate conduct with the aim of improving individual and population health. Gostin identifies three bases on which public health interventions are justified: (1) to prevent risks to others; (2) to protect incompetent persons; and (3) to prevent risks to self.[18] Gostin summarizes these justifications:

> The first justification is the standard, well-accepted idea that government may intervene to prevent harm to others or punish individuals for inflicting harm. The second justification supports government action to protect the health and safety of those who are incapable of safeguarding their own interests. The third justification, and by far the most controversial, is paternalism; the protection of the health or safety of

---

[16]   S.J. Olshansky *et al.*, "A Potential Decline in Life Expectancy in the United States in the 21st Century" (2005) 352 New Eng. J. Med. 1138.

[17]   See, *e.g.*, K. Booth, M. Pinkston & W. Poston, "Obesity and the Built Environment" (2005) 105 Journal of the American Dietetic Association 110 and Wendy Collins Perdue, Lesley A. Stone & Lawrence O. Gostin, "The Built Environment and its Relationship to the Public's Health: The Legal Framework" (2003) 93 American Journal of Public Health 1390.

[18]   Lawrence O. Gostin, "General Justifications for Public Health Regulation" (2007) 121 Public Health 829.

competent individuals irrespective of their own expressed wants and desires.[19]

Classic examples of public health powers involve regulating conduct to prevent spread of disease to others. Persons with communicable diseases have long been subject to restrictions on their liberty, such as compulsory screening for symptoms of disease and quarantine to prevent contact with others. Obesity, however, is not communicable in a traditional sense — though obesity does tend to spread through social networks[20] — and food consumption and physical activity are viewed as matters of personal choice, making government interventions contentious. As the Australian jurist, Jethro Brown, wrote in 1912, "it is one thing to insist that a man shall have his house connected with a system of deep drainage; it is quite another thing to insist that he shall practise calisthenics or that he shall go to bed at a reasonable hour".[21] Some contemporary legal scholars share this view, claiming that "[i]n the private realm of diet and exercise, the state should assert itself gently".[22]

Autonomous individuals make their own choices about food and physical activity, but numerous environmental factors influence and constrain these choices. The money, time and knowledge to make informed, healthy eating decisions are not equally distributed in populations. Foods we are advised to eat most frequently, such as fresh fruits and vegetables, are notoriously more expensive than many nutrient-poor, energy-dense foods. The additional cost of a healthier food basket has been quantified at almost $40 for a biweekly shopping list.[23] As noted above, the built environment — urban sprawl; access to green spaces and recreational opportunities; availability of pedestrian corridors and bicycle lanes; and location of food outlets — also affects food and activity

---

[19]   *Ibid.*

[20]   Nicholas A. Christakis & James H. Fowler, "The Spread of Obesity in a Large Social Network over 32 Years" (2007) 357 New England Journal of Medicine 370. The authors theorized (at 371): "To the extent that obesity is a product of voluntary choices or behaviors, the fact that people are embedded in social networks and are influenced by the evident appearance and behaviors of those around them suggests that weight gain in one person might influence weight gain in others. Having obese social contacts might change a person's tolerance for being obese or might influence his or her adoption of specific behaviors (e.g., smoking, eating, and exercising)." Their study found that a person's likelihood of becoming obese increased if a friend, sibling or spouse became obese (increases of 57 per cent, 40 per cent and 37 per cent, respectively).

[21]   Jethro Brown, *The Underlying Principles of Modern Legislation* (London: John Murray, 1914) at 169-70, quoted in Christopher Reynolds, *Public Health Law and Regulation* (Sydney: The Federation Press, 2004) at 207.

[22]   M. Gregg Bloche, "Obesity and the Struggle Within Ourselves" (2004–2005) 93 Geo. L.J. 1335 at 1353.

[23]   Karen M. Jetter & Diana L. Cassady, "The Availability and Cost of Healthier Food Alternatives" (2006) 30:1 American Journal of Preventive Medicine 38.

choices.[24] Increasingly, obesity is described as an environmental disease[25] and while "the individual is ultimately responsible for his lifestyle ... the importance and the influence of the environment on his behaviour"[26] must be recognized.

A comprehensive review of environmental influences on eating and physical activity summarizes recent changes that likely promote unhealthy weight gain:

They include increases in the availability and marketing of food products, particularly "fast food" and other prepackaged convenience foods that are eaten away from home, increased time spent in sedentary forms ... and changes in the dynamics of family life driven by increased affluence and social conditions, such as dramatic increases in the proportion of women who work. Although some recent environmental trends seem more favorable, such as the increased availability and use of facilities for physical fitness, the cumulative effect of recent changes in the environment are clearly disastrous from the perspective of obesity.[27]

---

[24]   For discussion, see, *e.g.*, Institute of Medicine, *Does the Built Environment Influence Physical Activity? Examining the Evidence — Special Report 282* (Washington, D.C.: National Academies Press, 2005); R. Ewing *et al.*, "Relationship between Urban Sprawl and Physical Activity, Obesity and Morbidity" (2003) 18:1 American Journal of Health Promotion 47; and Julie Samia Mair, Matthew W. Pierce & Stephen S. Teret, *The Use of Zoning to Restrict Fast Food Outlets: A Potential Strategy to Combat Obesity* (Center for Law & the Public's Health, Johns Hopkins and Georgetown Universities, 2005), online: <http://www.publichealthlaw.net/Zoning%20Fast%20Food%20Outlets.pdf>.

[25]   For example, the 2006 report of the British Columbia Select Standing Committee on Health states (at 13) that obesity is "an environmental disease formed by the interaction of a multitude of factors. Such factors range from the media and marketing messages that bombard children daily, to whether a child has access to safe areas to participate in physical activities, to a parent's ability to provide healthy food". See *A Strategy for Combatting Childhood Obesity and Physical Inactivity in British Columbia*, online: <http://www.leg.bc.ca/CMT/38thparl/session-2/health/reports/Rpt-Health-38-2-29Nov2006.pdf>.

[26]   Commission of the European Communities, *White Paper on a Strategy for Europe on Nutrition, Overweight and Obesity related Health Issues* (May 2007), at 3 online: <http://ec.europa.eu/health/ph_determinants/life_style/nutrition/documents/nutrition_wp_en.pdf>.

[27]   Simone A. French, Mary Story & Robert W. Jeffery, "Environmental Influences on Eating and Physical Activity" (2001) 22 Annual Review of Public Health 309 at 328. For further discussion of environmental influences on weight gain, see, *e.g.*, J.O. Hill & J.C. Peters, "Environmental Contributions to the Obesity Epidemic" (1998) 280 Science 1371. In regard to changing family dynamics, a recent study of 3,085 children born between 2000 and 2002 in the United Kingdom revealed that a child's chance of becoming overweight increased in proportion with every ten hours per week the mother worked outside the home. This relationship was only significant for households with annual income of USD $57,750 or higher. The authors conclude: "Long hours of maternal employment, rather than lack of money may impede young children's access to healthy foods and physical activity. Policies supporting work–life balance may help parents reduce potential barriers." See S.S. Hawkins, T.J. Cole & C. Law, "Maternal Employment and Early Childhood Overweight:

While modern environments of sedentary lifestyles and constant access to cheap, energy-dense food put almost everyone at risk for weight gain, some groups are particularly vulnerable to factors that promote obesity.[28] People with lower levels of income and education have higher rates of obesity[29] and, paradoxically, food insecurity is a risk factor for obesity.[30] Obesity rates have also increased dramatically among children, who often have little control over the food they eat and their opportunities for physical activity. Children depend on adults for food and parental food choices exert a strong influence on children's preferences for and attitudes about foods.[31]

Aboriginal populations in many countries also have dramatically higher rates of obesity. Aboriginal Canadians are almost twice as likely to be obese and have a high instance of diabetes.[32] In New Zealand, indigenous Maori and Pacific peoples have up to triple the risk of diabetes and younger onset of the disease as New Zealanders of European descent.[33] In the United States, American Indians have high rates of overweight and obesity, with highest prevalence among indigenous groups in Arizona where 80 per cent of women and nearly 70 per cent of men are overweight.[34]

Findings from the UK Millennium Cohort Study" (2008) 32 International Journal of Obesity 30 at abstract.

[28] We refer here not just to environmental factors, but to all factors, including biological and genetic factors that are not yet well understood. For discussion, see, e.g., Alfredo Martínez-Hernández, Luís Enríquez, María Jesús Moreno-Moreno & Amelia Martí, "Genetics of Obesity" (2007) 10 Public Health Nutrition 10a.

[29] Adam Drewnowski & S.E. Specter, "Poverty and Obesity: The Role of Energy Density and Energy Costs" (2004) 79:1 American Journal of Clinical Nutrition 6.

[30] See, e.g., P.P. Basiotis & M. Lino, "Food Insufficiency and Prevalence of Overweight among Adult Women" (2002) 26 Nutrition Insights 1.

[31] See, e.g., Leann L. Birch, "Development of Food Preferences" (1999) 19 Annual Review of Nutrition 41 and Chrisa Arcan et al., "Parental Eating Behaviours, Home Food Environment and Adolescent Intakes of Fruits, Vegetables and Dairy Foods: Longitudinal Findings from Project EAT" (2007) 10:11 Public Health Nutrition 1257. Interestingly, parental influences on children's physical activity have been found to be weak, especially in adolescent years. See, e.g., Norman Anderssen, Bente Wold & Torbjorn Torsheim, "Are Parental Health Habits Transmitted to Their Children? An Eight Year Longitudinal Study of Physical Activity in Adolescents and Their Parents" (2006) 29:4 Journal of Adolescence 513.

[32] Canadian Population Health Initiative, Improving the Health of Canadians (Ottawa: Canadian Institute for Health Information, 2004).

[33] New Zealand House of Representatives, Report of the Health Committee, Inquiry into Obesity and Type 2 Diabetes in New Zealand, 48th Parl. (August 2007) (Chair: Sue Kedgley) at 10.

[34] Thomas K. Welty et al., "Cariovascular Disease Risk Factors in American Indians: The Strong Heart Study" (1995) 142:3 American Journal of Epidemiology 269.

Current obesity trends, associated serious morbidity risks, consequent socio-economic costs and particular harms to vulnerable groups arguably warrant state intervention to address environmental factors that promote obesity. Characterizing obesity as a matter of individual choice and consequences will exacerbate the social and personal harms.[35] The question, then, is *how* governments ought to intervene. What are possible targets and types of interventions that may be used to address factors linked with obesity and, further, what evidence is available or needed to demonstrate their efficacy and effectiveness?

III. THE TARGETS AND TYPES OF PUBLIC HEALTH INTERVENTION

To address obesity, various domains may be the target of regulation, including the informational environment (do people have sufficient information to enable healthy lifestyle choices?); the built environment (do communities in which individuals live facilitate healthy lifestyle choices?); the educational environment (do school settings promote healthy weights for children?); and the socio-economic environment (do economic and other conditions help or hinder healthy choices?).[36] Fundamentally, it is argued that "[g]overnments can help to structure the physical and social environment to help people make healthier choices".[37]

Once a public health problem is identified, governments may select among eight types of public health interventions, ranging from least to most coercive: (1) do nothing or simply monitor a situation; (2) provide information; (3) enable choice; (4) guide choices through changing the default policy; (5) guide choices through incentives; (6) guide choices through disincentives; (7) restrict choice; and (8) eliminate choice.[38] Each

---

[35]   Others argue contrariwise that excessive government intervention, not obesity, is the real problem. Epstein writes: "In light of the enormous attention that the question of obesity has generated, who should we respond? Individually, not collectively, seems the better approach. Better a bit of self-control than a ton of state initiatives. In light of shaky science and inflated claims, a dose of individual self-control is the only viable option. It does not rest on some necessary truth about the autonomy of Kantian individuals, but simply on practical necessity. No sane person would trust his diet and lifestyle to a benevolent social planner." Richard A. Epstein, "What (Not) to Do About Obesity: A Moderate Aristotelian Answer" (2004–2005) 93 Geo. L.J. 1361 at 1385.

[36]   Lawrence O. Gostin, "Fast and Supersized: Is the Answer to Diet by Fiat?" (2005) Hastings Center Report (March-April) 11.

[37]   Lawrence O. Gostin, "General Justifications for Public Health Regulation" (2007) 121 Public Health 829 at 833. See also Lawrence O. Gostin, "Law as a Tool to Facilitate Healthier Lifestyles and Prevent Obesity" (2007) 297 Journal of the American Medical Association 87.

[38]   Nuffield Council on Bioethics, *Public Health: Ethical Issues* (London: Nuffield Council on Bioethics, 2007); see Box 3.2, "The Intervention Ladder".

of these types of interventions is relevant in measures to address environmental factors associated with obesity. In Canada, governmental bodies collect data to monitor trends in rates of overweight and obesity. For example, Statistics Canada's national Health Measures Survey collects height, weight and other measures to provide more accurate information that is "essential to evaluate the true extent of problems associated with such major health concerns as obesity, hypertension and cardiovascular disease".[39] Health Canada disseminates Canada's Food Guide to provide information about healthy nutrition choices.[40] Indian and Northern Affairs Canada funds a Food Mail program to help deliver nutritious, perishable foods (including fresh fruits, vegetables and dairy products) to isolated northern communities to enable healthier choices for residents.[41] In school settings, provincial governments and local school boards are changing default options for food served or sold in schools to guide students in making healthier choices. For example, milk and unsweetened fruit and vegetable juices may replace soft drinks in school vending machines.[42] Subsidizing the cost of healthier food and taxing energy-dense, nutrient-poor foods are examples of guiding choice through incentives and disincentives.[43] Statutory limits on the allowable content of trans fats in food products restricts industry choices about product formulation,[44] and statutory bans on food advertising during children's television programming eliminates industry choice to market their products through that medium.

---

[39] Statistics Canada, *Canadian Health Measures Survey. Information for Survey Participants* (2007), online: <http://www.statcan.ca/english/survey/household/measures/measures.htm#Q1>.

[40] Available online: Health Canada <http://www.hc-sc.gc.ca/fn-an/food-guide-aliment/index _e.html>.

[41] See online: Indian and Northern Affairs Canada <http://www.ainc-inac.gc.ca/ps/nap/air/ 1brofoomai_e.html>.

[42] See, *e.g.*, *Ontario's Healthy Foods for Healthy Schools Act, 2008*, S.O. 2008, c. 2 (which received Royal Assent 27 April 2008), that empowers the Minister of Education to set policies and regulations governing nutrition standards of foods in schools and regulates trans fat levels of foods sold in schools. See online: <http://www.elaws.gov.on.ca/html/ source/statutes/english/2008/elaws_src_s08002_e.htm>.

[43] For discussion, see, *e.g.*, Sean B. Cash, David Sunding & David Zilberman, "Fat Taxes and Thin Subsidies: Prices, Diet, and Health Outcomes" (2005) 2 Acta Agriculturæ Scandinavica, Section C — Food Economics 167.

[44] For further discussion of legal and policy responses to trans fats, see Nola M. Ries, "Food, Fat and the Law: A Comment on Trans Fat Bans and Public Health" (2007) 23 Windsor Rev. Legal Soc. Issues 17.

(a)   Regulatory Interventions to Address the Food Environment: Informing and Restricting

Numerous regulatory approaches may be used to address environmental factors associated with obesity.[45] This section explores in more detail several examples of legal intervention: (1) regulations that require disclosure of calorie and nutrient information of food products; (2) regulations that restrict food advertising targeted at children; and (3) price and access controls on food products. This section also provides a brief discussion of the use of litigation as a tool to address obesity, more specifically, to impose legal accountability on entities that are claimed to engage in activities that promote unhealthy body weight.

(b)   Provision of Information: Disclosure of Calorie and Nutrient Information

Food labelling generally has several objectives, including consumer protection, encouraging consumers to choose healthier foods and giving producers an incentive to introduce or reformulate products with better nutrition profiles. With a few exceptions, prepackaged foods sold in Canada must be labelled in accordance with the *Food and Drugs Act* and its regulations.[46] Foods may not be labelled, packaged or advertised in a way that is false, misleading or deceptive, or that is "likely to create an erroneous impression regarding its character, value, quantity, composition, merit or safety".[47] Nutrition labelling has been mandatory in Canada since 2003.[48] Nutrition labels in a prescribed format must provide calorie information per serving size and measures of 13 core nutrients, including their percentage of daily recommended intake.[49] The *Food and Drug Regulations* also regulate the claims that can appear on food labels. Nutrient content claims are claims about the amount of energy or nutrients found in foods (*e.g.*, "low fat" or "source of fibre"), and are only permitted on the label or in an advertisement if made in accordance with

---

[45]   For comprehensive analysis of legislative and policy actions in the United States aimed at controlling obesity and improving access to healthy food and opportunities for physical activity, see the National Conference of State Legislatures' database on Healthy Eating, Physical Activity and Food Systems to Support Healthy Communities, online: <http://www.ncsl.org/programs/health/KelloggHealthOverview.htm>.

[46]   *Food and Drugs Act*, R.S.C. 1985, c. F-27, s. 5(2); *Food and Drug Regulations*, C.R.C., c. 870, s. B.01.003.

[47]   *Food and Drugs Act*, R.S.C. 1985, c. F-27, s. 5(1).

[48]   Regulations Amending the Food and Drug Regulations (Nutrition Labelling, Nutrient Content Claims and Health Claims), S.O.R./2003-11.

[49]   See *Food and Drugs Regulations*, Sch. L for details on the prescribed "Food Facts Table".

the Regulations.[50] Health claims, or claims about the health benefits of consuming a food product, must also conform to the Regulations.[51] Examples of health claims are: "A healthy diet rich in a variety of vegetables and fruit may help reduce the risk of some types of cancer" or "A healthy diet low in saturated and trans fats may reduce the risk of heart disease".[52] For both nutrient content claims and health claims, the Regulations set out what claims are permissible, the conditions that must be met and the wording to be used.[53]

While these types of rules aim to provide factual, useful information to consumers in a consistent, comprehensible format, the impact of labels on healthier food choices — and healthier body weight — is debatable. Some studies have shown a correlation between nutrition label use and healthier diets[54] but, overall, evidence on the impact of labels is limited.[55] Although most people say they use nutrition labels, the evidence indicates that actual rates of use are lower and that much of this use does not actually affect purchasing decisions.[56] Common barriers to using nutrition

[50]   *Ibid.*, s. B.01.500*ff.* See *ibid.*, s. B.01.603 for a complete list of permitted statements and claims and conditions for their use.

[51]   *Ibid.*, s. B.01.600*ff.*

[52]   See *ibid.*, s. B.01.603.

[53]   *Ibid.*, ss. B.01.503(1), B.01.601. See also tables following s. B.01.513 (nutrient content claims) and s. B.01.603 (diet-related health claims).

[54]   Jayachandran N. Variyam, "Do Nutrition Labels Improve Dietary Outcomes?" (2007) Health Econ. [advance access]; Andreas C. Drichoutis, Panagiotis Lazaridis & Rodolfo M. Nayga, Jr., "Consumers' Use of Nutritional Labels: A Review of Research Studies and Issues" (2006) 10 Academy of Marketing Science Review 9 at 14-15, online: <http://www.amsreview.org/articles.htm>; Center for Science in the Public Interest, "Petition for Advance Notice of Potential Rulemaking on the Use of Symbols on the Principal Display Panel to Communicate the Healthfulness of Foods" (Submitted to the U.S. Department of Health and Human Services, U.S. Food and Drug Administration, 30 November 2006) at 5, online: <http://www.cspinet.org/new/pdf/healthy_symbol_petition.pdf>; U.S. Food and Drug Administration, *Calories Count: Report of the Working Group on Obesity* (2004) at 15, online: <http://www.cfsan.fda.gov/~dms/owg-toc.html>.

[55]   Gill Cowburn & Lynn Stockley, "Consumer Understanding and Use of Nutrition Labelling: A Systematic Review" (2005) 8 Public Health Nutrition 21 at 26-27; Ellen van Kleef, Hans C.M. van Trijp & Pieternell Luning, "Functional Foods: Health Claim-Food Product Compatibility and the Impact of Health Claim Framing on Consumer Evaluation" (2005) 44 Appetite 299 at 299; Cliona Ni Mhurchu & Delvina Gorton, "Nutrition Labels and Claims in New Zealand and Australia: A Review of Use and Understanding" (2007) 31 Australian and New Zealand Journal Public Health 105 at 111; A. Denny, "Stop, Think, Go? — Are Signposting Labelling Schemes the Way Forward?" (2006) 31 Nutrition Bulletin 84 at 86; Klaus G. Gruncrt & Josephine M. Wills, "A Review of European Research on Consumer Response to Nutrition Information on Food Labels" (2007) 15 J. Public Health 385.

[56]   Cliona Ni Mhurchu & Delvina Gorton, "Nutrition Labels and Claims in New Zealand and Australia: A Review of Use and Understanding" (2007) 31 Australian and New Zealand Journal Public Health 105 at 110; Gill Cowburn & Lynn Stockley, "Consumer Understanding and Use of Nutrition Labelling: A Systematic Review" (2005) 8 Public Health Nutrition 21 at 24, 26.

information are lack of time, education and knowledge about nutrition, and mistrust of the information provided.[57] Studies have shown that many consumers do not understand the information provided in nutrition information panels.[58] Levels of comprehension vary significantly according to the label format,[59] as well as personal characteristics such as age and level of education.[60] In its own focus group research, Health Canada found that consumers have difficulty understanding food labels: "Participants across the country are unsure of nutrition facts and of how to use the information that currently exists on food labels effectively. Additionally they bring a degree of skepticism to the label reading process: although they like the nutrition facts, nutrition claims need to be discounted as 'advertising' they say."[61]

The effectiveness of labelling schemes could be improved in several ways to increase impact on public health. Educational initiatives are likely to enhance consumers' understanding and use of existing nutrition labels.[62] It may also be possible to modify the mandatory nutrition

---

[57]   Cliona Ni Mhurchu & Delvina Gorton, "Nutrition Labels and Claims in New Zealand and Australia: A Review of Use and Understanding" (2007) 31 Australian and New Zealand Journal Public Health 105 at 110; Center for Science in the Public Interest, "Petition for Advance Notice of Potential Rulemaking on the Use of Symbols on the Principal Display Panel to Communicate the Healthfulness of Foods" (Submitted to the U.S. Department of Health and Human Services, U.S. Food and Drug Administration, 30 November 2006) at 6-7, online: <http://www.cspinet.org/new/pdf/healthy_symbol_petition.pdf>; Gill Cowburn & Lynn Stockley, "Consumer Understanding and Use of Nutrition Labelling: A Systematic Review" (2005) 8 Public Health Nutrition 21 at 24; Ann D. Sullivan, "Determining How Low-Income Food Shoppers Perceive, Understand, and Use Food Labels" (2003) 64 Canadian Journal Dietetic Practice and Research 25 at 26-27; George Baltas, "Nutrition Labelling: Issues and Policies" (2001) 35 European Journal of Marketing 708 at 710-11.

[58]   Gill Cowburn & Lynn Stockley, "Consumer Understanding and Use of Nutrition Labelling: A Systematic Review" (2005) 8 Public Health Nutrition 21 at 23; George Baltas, "Nutrition Labelling: Issues and Policies" (2001) 35 European Journal of Marketing 708 at 712-13.

[59]   Carol Byrd-Bredbenner, Angela Wong & Peta Cottee, "Consumer Understanding of US and EU Nutrition Labels" (2000) 102 British Food Journal 615; George Baltas, "Nutrition Labelling: Issues and Policies" (2001) 35 European Journal of Marketing 708 at 713.

[60]   Gill Cowburn & Lynn Stockley, "Consumer Understanding and Use of Nutrition Labelling: A Systematic Review" (2005) 8 Public Health Nutrition 21 at 25; George Baltas, "Nutrition Labelling: Issues and Policies" (2001) 35 European Journal of Marketing 708 at 713; Russell L. Rothman et al., "Patient Understanding of Food Labels: The Role of Literacy and Numeracy" (2006) 31 Am. J. Prev. Med. 391.

[61]   This finding is based on six focus groups in six cities and three additional focus groups in diabetics conducted in September 2000 among people aged 18 to 44 who were interested in health issues and responsible for grocery shopping: Health Canada, Food and Nutrition, "Research: Nutrition Label Message Testing", online: <http://www.hc-sc.gc.ca/fn-an/label-etiquet/nutrition/res-rech/mess_testing-verification_mess_e.html>.

[62]   Carol Byrd-Bredbenner, Angela Wong & Peta Cottee, "Consumer Understanding of US and EU Nutrition Labels" (2000) 102 British Food Journal 615 at 627; Cliona Ni Mhurchu & Delvina Gorton, "Nutrition Labels and Claims in New Zealand and Australia: A Review

information panels to make them more effective; for example, by requiring nutrient values to be listed both per serving and per 100g to make it easier for consumers to assess their total consumption and to compare products.[63] Stricter regulation and enforcement of the serving sizes used in nutrition information panels could also be important to ensuring that consumers accurately understand how much they are consuming.[64]

It has also been suggested that "front-of-package" labels on food products should be more strictly regulated. In Canada, the report of the federal Standing Committee on Health, *Healthy Weights for Healthy Kids*, recommended a "a mandatory, standardized, simple, front of package labelling requirement on pre-packaged foods for easy identification of nutritional value" to be phased in, beginning with foods primarily marketed to children.[65] In 2007, the United Kingdom Food Standards Agency ("FSA") implemented a voluntary "traffic light" system for front-of-package labelling, which includes a red, amber or green light for high, medium or low values of fats, saturated fat, salt and sugars.[66] For example, a food product high in fats and saturated fats in particular, low in sugar and moderate in salt, will bear two red symbols, one green symbol and an amber symbol. This system is said to provide consumers with at-a-glance information without having to scrutinize a label on the back of the product. Food industry opponents of the scheme argue it may encourage consumers to interpret red and amber lights as warnings and lead to crude categorization of food as either "good" or "bad" rather than sending a message that promotes consuming a range of foods in moderation.[67]

[   ] of Use and Understanding" (2007) 31 Australian and New Zealand Journal Public Health 105 at 108.

[63] C.S. Higginson *et al.*, "How Do Consumers Use Nutrition Label Information?" (2002) 32 Nutrition & Food Science 145 at 150, Beth Antonuk & Lauren G. Block, "The Effect of Single Serving Versus Entire Package Nutritional Information on Consumption Norms and Actual Consumption of a Snack Food" (2006) 38 Journal of Nutrition, Education and Behaviour 365.

[64] U.S. Food and Drug Administration, *Calories Count: Report of the Working Group on Obesity* (2004) at 18, online: <http://www.cfsan.fda.gov/~dms/owg-toc.html>; Allen Pelletier *et al.*, "Patients' Understanding and Use of Snack Food Package Nutrition Labels" (2004) 17 J. Am. Board Fam. Pract. 319.

[65] Canada, House of Commons, Standing Committee on Health, *Healthy Weights for Healthy Kids*, 39th Parl. 1st sess. (March 2007) (Chair: Rob Merrifield) at 22, online: <http://www.ccfn.ca/pdfs/HealthyWeightsForHealthyKids.pdf>.

[66] U.K. Food Standards Agency, "Front-of-Pack Traffic Light Signpost Labelling: Technical Guidance" (November 2007), online: <http://www.food.gov.uk/multimedia/pdfs/frontofpack guidance2.pdf>.

[67] See, *e.g.*, Gaynor Bussell, "Nutritional Profiling vs Guideline Daily Amounts as a Means of Helping Consumers Make Appropriate Food Choices" (2005) 35:5 Nutrition and Food Science 337.

There are two main rationales for adopting a simple, standardized, front-of-package labelling scheme. First, if designed appropriately, labels may be easier for consumers to use and understand. Second, there are concerns that consumers are being confused and possibly misled by the range of front-of-package labels that currently exist. Under the present law, food manufacturers are free to choose the information and images they put on the front of a food package (the nutrition label generally appearing on the back of the package), provided they adhere to the general regulations on health or nutrient content claims and the prohibition on false, misleading and deceptive promotion. As a result, there are many different label formats in the Canadian marketplace, including several schemes designed by manufacturers or non-government organizations (*e.g.*, the Canadian Heart and Stroke Foundation), designating "healthier" products according to various criteria. Some have argued these labelling schemes and logos are misleading or confusing, and may contribute to poor nutritional choices by consumers. For example, the Canadian Heart and Stroke Foundation's "Health Check" program has been criticized because some lower fat products that nonetheless have high sugar or sodium content are eligible to display the Health Check mark.[68] These concerns, if accurate, suggest the need for a more closely regulated or perhaps even a prescribed, mandatory front-of-package labelling scheme, as recommended by the Standing Committee on Health.[69] The question would still remain what type of scheme should be adopted — a matter of vigorous debate in the United Kingdom and Europe.[70]

Another area for potential reform is extending mandatory nutrition labelling to non-packaged foods, such as ready-to-eat foods (which are currently exempt[71]) or restaurant foods. Consumers often have little or no calorie and nutrient information at point-of-sale for foods purchased in restaurants, fast-food outlets, cafeterias and other food service facilities. This is a huge informational gap as the frequency of food consumption outside the home has increased dramatically in recent years. In the United States, people consume up to one-third of total daily calories from restaurant meals, and purchases of foods consumed away from home now

---

[68] Amanda Truscott, "Checking Up on Health Check" (2008) 178 C.M.A.J. 386.

[69] Canada, House of Commons, Standing Committee on Health, *Healthy Weights for Healthy Kids*, 39th Parl. 1st Sess. (March 2007) (Chair: Rob Merrifield) at 22-23, online: <http://www.ccfn.ca/pdfs/HealthyWeightsForHealthyKids.pdf>.

[70] See, *e.g.*, Rory Watson, "Europe Opts Against Traffic Light System for Food Labelling" (2008) 336 Brit. Med. J. 296; A. Denny, "Stop, Think, Go? — Are Signposting Labelling Schemes the Way Forward?" (2006) 31 Nutrition Bulletin 84; Gaynor Bussell, "Nutritional Profiling vs Guidelines Daily Amounts as a Means of Helping Consumers Make Appropriate Food Choices" (2005) 35 Nutrition and Food Science 337.

[71] *Food and Drug Regulations*, C.R.C., c. 870, s. B.01.401(2)(b)(vii).

account for half of all food expenditures.[72] Similar trends are evident in Canada,[73] and regular consumption of meals outside the home has been posited as a possible contributor to the obesity epidemic.[74] Many consumers — and even nutrition professionals — underestimate the number of calories in restaurant meals.[75] While some restaurants provide nutrition information on a voluntary basis, mandatory disclosure has been proposed.[76] Advocates of extending mandatory disclosure to restaurants argue:

> As the rate of, and number of, cases of obesity increase, legislation should dictate that menus disclose fat, calories and cholesterol content of food items. Legislation must protect consumers from themselves because as evidenced by the rising number of health complications, partially due to poor eating habits, consumers are continually showing that they are unable or do not have the discipline to protect themselves from their behaviors.[77]

To address the "relentlessly upward"[78] trajectory of the numbers overweight and obese residents, the City of New York amended its Health

---

[72] Hayden Stewart, Noel Blisard & Dean Jolliffe, *Let's Eat Out: Americans Weigh Taste, Convenience and Nutrition* (October 2006) Economic Information Bulletin No. 19 (United States Department of Agriculture, Economic Research Service), online: <http://ers.usda.gov/publications/eib19/eib19.pdf>.

[73] Trans Fat Task Force, *TRANSforming the Food Supply: Report of the Trans Fat Task Force* (June 2006), online: Health Canada <http://www.hc-sc.gc.ca/fn-an/alt_formats/hpfb-dgpsa/pdf/nutrition/tf-gt_rep-rap_e.pdf>.

[74] Scot Burton *et al.*, "Attacking the Obesity Epidemic: The Potential Health Benefits of Providing Nutrition Information in Restaurants" (2006) 96 Am. J. Pub. Health 1669 at 1669.

[75] See, *e.g.*, Brian Wansink & Pierre Chandon, "Meal Size, not Body Size, Explains Errors in Estimating the Calorie Content of Meals" (2006) 145:5 Annals of Internal Medicine 326; Lisa R. Young & Marion Nestle, "Portion Sizes and Obesity: Responses of Fast-Food Companies" (2007) 28 Journal of Public Health Policy 238; and Lisa R. Young & Marion Nestle, "Portion Sizes in Dietary Assessment: Issues and Policy Implications" (1995) 53 Nutrition Reviews 149. For a study testing dieticians' ability to estimate calorie content of restaurant meals, see *e.g.*, J. Backstrand, M.G. Wootan, L.R. Young & J. Hurley, *Fat Chance* (Washington, D.C.: Center for Science in the Public Interest, 1997).

[76] The most recent bill in Canada was Bill C-283, *An Act to Amend the Food and Drugs Act (Food Labelling)*, 1st Sess., 39th Parl., (negatived 8 November 2006). For legislative initiatives in the United States, see The Keystone Center, *The Keystone Forum on Away-From-Home Foods: Opportunities for Preventing Weight Gain and Obesity* (Washington, D.C.: The Keystone Center, 2006) at 74, online: <http://www.keystone.org/spp/documents/Forum_Report_FINAL_5-30-06.pdf>.

[77] Lionel Thomas & Juline E. Mills, "Consumer Knowledge and Expectations of Restaurant Menus and their Governing Legislation: A Qualitative Assessment" (2006) 17 Journal of Foodservice Business Research 6 at 19.

[78] New York City Department of Health and Mental Hygiene, Board of Health, *Notice of Intention to Repeal and Reenact §81.50 of the New York City Health Code: Notice of Public Hearing* (18 October 2007), online: <http://www.nyc.gov/html/doh/downloads/pdf/public/notice-intention-hc-art81-50-1007.pdf>.

Code to require restaurants that already make calorie information publicly available (*e.g.*, on a company website or tray liners) to post this information on menus and menu boards.[79] The regulation initially took effect July 1, 2007, but was successfully challenged by the New York State Restaurant Association on the grounds that it was pre-empted by federal law.[80] Amended regulations came into effect in the spring of 2008 that require specified types of food service establishments to post calorie information.[81] The Department of Health took this step to address the "calorie information gap",[82] arguing that more accessible calorie disclosure "would enable New Yorkers to make more informed, healthier choices and can reasonably be expected to reduce obesity and the many related health problems which obesity causes".[83] A 2007 survey of major restaurant chains in the city found the average calorie content of a lunchtime meal purchase to exceed 800 calories, with approximately one-third of customers purchasing over 1,000 calories,[84] amounts that provide at least half of daily calorie needs for many people.

Surveys indicate many consumers favour more accessible disclosure of calorie and nutrient information in food service outlets.[85] Yet, if restaurants are required to disclose calorie information on menus and menu boards, the question remains whether consumers will actually understand and use this information to choose meals with fewer calories. Some preliminary studies suggest that consumers who see calorie

---

[79] For a summary of other state and local legislation, see Center for Science in the Public Interest, "Nutrition Labeling in Chain Restaurants: State and Local Bills/Regulations – 2007-2008" (2008), online: <http://www.cspinet.org/nutritionpolicy/MenuLabelingBills2007-2008.pdf>.

[80] *New York State Restaurant Association v. New York City Board of Health, et al.* (509 F. Supp. 2d 351 (S.D.N.Y. 2007). At the time of the legal challenge to New York City's regulation, 17 similar regulations were in force or under consideration throughout the United States.

[81] See New York City Department of Health and Mental Hygiene, Board of Health, *Notice of Adoption of a Resolution to Repeal and Reenact §81.50 of the New York City Health Code* (January 2008), online: <http://www.nyc.gov/html/doh/downloads/pdf/public/notice-adoption-hc-art81-50-0108.pdf>.

[82] *Ibid.*, at 8.

[83] *Ibid.*, at 2.

[84] *Ibid.*, at 4.

[85] Lionel Thomas & Juline E. Mills, "Consumer Knowledge and Expectations of Restaurant Menus and their Governing Legislation: A Qualitative Assessment" (2006) 17 Journal of Foodservice Business Research 6 and D.A. Carange, M.T. Conklin & C.U. Lambert, "Effect of Nutritional Information in Perceptions of Food Quality, Consumption Behaviour and Purchase Intentions" (2004) 7 Journal of Foodservice Business Research 43. *The New York Times* reported that a 2005 survey conducted by the food service company, Aramark, found that 83 per cent of respondents (N=5297) wanted better disclosure of nutrition information in restaurants: see Roni Caryn Rabin, "Calorie Labels May Clarify Options, Not Actions" *The New York Times* (17 July 2007), online: <http://www.nytimes.com/2007/07/17/health/nutrition/17cons.html?_r=1&oref=slogin>.

information posted at the point of purchase in a fast-food outlet select meals with fewer calories.[86] Following the enactment of mandatory labelling laws in the United States, sales of some high-fat products declined significantly, suggesting consumers used the label information in their purchase decisions.[87] Disclosure of calorie information will, however, only be useful if consumers have an understanding of their appropriate daily calorie intake to maintain a healthy weight.

The industry has resisted mandatory disclosure proposals, arguing it is impractical and too costly, particularly because of the variation in ingredients, preparation and portion sizes.[88] Given these concerns, current proposals focus on fast-food chain restaurants because their menus and food preparation are more standardized. However, even in this context, the industry has generally opposed mandatory labelling, preferring voluntary initiatives.[89]

(c) Control of Information: Restricting Food Advertising Targeted at Children

Children and youth represent a significant portion of the food and beverage market. In 2002 in the United States, sales of food and beverages to young people exceeded $27 billion.[90] In 2004, food and beverage advertising expenditures directed at children and youth amounted to $15 billion, a substantial increase from approximately $2 billion in 1999.[91] Children exert

---

[86] New York City Department of Health and Mental Hygiene, Board of Health, *Notice of Intention to Repeal and Reenact §81.50 of the New York City Health Code: Notice of Public Hearing* (18 October 2007), online: <http://www.nyc.gov/html/doh/downloads/pdf/public/notice-intention-hc-art81-50-1007.pdf> at 6. A study of 1,816 Subway customers at 47 locations throughout New York City indicated that those who saw the posted calorie information selected meals with fewer calories, though the calorie reduction ranged from 48 and 92 fewer calories on average.

[87] Alan D. Mathios, "The Impact of Mandatory Disclosure Laws on Product Choices: An Analysis of the Salad Dressing Market" (2000) 43:2 J.L. & Econ. 651.

[88] See, *e.g.*, The Keystone Center, *The Keystone Forum on Away-From-Home Foods: Opportunities for Preventing Weight Gain and Obesity* (Washington, D.C.: The Keystone Center, 2006) at 71, online: <http://www.keystone.org/spp/documents/Forum_Report_FINAL_5-30-06.pdf>; Carl A. Boger, Jr., "Food Labeling for Restaurants: Fact versus Fiction" (1995) 36:3 Cornell Hotel & Restaurant Administration Quarterly 62 at 67-69; Barbara A. Almanza, Douglas Nelson & Stella Chai, "Obstacles to Nutrition Labeling in Restaurants" (1997) 97 J. Am. Dietetic Assoc. 157 at 159-61.

[89] Canadian Restaurant and Foodservices Association, News Release, "Menu Labelling Vote Set for Nov. 8" (7 November 2006), online: <http://www.crfa.ca/news/2006/menu_labelling_vote_set_for_nov_8.asp>.

[90] Jeffrey P. Koplan, Catharyn T. Liverman & Vivica I. Kraak, eds., *Preventing Childhood Obesity: Health in the Balance* (Washington, D.C.: The National Academies Press, 2005) at 153 and 172.

[91] Juliet B. Schor & Margaret Ford, "From Tastes Great to Cool: Children's Food Marketing and the Rise of the Symbolic" (2007) 35:1 J.L. Med. & Ethics 10 at 11.

important influence over parental food (and other product) purchasing decisions; one estimate suggests that, in 2002, "children aged four to twelve directly influenced $310 billion of adult purchasing and evoked another $340 billion".[92] Television remains the most popular medium for food advertising, though Internet sites, event sponsorship and product placement in children's movies are also important marketing tools.[93]

A major study examining the daily number of food ads children see on TV found that two- to seven-year-olds see 12 ads each day, eight- to twelve-year-olds see 21 ads and thirteen- to seventeen-year-olds see 17 ads each day.[94] Nearly three-quarters of ads are for candy, snacks, cereals and fast food that are high in fat, sugar and salt (often referred to as "HFSS foods"). With the exception of a few ads for fruit juice, fruits and vegetables are not part of children's food advertising. Pre-teen groups see only one public service announcement related to nutrition and fitness every two or three days and teens see less than one such announcement each week. This study concludes that "food marketing is a predominant part of the television advertising landscape for children, and that young people's exposure to such messages is substantial, while their exposure to countervailing health messages on TV is minimal".[95]

The pervasiveness of advertising of HFSS foods has prompted calls for legislative restrictions on television advertising directed at children. In Canada, various organizations including the Center for Science in the Public Interest and the Heart and Stroke Foundation advocate regulatory limits on advertising aimed at children[96] and, in 2004, a member of the Senate attempted (unsuccessfully) to stimulate legislative reform "to curb child-directed advertising that encourages poor nutrition and physical inactivity".[97] Québec is unique in Canada in prohibiting commercial advertising directed at children under age 13.[98] In the rest of Canada, the

---

[92]   *Ibid.*, at 11.

[93]   *Ibid.*

[94]   The Henry J. Kaiser Family Foundation, *Food for Thought: Television Food Advertising to Children in the United States* (March 2007) at 15, online: <http://www.kff.org/entmedia/upload/7618.pdf>.

[95]   *Ibid.*, at 4. A June 2007 Federal Trade Commission report into children's exposure to TV ads reported similar statistics, but states that exposure has not increased since a similar study done in 1977: Federal Trade Commission, *Children's Exposure to TV Advertising in 1977 and 2004: Information for the Obesity Debate*. This report notes that ads for sedentary entertainment (such as movies and computer games) have increased substantially.

[96]   Bill Jeffery, "The Supreme Court of Canada's Appraisal of the 1980 Ban on Advertising to Children in Quebec: Implications for 'Misleading' Advertising Elsewhere" (2006) 39 Loyola Law Review 237 at 243.

[97]   Hon. Mira Spivak, Senate Debates (11 May 2004).

[98]   *Consumer Protection Act*, R.S.Q. c. P-40.1, ss. 248, 249. For further commentary on Québec's legislation, see Bill Jeffery, "The Supreme Court of Canada's Appraisal of the 1980 Ban on Advertising to Children in Quebec: Implications for 'Misleading' Advertising Elsewhere" (2006) 39 Loyola Law Review 237 at 243.

advertising industry follows a self-regulatory Broadcast Code for Advertising to Children ("Children's Code")[99] and the Canadian Code of Advertising Standards.[100] The Children's Code applies to commercial messages shown during children's (those under 12) programming and also to ads aimed at children that air during other programs. The Children's Code stipulates that ads "must not *directly* urge children to purchase or urge them to ask their parents to make inquiries or purchases".[101] The Children's Code also restricts product endorsements by cartoon characters, puppets and persons well known to children, though these may appear in the ad, give factual (*i.e.* not promotional) statements, as well as educational messages about nutrition.[102] The Canadian Code of Advertising Standards requires that "advertising that is directed to children must not exploit their credulity, lack of experience or their sense of loyalty, and must not present information or illustrations that might result in their physical, emotional or moral harm".[103]

It has been argued that these industry codes are "wholly inadequate for safeguarding children's interests";[104] although the Canadian Radio-television and Telecommunications Commission ("CRTC") requires broadcasters to comply with the Children's Code as a condition of licence, "there is no evidence on record that the CRTC has ever considered violations of the Children's Code to determine whether a license should be renewed, revoked, or subjected to additional terms".[105] In its 2007 report, *Healthy Weights for Healthy Kids*,[106] the federal Standing Committee on Health endorsed a need to evaluate the adequacy of industry self-regulation of advertising directed at children.[107]

---

[99] Advertising Standards Canada & Canadian Association of Broadcasters, *The Broadcast Code for Advertising to Children* (April 2007), online: Advertising Standards Canada <http://www.adstandards.com/en/clearance/clearanceAreas/childrensBroadcastCode.pdf>.

[100] Advertising Standards Canada, *Canadian Code of Advertising Standards* (November 2007), online: <http://www.adstandards.com/en/Standards/adStandards.pdf>.

[101] Advertising Standards Canada & Canadian Association of Broadcasters, *The Broadcast Code for Advertising to Children* (April 2007) at Clause 5(a) [emphasis in original], online: Advertising Standards Canada <http://www.adstandards.com/en/clearance/clearanceAreas/childrensBroadcastCode.pdf>.

[102] *Ibid.*, at Clause 7.

[103] Advertising Standards Canada, *Canadian Code of Advertising Standards* (November 2007) at Clause 12, online: <http://www.adstandards.com/en/Standards/adStandards.pdf>.

[104] Bill Jeffery, "The Supreme Court of Canada's Appraisal of the 1980 Ban on Advertising to Children in Quebec: Implications for 'Misleading' Advertising Elsewhere" (2006) 39 Loyola Law Review 237.

[105] *Ibid.*, at 249.

[106] Canada, House of Commons, Standing Committee on Health, *Healthy Weights for Healthy Kids*, 39th Parl., 1st Sess. (March 2007) (Chair: Rob Merrifield), online: <http://www.ccfn.ca/pdfs/HealthyWeightsForHealthyKids.pdf>.

[107] There is, however, no indication of impending regulatory change in Canada. The federal government's response to the Standing Committee recommendations regarding advertising to

The situation in the United Kingdom is different: ads for foods and beverages high in fat, sugar and salt are restricted during television programming aimed at viewers younger than 16.[108] Effective January 1, 2008, ads for HFSS foods are prohibited during television programs aimed at children aged four to 15. This follows a July 1, 2007 ban on HFSS food ads during children's programming, including programs for pre-school children and during shows aimed at children between ages four and nine.[109]

Despite the evidence about prevalence of food advertising aimed at children, its actual influence on children's food preferences — and, more to the point, its impact on childhood obesity — is disputed. Will restrictions or bans on television ads for HFSS foods make children more likely to prefer and choose healthier foods and help prevent children from becoming overweight or obese? After a comprehensive review of available research, the United States Institute of Medicine concluded in a 2006 report that "[t]elevision advertising influences the food preferences, purchase requests, and diets, at least of children under age 12 years, and is associated with the increased rates of obesity among children and youth".[110] This contrasts with the conclusion of a 2004 U.S. paper: "Overall, our review of the available public evidence suggests that currently there is little theoretical or empirical foundation to support the 'advertising causes obesity' thesis or the inference that restrictions on

children states: "The Government of Canada understands the concerns related to marketing to children, and is undertaking efforts to further explore this issue. The Public Health Agency of Canada is currently examining the various methods used by marketers to reach children and the current situation in Canada. Different models for reducing the influence of marketing on children will be considered ... The feasibility and effectiveness of [regulatory] approaches, as well as self-regulation ... will be assessed." See Canada, *Government Response to the Seventh Report of the Standing Committee on Health: Healthy Weights for Healthy Kids*, online: <http://cmte. parl.gc.ca/cmte/CommitteePublication.aspx?SourceId=213785>.

[108] Office of Communications, *Television Advertising of Food and Drink Products to Children: Final Statement* (22 February 2007), online: <http://www.ofcom.org.uk/consult/condocs/ foodads_new/statement/statement.pdf>. Several other European countries also restrict television ads aimed at children. Since 1991, Swedish law has prohibited TV and radio ads targeted to children younger than 12, and Belgian law bans commercials during children's programming: Mary Story & Simone French, "Food Advertising and Marketing Directed at Children and Adolescents in the US" (2004) 1 International Journal of Behavioral Nutrition and Physical Activity 3.

[109] A January 2008 report by the Advertising Standards Authority revealed high compliance (99.2 per cent of ads) with these regulatory changes: Advertising Standards Authority, *Compliance Report — Food and Soft Drink Advertising Survey 2007* (January 2008), online: <http://www.asa.org.uk/NR/rdonlyres/120B91FD-FB23-4551-A554-776822DEE333/ 0/FoodandSoftDrinkAdvertisingSurvey2007.pdf>.

[110] Institute of Medicine, *Food Marketing to Children and Youth: Threat or Opportunity?* (Washington, D.C.: National Academies Press, 2006).

food advertising would meaningfully reduce the incidence of childhood obesity."[111]

Even the telecommunications regulator that will enforce the new restrictions in the United Kingdom acknowledges that "multiple factors account for childhood obesity. Television viewing/advertising is one among many influences ... other factors include social, environmental and cultural factors, all of which interact in complex ways not yet well understood ... a total ban on food advertising would be neither proportionate nor, in isolation, effective".[112]

In addition to debate about the efficacy of advertising restrictions, another drawback is their potential infringement of constitutionally protected free speech rights, such as rights protected under s. 2(b) of the *Canadian Charter of Rights and Freedoms*.[113] Québec's ban on commercial advertising directed at children aged 13 and younger was found by the majority of the Supreme Court of Canada to be a justifiable limitation on free speech rights,[114] but any new attempt to restrict advertising would likely be subject to constitutional challenge. Justifying restrictions on the grounds of mitigating childhood obesity could be a difficult argument, particularly considering conflicting evidence about the practical impact of ad restrictions on children's food choices and body weight.

Heightened concern about childhood obesity, criticism of corporate promotion of HFSS foods and fear of regulation have, nonetheless, recently prompted food companies and industry associations to adopt voluntary measures to limit advertising to children and to promote healthy eating and physical activity. The U.S. Children's Food and Beverage

---

[111]   Todd J. Zywicki, Debra Holt & Maureen K. Ohlhausen, "Obesity and Advertising Policy" (2004) 12 Geo. Mason L. Rev. 979. For additional analysis of advertising and obesity in children, see Debra M. Desrochers & Debra J. Holt, "Children's Exposure to Television Advertising: Implications for Childhood Obesity" (2007) 26:2 Journal of Public Policy and Marketing 182.

[112]   Office of Communications, *Television Advertising of Food and Drink Products to Children: Final Statement* (22 February 2007) at 2, online: <http://www.ofcom.org.uk/consult/condocs/foodads_new/statement/statement.pdf>.

[113]   *Canadian Charter of Rights and Freedoms*, Part I of the *Constitution Act, 1982*, being Schedule B to the *Canada Act 1982* (U.K.), 1982, c. 11. Section 2(b) provides: "Everyone has the following fundamental freedoms: ... (b) freedom of thought, belief, opinion and expression, including freedom of the press and other media of communication ... "

[114]   *Irwin Toy Ltd. v. Québec (Attorney General)*, [1989] S.C.J. No. 36, [1989] 1 S.C.R. 927 (S.C.C.). For discussion of constitutionality of statutory limits on tobacco advertising, see *RJR-MacDonald Inc. v. Canada (Attorney General)*, [1995] S.C.J. No. 68, [1995] 3 S.C.R. 199 (S.C.C.) and *Canada (Attorney General) v. JTI-Macdonald Corp.*, [2007] S.C.J. No. 30, 2007 SCC 30 (S.C.C.). Statutory prohibitions against direct-to-consumer advertising of prescription pharmaceuticals in Canada are a current target of constitutional challenge, brought by CanWest Global Communication: for discussion, see Alicia Priest, "CanWest Set to Challenge Ban on DTCA" (2007) 126:1 C.M.A.J. 19.

Advertising Initiative, comprised of representatives from ten of the largest food companies in the U.S., has pledged to allocate half of all television, radio, print and Internet advertising aimed at children under 12 to promotion of healthier foods and lifestyles.[115] Major food companies operating in Canada and the European Community have announced similar self-regulatory initiatives.[116]

Restrictions on child-directed advertising seek to shield children from messages that may encourage poor food choices. However, industry may point to compliance with self-regulatory codes to oppose governmental regulation. As a more coercive and legally contentious intervention, some governments may hesitate to regulate in this area.[117]

(d) Promoting Healthier Choices: Price and Access Strategies to Encourage Healthier Food Consumption

A growing body of evidence suggests that socio-economic status affects food consumption patterns and the risk of obesity.[118] Lower income households facing food insecurity and having limited amounts of money to spend on food tend to buy energy-dense foods that are also typically nutrient-poor.[119] Healthier diets with a greater proportion of fruits, vegetables and lower-fat protein sources may not be affordable for many lower-income households.[120] Some studies have also shown that demand

---

[115] The Initiative is available online: <http://www.us.bbb.org/WWWRoot/storage/16/documents/InitiativeProgramDocument.pdf>.

[116] For the Canadian initiative, see Advertising Standards Canada, online: <http://www.adstandards.com/en/clearance/clearanceAreas/childrensInitiative.asp>. For the European initiative, see Jenny Wiggins & Andrew Bounds, "Companies move to halt junk food advertising" *Financial Times* (11 December 2007). See also Confederation of the Food and Drink Industries: <http://www.active-lifestyle.eu/asp/our_actions/l1.asp?doc_id=16>.

[117] In its comprehensive report on food advertising directed at children, the U.S. Institute of Medicine recommended that if self-regulatory models fail to produce a decline in advertising of low-nutrition foods, governments should restrict or prohibit advertising: Institute of Medicine, *Food Marketing to Children and Youth: Threat or Opportunity?* (Washington, D.C.: National Academies Press, 2006).

[118] See, *e.g.*, Canada, House of Commons, Standing Committee on Health, *Healthy Weights for Healthy Kids*, 39th Parl., 1st Sess. (March 2007) (Chair: Rob Merrifield) at 5-6, online: <http://www.ccfn.ca/pdfs/HealthyWeightsForHealthyKids.pdf>; Elaine Power, "Determinants of Healthy Eating Among Low-income Canadians" (2005) 3 Can. J. Public Health S37 (Supp.); Adam Drewnowski, "Obesity and the Food Environment: Dietary Energy Density and Diet Costs" (2004) 27(3S) Am. J. Preventive Medicine 154.

[119] Adam Drewnowski & Nicole Darmon, "The Economics of Obesity: Dietary Energy Density and Energy Cost" (2005) 82 Am. J. Clinical Nutrition 265S (Supp.); Adam Drewnowski, "Obesity and the Food Environment: Dietary Energy Density and Diet Costs" (2004) 27(3S) Am. J. Preventative Medicine 154.

[120] Canada, House of Commons, Standing Committee on Health, *Healthy Weights for Healthy Kids*, 39th Parl. 1st Sess. (March 2007) (Chair: Rob Merrifield) at 5, online: <http://www.ccfn.ca/

for different types of food products varies according to price, with the magnitude of this effect depending in some cases on income and age.[121] All of this suggests that manipulating the price of food products could be one way of influencing consumption patterns and thereby decrease rates of obesity.

Price manipulation could take place by means of taxation, which would increase the cost of food products to discourage their consumption, or subsidies, which would have the opposite effect. The best-known policy proposals have been for a "fat tax" or "junk food tax" that would be added to the price of foods that are high in fat, sugar or calories; or to foods in particular categories, such as snack foods, soft drinks or fast food.[122] A number of U.S. cities and states have implemented "junk food" taxes, though the aim of many of these has focused on raising revenue rather than discouraging consumption, and they have been strongly opposed by the food and beverage industry.[123] Alternatively, "thin" subsidies or healthy food subsidies could be used to lower the price of fruits and vegetables or lower fat and lower calorie versions of popular food products.[124] The application of sales taxes to food products generally has public revenue rather than public health objectives, but can be

---

pdfs/HealthyWeightsForHealthyKids.pdf>; Elaine Power, "Determinants of Healthy Eating Among Low-income Canadians" (2005) 3 Can. J. Public Health S37 at S38 (Supp.); Karen M. Jetter & Diana L. Cassady, "The Availability and Cost of Healthier Food Alternatives" (2006) 30 Am. J. Preventive Medicine 38; Jamy D. Ard et al., "The Impact of Cost on the Availability of Fruits and Vegetables in the Homes of Schoolchildren in Birmingham, Alabama" (2007) 97 Am. J. Public Health 367.

[121] Sinne Smed, Jørgen D. Jensen & Sigrid Denver, "Socio-economic Characteristics and the Effect of Taxation as a Health Policy Instrument" (2007) 32 Food Policy 624; Simone A. French et al., "Pricing and Promotion Effects on Low-Fat Vending Snack Purchases: The CHIPS Study" (2001) 91 Am. J. Pub. H. 112.

[122] Michael F. Jacobson & Kelly D. Brownell, "Small Taxes on Soft Drinks and Snack Foods to Promote Health" (2000) 90 Am. J. Public Health 854; Sinne Smed, Jørgen D. Jensen & Sigrid Denver, "Socio-economic Characteristics and the Effect of Taxation as a Health Policy Instrument" (2007) 32 Food Policy 624; Christiane Schroeter, Jayson Lusk & Wallace Tyner, "Determining the Impact of Food Price and Income Changes on Body Weight" (2008) 27 J. Health Economics 45; Andrew Leicester & Frank Windmeijer, "The 'Fat Tax': Economic Incentives to Reduce Obesity" (Institute for Fiscal Studies, Briefing Note No. 49) at 8-9, online: <http://www.ifs.org.uk/bns/bn49.pdf>.

[123] Jeff Strnad, "Conceptualizing the 'Fat Tax': The Role of Food Taxes in Developed Economies" (2004–2005) 78 S. Cal. L. Rev. 1221 at 1224-25; Martin Caraher & Gill Cowburn, "Taxing Food: Implications for Public Health Nutrition" (2005) 8 Public Health Nutrition 1242 at 1245; Michael F. Jacobson & Kelly D. Brownell, "Small Taxes on Soft Drinks and Snack Foods to Promote Health" (2000) 90 Am. J. Public Health 854 at 855-56.

[124] See, e.g., Sean B. Cash, David L. Sunding & David Zilberman, "Fat Taxes and Thin Subsidies: Prices, Diet, and Health Outcomes" (2005) 2 Food Economics: Acta Agriculturoe Scandinavica, Section C — Food Economics 167; Simone A. French et al., "Pricing and Promotion Effects on Low-Fat Vending Snack Purchases: The CHIPS Study" (2001) 91 Am. J. Pub. H. 112.

adjusted to provide either an additional tax (through higher rates on certain products) or a subsidy (through exemptions, zero ratings or lower rates) to influence consumption.[125] Revenue from additional taxes on some foods could be used to subsidise the price of others, or it could be used to fund other obesity prevention initiatives.[126]

Both taxes and subsidies could be applied at the production or manufacturing stage, at the point of sale or at some stage in between, such as marketing and distribution.[127] It has been suggested that taxes and subsidies could be directed at food manufacturers to encourage them to produce healthier foods, which could have a broad population health impact.[128] Price manipulation at the point of sale may be more feasible and effective in relatively closed environments such as schools or workplaces, where it is possible to exercise greater control over the range of products available and their relative prices.[129]

There are mixed views as to the feasibility and desirability of using price manipulation to encourage healthier diets. Taxation and subsidization will only have the desired public health impact if they actually affect rates of consumption of particular types of foods. There is some limited evidence supporting this assumption,[130] but predictions about the impact of these interventions are largely based on economic models,[131] and accurate predictions are difficult because of the complexity of food consumption patterns. Both elasticity (the change in demand for a particular product when its price changes) and cross-elasticity (the change in demand for

---

[125]   Martin Caraher & Gill Cowburn, "Taxing Food: Implications for Public Health Nutrition" (2005) 8 Public Health Nutrition 1242 at 1244; Tom Marshall, "Exploring a Fiscal Food Policy: The Case of Diet and Ischaemic Heart Disease" (2000) 320 British Med. J. 301.

[126]   R.C. Davey, "The Obesity Epidemic: Too Much Food for Thought?" (2004) 38 Br. J. Sports Med. 360 at 362; Michael F. Jacobson & Kelly D. Brownell, "Small Taxes on Soft Drinks and Snack Foods to Promote Health" (2000) 90 Am. J. Public Health 854 at 856-57; Andrew Leicester & Frank Windmeijer, "The 'Fat Tax': Economic Incentives to Reduce Obesity" (Institute for Fiscal Studies, Briefing Note No. 49) at 10, online: <http://www.ifs.org.uk/bns/bn49.pdf>.

[127]   Regarding taxation of advertising of food to children, see Valere Byrd Fulwider, "Future Benefits? Tax Policy, Advertising, and the Epidemic of Obesity in Children" (2003–2004) 20 J. Contemp. Health L. & Pol'y 217.

[128]   Martin Caraher & Gill Cowburn, "Taxing Food: Implications for Public Health Nutrition" (2005) 8 Public Health Nutrition 1242 at 1248.

[129]   Ibid., at 1247.

[130]   See, e.g., the surveys in Andrew Leicester & Frank Windmeijer, "The 'Fat Tax': Economic Incentives to Reduce Obesity" (Institute for Fiscal Studies, Briefing Note No. 49 at 9-10), online: <http://www.ifs.org.uk/bns/bn49.pdf>; Myles S. Faith et al., "Toward the Reduction of Population Obesity: Macrolevel Environmental Approaches to the Problems of Food, Eating and Obesity" (2007) 133 Psych. Bulletin 205 at 207-209.

[131]   See, e.g., Andrew Leicester & Frank Windmeijer, "The 'Fat Tax': Economic Incentives to Reduce Obesity" (Institute for Fiscal Studies, Briefing Note No. 49) at 11-17, online: <http://www.ifs.org.uk/bns/bn49.pdf>.

other products) need to be considered.[132] There is the potential that introducing a tax on a target food type may have unintended impacts on the consumption of others,[133] though this could be minimized by introducing a tax and subsidy regime that addresses a range of products.[134] Various studies have come to quite different conclusions about the potential impact of price interventions.[135] To be cost effective, these interventions would need to be carefully designed and avoid placing a large burden either on consumers or on the public purse.[136]

Not surprisingly, the evidence indicates that households with lower incomes will be more sensitive to price increases. This suggests that selective taxation might be effective in changing consumption patterns in lower income groups,[137] which may be desirable since they are also generally at higher risk of obesity. However, it also means that taxation could have a regressive impact, which many will perceive as unfair.[138] For this and other reasons, additional taxes on food may be politically unpopular,[139] though Jacobson and Brownell argue, based on public opinion polling, that "small taxes on soft drinks, candy, gum, and snack foods are politically feasible and, when revenues are applied to health programs, likely to be supported by many consumers".[140] Experience in the United States suggests that the food and beverage industry is likely to be strongly opposed to taxation. Subsidies would avoid the regressive

---

[132] Oliver Mytton et al., "Could Targeted Food Taxes Improve Health?" (2007) 61 J. Epidemiol. Community Health 689 at 693.

[133] Ibid.

[134] Sinne Smed, Jørgen D. Jensen & Sigrid Denver, "Socio-economic Characteristics and the Effect of Taxation as a Health Policy Instrument" (2007) 32 Food Policy 624 at 636.

[135] Compare, e.g., Tom Marshall, "Exploring a Fiscal Food Policy: The Case of Diet and Ischaemic Heart Disease" (2000) 320 British Med. J. 301; Oliver Mytton et al., "Could Targeted Food Taxes Improve Health?" (2007) 61 J. Epidemiol. Community Health 689.

[136] Jørgen D. Jensen & Sinne Smed, "Cost-effective Design of Economic Instruments in Nutrition Policy" (2007) 4 Int'l J. Behavioral Nutrition & Physical Activity 1 at 5-8.

[137] R.C. Davey, "The Obesity Epidemic: Too Much Food for Thought?" (2004) 38 Br. J. Sports Med. 360 at 362; Oliver Mytton et al., "Could Targeted Food Taxes Improve Health?" (2007) 61 J. Epidemiol. Community Health 689 at 693; Tom Marshall, "Exploring a Fiscal Food Policy: The Case of Diet and Ischaemic Heart Disease" (2000) 320 British Med. J. 301 at 303.

[138] Andrew Leicester & Frank Windmeijer, "The 'Fat Tax': Economic Incentives to Reduce Obesity" (Institute for Fiscal Studies, Briefing Note No. 49) at 12, 16-17, online: <http://www.ifs.org.uk/bns/bn49.pdf>; Oliver Mytton et al., "Could Targeted Food Taxes Improve Health?" (2007) 61 J. Epidemiol. Community Health 689 at 693; Tom Marshall, "Exploring a Fiscal Food Policy: The Case of Diet and Ischaemic Heart Disease" (2000) 320 British Med. J. 301 at 303; Lawrence O. Gostin, "Law as a Tool to Facilitate Healthier Lifestyles and Prevent Obesity" (2007) 297 J. Am. Med. Assoc. 87 at 88.

[139] Martin Caraher & Gill Cowburn, "Taxing Food: Implications for Public Health Nutrition" (2005) 8 Public Health Nutrition 1242 at 1247-48.

[140] Michael F. Jacobson & Kelly D. Brownell, "Small Taxes on Soft Drinks and Snack Foods to Promote Health" (2000) 90 Am. J. Public Health 854 at 857.

impacts of taxation[141] and are more likely to be favourably received by industry, but the need to invest money up-front to implement subsidies may present a political barrier.

Subsidies and other programs can also be used to address the related problem of restricted access to affordable healthy food in particular communities, especially remote communities. In Canada, the Food Mail Program, also known as the Northern Air Stage Program, aims to make nutritious perishable food and other essential items more affordable in isolated northern communities.[142] Indian and Northern Affairs Canada manages the program and provides funding to Canada Post to help subsidize the cost of shipping eligible items. Eligible food items include nutritious perishable food such as fresh and frozen fruit and vegetables, milk, cheese, eggs, bread and meat; and non-perishable food such as canned food, cereal, pasta and baking supplies. Foods of little nutritional value such as pop, chips and candy; convenience perishable foods such as prepared sandwiches and fried chicken; and alcohol are not eligible. Other programs help to offset the amount of food that must be purchased in northern communities. For example, the Nunavut Harvester Support Program provides financial assistance to eligible residents of Nunavut who need equipment and supplies for hunting.[143] Similar programs are available in James Bay and Northern Québec.[144] Facilitating healthier eating and supporting traditional livelihoods in remote communities clearly also raise a range of much broader and challenging issues, including Aboriginal rights and environmental protection. More generally, using subsidies and taxation to influence food prices may be seen as a potentially effective but very limited way of addressing disparities in health and socioeconomic status.

(e)   Private Enforcement: Obesity-Related Litigation

The value of litigation as a public health strategy has been a matter of debate.[145] In the context of tobacco control, litigation has arguably

---

[141] Sean B. Cash, David L. Sunding & David Zilberman, "Fat Taxes and Thin Subsidies: Prices, Diet, and Health Outcomes" (2005) 2 Food Economics: Acta Agriculturoe Scandinavica, Section C — Food Economics 167 at 168.

[142] Indian and Northern Affairs Canada, "Food Mail Program Brochure", online: <http://www.ainc-inac.gc.ca/ps/nap/air/1brofoomai_e.html>.

[143] Nunavut Tunngavik Inc., "Nunavut Harvesters Support Program Description", online: <http://www.tunngavik.com/english/pdfs-english/NHSP/NHSP%20Program%20Description%20ENG.pdf>.

[144] Indian and Northern Affairs Canada, "Hunter and Trapper Income Support Programs", online: <http://www.ainc-inac.gc.ca/ch/rcap/sg/sj35_e.html>.

[145] See, e.g., Peter D. Jacobson & Soheil Soliman, "Litigation as Public Health Policy: Theory or Reality?" (2002) 30 J.L. Med. & Ethics 224; Benedickt Fischer & Jurgen Rehm, "Some Reflections on the Relationship of Risk, Harm and Responsibility in Recent Tobacco

served several purposes, including compensating affected individuals and governments, deterring industry misconduct, indirectly increasing product costs, raising public awareness, and providing access to internal industry documents through the discovery process.[146] Some advocates believe that similar benefits may be gained through litigation targeting the food industry and its role in obesity.[147] They point to parallels between tobacco and certain food products, such as similar marketing strategies, allegations of misleading conduct by their manufacturers, the importance of consumption habits formed during childhood or adolescence, and the high health and economic costs that can be associated with their consumption.[148] However, there are also obvious differences between tobacco and food products, leading some to question the comparison: food consumption is essential and has some health benefits, even when the food is relatively unhealthy; people generally eat food from a variety of different sources, making it very difficult to attribute causation of obesity to any particular product or manufacturer; and the role of personal and parental responsibility is seen differently in the context of obesity.[149]

The term "obesity litigation" has been used to refer to a range of distinct claims, each of which "has different policy implications for obesity and for the legal system".[150] There are two main types of claims that are most likely to be pursued in this context, both of which could be pursued in either an individual or a class action. The first is personal injury claims, which would argue that the manufacturer negligently marketed a dangerous or defective product and failed to warn consumers of its hazards, causing injury to consumers.[151] The second type of claim is based on consumer protection law, and would involve arguing that the

---

Lawsuits, and Implications for Public Health" (2001) 92 Can. J. Public Health 7; Roberta Ferrence *et al.*, "Tobacco Industry Litigation and the Role of Government: A Public Health Perspective" (2001) 92 Can. J. Public Health 89.

[146] Jon S. Vernick, Lainie Rutkow & Stephen P. Teret, "Public Health Benefits of Recent Litigation Against the Tobacco Industry" (2007) 298 J. Am. Med. Assn. 86.

[147] Richard A. Daynard, P. Tim Howard & Cara L. Wilking, "Private Enforcement: Litigation as a Tool to Prevent Obesity" (2004) 25 J. Public Health Pol'y 408.

[148] *Ibid.*, at 408; Brooke Courtenay, "Is Obesity Really the Next Tobacco? Lessons Learned from Tobacco for Obesity Litigation" (2006) 15 Annals Health L. 61 at 63, 92-93; Alyse Meislik, "Weighing In On the Scales of Justice: The Obesity Epidemic and Litigation Against the Food Industry" (2004) 46 Ariz. L. Rev. 781 at 785-87, 804-806.

[149] Courtenay, *ibid.*, at 94-96; Meislik, *ibid.*, at 808; Joseph P. McMenamin & Andrea D. Tiglio, "Not the Next Tobacco: Defenses to Obesity Claims" (2006) 61 Food & Drug L. J. 445 at 446-47.

[150] Theodore H. Frank, "A Taxonomy of Obesity Litigation" (2005–2006) 28 U.A.L.R. L. Rev. 427 at 429.

[151] Richard A. Daynard, P. Tim Howard & Cara L. Wilking, "Private Enforcement: Litigation as a Tool to Prevent Obesity" (2004) 25 J. Public Health Pol'y 408 at 411-13; Charles E. Cantú, "Fattening Foods: Under Products Liability Litigation is the Big Mac Defective?" (2005) 1 J. Food L. & Pol'y 165.

manufacturer engaged in unfair, misleading or deceptive practices in marketing their products. These claims are typically based on a statutory cause of action, which may not require the plaintiff to prove that impugned practices caused injury.[152] These claims are thought to be more promising in the obesity context, since they relieve the plaintiff of the burden of proving that the manufacturer caused his or her obesity or associated health problems; however, any resulting damages will likely be small.[153]

The best-known examples of obesity litigation are the American cases of *Barber v. McDonald's Corp.*,[154] a proposed class action commenced and discontinued in 2002, and *Pelman v. McDonald's Corp.*[155] The initial claim in *Pelman* was filed by the parents of two minors, alleging both negligence and violations of consumer protection legislation. This claim was dismissed, but the plaintiffs were permitted to file an amended claim, focusing on the consumer protection arguments regarding deceptive advertising. When this claim in turn was dismissed, the plaintiffs successfully appealed, but then McDonald's filed a motion for a more detailed statement of the claim, which was partly granted. The court ordered the plaintiffs to identify the advertisements or other statements that were alleged to be deceptive and the injuries allegedly suffered.[156] A further motion to dismiss the claim was granted in part but left a limited set of claims to proceed, ordering McDonald's to respond to the statement of claim.[157] Although the ultimate outcome remains uncertain and many obstacles remain, the decisions in this case have provided useful guidance about the way in which claims should be framed to have any prospect of success, and are believed to show some potential for public health-based arguments in obesity litigation.[158]

---

[152]   Daynard, Howard & Wilking, *ibid.*, at 410-11.

[153]   *Ibid.*, at 411; Brooke Courtenay, "Is Obesity Really the Next Tobacco? Lessons Learned from Tobacco for Obesity Litigation" (2006) 15 Annals Health L. 61 at 98-99.

[154]   *Barber v. McDonald's Corp.*, N.Y. Sup. Ct., complaint filed 23 July 2002.

[155]   237 F. Supp. 2d 512 (S.D.N.Y. 2003); 2003 U.S. Dist. LEXIS 15202 (S.D.N.Y.); 396 F. 3d 508 (2d Cir. 2005); 396 F. Supp. 2d 439 (S.D.N.Y. 2005); 452 F. Supp. 2d 320 (S.D.N.Y. 2006).

[156]   *Pelman v. McDonald's Corp.*, 396 F. Supp. 2d 439 (S.D.N.Y. 2005). For a review of the litigation and discussion of this decision and its implications, see Jason A. Smith, "Setting the Stage for Public Health: The Role of Litigation in Controlling Obesity" (2005–2006) 28 U.A.L.R. L. Rev. 443 at 449-52.

[157]   *Pelman v. McDonald's Corp.*, 452 F. Supp. 2d 320 (S.D.N.Y. 2006).

[158]   Jason A. Smith, "Setting the Stage for Public Health: The Role of Litigation in Controlling Obesity" (2005–2006) 28 U.A.L.R. L. Rev. 443 at 449-52; Andrea Freeman, "Fast Food: Oppression Through Poor Nutrition" (2007) 95 California L. Rev. 2221 at 2247-48.

Despite the existence of potential causes of action, "food litigation has been largely unsuccessful and politically unpopular".[159] The prospects for successful claims do not appear to be very strong, particularly given the difficulty of establishing causation in these lawsuits.[160] In the United States, a number of jurisdictions have also passed legislation blocking or limiting litigation against the food industry (so-called "cheeseburger bills"), further diminishing the chances of success in that country.[161] However, it appears that litigation may have had some limited effect. There is some evidence that actual or threatened lawsuits have prompted food companies to change their practices.[162] For example, in 2007, Kellogg settled a lawsuit brought by a group of parents and organizations, agreeing to certain limits on its advertising practices and nutrition standards for foods advertised to children.[163] A claim against Kentucky Fried Chicken was withdrawn after the company agreed to switch to a trans fat-free frying oil.[164] These developments suggest that, in this context as in others, the impact of public health litigation cannot be measured solely by the ultimate success of legal claims.

IV. CONCLUSIONS

Contemporary public health problems "are complex systems problems, with equally complex solutions; there are problems that have the potential to affect all individuals at different levels, affecting health, the sustainability of health services, and potentially the long-term economic prosperity of the country".[165] Obesity is a clear example of a complex problem where there are no clear and easy regulatory and policy solutions, since so many

---

[159] Lawrence O. Gostin, "Law as a Tool to Facilitate Healthier Lifestyles and Prevent Obesity" (2007) 297 J. Am. Med. Assn. 87 at 87.

[160] Brooke Courtenay, "Is Obesity Really the Next Tobacco? Lessons Learned from Tobacco for Obesity Litigation" (2006) 15 Annals Health L. 61 at 99 100.

[161] See David Burnett, "Fast-food Lawsuits and the Cheeseburger Bill: Critiquing Congress's Response to the Obesity Epidemic" (2007) 14 Va. J. Soc. Pol'y & L. 357. These statutes do not generally preclude claims based on consumer protection law, however: Dustin A. Frazier, "The Link Between Fast Food and the Obesity Epidemic" (2007) 17 Health Matrix 291 at 304-305.

[162] Alyse Meislik, "Weighing In On the Scales of Justice: The Obesity Epidemic and Litigation Against the Food Industry" (2004) 46 Ariz. L. Rev. 781 at 783, 795, 799-801; Richard A. Daynard, P. Tim Howard & Cara L. Wilking, "Private Enforcement: Litigation as a Tool to Prevent Obesity" (2004) 25 J. Public Health Pol'y 408 at 409-10.

[163] Center for Science in the Public Interest, News Release, "Kellogg Makes Historic Settlement Agreement, Adopting Nutrition Standards for Marketing Foods to Children" (14 June 2007), online: <http://www.cspinet.org/new/200706141.html>.

[164] Center for Science in the Public Interest, News Release "CSPI Withdraws from Lawsuit After KFC Cuts Trans Fat" (30 October 2006), online: <http://www.cspinet.org/new/200610301.html>.

[165] Fiona Adshead & Allison Thorpe, "The Role of the Government in Public Health: A National Perspective" (2007) 121 Public Health 835 at 836.

environmental factors influence food and physical activity behaviours. Specific regulatory measures to address obesity are likely to face opposition, from those who claim measures are unduly paternalistic and impose unjustifiable burdens to those who claim regulations do not go far enough to counter the influence of our obesogenic environments.

It has been aptly noted that regulatory measures intended to address obesity may result in "a staggering patchwork of different laws regarding policy areas that had until recently received little regulatory attention".[166] Further, it is contended that "adverse effects of specific dietary practices or foods have not yet been definitively linked to obesity. Therefore, many regulatory strategies that might affect food consumption cannot yet be justified. The identification of these linkages must remain a high priority".[167] The serious health, social and economic costs associated with current numbers at overweight and obese people demand attention to the environmental factors that promote unhealthy weight gain. Regulatory intervention to address the problem is warranted, but the follow-on issue is to identify what specific measures should be adopted. Taken individually, specific regulatory interventions — like the disclosure of calorie and nutrient information on food labels and menus; limits on TV food advertising directed at children; and food price manipulation — may have little measurable impact on obesity in populations. But as three strategies among others, they may contribute to cumulative benefits.

Regulating to address factors associated with overweight and obesity is a relatively novel area of public health intervention that, not surprisingly, generates disagreement about the appropriate role of the state. New and different interventions often stir controversy: England's liquor licensing laws in the 1870s that restricted business hours for pubs and banned children from imbibing spirits in them were decried by those who argued English citizens were better "free than ... compulsorily sober".[168] Today, public health interventions across many areas of policy and behaviour are commonplace and unquestioned. With the aim of reversing (or at least slowing) current obesity trends, the number and types of interventions to promote healthier eating and physical activity are growing, though governments acknowledge that "[t]o demonize eating is not an option" and they cannot order people "to embrace sports or go for a long walk

---

[166]   Sean B. Cash, David Sunding & David Zilberman, "Fat Taxes and Thin Subsidies: Prices, Diet, and Health Outcomes" (2005) 2 Acta Agriculturæ Scandinavica, Section C — Food Economics 167 at 168.

[167]   Shawna L. Mercer, "Drawing Possible Lessons for Obesity Prevention and Control from the Tobacco Control Experience" in David Crawford & Robert W. Jeffery, eds., *Obesity Prevention and Public Health* (New York: Oxford University Press, 2005) at 241.

[168]   Karen Jochelson, "Nanny or Steward? The Role of Government in Public Health" (2006) 120 Public Health 1149 at 1150.

every day".[169] Governments can, however, choose among a range of public health interventions to address obesogenic aspects of modern environments and, in doing so, ought to remain mindful of the need to evaluate those interventions to identify if and how they influence targeted behaviour (such as individual food choices and physical activity or commercial food product development, pricing and marketing) and help control rates of obesity.

---

[169]   British Columbia Select Standing Committee on Health, *A Strategy for Combatting Childhood Obesity and Physical Inactivity in British Columbia* at 1, online: <http://www.leg.bc.ca/ CMT/38thparl/session-2/health/reports/Rpt-Health-38-2-29Nov2006.pdf>.

10

The Intersection of Aboriginal Public Health with Canadian Law and Policy

Constance MacIntosh[*]

I. INTRODUCTION

This chapter presents an overview of law, policy and practices concerning the population health of Aboriginal Canadians. Any consideration of these matters requires coming to terms with the overall living conditions of Aboriginal peoples. These conditions reflect long-standing and shifting relations of power within the Canadian state, and its jurisdictional presumptions and arrangements.

This chapter is divided into several sections. The first section of this chapter provides a general description of the socio-legal categories that are drawn upon in health policy, programming and legislation regarding Aboriginal peoples. It then turns to a brief discussion of Aboriginal conceptions of good health.

The second section provides an overview of the health status of Aboriginal populations. It focuses upon epidemiological data, drawing comparisons between Aboriginal and non-Aboriginal populations, as well as between populations of Aboriginal peoples. This section also discusses how law and policy informs both research with Aboriginal populations as well as the practical delivery of community health programming and services.

---

[*] The author is grateful to Dr. Brian Noble, for providing thoughtful comments on earlier drafts of this chapter.

The third section moves into three detailed case studies of environmental determinants of health that are particularly pressing for the Aboriginal population: quality and availability of housing, quality of drinking water, and quality of "country food". These case studies illustrate the operation of law and policy at various levels of jurisdiction: federal, provincial-federal, and domestic-international. They also illustrate how claims to Aboriginal treaty rights, and the legal implications of the special fiduciary relationship between the Crown and Aboriginal peoples, may shape or create barriers to proposed state action. This section is rounded out by a discussion of conflicting claims of jurisdiction over public health as between provincial and First Nation governments. This discussion is grounded through a case study regarding the application of provincial smoking bans to on-reserve establishments, such as casinos.

Where the third section assesses how the state protects or promotes Aboriginal community health, the fourth section considers how the state regulates traditional Aboriginal health practices. Three topics are considered: traditional midwifery, traditional healers and traditional medicines. Interwoven within this chapter are assessments of how Aboriginal rights may affect the lawfulness of existing and proposed legislation.

Section five concludes this chapter by delving into law and policy regarding the transfer of control over public health to Aboriginal communities. Both treaty-based, as well as policy-based, transfers are considered. This section ends with a discussion of the public health consequences of Aboriginal communities having control over their health programming.

(a) An Overview of the Aboriginal Population

Approximately 4 per cent of the Canadian population — about 1.3 million people — identify themselves as having Aboriginal ancestry.[1] Of these individuals, about 49 per cent live in urban areas, about 31 per cent live on one of Canada's 2,360 reserves, and the remainder live in other rural areas.[2]

The Aboriginal population is quite diverse, including approximately 50 linguistically distinct groups, each with their own culture, and each claiming a traditional land base.[3] Canadian legislation and policy

---

[1]   Canadian Population Health Initiative, *Improving the Health of Canadians* (Ottawa: Canadian Institute for Health Information, 2004) at 76.

[2]   D. Elliot, *Law and Aboriginal Peoples in Canada, 5th Ed.* (North York: Captus Press, 2005) at 14.

[3]   Canadian Population Health Initiative, *Improving the Health of Canadians* (Ottawa: Canadian Institute for Health Information, 2004) at 76.

reference several "categories" of Aboriginal peoples, which cannot possibly capture this diversity, and indeed have little or no correlation with culturally meaningful groupings. Nonetheless, these socio-legal categories often frame the collection and organization of data, which is in turn used to make programming and policy decisions about health services and delivery for Aboriginal peoples. As a consequence, it is essential to understand how these categories include or exclude segments of the Aboriginal population.

The majority of people who self-identify as Aboriginal, about 805,700,[4] fall into the federally created category of "Registered Indians" (also known as "Status Indians"). That is, they are members of First Nations who meet certain criteria as set out in the federal *Indian Act*,[5] and as a consequence can be registered on a list maintained by Indian and Northern Affairs Canada ("INAC").[6] The criteria are complex, and relate to parentage. They are divorced from any culturally informed sense of Aboriginality or community. As a matter of policy, certain federally administered health and social benefits, which are above and beyond those provided by provinces to all residents, are potentially available to those Aboriginal people who are registered on INAC's list. These include vision and dental care, as well as medical products, drugs and services.

Approximately 30 per cent of all Aboriginal peoples who self-identify as Aboriginal, and as a member of a First Nation, either do not meet the statutory criteria for registration or do meet the criteria but have chosen not to apply to be registered.[7] The members of this population, who used to be referred to commonly as "non-Status Indians", are not recognized under the *Indian Act*.

Prior to 1985, eligibility for registration was determined by paternity, and could be gained or lost through marriage. As a result, Status women who married non-Status men were removed from the registry, and lost their benefits. The children of these women were also ineligible to register for status. However, where a Status man married a non-Status woman, that woman gained the right to register for status, as did their children.

---

[4] *Report on Plans and Priorities: 2007–2008 Estimates* (Ottawa: Indian and Northern Affairs Canada, 2007) at 9.

[5] *Indian Act*, R.S.C. 1985, c. I-5, ss. 6-7.

[6] *Ibid.*, s. 5.

[7] Canada, Standing Senate Committee on Social Affairs, Science and Technology, *The Health of Canadians — the Federal Role (Interim Report: Volume Four — Issues and Options)* (Ottawa: Standing Senate Committee on Social Affairs, Science and Technology, 2001) at 129 (Chair: Hon. M. Kirby) ["*The Kirby Report*"].

These sexually discriminatory provisions were largely reformed in 1985, pursuant to Bill C-31.[8] The bill allowed many of the women who had lost status to regain it, and allowed some of their descendants to register for status as well.[9] Portions of the bill which had the effect of treating descendants differently based upon whether they traced their ancestry through the maternal or paternal line were harshly criticized, but remained in effect until struck under a *Charter* challenge in 2007.[10] Bill C-31 was also intended to counter the consequences of other legislation under which Aboriginal people had lost status. For example, they had to "enfranchise" and denounce their status in law if they wished to obtain the right to vote, to serve in the military or to train for certain professions, such as medicine or law. Under Bill C-31, many of these individuals, and some of their descendants, became eligible to be registered for status once again.

Between 1985 and 2002, over 114,000 people applied for and were granted Status pursuant to the terms of Bill C-31.[11] Although this increase in population resulted in increased demand for the on-reserve housing and health services which are administered under Band Councils, additional resources were not committed to reflect this increase in population.

Another Aboriginal population is the Inuit, who number approximately 56,000.[12] About 20 per cent of this population live in urban areas in southern Canada, while the majority lives primarily in four Arctic coastal regions: northern and southeastern Labrador, Nunavik in northern Québec, Nunavut, and Inuvialuit in the northwestern portion of the Northwest Territories.[13] The eight main tribal groups of the Inuit speak a common language, Inuktituk, of which there are six different dialects. Inuit are excluded from registration under the *Indian Act*, although there are several federal health and social services programs for Inuit people.

The last key socio-legal category is Métis. "Métis" refers to the population that formed communities comprised of descendants from

---

8   *An Act to Amend the Indian Act*, R.S.C. 1985, c. 32 (1st Supp.), amending R.S.C. 1985, c. I-5 ["Bill C-31"]. Bill C-31 primarily modified ss. 6 and 7 of the *Indian Act*, R.S.C. 1985, c. I-5.

9   One of the other changes brought about by Bill C-31, *ibid.*, is that it is no longer possible for women to gain a right to register by virtue of marrying a man with Status.

10   *McIvor v. Canada (Registrar, Indian and Northern Affairs)*, [2007] B.C.J. No. 1259, 2007 BCSC 827 (B.C.S.C.). This decision has been appealed.

11   S. Clatworthy, *Indian Registration, Membership and Population Changes in First Nation Communities* (Ottawa: Indian and Northern Affairs Canada, 2005) at 1.

12   J. Frideres & R. Gadacz, *Aboriginal Peoples in Canada*, 6th ed. (Toronto: Prentice Hall, 2001) at 29.

13   Statistics Canada, *Aboriginal Peoples Survey 2001 — initial findings: Well-being of the non-reserve Aboriginal Population* by V. O'Donnell & H. Tait (Ottawa: Minister of Industry, 2003) at 8.

marriages between Aboriginal people and those of European descent. These communities were and are located primarily in Ontario, Manitoba, Saskatchewan and Alberta. These communities only have constitutional status if they "developed their own customs, way of life, and recognizable group identity separate from their Indian or Inuit and European forebears ... prior to the entrenchment of European control".[14] There are currently over 300,000 Métis people living in Canada.[15] Once again, Métis people usually do not qualify for registration under the *Indian Act* and so, as a matter of policy, do not receive comprehensive health or social benefits from the federal government.

(b) Aboriginal Conceptions of Good Health

The perspective of many Aboriginal peoples as to how to measure and promote health resonates with the population health approach. The Royal Commission on Aboriginal Peoples cited Henry Zoe, who summed up the Aboriginal perception of health as follows:

> For a person to be healthy, [he or she] must be adequately fed, be educated, have access to medical facilities, have access to spiritual comfort, live in a warm and comfortable house with clean water and safe sewage disposal, be secure in cultural identity, have an opportunity to excel in meaningful endeavor, and so on. These are not separate needs; they are all aspects of the whole.[16]

The National Aboriginal Health Organization similarly concluded that from an indigenous perspective, health is generally not seen as separate and distinct from other aspects of life, and engages with physical, mental, emotional, social and spiritual factors.[17]

---

[14] *R. v. Powley*, [2003] S.C.J. No. 43, [2003] 2 S.C.R. 207, 2003 SCC 43 at para. 10 (S.C.C.).

[15] Métis National Council, *HIV/AIDS: The Basic Facts for Métis Communities* (Ottawa: Métis National Council, 2003) at 1.

[16] Canada, Royal Commission on Aboriginal Peoples, *Report of the Royal Commission on Aboriginal Peoples: Volume 3 Gathering Strength* (Ottawa: Minister of Supply and Services, 1996) at 206 ["*Royal Commission Report*"]. Henry Zoe testified before the Royal Commission in Yellowknife. Although all Aboriginal peoples and cultures are different from one another, it is the author's opinion that this statement captures a perspective that can legitimately be attributed to most Aboriginal peoples in Canada.

[17] National Aboriginal Health Organization, *Ways of Knowing: A Framework for Health Research* by Policy Research Unit (Ottawa: National Aboriginal Health Organization, 2003) at 5. For further analysis of indigenous perspectives on health, see Assembly of First Nations, *First Nations Regional Longitudinal Health Study (RHS) 2002/03: Results for Adults, Youth and Children Living in First Nations Communities* (Ottawa: Assembly of First Nations/First Nations Information Governance Committee, 2007) at 1-4.

II. THE POPULATION HEALTH OF ABORIGINAL CANADIANS

This section presents a sampling of epidemiological data, selected to provide an overview of the health status of Aboriginal peoples. The conclusions of several national reports are briefly described, and specific data is referenced to illustrate rates of infectious diseases, non-communicable chronic illnesses and injuries. To maintain a broad perspective on the meaning of health, unemployment rates, income and educational attainment are also described. Having established these baseline conditions, this section then moves to a consideration of public and community health services. The delivery of these services is complicated by issues of jurisdictional and constitutional interpretation, as well as gaps in research data. This section closes with a consideration of protocols regarding health-based research with Aboriginal populations.

(a) Epidemiological Data

In his 2002 report on health, Roy Romanow asserted that the "deep and continuing disparities" between the health of Aboriginal and non-Aboriginal populations is "simply unacceptable".[18] Two years earlier, the Senate committee chaired by Senator Kirby, had similarly observed that "the state of health of Aboriginal Canadians and the socio-economic conditions in which they live remain deplorable".[19] Romanow's and Kirby's conclusions were quite similar to those described in 1996, when the Royal Commission on Aboriginal Peoples found that "despite the large sums spent by Canadian governments to provide [medical] services, Aboriginal people still suffer from unacceptable rates of illness and disease".[20]

The most recent comprehensive report on public health, the Naylor Report,[21] indicates that this situation remains unchanged. Upon comparing the health status indicators for Canada's First Nations and Inuit peoples

---

[18]   Commission on the Future of Health Care in Canada, *Building on Values: The Future of Health Care in Canada — Final Report* (Saskatoon: Commission on the Future of Health Care in Canada, 2002) at 211 (Commissioner: R.J. Romanow).

[19]   Canada, Standing Senate Committee on Social Affairs, Science and Technology, *The Health of Canadians — the Federal Role (Interim Report: Volume Four — Issues and Options)* (Ottawa: Standing Senate Committee on Social Affairs, Science and Technology, 2001) at 129 (Chair: Hon. M. Kirby).

[20]   Canada, Royal Commission on Aboriginal Peoples, *Report of the Royal Commission on Aboriginal Peoples: Volume 3 Gathering Strength* (Ottawa: Minister of Supply and Services, 1996) at 119.

[21]   National Advisory Committee on SARS and Public Health, *Learning from SARS: Renewal of Public Health in Canada* (Ottawa: Health Canada, 2003) (Chair: Dr. D. Naylor) ["Naylor Report"].

with those of the non-Aboriginal population, the Naylor Report described the disparity as "a national disgrace".[22]

This disparity can be seen both in rates of infectious diseases as well as non-communicable illnesses. For example, compared to non-Aboriginal Canadians, the rate of tuberculosis experienced by Status members of First Nations is 23 times higher, while the rate for the Inuit population is 70 times higher.[23] Chronic diseases are similarly present at elevated rates. Heart problems are experienced within the Aboriginal population at approximately three times the rate of non-Aboriginal people, and diabetes at approximately three to four times the rate. As well, Aboriginal peoples are twice as likely to be obese as non-Aboriginal Canadians.[24]

Status members of First Nations also have a shorter life expectancy than non-Aboriginal Canadians (five years less for women, seven years less for men), as do Inuit peoples (14 years less for women, six years less for men).[25] This shorter life expectancy reflects not just higher incidences of disease, but also disturbing trends regarding rates of death by accident or suicide. Overall, the Status population has twice the suicide rate of non-Aboriginal Canadians, while Inuit communities experience six times the suicide rate.[26] Where injury only accounts for the cause of death for 8.6 per cent of the male Canadian population, and 5.2 per cent of the female population, it accounts for a staggering 33.5 per cent of male deaths and 18.2 per cent of female deaths among registered members of First Nations.[27] Injuries contribute to premature death among the on-reserve Status Indian population at a rate four times higher than that of the Canadian population as a whole,[28] perhaps reflecting the four-fold greater risk of severe trauma experienced by Aboriginal Canadians generally.[29]

Fatal injuries result from four main sources: motor vehicle accidents (with alcohol as a major contributing factor), drownings, house fires and

---

[22]   *Ibid.*, at 79.

[23]   Canadian Population Health Initiative, *Improving the Health of Canadians* (Ottawa: Canadian Institute for Health Information, 2004) at 83.

[24]   *Ibid.*, at 83.

[25]   *Ibid.*, at 81.

[26]   *Ibid.*, at 81.

[27]   Canada, Royal Commission on Aboriginal Peoples, *Report of the Royal Commission on Aboriginal Peoples: Volume 3 Gathering Strength* (Ottawa: Minister of Supply and Services, 1996) at 122.

[28]   Canadian Population Health Initiative, *Improving the Health of Canadians* (Ottawa: Canadian Institute for Health Information, 2004) at 81.

[29]   S. Karmali *et al.*, "Epidemiology of Severe Trauma Among Status Aboriginal Canadians: A Population-Based Study" (2005) 172(8) C.M.A.J. 1007 at 1009.

gunshot wounds.[30] These high rates of injury reflect adverse psycho-social and economic factors that are often present in Aboriginal communities. The unemployment rate for Status Indians is about three times higher than the Canadian average (29 per cent compared to 10 per cent), with the highest unemployment experienced by Status youth between the ages of 15 and 24, which hovers at 41 per cent.[31] Given these figures, it is not surprising that in 1997–1998 social assistance rates were around 46 per cent, a figure four times above the Canadian average.[32] Income rates are low, and only rising incrementally — for registered on-reserve members of First Nations, the average income in 1990 was $11,941, and in 1995 was only $14,833.[33] The rate of improvement has slowed, as by 2000 median personal income was only $15,667, in stark contrast to the Canadian average of $40,000 for men and $24,000 for women.[34] Data regarding educational attainment is also discouraging: while 79 per cent of Canadians complete high school, only 48 per cent of Aboriginal people with status do so.[35]

Reckless and self-destructive behaviour (such as drunk driving) has been linked with feelings of grief, anger and hopelessness that much of the Aboriginal population experiences. Similarly, the increased likelihood of household fires has been linked with the correlates of poverty (including substandard housing).[36] It is not surprising that the Royal Commission concluded the Aboriginal population will not achieve good health until extremely broad social and political factors are addressed.[37] Some of these factors, such as housing and the desire for self-government, are discussed below.

---

[30]   Canada, Royal Commission on Aboriginal Peoples, *Report of the Royal Commission on Aboriginal Peoples: Volume 3 Gathering Strength* (Ottawa: Minister of Supply and Services, 1996) at 153.

[31]   First Nations and Inuit Health Branch, Health Canada, *A Statistical Profile on the Health of First Nations in Canada* (Ottawa: Health Canada, 2003) at 64.

[32]   National Aboriginal Health Organization, *Improving Population Health, Health Promotion, Disease Prevention and Health Protection Services and Programs for Aboriginal People* by D. Kinnon (Ottawa, National Aboriginal Health Organization, 2002) at 10.

[33]   First Nations and Inuit Health Branch, Health Canada, *A Statistical Profile on the Health of First Nations in Canada* (Ottawa: Health Canada, 2003) at 64.

[34]   Assembly of First Nations, *First Nations Regional Longitudinal Health Survey (RHS) 2002/03: Results for Adults, Youth and Children Living in First Nations Communities* (Ottawa: Assembly of First Nations/First Nations Information Governance Committee, 2007) at 28.

[35]   *Ibid.*, at 26.

[36]   Canada, Royal Commission on Aboriginal Peoples, *Report of the Royal Commission on Aboriginal Peoples: Volume 3 Gathering Strength* (Ottawa: Minister of Supply and Services, 1996) at 155.

[37]   *Ibid.*, at 109.

(b) Public and Community Health Services

Given such appalling health and social data, one might be led to think that governments are not allocating sufficient resources to Aboriginal health services. In fact, spending on Aboriginal health matters is quite high. The fundamental inadequacy reflects historically and legally entrenched divisions of powers and responsibilities, the marriage of these divisions through policy to socio-legal categorizations of Aboriginal peoples, and the complexity of recovering from the ongoing social, cultural and economic consequences of colonialism. This final point is taken up in the last substantive section of this chapter.

As to the first two points, community health programs and services are delivered to Aboriginal peoples through a complex myriad of mechanisms and jurisdictionally separated agencies, provincial departments and federal Ministries. In practice, there is often little co-ordination among these participants.[38] The pattern of delivery reflects, to some extent, the division of powers mandated by the Canadian *Constitution Act, 1867*.[39] The Constitution assigns various heads of power between the federal and provincial governments. In s. 91(24), the federal government is assigned authority over "Indians and lands reserved for Indians",[40] while provinces are considered to have been assigned jurisdiction over health pursuant to other sections of the Constitution. The constitutional designation of "Indians" — a *category of people* (as opposed to a topic) being specifically assigned to a certain level of government regardless of their place of residence — is problematic, both conceptually and pragmatically. One question this assignment of categories begs is whether the health of Aboriginal people is a "health issue" (and thus within provincial jurisdiction) or an "Indian issue" (and thus within federal jurisdiction). And, of course, there is the further question of to whom the term "Indian" refers in the context of s. 91(24) of the *Constitution Act, 1867.*

These questions have not been answered in a direct or systematic fashion. Canada has generally interpreted its constitutional obligation to extend only to registered members of First Nations, and Inuit peoples.[41]

---

[38] M. Maar, "Clearing the Path for Community Health Empowerment: Integrating Health Care Services at an Aboriginal Health Access Centre in Rural North Central Ontario" (2004) 1 Journal of Aboriginal Health 54 at 56.

[39] *Constitution Act, 1867* (U.K.), 30 & 31 Vict., c. 3, reprinted in R.S.C. 1985, App. II, No. 5.

[40] *Ibid.*, s. 91(24).

[41] The Supreme Court of Canada determined in 1939 that Inuit peoples were entailed within the jurisdiction granted under s. 91(24). *Reference Re Eskimos*, [1939] S.C.J. No. 5, [1939] S.C.R. 104 (S.C.C.). Although there has been no judicial determination of whether this section also encompasses Métis people, or other members of First Nations without Status, this position is certainly arguable given the reasoning of the Court in this case.

Health Canada thus manages health programming for these populations while provinces are assumed to have jurisdiction — and so authority — to address the needs of the remainder of the Aboriginal population.

In practice, provinces are inconsistent in responding to the unique health needs of Aboriginal peoples. Ontario has developed distinctive programs for Aboriginal communities, such as an HIV/AIDS program. Other provinces, such as Nova Scotia, regard Aboriginal health as within federal jurisdiction, so do not generally support programs designed specifically for the provincial Aboriginal population. As well, there is often uncertainty between federal and provincial service providers as to who is responsible for Status members of First Nations who live off-reserve, especially those who reside in urban cores.

The overall result is that health care programming and delivery depends upon a mix of eligibility factors, including ancestry (*e.g.*, Inuit versus Métis), eligibility for registration (*e.g.*, Status or non-Status), place of residence (on- or off-reserve), and province of residence (*e.g.*, Ontario or Nova Scotia). These factors combine to produce silos of delivery characterized by duplication and gaps in services.[42]

Health Canada's programming activity for Aboriginal peoples is directed through the First Nations and Inuit Health Branch ("FNIHB"). FNIHB's main areas of activity include providing community-based health promotion and primary care for on-reserve and Inuit communities, and administering some non-insured health benefits (such as medication and medical devices) for all status members of First Nations.[43]

Health Canada also delivers a number of programs targeted at specific community health issues, such as diabetes and drug and alcohol addiction. A key component of Health Canada's public health activities is the placement of Community Health Representatives ("CHR") in approximately 577 bands and Inuit organizations. The CHR's primary roles are to link the various community health programming activities, to work with the community to identify its health care needs, to provide culturally appropriate health education and promotion, and to assist community members to access and fully utilize existing health services.

Health Canada's Population and Public Health Branch provides limited programs that target Métis people and off-reserve members of First Nations. For example, there is an off-reserve component of Health Canada's

---

[42]   These issues are discussed in detail in Constance MacIntosh, "Jurisdictional Roulette: Constitutional and Structural Barriers to Aboriginal Access to Health" in C. Flood, ed., *The Frontiers of Fairness* (Toronto: University of Toronto Press, 2006).

[43]   National Aboriginal Health Organization, *Improving Population Health, Health Promotion, Disease Prevention and Health Protection Services and Programs for Aboriginal People* by D. Kinnon (Ottawa, National Aboriginal Health Organization, 2002) at 26.

Aboriginal Diabetes Initiative, Aboriginal Head Start,[44] and Healthy Start. Healthy Start is intended to improve the poor health outcomes of newborn Aboriginal children, by working with pregnant Aboriginal women on issues such as nutrition.

For the most part, non-Status members of First Nations, members of First Nations with Status but who live off-reserve, and Métis people, must rely on provincial community health programs and services, which are seldom tailored to be culturally appropriate for these populations, and are almost never created to address issues unique to the Aboriginal population. However, provinces do in some instances consider Aboriginal peoples as one of the target groups to be served by certain health strategies.

(c) Research Gaps

Many studies have been produced to identify the population health issues of Aboriginal peoples. However, these studies tend to focus upon registered members of First Nations who also claim reserves as their residences.[45] This group only represents about one-third of the Aboriginal population. There is a dearth of materials relating to Aboriginal peoples who live off-reserves in other rural areas, and Aboriginal peoples who live in urban areas. In studies published on Medline from 1992–2001, 158 papers referred to First Nations but only two dealt specifically with Aboriginal peoples living off-reserve, and only five addressed urban Aboriginal populations.[46] There is at present almost no data-based health

---

[44]   Aboriginal Head Start is a program aimed at pre-school Aboriginal children. It emphasizes health promotion, nutrition and building family support, and exposes the children to stimulation and socialization.

[45]   For example, in the Centres of Excellence for Women's Health synthesis report on all work done by the centres on Aboriginal women's health, none of the studies appear to have included non-Status Indians. Most of the studies only addressed the health of Status Indians, although some also considered Métis and Inuit peoples. See Centres of Excellence for Women's Health, *Aboriginal Women's Health Research Synthesis Project: Final Report* by M. Stout, G. Kipling & R. Stout (Ottawa: Centres of Excellence for Women's Health, 2001). Health Canada has similarly produced reports that tend to only assess Status Indians and Inuit peoples. See *e.g.*, Health Canada, *A Second Diagnostic on the Health of First Nations and Inuit Peoples in Canada, 1999* by Medical Services Branch (Ottawa: Health Canada, 1999); see also First Nations and Inuit Health Branch, Health Canada, *A Statistical Profile on the Health of First Nations in Canada* (Ottawa: Health Canada, 2003) at 64. One notable exception is Statistics Canada's report compiled from census data on Aboriginal peoples who live off-reserve. See Statistics Canada, *Aboriginal Peoples Survey 2001 — initial findings: Well-being of the non-reserve Aboriginal Population* by V. O'Donnell & H. Tait (Ottawa: Minister of Industry, 2003) at 8. Unfortunately the data in this report cannot be compared to existing data regarding the Status First Nation population, because the report is Status blind — so the health situation of persons with Status who live off-reserve would be double-counted, appearing both in Status-only reports, as well as in this report.

[46]   See T. Young "Review of research on aboriginal populations in Canada: relevance to their health needs" (23 August 2002) 327 British Medical Journal 419 at 420.

research regarding Métis people.[47] This gap has been attributed to the absence of a Métis registry, and the absence of an organization or level of government charged to deliver or fund health services directed to Métis people.[48]

This is not to suggest that there is sufficient population health data regarding the on-reserve registered population, but to highlight the startling fact that the majority of the Aboriginal population — around 66 per cent — remains somewhat invisible in the population health literature.

(d) Research Ethics and Protocols

Protocols for health-related research involving Aboriginal populations have undergone considerable transformations over the last ten years. These transformations respond to the fact that ethical safeguards were often inadequately addressed in the past, resulting in some research having had a rather exploitative character. There has also been an acknowledgement that Aboriginal perspectives of health were often missing from health research studies, which raised questions about relevance to and benefit for the subject community. A final motivation for change has been the growing assertions by Aboriginal peoples of an inherent right to control knowledge and information about themselves and their communities, assertions which are acted upon when researchers come calling.[49]

Both federal as well as First Nation governments have established protocols which are intended to address the above issues and also reflect the unique cultural and political character and concerns of Aboriginal peoples and communities. For example, in Nova Scotia the Mi'kmaq Nation has developed the Mi'kmaq Research Principles and Protocols, under which any party seeking to conduct research within Mi'kmaw communities must submit an application to the Mi'kmaq Ethics Watch. The Watch evaluates the application and decides whether to require revisions, reject or permit the research (subject to local community approval as well).

---

[47]   Human Resources Development Canada, Manitoba Aboriginal Affairs Secretariat, Manitoba Family Services and Housing, *Aboriginal People in Manitoba 2000* by B. Hallett (Manitoba Department of Northern Affairs, 2000) at 45.

[48]   *Ibid.*, at 45. See also National Aboriginal Health Organization, *Ways of Knowing: A Framework for Health Research* by Policy Research Unit (Ottawa: National Aboriginal Health Organization, 2003) at 7.

[49]   C. MacIntosh, "Indigenous Self-Determination and Research on Human Genetic Material: A Consideration of the Relevance of Debates on Patents and Informed Consent, and the Political Demands on Researchers" (2005) 13 Health L.J. 213 at 247-51.

On a federal level, the Canadian Institutes of Health Research ("CIHR") has released its Guidelines for Health Research Involving Aboriginal people. The Guidelines indicate that where research is funded by CIHR, the researcher is contractually bound to abide by them.[50] The Guidelines are grounded in recognizing and deferring to Aboriginal jurisdiction, as well as Aboriginal values and traditions, and require researchers to allow the community to determine its level of participation in any given project. For example, the Guidelines require researchers to recognize the right of communities to impose their own research protocols, and to participate in data interpretation. They also require a research agreement be developed which incorporates and respects the Aboriginal community's views regarding accountability and responsibilities associated with knowledge transfer. In practice, these initiatives will likely result in health researchers needing to engage Aboriginal communities long before they seek to actually do research, and to expect that project design may be highly collaborative. In turn, this will likely reduce the number of scholars able to engage in health research. Scholars and other researchers are pressured to produce research results and publications/reports on a timely basis, and may not feel able to risk spending the time to develop a long-term collaborative relationship which may not culminate in a research project which attracts funding or meets the requirements of the researcher's sponsor. However, these protocols will likely also result in improvements in the quality and relevance of the health research which is performed.

III. ENVIRONMENTAL DETERMINANTS OF ABORIGINAL POPULATION HEALTH: EXAMPLES OF LAW AND POLICY AT VARIOUS LEVELS OF JURISDICTION

One determinant of health which is also recognized as relevant within Aboriginal perspectives on well-being is the state of the physical environment. The following section discusses three environmental factors that inform Aboriginal population health, and which engage law and policy at different levels of jurisdiction. These three factors are quality of housing (federal jurisdiction), drinking water (federal-provincial jurisdiction), and "country food" (federal and international jurisdiction). It then turns to jurisdictional conflicts over who occupies the field regarding public health on reserves, as between provincial and First Nation governments. The case study for this conflict is the applicability of

---

[50]   Canadian Institutes of Health Research, Canadian Institutes of Health Research *Guidelines for Health Research Involving Aboriginal People* (Ottawa: Canadian Institutes of Health Research, 2007) at 12-13.

provincial smoking bans to on-reserve casinos. Together, these discussions and examples illustrate some of the economic, political, legal and structural elements that inform the population health of Aboriginal peoples, and the complex issues raised by existing and proposed responses.

(a) Housing

This subsection commences with a review of data regarding the quality of housing, and the prevalence of overcrowding in Aboriginal households. There is then an examination of Aboriginal claims regarding a right to housing, based on treaties or the fiduciary relationship between the Crown and Aboriginal peoples. Finally, there is an overview of existing federal housing policies and programs.

(i)   Housing Conditions of Aboriginal Peoples

Housing conditions are critical for community health. Poor or inadequate housing is associated with a plethora of health and social problems, including increases in transmission of infectious disease, risk of injury, mental health problems, family tension and violence.[51] As described above in the epidemiological data, all these conditions are present at elevated levels among the Aboriginal population.

Aboriginal peoples who live on reserves are able to benefit from some federal need-based assistance programs, and Band Councils receive some federal funding for housing. The adequacy of these programs has been questioned. In particular, the accusation has been leveled that the programs do not provide Aboriginal people who live on reserves with housing assistance to the same degree as it does to other Canadians.[52]

Housing on reserves is, on average, poor both in terms of overcrowding and quality. Although the homes of Aboriginal Canadians tend to be smaller than those of non-Aboriginal Canadians, on average

---

[51] Indian and Northern Affairs Canada, "First Nations Housing" (20 December 2002), online: <http://www.ainc-inac.gc.ca/pr/info/info104_e.html>; Statistics Canada, *Aboriginal Peoples Survey 2001 — initial findings: Well-being of the non-reserve Aboriginal Population* by V. O'Donnell & H. Tait (Ottawa: Minister of Industry, 2003) at 24.

[52] Canada, Royal Commission on Aboriginal Peoples, *Report of the Royal Commission on Aboriginal Peoples: Volume 3 Gathering Strength* (Ottawa: Minister of Supply and Services, 1996) at 376. The Report finds that the level of financial support for social housing for low-income reserve residents has not been as generous as that offered elsewhere in Canada since 1986, that the shelter component of social assistance has been withheld from reserve residents unless they occupy social housing, and that whereas capital subsidies have been sufficient to generally meet the needs of other Canadians for adequate housing, the subsidies for low-income Aboriginal people living on-reserve have not been provided to the same level.

there are more people living in Aboriginal households. About 17 per cent of dwellings on reserves are considered overcrowded; that is, there is more than one person per room in the house.[53] Of particular concern is the correlation between crowding and homes that themselves are more likely to require major repairs.[54] Overcrowding along with inadequate ventilation and lack of maintenance has resulted in poor indoor air quality, and a plethora of harmful molds, in many on-reserve houses,[55] with 44 per cent of adult respondents to the National Aboriginal Health Organization's 2002–2003 regional health survey ("RHS") indicating mold or mildew in their homes the year prior to the survey.[56] These general conditions have led federal health officials to warn that overcrowding has made Canadian reserves "breeding grounds" for outbreaks of infectious disease.[57] Recent research confirms that overcrowding is an even more pressing issue in the Arctic. Overall, 53 per cent of Inuit live in crowded conditions — from 28 per cent in Labrador to 68 per cent in Nunavik.[58]

As to quality of the structures, as of 1991, 38.7 per cent of on-reserve housing either needed to be replaced, or else required major repairs to be inhabitable, as did 15 per cent to 18 per cent of the housing inhabited by Inuit, Métis, or off-reserve registered members of First Nations.[59] These figures contrast with those relating to non-Aboriginal people, of whom 9.8 per cent live in homes in need of major repair.[60] A

---

[53] National Aboriginal Health Organization, *First Nations Regional Longitudinal Health Survey (RHS) 2002/03: Report on First Nations' Housing* (Ottawa: National Aboriginal Health Organization, 2006) at 4.

[54] *Ibid.*

[55] Indian and Northern Affairs Canada, "First Nations Housing" (20 December 2002), online: <http://www.ainc-inac.gc.ca/pr/info/info104_e.html>; Statistics Canada, *Aboriginal Peoples Survey 2001 — initial findings: Well-being of the non-reserve Aboriginal Population* by V. O'Donnell & H. Tait (Ottawa: Minister of Industry, 2003) at 24.

[56] National Aboriginal Health Organization, *First Nations Regional Longitudinal Health Survey (RHS) 2002/03: Report on First Nations' Housing* (Ottawa: National Aboriginal Health Organization, 2006) at 10.

[57] B. Laghi, "Epidemic feared if SARS spreads to native reserves" *The Globe and Mail* (16 June 2003) A1.

[58] Statistics Canada, *Aboriginal Peoples Survey 2001 — initial findings: Well-being of the non-reserve Aboriginal Population* by V. O'Donnell & H. Tait (Ottawa: Minister of Industry, 2003) at 25.

[59] Canada, Royal Commission on Aboriginal Peoples, *Report of the Royal Commission on Aboriginal Peoples: Volume 3 Gathering Strength* (Ottawa: Minister of Supply and Services, 1996) at 368. The Commission compiled these figures from several different sources. Major repairs include defective plumbing, electrical wiring, structural problems with floors, *etc.*

[60] *Ibid.*, at 367. Regarding sewage, the results of a 1991 survey were that nearly 20 per cent of houses on reserves failed to have flush toilets, and 14 per cent had no indoor plumbing whatsoever. *Ibid.*, at 368-69. INAC currently considers there to be adequate sewage systems in place for 93.8 per cent of on-reserve homes. See First Nations and Inuit Health Branch, Health Canada, *A Statistical Profile on the Health of First Nations in Canada* (Ottawa: Health Canada, 2003) at 67.

1996 census similarly determined that only about half of on-reserve and non-reserve native homes met Canada's housing standards.[61] As of the 2002–2003 RHS, this situation had only slightly improved, with 33.6 per cent of respondents indicating their homes needed major repairs. It is clear that Aboriginal peoples' housing has tended and continues to be both substandard and crowded.

(ii)   Aboriginal Claims to a Unique Right to Housing

Some Aboriginal organizations and communities have alleged that this standard and quality of housing places Canada in breach of a purported lawful obligation to ensure Aboriginal peoples have adequate shelter. For example, the national political representative organization for First Nations in Canada, the Assembly of First Nations ("AFN") stated that "housing is a federal responsibility which flows from the special relationship [which First Nations have] with the Crown ... and treaty agreements themselves".[62] The Federation of Saskatchewan Indian Nations ("FSIN") similarly argues that shelter "is a treaty right, and forms part of the federal trust and fiduciary responsibility".[63]

The AFN and FSIN both rely on treaties and the fiduciary character of the Crown-Aboriginal relationship as a source for a federal legal obligation to provide adequate housing. In this context, treaties are written and signed agreements that reflect understandings of how the British Crown[64] and Aboriginal nations would co-exist in what is now Canada. These agreements often include terms that characterize the relationship, impose specific obligations, and refer to the surrender, modification or protection of existing rights. There are no treaties that expressly *state* that the Crown will provide Aboriginal parties with shelter, nor has such a claim been litigated. Justice La Forest of the Supreme Court of Canada made one of the few judicial comments on shelter and treaty rights when he described housing as an example of an ancillary obligation that could

---

[61]   Canada Mortgage and Housing Corporation, "Special Studies on 1996 Census Data: Housing Conditions of Native Households" by P. Spurr *et al.* (2001) 55-6 Research Highlights: Socio-economic Series 1 at 4, online: <http://www.cmhc-schl.gc.ca/publications/en/rh-pr/socio/socio055-6.pdf>.

[62]   Assembly of First Nations, "Address" (Presentation to the Standing Committee on Aboriginal Affairs on First Nations' Housing, 18 February 1992) [unpublished], cited in Canada, Royal Commission on Aboriginal Peoples, *Report of the Royal Commission on Aboriginal Peoples: Volume 3 Gathering Strength* (Ottawa: Minister of Supply and Services, 1996) at 373-74.

[63]   Cited in *Royal Commission Report, ibid.*, at 374.

[64]   In 1981, the English Court of Appeal conclusively determined that any obligations the British Crown may have to Aboriginal peoples in Canada had become Canada's obligations when the Crown became separate and divisible for each self-governing domain of the former British Commonwealth. *R. v. The Secretary of State for Foreign and Commonwealth Affairs*, [1981] 4 C.N.L.R. 86 (C.A. U.K.).

arise under more general treaty promises.[65] Unfortunately, La Forest J. did not elaborate on this point.

Given this context, much of the strength in the AFN and FSIN's position derives from the unique body of jurisprudence that has developed regarding the interpretation of Crown-Aboriginal treaties in Canada. For example, silence within a treaty document itself is not considered determinative of the scope of treaty obligations. Rather, courts must give weight to any oral undertakings made when the treaty was entered into, even absent any ambiguity on the face of the document. Courts are also to consider the historic and cultural context of the treaty when giving meaning to any written or oral undertakings, to construe any rights described in a treaty in a liberal and dynamic fashion, and to interpret ambiguity in favour of the Aboriginal party.[66] Given these principles, a claim to a right to housing may be viable before the courts. The likelihood of a treaty-based claim to shelter succeeding would depend upon the persuasiveness of extrinsic evidence, including oral history, colonial documents, and the general events surrounding the signing of the treaty.

The second line of argument the AFN and the FSIN refer to is based on the fiduciary character[67] of the Crown-Aboriginal relationship. This feature is primarily the result of the Crown having taken discretionary control over many aspects of Aboriginal people's lives.[68] In some instances this control was assumed and asserted by the Crown, who described Aboriginal peoples as its "wards", while in other instances it was negotiated through agreements such as treaties. The fiduciary character of the relationship has significant legal consequences: it implies not only political obligations that ought to manifest through policy, but also sets lawful standards for government actions that affect Aboriginal people in a broad range of circumstances.[69] The centrality of this concept for the Crown-Aboriginal relationship is signalled through its incorporation as the key interpretive principle for s. 35(1) of the

---

[65]   *Mitchell v. Peguis Indian Band*, [1990] S.C.J. No. 63, 71 D.L.R. (4th) 193 at 230 (S.C.C.).

[66]   *R. v. Marshall*, [1999] S.C.J. No. 55, [1999] 3 S.C.R. 456 at paras. 9-14 (S.C.C.). Many of these principles were developed to reflect the fact that although treaties were negotiated orally, the Crown representatives wrote the terms of the treaties, and the Aboriginal signatories were not literate and so were unable to verify that the document reflected their understanding of the agreement. As well, much of the negotiations took place through the use of interpreters of unknown quality.

[67]   The concept of a "fiduciary" arises out of trust law, where one party (the fiduciary) is empowered to make decisions regarding the interests of another (the beneficiary). The fiduciary is held to a high standard of behaviour, and is required to always act in the best interest of the beneficiary.

[68]   *Wewaykum Indian Band v. Canada*, [2002] S.C.J. No. 79, [2002] 4 S.C.R. 245, 2002 SCC 79 at paras. 79-80 (S.C.C.).

[69]   R. Mainville, *An Overview of Aboriginal and Treaty Rights and Compensation for their Breach* (Saskatoon: Purich Publishing, 2001) at 53-54.

Constitution Act, 1982. This provision recognizes and affirms the existence of existing treaty and Aboriginal rights. The Supreme Court of Canada wrote in *R. v. Sparrow*:

> In our opinion, . . . a general guiding principle for s. 35(1) [is that] . . . the Government has the responsibility to act in a fiduciary capacity with respect to aboriginal peoples. The relationship between the Government and aboriginals is trust-like, rather than adversarial, and contemporary recognition and affirmation of aboriginal rights must be defined in light of this historic relationship.[70]

Thus, as well as serving as an *interpretive principle* for understanding the meaning of treaty terms, the fiduciary relationship may also impose *lawfully enforceable obligations* upon the Crown whenever it asserts a discretionary power over the rights or interests of Aboriginal people. The fiduciary relationship was key to the Royal Commission's conclusion that Canada does have a lawful obligation to address Aboriginal housing.

Given Canada's historic and continuing fiduciary obligation to protect Aboriginal lands and resources, the Royal Commission was struck by Canada's role in undermining Aboriginal self-sufficiency through dispossession from their land base. The Royal Commission considered that given this role, and Canada's current policy commitment to facilitate Aboriginal self-government and self-sufficiency,[71] Canada is required to bear the main burden of financing adequate shelter for Aboriginal communities until their economic base is restored.[72] In a nutshell, it would be disingenuous for Canada to promote a policy of Aboriginal communities taking control over an infrastructure that is in desperate need of extensive and costly repair as an answer to calls for self-determination.[73] A second argument on this point is that having asserted

---

[70]   *R. v. Sparrow*, [1990] S.C.J. No. 49, [1990] 1 S.C.R. 1075 at 1108 (S.C.C.).

[71]   The federal government has stated that two of its policy goals are to enable Aboriginal people to govern themselves, and to empower Aboriginal peoples to become self-reliant. See Indian and Northern Affairs Canada, *Federal Policy Guide: Aboriginal Self Government* (Ottawa: Minister of Public Works and Government Services Canada, 1994) at 2.

[72]   Canada, Royal Commission on Aboriginal Peoples, *Report of the Royal Commission on Aboriginal Peoples: Volume 3 Gathering Strength* (Ottawa: Minister of Supply and Services, 1996) at 375-77.

[73]   The Royal Commission also found that Canada's international legal commitments were relevant, including its status as a signatory of the International Covenant on the Economic, Social and Cultural Rights. This Covenant was adopted by the General Assembly of the United Nations on 16 December 1966. Article 11 of this instrument recognizes "the right to an adequate standard of living ... including adequate ... housing; and the right to the continuous improvement of living conditions". Implementation of the Covenant is based on the principle that states are to undertake progressive steps to meet their obligations. The Royal Commission found this Article of the Covenant required Canada to take necessary action to ensure all Canadians have adequate housing. Although this argument has moral

control over where many Aboriginals are to live, for this exercise of discretion to be practiced with honour, the Crown is obliged to ensure that reserves are livable places.

Canada does not recognize a treaty right to housing, or a fiduciary obligation to address housing needs. Rather, it takes the position that any housing assistance it provides to Aboriginal peoples is based solely on voluntarily assumed social policy objectives.[74] As discussed below, Canada has indeed been active on the policy front, in spite of its unwillingness to acknowledge treaty and fiduciary based obligations.

(iii) Federal Housing Policies and Programs

In response to the Royal Commission's general observations regarding the poor quality of Aboriginal housing, Ottawa introduced a new policy framework.[75] This policy involves transferring a considerable amount of control and funding to Aboriginal peoples so they can identify their own priorities and direct decisions about their communities. One key feature was the introduction of flexibility as to how housing funding could be used by Band Councils. Prior to the introduction of the new policy, housing funds from INAC could only be used for new construction, or for renovations. It could not be used for maintenance or insurance.[76]

The funding criteria require First Nations to develop cost-shared programs, where the housing costs for each project are shared between the government and either a private party or else the First Nation itself. Financing the construction of new homes and major repairs has been, and continues to be, a significant concern for on-reserve residents. Crown ownership of the underlying title of reserve lands, the tenure in homes usually resting with the Band, and the statutory prohibition against reserve property being seized, have left private financial institutions hesitant to grant housing loans and mortgages, and individual Aboriginal peoples hesitant to burden themselves with such a loan.

Another hurdle, which has yet to be overcome, is the differing views as to whether Canada has treaty obligations to provide housing. Disputes over this issue have had serious consequences in some on-reserve communities. Some communities refuse to participate in the cost-share housing programs, and residents of some on-reserve subsidized housing

---

strength, it has questionable legal strength, as the Covenant only requires Canada to take progressive steps towards this goal — there is no obligation to actually achieve it.

[74]   Auditor General, *Report of the Auditor General of Canada April 2003* (Ottawa, 2003) at 6.34-6.35; Indian and Northern Affairs Canada, *On-Reserve Housing Policy Impact Assessment 1996-2000* by N. Koeck (Ottawa, 2000) at 20.

[75]   See Koeck, *ibid.*

[76]   *Ibid.*, at 2.

have refused to pay rent, on the grounds that they have a lawful entitlement to shelter.[77] Although this position may be legally supportable, individuals within communities continue to suffer overcrowded and substandard housing while both Canada and Aboriginal communities extend their dispute.

Among those First Nations who have chosen to participate in the program, most who participated in a 2000 survey felt the program was significantly underfunded. In particular, while the housing situation was undeniably improving, current funding levels were inadequate to address the backlog of housing need that has resulted from decades of sub-standard housing, overcrowding, the rate of new family formation, and requests by people who regained status under Bill C-31 to once again have a place to live on their home reserve.[78] In practice, the existence of long waiting lists for homes limits the ability of Band Councils to direct funds into maintenance and repair.[79]

Despite these legal uncertainties and tensions, the on-reserve housing situation improved considerably between 1996 and 2000. By 2000, over 61 per cent of eligible First Nations had chosen to operate under the 1996 On-Reserve Housing Policy.[80] The total number of houses increased by 13 per cent, and the number of houses considered to be in "adequate" condition increased by more than 11,000.[81] However, 11 per cent of on-reserve homes are still considered overcrowded (compared to a Canadian average of 1 per cent).[82] Reliable data is not available to assess how these shifts have impacted the health of the Aboriginal population.[83]

Unfortunately, this program was only made available for registered members of First Nations who live on reserves. It does not extend to off-reserve members of First Nations, or Inuit and Métis, 24 per cent of

---

[77]   Canada, Royal Commission on Aboriginal Peoples, *Report of the Royal Commission on Aboriginal Peoples: Volume 3 Gathering Strength* (Ottawa: Minister of Supply and Services, 1996) at 374; Indian and Northern Affairs Canada, *On-Reserve Housing Policy Impact Assessment 1996-2000* by N. Koeck (Ottawa, 2000) at 20.

[78]   Koeck, *ibid.*, at 11.

[79]   *Ibid.*, at 19.

[80]   *Ibid.*, at 9.

[81]   Indian and Northern Affairs Canada, "First Nations Housing" (20 December 2002), online: <http://www.ainc-inac.gc.ca/pr/info/info104_e.html>; Statistics Canada, *Aboriginal Peoples Survey 2001 — initial findings: Well-being of the non-reserve Aboriginal Population* by V. O'Donnell & H. Tait (Ottawa: Minister of Industry, 2003) at 24.

[82]   *Ibid.*

[83]   M. Maar, "Clearing the Path for Community Health Empowerment: Integrating Health Care Services at an Aboriginal Health Access Centre in Rural North Central Ontario" (2004) 1 Journal of Aboriginal Health 54 at 59.

whom, in 2001, were considered to be in core housing need.[84] No data appears to be available to indicate whether there has been any general improvement for non-reserve or non-Status Indians, Inuit or Métis communities, although Canada has initiated various short-term investments into housing needs for the North and for urban homeless Aboriginal people.

(b) Water Safety: A Provincial-Federal Jurisdictional Void

Another key issue for community health is the quality of drinking water. The discussion below first presents data on water quality, and then considers the question of whether any regulatory regime protects the health of Aboriginal peoples from contaminated drinking water on reserves.

In some cases, the living conditions in reserve communities have been compared to those in developing countries. Although this comparison seems drastic, a 1991 survey revealed that 24 per cent of homes located on reserves did not have drinkable water.[85] Recent data is not as dire, but remains unacceptable. In 2006, about 12 per cent of reserve communities were under boil water orders or advisories at any given time. Some of these orders had become the status quo — of the 76 communities with orders in place in March 2006, 50 of these orders had lasted for over a year, and seven for more than five years.[86] These are extraordinarily long periods of time for a community to be without safe tap water.

Following the deaths due to contaminated water in Walkerton, a report was commissioned to consider the quality of water throughout the province of Ontario (the "O'Connor Report"). The O'Connor Report assessed the status and quality of on-reserve water systems in Ontario, and found that as of 2000, 12 per cent posed *immediate health risks.*[87] Water treatment facilities and infrastructure are generally inadequate — on-site studies by INAC in 2001 and 2003 both found that approximately 75 per cent of reserve communities were at risk of their water treatment facilities

---

[84]   Indian and Northern Affairs Canada, "Fact Sheet: Aboriginal Housing, (October 2006), online: <http://www.ainc-inac.gc.ca/pr/info/fnsocec/abhsg_e.html>.

[85]   Canada, Royal Commission on Aboriginal Peoples, *Report of the Royal Commission on Aboriginal Peoples: Volume 3 Gathering Strength* (Ottawa: Minister of Supply and Services, 1996) at 368-69.

[86]   Health Canada, "First Nations, Inuit and Aboriginal Health: Drinking Water Advisories", online: <http://www.hc-sc.gc.ca/fnih-spni/promotion/water-eau/advis-avis_concern-eng.php>; "Cleaner Water for Natives" *The National Post* (6 March 2006).

[87]   This figure is an improvement from 1995, when 22 per cent were considered high risk. See Ontario, Walkerton Commission of Inquiry, *Report of the Walkerton Inquiry: A Strategy for Safe Drinking Water (Part Two)* (Ontario Ministry of the Attorney General: Queen's Printer for Ontario, 2002) (Commissioner: D. O'Connor) at 488.

failing due to facility conditions. The 2003 study also determined that only about 11 per cent of the facility operators met industry standards in terms of training and qualifications.[88]

The legal and policy issues that must be engaged to address water quality on reserves are complex.[89] Although provinces have water protection regulations, these regulations are not usually considered to extend to water located on reserve lands. Their operation is assumed to be excluded due to jurisdictional boundaries, as reserve land comprises pockets of federal land located within provinces.[90] However, water — and water-borne pollutants — do not respect jurisdictional boundaries. The researchers for the O'Connor Report were unable to find any legally enforceable federal or provincial standards relating to drinking water on reserves.[91]

It may be that provincial water quality regulations of general application *could* apply on reserves. This may be permissible pursuant to s. 88 of the *Indian Act*,[92] under which all provincial laws of general application "are applicable to and in respect of Indians in the province".[93] Although this line of reasoning has some appeal, s. 88 only makes reference to permitting the operation of provincial laws that are applicable to "*Indians*" (*i.e.*, the human population) and not to "*land* reserved for Indians". This distinction was found to be legally relevant by the British Columbia Court of Appeal. This court found that s. 88 could not result in provincial forestry legislation applying to on-reserve land.[94] By analogy, it seems likely that provincial water legislation — with its quality controls and remedies — may not be operable on reserve land.

---

[88]   Indian and Northern Affairs Canada, *National Assessment of Water and Wastewater Systems in First Nations Communities: Summary Report* (Ottawa: Indian and Northern Affairs Canada, 2003) at 10; Commissioner of the Environment and Sustainable Development, *Report of the Commissioner of the Environment and Sustainable Development to the House of Commons* (Ottawa: Minister of Public Works and Government Services Canada, 2005) at para 5.13.

[89]   For an in-depth analysis of reserve water issues, see C. MacIntosh, "Testing the Waters: Jurisdictional and Policy Aspects of the Continuing Failure to Remedy Drinking Water Quality on First Nations Reserves" (2008) 39.1 Ottawa L.R. 65.

[90]   *Constitution Act, 1867* (U.K.), 30 & 31 Vict., c. 3, s. 91(24), reprinted in R.S.C. 1985, App. II, No. 5.

[91]   Ontario, Walkerton Commission of Inquiry, *Report of the Walkerton Inquiry: A Strategy for Safe Drinking Water (Part Two)* (Ontario Ministry of the Attorney General: Queen's Printer for Ontario, 2002) (Commissioner: D. O'Connor) at 490.

[92]   R.S.C. 1985, c. I-5.

[93]   Section 88 imposes some express restrictions, and excludes provincial laws which conflict with federal law or impinge on treaty rights.

[94]   *Paul v. British Columbia (Forest Appeals Commission)*, [2001] B.C.J. No. 1227, 2001 BCCA 411 (B.C.C.A.), rev'd [2003] S.C.J. No. 34 (S.C.C.). See also *Re Stony Plain Indian Reserve No. 135*, [1981] A.J. No. 1007, [1982] 1 C.N.L.R. 133 (Alta. C.A.).

O'Connor's key policy recommendation on this jurisdictional quandary is that First Nations and Canada formally adopt drinking water standards for reserves that are the same as or at a higher level than those off-reserve,[95] and that these standards be made legally enforceable.[96] Such standards would clearly be of benefit to all First Nations, not only to those located in Ontario.

Meanwhile, the Canadian government continues to operate via guidelines, with the most notable recent example being the *Protocol for Safe Drinking Water in First Nation Communities.*[97] This policy document describes recommended practices, and asserts that INAC or First Nations are responsible for different matters.   These assertions are seldom buttressed by legal argument, but occasionally reflect contractual arrangements.   The Canadian government has taken steps towards assessing how various regulatory options would play out, and commissioned an Expert Panel which reported in 2006.[98] The Panel rejected the option of assuming that provincial laws of general application could apply through s. 88 of the *Indian Act* due to legal uncertainty, and found the option of merely modifying existing federal legislation inadequate. It identified the enactment of a fresh federal regulatory regime as the most practical and legally certain route, but also found the notion of starting with indigenous customary law and building a regime which would then be enshrined in federal law to be a strong option. The other option which the Panel considered viable was to referentially incorporate provincial law into federal law. In all cases, the Panel identified a series of benefits and drawbacks. It also concluded that merely enacting a regulatory regime will not fix the problem, and that several preconditions must be addressed.[99] First, a regime must be both lawful and have legitimacy from the Aboriginal perspective, and so must be developed in consultation with First Nations. Second, a regime must have support to make it effective, and so must be accompanied by an infusion of resources and capacity development. To date, the Panel's report has not been acted upon: the status quo continues.

[95]   Ontario, Walkerton Commission of Inquiry, *Report of the Walkerton Inquiry: A Strategy for Safe Drinking Water (Part Two)* (Ontario Ministry of the Attorney General: Queen's Printer for Ontario, 2002) (Commissioner: D. O'Connor) at 495-96.

[96]   *Ibid.*, at 495-96.

[97]   Indian and Northern Affairs Canada, *Protocol for Safe Drinking Water in First Nations Communities (Standards for Design, Construction, Operation, Maintenance and Monitoring of Drinking Water Systems)* (Ottawa: Indian and Northern Affairs Canada, 2006).

[98]   Expert Panel on Safe Drinking Water for First Nations, *Report of the Expert Panel on Safe Drinking Water for First Nations* (Ottawa: Minister of Public Works and Government Services Canada, 2006).

[99]   *Ibid.*, at 49-51.

(c) Country Food and Contaminants

Just as regulatory practices related to housing and water affect Aboriginal conditions of health, so, too, do general environmental laws impact the health of Aboriginal peoples. The final case study on environmental determinants of Aboriginal health considers the cultural practice of consuming "country foods", and the health threat this practice entails due to the chemical contamination of this food source. This section then turns to an examination of domestic and international law and policy that respond to the matter of contaminants in the food chain.

(i)   Country Food and Community Well-Being

The population health of all Canadians is vulnerable to shifting housing and water conditions. There are, however, some unique environmental factors that have a more direct and significant effect on the population health of Aboriginal peoples. The availability and quality of "country food" — mammals, fish, birds, and plants that are locally harvested from wild stock — is one of these factors. The most comprehensive data regarding country food consumption relates to the 56,000 Aboriginal peoples (primarily Inuit and Dene) who live in the Arctic region. This area includes Nunavut, the Northwest Territories, Nunavik in Northern Québec, and the Yukon.

Approximately 91 per cent of all Arctic Aboriginal households consume traditionally harvested foods, and 22 per cent report that country food is their only source for meat and fish.[100] In more remote areas, approximately 40 per cent of food energy is from country food.[101]

Country foods are essential for the health of these peoples on many levels. Firstly, they "play a vital role in the social, cultural, ... and spiritual well-being of Aboriginal peoples".[102] The exchange and consumption of country foods, including specific portions of certain animals, involve complex socio-economic rules and procedures that bind families and communities, and underwrite the entire structural organization of these Aboriginal societies.[103]

---

[100] Indian and Northern Affairs Canada, *Canadian Arctic Contaminants Assessment Report II: Knowledge in Action* by J. Van Oostdam *et al.* (Ottawa: Indian and Northern Affairs Canada, 2003) at 5, online: <http://www.ainc-inac.gc.ca/ncp/pub/knotoc_e.html>.

[101] Indian and Northern Affairs Canada, *Canadian Arctic Contaminations: Assessment Report II: Human Health* by J. Van Oostdam *et al.* (Ottawa: Indian and Northern Affairs Canada, 2003) at 13.

[102] *Ibid.*, at 6.

[103] *Ibid.*, at 4.

There are also economic and nutritional factors to consider. The cost of "market" food to provide a nutritious diet is prohibitively high in many northern communities, due to a combination of low incomes and low employment rates as well as extra costs incurred by transportation.[104] The nutritional benefits of country food are well-documented. This food has been described as possessing "remarkable nutrient properties".[105] Many country foods are high in vitamin C, omega fatty acids, vitamins A, D, and E, as well as iron, zinc, selenium, copper, magnesium and manganese.[106] In contrast, market food available in the North is high in saturated fat and sucrose.[107] In communities where there have been shifts away from country foods to market foods, there has been a noticeable rise in obesity, diabetes, and cardiovascular disease.[108] Country foods are necessary both for personal physical health and for the community well-being of Inuit and Dene people.

However, the consumption of country food also exposes Aboriginal peoples to contaminants that have entered the wild food chain. The two categories of contaminants of major concern in the Canadian North are persistent organic pollutants ("POPs")[109] (such as PCBs and DDT), and heavy metals (such as mercury and lead). These types of contaminants (1) remain intact for extended periods of time, (2) are toxic, (3) are bioaccumulative, and (4) are prone to long-range transport (e.g., on winds). Many key country foods, such as fish, and land and marine animals, are long-lived and positioned at the higher trophic levels of the food chain. As a consequence, contaminants may "bioaccumulate" in the bodies of fish and animals. An Aboriginal person who consumes country food is potentially exposed to concentrated levels of these contaminants. Recent data appears to bear out this possibility.

In most Kivalliq and Baffin communities, more than 25 per cent of the population takes in levels of mercury that are above the margin considered to be safe.[110] Mercury is a highly toxic environmental neurotoxin that can cause irreversible damage to the human nervous system. Mercury is passed through the umbilical cord at the same rate as it

---

[104] *Ibid.*, at 6.

[105] *Ibid.*, at 71.

[106] *Ibid.*, at 71.

[107] *Ibid.*, at 69.

[108] *Ibid.*, at 71.

[109] POPs are human-made chemicals that are either industrial by-products, or else generated as pesticides. Indian and Northern Affairs Canada, *Canadian Arctic Contaminants Assessment Report II: Knowledge in Action* by J. Van Oostdam *et al.* (Ottawa: Indian and Northern Affairs Canada, 2003) at 3, online: <http://www.ainc-inac.gc.ca/ncp/pub/pdf/knotoc_e.html>.

[110] Indian and Northern Affairs Canada, *Canadian Arctic Contaminations: Assessment Report II: Human Health* by J. Van Oostdam *et al.* (Ottawa: Indian and Northern Affairs Canada, 2003) at 56.

is taken in by pregnant women. Prenatal exposure to elevated mercury levels is associated with children who demonstrate neurobehavioural deficits in areas such as fine motor functions, attention, language ability, visual-spatial abilities, and verbal memory.[111] Recent data indicates that 80 per cent of pregnant women in Nunavik and 68 per cent in Baffin have mercury blood levels that exceed safety guidelines.[112]

Nearly one-half of pregnant women in Baffin, Kivalliq and Nunavik have intake levels of PCBs through country food that are above Health Canada's "level of concern".[113] Pre-natal PCB exposure is associated with low birth weight, pre-term births,[114] slow reflexes and growth, poor visual recognition, poor intellectual function, and deficits in psychomotor development,[115] as well as weak immune responses leading to greater susceptibility to infectious disease, especially respiratory illness.[116] Adult exposure to PCBs is linked to health problems such as low bone density, which has placed an estimated 19 per cent of Inuit women at high risk of osteoporosis fracture.[117]

This epidemiological data was described in terms of its lived impact on individuals within the Arctic Aboriginal population as follows:

> ... imagine for a moment if you will the emotions we now feel; shock, panic, grief — as we discover that the food which for generations nourished us and keeps us whole physically and spiritually, is now poisoning us. You go to the supermarket for food. We go out on the land to hunt, fish, trap, and gather. The environment is our supermarket ... As we put babies to our breasts we feed them a noxious chemical cocktail that foreshadows neurological disorders, cancers, kidney failure, and reproductive dysfunction. That Inuit mothers — far from areas where POPs are manufactured and used, have to think twice before breast-feeding their infants is surely a wake-up call to the world.[118]

---

[111] *Ibid.*, at 57.

[112] Indian and Northern Affairs Canada, *Highlights of the Canadian Arctic Contaminations: Assessment Report II* by J. Van Oostdam *et al.* (Ottawa, Indian and Northern Affairs Canada, 2003) at 7.

[113] *Ibid.*, at 7.

[114] Indian and Northern Affairs Canada, *Canadian Arctic Contaminations: Assessment Report II: Human Health* by J. Van Oostdam *et al.* (Ottawa: Indian and Northern Affairs Canada, 2003) at 57.

[115] *Ibid.*, at 50.

[116] *Ibid.*, at 46.

[117] *Ibid.*, at 55.

[118] From a speech given by the President of the Inuit Circumpolar Conference Canada, speaking on behalf of Canadian Arctic Indigenous Peoples Against POPs, at the Nairobi meeting of the working group on POPs. The text from the speech is reproduced in Indian and Northern Affairs Canada, *Canadian Arctic Contaminants Assessment Report II: Knowledge in Action* by J. Van Oostdam *et al.* (Ottawa: Indian and Northern Affairs Canada, 2003) at 79, online: <http://www.ainc-inac.gc.ca/ncp/pub/knotoc_e.html>.

(ii) Domestic Law and Policy

Canada has taken steps, both in law and in policy, to address the issue of contaminants in country foods. In particular, in 1991 the Northern Contaminants Program ("NCP") was developed within Indian and Northern Affairs Canada. One of its key objectives is "to reduce and wherever possible eliminate contaminants in traditionally harvested foods, while providing information that assists informed decision-making by individuals and communities in their food use".[119]

Following on reports developed by the NCP, Canada has enacted a number of domestic policies and legislative instruments directed at reducing the presence of contaminants in the Arctic food chain. A key document is the Toxic Substances Management Policy ("TSMP"). Under the TSMP, any substances that are toxic, persistent, bioaccumulative, and primarily resulting from human activity are targeted for "virtual elimination from the environment".[120] On the legislative level, the *Canadian Environmental Protection Act* has reporting requirements that have resulted in risk assessments for existing substances in commerce. They are assessed to determine whether they are persistent and bioaccumulative, and, if so, whether the substance is toxic.[121] If found toxic, the substance will be subject to measures to reduce impact on human health.

(iii) International Law and Policy

An effective response to contaminants in country food requires more than federal and provincial/territorial action. As contaminants travel on the wind and through the water, eliminating the presence of contaminants requires changes, both to international law and policy, and to domestic legislation and practice in other countries.[122]

Canada has been a participant in advocating for such change, partially as a response to pressure from Arctic Aboriginal peoples. For example, the Inuit Circumpolar Conference Canada, Inuit Tapirisat of Canada, Dene Nation, and Council for Yukon First Nations formed a coalition in 1997 called CAIPAP: Canadian Arctic Indigenous Peoples Against POPs.[123] CAIPAP's objective was to influence Canada's position

---

[119]   *Ibid.*, at 17.

[120]   *Ibid.*, at 73.

[121]   *Ibid.*

[122]   *Ibid.*, at 2.

[123]   *Ibid.*, at 79.

in negotiating the terms of the Stockholm Convention on Persistent Organic Pollutants.[124]

As finally drafted, this international Convention acknowledges that Arctic Aboriginal peoples are particularly at risk due to biomagnification of POPs through the consumption of Arctic fish and animals.[125] It also expressly recognizes that "contamination of their traditional foods is a public health issue". The objective of the instrument is to "protect human health",[126] and it requires states to restrict, phase out and ban the production and use of POPs, pesticides and industrial chemicals, to prevent or avoid the generation of POPs as industrial byproducts,[127] and to properly dispose of existing stocks of POPs.[128]

Part of the complexity of eliminating contaminants relates to the fact that some countries currently have no viable choice but to make use of them — for example, DDT is the primary means of malaria control in some developing countries.[129] Canada and other countries have responded by committing funds to create alternative methods of control.[130]

Canada ratified the *Stockholm Convention* in 1998, and it came into effect on May 17, 2004.[131] It is unclear how long it will take for levels of contamination in local fish and animals to reach levels that are safe for Aboriginal peoples to consume. However, it is clear this issue is impossible to address without international co-operation.

These three examples of environmental determinants of Aboriginal population health demonstrate the complexity of effectively addressing the gap in health between Aboriginal and non-Aboriginal populations. In some cases, the gap can potentially be closed through policy adjustments and cash infusions (*e.g.*, housing) or by filling a legislative void (*e.g.*,

---

[124] *Stockholm Convention on Persistent Organic Pollutants*, 9 March 2001, UN Doc. UNEP/POPS/CONF/2, 40 I.L.M. 532, online: Stockholm Convention on Persistent Organic Pollutants <http://www.pops.int/documents/convtext/convtext_en.pdf>.

[125] *Ibid.*, Preamble.

[126] *Ibid.*, art. 1.

[127] *Ibid.*, arts. 3, 5.

[128] *Ibid.*, art. 6.

[129] Indian and Northern Affairs Canada, *Canadian Arctic Contaminants Assessment Report II: Knowledge in Action* by J. Van Oostdam *et al.* (Ottawa: Indian and Northern Affairs Canada, 2003) at 2, 17, online: <http://www.ainc-inac.gc.ca/ncp/pub/knotoc_e.html>. These countries continue to use DDT because it is the most cost-effective chemical to prevent malaria, and the countries either do not have the funds to use alternative methods, and/or do not have the capacity to develop alternate methods themselves.

[130] *Ibid.*, at 80.

[131] United Nations Environment Program, "Press Release: Stockholm Convention on POPs to become international law, launching a global campaign to eliminate 12 hazardous chemicals" Stockholm (14 May 2004), online: <http://www.pops.int/documents/press/EIF/pr5-04POPsEIF-E.pdf>.

water quality). In other situations, international legislative co-ordination and co-operation is required (*e.g.*, country food). In most cases, any initiative is unlikely to be effective if it is developed without extensive participation and direction from Aboriginal populations.

(d) Provincial Public Health Legislation and Reserve Lands: Tensions over Jurisdiction

This subsection considers whether provincial public health legislation applies on reserve land located within any given province, using the case study of provincial bans on smoking in public places. This issue highlights how the uncertain scope of Aboriginal rights to self-determination, coupled with the federal-provincial division of powers, complicates public health initiatives even where all parties share the same ultimate goal of improving health.

Over the last few years, most Canadian provinces have enacted public health legislation which restricts smoking in public places.[132] The question has arisen as to whether such legislation can lawfully extend to on-reserve establishments, such as casinos. As discussed above in the context of water quality, jurisdictional assignment under s. 91(24) of the *Constitution Act, 1867* for "lands reserved for the Indians" to the federal government, and the limitations of incorporating provincial laws under s. 88 of the *Indian Act* to make them applicable on reserve lands, create a nuanced legal landscape.[133] Just as in the case of water, the answer to whether anti-smoking legislation applies to reserve-based casinos largely turns on how that legislation is characterized. If it is public health legislation, and there is no federal conflicting legislation, then it would extend to on-reserve casinos as long as the law is one of general application,[134] which it likely would be. However, if the legislation is characterized as regulating land use, then s. 88 could not effectively incorporate the law to render it applicable to reserve-based casinos due to s. 88's lack of reference to the second branch of s. 91(24); "lands reserved for the Indians".[135]

If such legislation carries the first characterization, there are still at least two matters to consider. First, Aboriginal interests in land inherently

---

[132] E.g., *Non-Smokers Health Protection Act*, C.C.S.M. c. N92; *Smoke-free Environment Act, 2005*, S.N.L. 2005, c. S-16.2, *Smoke-free Ontario Act*, S.O. 1994, c. 10; *Tobacco Control Act*, S.S. 2001, c. T-14.1.

[133] These arguments are considered to some degree in *R. v. Jenkinson; R. v Creekside Hideaway Hotel Ltd.*, [2006] M.J. No. 250, 2006 MBQB 185, 273 DLR (4th) 524 (Man. Q.B.), rev'd [2008] M.J. No. 78, 2008 MBCA 28 (Man. C.A.).

[134] *Four B Manufacturing v. UGW*, [1979] S.C.J. No. 138, [1980] 1 S.C.R. 1031 (S.C.C.).

[135] *Derrickson v. Derrickson*, [1986] S.C.J. No. 16, [1986] 1 S.C.R. 285 at 295 (S.C.C.).

include a governance aspect.[136] As a result, it is arguable that regardless of the presumptions that underlie a division of powers analysis,[137] Aboriginal communities maintain inherent decision-making powers that could preclude the imposition of provincial law.

A second and related issue is that the *Indian Act* recognizes the power of Band Councils to pass by-laws providing for "the health of residents on the reserve".[138] Such powers were granted or recognized by Canada "to provide a mechanism by which Band Councils could assume management over certain activities within the territorial limits of their constituencies".[139] As a result, even if provincial anti-smoking legislation was characterized as public health legislation of general application, and found applicable, a Band Council could choose whether to permit it to apply within the reserve. By not taking any action, the provincial law would apply. However, if a Band Council chose to pass its own by-law and that by-law conflicted with the provincial law, the paramountcy principle would result in the provincial law being ousted.

IV. ABORIGINAL CULTURAL PRACTICES: THE REGULATION OF TRADITIONAL HEALERS AND MIDWIVES

As discussed above, the population health model Canada adopted in the mid-1990s recognized culture as a key determinant of health. Culture shapes how people interact with the health care system. This includes whether or how they participate in prevention and health promotion programs, access health information, make lifestyle choices, as well as how they understand and prioritize issues of health and illness.[140] One of the regular critiques of existing health services is that they are not conceived of, nor designed, in a fashion that is culturally appropriate for most Aboriginal peoples.

The Royal Commission on Aboriginal Peoples concluded that health systems will only work for Aboriginal peoples if they are free to diverge from the bio-medical model.[141] One proposed "divergence" is to promote

---

[136] *Delgamuukw v. British Columbia*, [1997] S.C.J. No. 108, 153 D.L.R. (4th) 193 at para. 182 (S.C.C.).

[137] *E.g.*, see *Campbell v. British Columbia*, [2000] B.C.J. No. 1524, 2000 BCSC 1123 (B.C.S.C.).

[138] *Indian Act*, R.S.C. 1985, c. I-5, s. 81(1)(*a*).

[139] *R. v. Lewis*, [1996] S.C.J. No. 46, [1996] 1 S.C.R. 921 at para. 80 (S.C.C.).

[140] T. Speck, "The Importance of Culture to Aboriginal Health and Health Care" (2003) 5 Health Policy Research 20 at 20.

[141] Canada, Royal Commission on Aboriginal Peoples, *Report of the Royal Commission on Aboriginal Peoples: Volume 3 Gathering Strength* (Ottawa: Minister of Supply and Services, 1996) at 228-29.

and support traditional healing practices,[142] including traditional midwifery. Engaging in such practices is expected to improve population health outcomes in a variety of situations through positive impacts on physical, social and spiritual well-being.[143]

As traditional healing practices may have a medical component, matters of state regulation must be addressed. Provinces are considered to have the right, pursuant to the constitutional division of powers, to regulate the practice of medicine. It is unclear whether this power lawfully extends to Aboriginal peoples practicing traditional medicine on reserves.[144]

Provincial regulations that would appear to regulate traditional midwives and healers are discussed below, as well as whether there is an Aboriginal right to practice traditional healing. As a part of this discussion, this section considers contemporary treaties and other agreements that expressly recognize Aboriginal jurisdiction to regulate traditional Aboriginal healers. The section then turns to an assessment of Canada's policy decision to provide financial support to those seeking treatment from a traditional healer. The final issue discussed in this section is the regulation of substances used by traditional healers. There is a review both of existing and proposed legislation.

(a) The Regulation of Traditional Midwifery

In Canada, birthing was shifted from an event that was usually attended by a midwife at the home of the pregnant woman, to a hospital based event with a physician attending. This shift in location, as well as the medicalization of the birth process, has had dramatic effects upon Aboriginal women. As many Aboriginal communities have been and are located far away from hospitals with birthing units, women have been forced to travel great distances several weeks before their babies are due, and then forced to wait in the hospital, away from family and friends. Instead of being attended by the community members who supported the woman during her pregnancy, the woman would be a "one-off" patient for an unknown physician who is likely from a different culture. These women would not have been able to benefit from the experience of midwives located in their home communities, who would have had culturally meaningful and appropriate practices to give comfort and assist the birthing process.

---

[142]   *Ibid.*, at 290.

[143]   *Ibid.*, at 352.

[144]   *R. v. Hill*, [1907] O.J. No. 78, 15 O.L.R. 406 at paras. 19, 34-35 (Ont. C.A.).

The problems inherent in such an approach, including unnecessary cost and personal stress, have come to be generally recognized. Midwifery is becoming a commonly accepted alternative to hospitalization for low risk births.

Most provinces recognize midwifery as a legitimate medical practice, and have chosen to regulate it.[145] These regulations require midwives to be licensed. Licensing, in turn, depends on meeting specific educational and training requirements. Only Ontario has created a blanket recognition in its *Midwifery Act*[146] for Aboriginal persons who provide "traditional midwifery services".[147] Such individuals do not require licensing. Only one other province recognizes Aboriginal midwives as legitimate. Québec's *Midwives Act* permits persons without provincial licences to practice midwifery if an agreement to this effect is formed between the province and an Aboriginal community.[148] This approach is one which respects and defers to an Aboriginal community's assessment of the integrity of the knowledge of its midwives. Other provinces recognize no exceptions, which implies that Aboriginal midwives in these provinces may be providing their services, and so practising medicine, illegally.

(b) The Regulation of Traditional Healers

As noted above, provinces regulate the practice of medicine. All provinces make it an offence to practise medicine — and medicine is broadly defined — except under licensing from the self-governing body of physicians. Only Ontario acknowledges the existence of traditional Aboriginal healers in its statute. It expressly exempts them from provincial regulation,[149] as long as the healing services are only provided to Aboriginal patients, or to members of Aboriginal communities.[150] In other jurisdictions, laws that protect the public through regulating the practice of medicine may put traditional healers in jeopardy of violating the law. A defence against such charges would require either proving that the accused possessed an Aboriginal right to practice traditional healing or

---

[145]   See *e.g.*, *Midwifery Act*, R.S.N.L. 1990, c. M-11; *The Midwifery Act*, C.C.S.M. c. M125; *The Midwifery Act*, S.S. 1999, c. M-14.1.

[146]   *Midwifery Act, 1991*, S.O. 1991, c. 31.

[147]   *Ibid.*, s. 8(3). See also *Regulated Health Professions Act, 1991*, S.O. 1991, c. 18, s. 35(1)(b).

[148]   R.S.Q. c. S-0.1, s. 12(2).

[149]   *Regulated Health Professions Act, 1991*, S.O. 1991, c. 18, s. 35.

[150]   The Yukon Transfer Agreement takes a slightly different approach, and makes provision for traditional medicine to be delivered at the Whitehorse General Hospital. T. Speck, "The Importance of Culture to Aboriginal Health and Health Care" (2003) 5 Health Policy Research 20 at 21.

that the regulation was *ultra vires* provincial authority as it directly affects "Indianness", a matter within federal jurisdiction pursuant to s. 91(24).[151]

The term "Aboriginal right" is a legal turn of phrase. It is used to identify practices or activities that are distinctive and integral to an Aboriginal culture, have a pre-contact origin, and have been practiced with some continuity to the present. It is difficult to conceive of a court concluding that traditional Aboriginal healing practices do not meet this *prima facie* test.

Although Aboriginal rights existed at common law, their status was not formally recognized by Canada until 1982.[152] At this time, Canada went beyond merely acknowledging the existence of these rights: Canada afforded them constitutional protection through their inclusion in s. 35(1) of the *Constitution Act, 1982*, which states that existing Aboriginal rights are "recognized and affirmed". This provision has been judicially interpreted to mean that if an Aboriginal right was not extinguished prior to 1982, then it can only be lawfully impaired if the regulatory regime meets a test of justification.

For legislation to have already extinguished the right of a member of an Aboriginal community to practice traditional healing, the legislation must expressly demonstrate a "clear and plain intention" to do so. As discussed above, s. 91(24) of the *Constitution Act, 1867* assigns jurisdiction over "Indians" to the federal government. According to the doctrine of interjurisdictional immunity, given that "Indians" are assigned to the federal government, provincial laws can only affect "Indians" if the laws are of general application — that is, provinces cannot pass laws directed at regulating Aboriginal peoples.[153] Therefore if a provincial law demonstrated the "clear and plain intention" required to extinguish an Aboriginal right, then that law would be directed at Aboriginal peoples, and so would be *ultra vires*, and of no effect. As noted above, only *provinces*, and not the federal government, have passed laws regulating who may practice medicine. As a consequence, there is no legislation regulating the practice of medicine that could have had the effect of extinguishing Aboriginal rights prior to 1982.

---

[151]   There has not been any litigation on these matters in Canada.

[152]   Courts have determined that the common law doctrine of Aboriginal rights arose as a normative order to reconcile the fact that when Europeans arrived in North America and asserted rights of sovereignty, Aboriginal peoples were already occupying the land and engaging in practices — many of which were not necessarily impaired or otherwise extinguished by European claims to sovereignty. The leading case regarding the common law basis and constitutionalization of Aboriginal rights is *R. v. Sappier; R. v. Grey*, [2006] S.C.J. No. 54, [2006] 2 S.C.R. 686 (S.C.C.).

[153]   *Delgamuukw v. British Columbia*, [1997] S.C.J. No. 108 at paras. 178-81 (S.C.C.). On interjurisdictional immunity generally, see P. Hogg, *Constitutional Law of Canada, 1997 Student Edition* (Toronto: Carswell, 1997) at 361-70, 566-67.

However, provincial law can indirectly *affect* Aboriginal rights. If a law does so, its validity depends upon meeting a justification test. The central elements of the test for justifying an impairment include the state proving that the regulatory activity engages a valid and compelling legislative objective, and proving that the infringement of the Aboriginal right is formulated to reflect the special fiduciary relationship between Aboriginal peoples and the Crown. This second element usually requires the state to bring evidence that it consulted with the Aboriginal peoples whose claimed rights would be impacted, took steps to accommodate their concerns, and impaired the claimed right as minimally as possible.[154]

The public safety goals of regulating the practice of medicine provide a compelling legislative objective. However, no province (other than Ontario) appears to have engaged in the required processes of consultation or accommodation. In the absence of such processes, it is likely that as a matter of law traditional Aboriginal healers would be able to defend themselves against charges of practising medicine without a provincial licence due to the failure to consult.

Recent treaties appear to reflect state support for traditional healers being regulated by Aboriginal communities themselves. In the 1999 treaty between Canada, British Columbia and the Nisga'a First Nation, the federal and provincial governments recognized the authority of the Nisga'a to regulate traditional healers.[155] In the Nisga'a Agreement, the licensing process for healers must include measures respecting competence, ethics and quality of practice.[156] Similarly, in the Labrador Inuit Land Claims Agreement, which was ratified by the Inuit on May 27, 2004, the newly created Nunatsiavut Government has the express power to make laws regarding traditional healing and medicine and community healing, "including the qualifications of practitioners of traditional healing and medicine".[157]

Outside of these few agreements, in which health is rolled into a general governmental package, the question of whether or how to regulate traditional healers, and their practices, is an awkward one. There is a polarization of views among Aboriginal peoples regarding whether there should be any form of regulation. Some traditional practitioners view formal regulation as culturally inappropriate, and argue that customary practice and informal norms will protect against fraudulent or harmful

---

[154] *Wewaykum Indian Band v. Canada*, [2002] S.C.J. No. 79 at paras. 79-80 (S.C.C.).

[155] *Nisga'a Final Agreement Act*, S.B.C. 1999, c. 2, ss. 86-88.

[156] *Ibid.*, s. 88.

[157] *Labrador Inuit Land Claims Agreement*, S.N.L. 2004, c. L-3.1 Part 17.13.1(h).

activities.[158] These mechanisms, which rely on community censure, cannot be assumed to be effective in all contexts, especially where the practitioner practises outside of his or her home community.[159] One suggestion is to develop a system of professional accountability for traditional healers, in which that system is developed internally and is self-regulating, similar to other health professions.[160] Under such a system, both the professional society as well as criminal justice would be available to punish rogue individuals.

Despite the ambiguous and inconsistent positions which the provinces and Canada occupy regarding the lawfulness of Aboriginal healing practices, Canada has made the policy decision to provide some financial support for those seeking traditional treatment. The Non-insured Health Benefits Program includes funding to cover some of the costs associated with travel that may be involved for an Aboriginal person to be treated by a traditional healer.[161] Eligible costs may include meals, transportation and accommodation.[162]

Although this financial assistance is clearly an endorsement of traditional healing practices, it is subject to a number of limitations that may render it unsatisfactory to many Aboriginal peoples. First, only registered members of First Nations and Inuit are eligible for this funding — the populations of unregistered members of First Nations, and Métis people, are excluded.[163] Second, no financial assistance is available to cover honoraria for the healer, nor any ceremonial expenses.[164] Third, although the Non-insured Health Benefits Program covers the costs of many medicines, including "over-the-counter" drugs as long as they are prescribed, medicines which are used or prescribed by a traditional healer are not eligible for coverage.[165]

[158]   Canada, Royal Commission on Aboriginal Peoples, *Report of the Royal Commission on Aboriginal Peoples: Volume 3 Gathering Strength* (Ottawa: Minister of Supply and Services, 1996) at 355.
[159]   There have been instances of persons claiming to practice traditional Aboriginal healing in an urban context, where the "healer" and patient were strangers, and the healer used the opportunity of "healing ceremonies" to sexually abuse the patient. In such situations, there may not be a community that can effectively censure rogue individuals or protect vulnerable persons. See *e.g.*, *R. v. Mianskum*, [2000] O.J. No. 5807 (Ont. S.C.J.).
[160]   Canada, Royal Commission on Aboriginal Peoples, *Report of the Royal Commission on Aboriginal Peoples: Volume 3 Gathering Strength* (Ottawa: Minister of Supply and Services, 1996) at 356.
[161]   Health Canada, *Non-Insured Health Benefits: Medical Transportation Policy Framework, July 2005* (Ottawa: Health Canada, 2005) at 15, online: <http://www.hc-sc.gc.ca/fniah-spnia/alt_formats/fnihb-dgspni/pdf/pubs/medtransp/2005_med-transp-frame-cadre-eng.pdf>.
[162]   *Ibid.*, at 5.
[163]   *Ibid.*, at 23.
[164]   *Ibid.*, at 15.
[165]   *Ibid.*

The fourth major limitation which may be unsatisfactory to Aboriginal peoples is the process for having the expenses approved. Medical transportation services to access a traditional healer must be approved in advance by the appropriate Health Canada funded First Nations/Inuit Health Authority. The Authority is required to consider certain criteria when making a funding decision. One of these criteria is that a licensed physician has confirmed that the individual has a "medical condition".[166] In a review of access to traditional healing services, it was observed that support for accessing traditional healers was "arbitrary, unsystematic and controlled (through the referral process) by doctors who may be unsympathetic or ignorant".[167] It is not surprising that a bio-medical practitioner may have difficulty assessing whether a "medical condition" exists that would be assuaged through the complex social, cultural and physical nexus of well-being engaged by traditional healing practices.[168] Indeed, this nexus would not normally be entailed by the bio-medical concept as a "medical condition". As a consequence, although Canada does not formally regulate traditional healers, it does impose a system where the decision of individual bio-medical doctors may be determinative of whether an Aboriginal person is able to access such healers.

(c)   The Regulation of Traditional Medicines and Other Substances

Although provinces other than Ontario have not exempted traditional healers from regulation, or even mentioned them in existing regulations, Nova Scotia, Saskatchewan and Manitoba have adopted legislative provisions that permit giving tobacco to youth for use in traditional Aboriginal spiritual or cultural practices.[169] It is debatable whether the term "spiritual or cultural practices" is intended to include traditional healing practices. If it does include this aspect, then such healing practices would implicitly have obtained provincial sanction.

---

[166] *Ibid.*, at para. 15. If there is no licensed physician routinely available in the community, then the individual must seek confirmation from a community health professional or from a representative of the First Nations and Inuit Health Branch of Health Canada.

[167] Canada, Royal Commission on Aboriginal Peoples, *Report of the Royal Commission on Aboriginal Peoples: Volume 3 Gathering Strength* (Ottawa: Minister of Supply and Services, 1996) at 354.

[168] L. Lemchuk-Favel & R. Jock, "Aboriginal Health Systems in Canada: Nine Case Studies" (2004) 1 Journal of Aboriginal Health 28 at 29.

[169] *Smoke-free Places Act*, S.N.S. 2002, c. 12, s. 3(2); *Tobacco Control Act*, S.S. 2001, c. T-14.1, s. 4(5); and *Non-Smokers Health Protection Act*, C.C.S.M. c. 92, s. 7(2)(b).

Saskatchewan also has a general provision permitting the use of tobacco for traditional ceremonies in public places,[170] while Nova Scotia has a blanket clause that specifies its smoking regulations do not affect the rights of Aboriginal people respecting traditional cultural practices or ceremonies.[171]

Ontario has expressly recognized that tobacco is often used as an element of "Aboriginal culture and spirituality".[172] Its *Tobacco Control Act* permits giving tobacco to Aboriginal youth under the age of 19 if the tobacco is to be used in traditional ceremonies, allows the ceremonial use of tobacco in places otherwise designated "smoke-free", and requires health facilities to provide areas where tobacco can be burned as part of a traditional healing ceremony (other than general smoking rooms).[173]

These exemptions regarding tobacco do not extend to other substances. Indeed, although the *Nisga'a Treaty* and the *Inuit Agreement* recognize the right of the Aboriginal Nations to regulate traditional healers, these agreements expressly exclude the authority of the Aboriginal nation to regulate the use of any products or substances that are regulated under federal or provincial laws of general application.[174] It would appear that Canada does not see the right to regulate traditional healing products as ancillary to the right to regulate the profession. Canada's proposed new health protection legislation[175] would regulate "natural health products", a term that is defined to include "substances used as traditional medicines".[176] The Legislative Proposal provides specific examples of "traditional medicines", including "North American Aboriginal medicine".[177]

This measure appears to indicate that the Ministry of Health has recanted the position it took just a few years ago. When the *Natural Health Products Regulations*[178] were drafted, the definition section was expressly crafted to exclude the application of the regulations to traditional healers who compounded products at the request of their

---

[170] *Tobacco Control Act*, S.S. 2001, c. T-14.1, s. 11(3)(d).
[171] *Smoke-free Places Act*, S.N.S., 2002, c. 12, s. 3(2).
[172] *Tobacco Control Act, 1994*, S.O. 1994, c. 10, s. 13(1).
[173] *Ibid.*, s. 13(2)-(4).
[174] *Nisga'a Final Agreement Act*, S.B.C. 1999, c. 2, s. 86; *Labrador Inuit Land Claims Agreement*, S.N.L. 2004, c. L-3.1 Part 17.13.1(h).
[175] Health Canada, *Health Protection Legislative Renewal: Detailed Legislative Proposal* (Ottawa, Minister of Health, 2003).
[176] *Ibid.*, at para. B7.4.2.4.
[177] *Ibid.*, at B7.4.2.4. A federal bill was tabled on 8 April 2008, but has not yet gone through Second Reading. See Bill C-51, *An Act to amend the Food and Drugs Act and to make consequential amendments to other Acts*, 2nd Sess., 39th Parl., 2008.
[178] S.O.R./2003-196.

patient.[179] This exclusion was drafted in response to concerns raised at a roundtable between representatives of the Natural Health Products Directorate and a number of Aboriginal peoples, in which the Aboriginal participants were concerned that the regulations would unduly restrict the practices of traditional healers.[180] The proposed new health protection legislation would revoke these regulations.[181]

As a consequence, under the proposed new legislation, products used by traditional healers — even those whose practices are regulated by the Aboriginal Nations — would be subject to scrutiny pursuant to Canada's proposed new regulatory regime. The regime would prohibit the use of "North American Aboriginal medicine" unless evidence is brought to Health Canada to demonstrate the product's efficacy "based solely on science and objective information".[182] Once again, one of the policy questions this raises is whether efficacy ought to be assessed based on a bio-medical model, or through a methodology that is developed and approved by Aboriginal communities (which might include a bio-medical component). The Royal Commission had admonished that health systems will only work for Aboriginal peoples if they are free to diverge from the bio-medical model.[183] As a result, Canada's initiatives to protect all members of the public, including Aboriginal peoples, risk creating considerable political and legal tension with Aboriginal communities.

The proposed state regulation of medicinal products used in traditional healing practices could be an unlawful violation of Aboriginal rights.[184] The use of traditional medicinal products as an element of traditional healing practices would, in most cases, qualify as an Aboriginal right, as long as historic and ethnographic evidence is available to substantiate the specific claim.

Canada would have little difficulty meeting the first component of the justification analysis: the proposed legislation clearly has the valid and compelling objective of protecting the public from fraudulent product claims. However, at the present stage, it does not appear that Canada could meet the second component of the justification test. There is no

---

[179] *Ibid.*, s. 1. See the definition of "Manufacturer".

[180] T. Speck, "The Importance of Culture to Aboriginal Health and Health Care" (2003) 5 Health Policy Research 20 at 22.

[181] The new legislation would revoke a number of statutes and their affiliated regulations, including the *Food and Drugs Act*, S.C. 1999, c. 33.

[182] Health Canada, *Health Protection Legislative Renewal: Detailed Legislative Proposal* (Ottawa, Minister of Health, 2003) at para. B11.2.2.

[183] Canada, Royal Commission on Aboriginal Peoples, *Report of the Royal Commission on Aboriginal Peoples: Volume 3 Gathering Strength* (Ottawa: Minister of Supply and Services, 1996) at 228-29.

[184] See discussion above regarding Aboriginal rights in Section III (d).

evidence that Canada consulted with Aboriginal peoples in its decision to regulate traditional medicines, much less took any steps to accommodate or substantially address Aboriginal concerns regarding the regulation's impact on their rights.

According to a draft report issued by the National Aboriginal Health Organization, "the federal government has stated that it will acknowledge no Aboriginal right [to use traditional medicines] — even in the clearest of cases, and that it will rely exclusively on the courts to make the determination".[185] Such a position, where Canada has denied the existence of the right, does not suggest Canada has taken steps to accommodate the practice of the right, or Aboriginal people's related concerns. As a consequence, such regulations could be found to violate s. 35 of the *Constitution Act, 1982*.

V. TRANSFER OF CONTROL OVER PUBLIC HEALTH

This last substantive section considers the transfer of control over health to Aboriginal communities. Reference is first made to the most common routes for transferring control, and then there is a discussion of the public health consequences of these transfers.

(a) Routes of Control

Canada has recognized the authority of First Nations to pass by-laws relating to some community health matters, as set out in the *Indian Act*. In particular, they may pass by-laws relating to the health of residents on reserve, and to prevent the speading of contagious and infectious disease,[186] and for the construction and regulation of the use of public wells, cisterns, reservoirs and other water supplies.[187] However, by-laws must be submitted to Canada for approval, and Canada can disallow any by-law. In practice, the power to pass by-laws has had limited impact on Aboriginal health.

Aboriginal communities have gained more significant and direct control over health through two key routes. The first route, in which control over some aspects of health programming is contained within a larger governance envelope, usually involves the settlement of self-government and land claims agreements. For example, the first independent Aboriginal health and social services board was created as a

---

[185] National Aboriginal Health Organization, *Federal Proposal for a New Canada Health Protection Act, Briefing Note (External) (Draft)* (Ottawa: National Aboriginal Health Organization, 15 April 2004) at 6.

[186] *Indian Act*, R.S.C. 1985, c. I-5, s. 81(1)(*a*).

[187] *Ibid.*, s. 81(1)(l).

part of the James Bay and Northern Quebec Agreement of 1975.[188] Both the *Nisga'a Agreement* and the *Labrador Inuit Agreement* described earlier also included health programming. These agreements are complex and took decades to negotiate.

A second route is offered through Canada's Health Services Transfer Policy, which has been operational since 1989. This option can be put in place within a span of just a few years, but only involves the transfer of administrative control over some community health services from Health Canada to First Nations. The rate of community participation is quite high: 83 per cent of eligible communities opted in by March 2008, with approximately two-thirds having entered into a Health Services Transfer Agreement, and one-third having entered into an alternative arrangement which involves assuming a lesser degree of responsibility (and control).[189] The program has facilitated several community success stories.[190] In general, all participating communities have benefited from flexibility in the use of program funds, and some freedom to adapt community health services to better meet local needs and priorities.[191]

The program has also received some serious criticism.[192] The control communities exercise is largely administrative in character. Communities are expected to design and deliver programs that operate within often rigid parameters.[193] As well, the funding envelope is based on expenditure the year prior to when the community enters transfer, and is only increased by standardized indexing, not the rates at which services are accessed. Funding is not modified in response to actual use or need, or increases in the service population, potentially creating a deficit situation. Finally, and perhaps most importantly, the transfer can only encompass those areas of health that are currently delivered through FNIHB.[194] Thus, control over programming that targets other determinants of health such as community

---

[188] Canada, Royal Commission on Aboriginal Peoples, *Report of the Royal Commission on Aboriginal Peoples: Volume 3 Gathering Strength* (Ottawa: Minister of Supply and Services, 1996) at 116.

[189] Health Canada, First Nations & Inuit Health, "Transfer Status as of March 2008", online: <http:/www.hc-sc.gc.ca/fnih-spni/finance/agree-accord/trans_rpt_stats_e.html>.

[190] L. Lemchuk-Favel & R. Jock, "Aboriginal Health Systems in Canada: Nine Case Studies" (2004) 1 Journal of Aboriginal Health 28 at 45-46.

[191] Canada, Royal Commission on Aboriginal Peoples, *Report of the Royal Commission on Aboriginal Peoples: Volume 3 Gathering Strength* (Ottawa: Minister of Supply and Services, 1996) at 117.

[192] *E.g.*, see C. MacIntosh, "Envisioning the Future of Aboriginal Health under the Health Transfer Process" (2008) Health L.J. [forthcoming].

[193] M. Maar, "Clearing the Path for Community Health Empowerment: Integrating Health Care Services at an Aboriginal Health Access Centre in Rural North Central Ontario" (2004) 1 Journal of Aboriginal Health 54 at 58.

[194] D. Gregory *et al.*, "Canada's Indian Health Transfer Policy: The Gull Bay Experience" (1992) 51(3) Human Organization 214 at 216-17.

conditions, deficient housing, environmental factors and community development, are not included in the transfer. Although the objective is to promote community health through community control, many of the determinants of community health remain out of reach of the community, and the community is defined to include funding for community members who live on-reserve and have status, a definition which is clearly at odds with how most Aboriginal communities understand themselves.

(b)   Public Health Consequences of Community Control

The National Aboriginal Health Organization ("NAHO") links the poor health status of the Aboriginal population both to features of the current health service system, as well as broad social, political and environmental factors. These factors include cultural suppression, the effects of colonization, family and community dislocation, poverty, and unhealthy physical environments.[195] NAHO argues these factors can only be addressed within a larger project of Aboriginal communities exercising self-determination:

> A return to self-determination and self-sufficiency, including the exercise of inherent rights, self-government, economic stability, [and] sound community infrastructure … are central to improving the health status of Aboriginal Peoples in Canada.[196]

It is commonly accepted that those populations who have direct control over their own lives, as well as the resources required for meaningful participation in decision-making processes, tend to have better health outcomes than those who have little control.[197] Indeed, the Royal Commission, and others, have concluded that community control is essential for improving the health of Aboriginal Canadians.[198]

There have been very few studies on the impact of Aboriginal community control on population health, and as such, it has proven extremely challenging to provide an objective assessment due to the lack of baseline data and the complex factors which combine to influence

---

[195]   National Aboriginal Health Organization, *Ways of Knowing: A Framework for Health Research* by Policy Research Unit (Ottawa: National Aboriginal Health Organization, 2003) at 12.

[196]   *Ibid.*, at 12.

[197]   *Ibid.*, at 13.

[198]   See *e.g.*, Canada, Royal Commission on Aboriginal Peoples, *Report of the Royal Commission on Aboriginal Peoples: Volume 3 Gathering Strength* (Ottawa: Minister of Supply and Services, 1996) at 108; L. Lemchuk-Favel & R. Jock, "Aboriginal Health Systems in Canada: Nine Case Studies" (2004) J. Aboriginal Health 28 at 28-30, 33; Assembly of First Nations, *First Nations Public Health: A Framework for Improving the Health of Our People and Our Communities* (November 2006) at 24.

health outcomes.[199] There has, however, been one set of researchers who have twice studied suicide rates in Aboriginal communities in British Columbia. Suicide is a serious problem within the Aboriginal population. Data from Health Canada's *Second Diagnostic on the Health of First Nations and Inuit People in Canada* indicated that, in 1997, the suicide rate for Inuit in the Northwest Territories was six times higher than the national rate, and that the Status population in British Columbia had a suicide rate about three times higher than the national average.[200] The researchers set out to assess how those rates changed when certain other factors relating to levels of community control were present.[201]

Both of their studies considered suicide rates in British Columbia over a five-year period, and correlated suicide data with other factors. The first study assessed the presence of six specific indicators of community control: completed land claims; self-governance powers including economic and political independence; band-controlled education; band-controlled police and fire services; permanent in-community health care providers; and a facility designated for cultural use. The researchers found that there were *no* suicides in communities where all six factors were present over the five-year period of study, but that communities where *none* of the factors were present had suicide rates of 137.5 *per* 100,000. (The Canadian average is 13 *per* 100,000.)[202] The researchers determined that the suicide rates did not shift significantly unless at least three of the factors of community control were present. The factor which correlated with the most dramatic statistical shift was the Aboriginal community having completed a land claim agreement.

The second study developed upon the first, and expanded the factors under consideration to include remoteness, wealth and education, among others.[203] The researchers' findings were consistent with their earlier

---

[199]   C. MacIntosh, "Visioning the Future of Aboriginal Health under Health Transfer" (2008) Health L.J. [forthcoming]; J. Lavoie "From the Local to the National: Opportunities and Challenges Associated with First Nation Health Transfer Evaluations" (2008) Canadian J. of Program Evaluation [forthcoming].

[200]   Health Canada, *A Second Diagnostic on the Health of First Nations and Inuit Peoples in Canada, 1999* by Medical Services Branch (Ottawa: Health Canada, 1999) at para. 7.1.

[201]   M.J. Chandler & C. Lalonde, "Cultural Continuity as a Hedge Against Suicide in Canada's First Nations" (1998) 35 Transcultural Psychiatry 191; M. Chandler & C. Lalonde, "Cultural Continuity as a Moderator of Suicide Risk Among Canada's First Nations" in L. Kirmayer & G. Valaskakis, eds., *Healing Traditions: The Mental Health of Aboriginal Peoples in Canada* (Vancouver: University of British Columbia Press) [forthcoming].

[202]   Health Canada, *A Second Diagnostic on the Health of First Nations and Inuit Peoples in Canada, 1999* by Medical Services Branch (Ottawa: Health Canada, 1999) at para. 7.1. This figure is for 1996.

[203]   M. Chandler & C. Lalonde, "Cultural Continuity as a Moderator of Suicide Risk Among Canada's First Nations" in L. Kirmayer & G. Valaskakis, eds., *Healing Traditions: The*

study. These new factors were not found to have statistically significant relationships with suicide rates. Instead, the rates were "strongly related" to factors associated with "cultural continuity", including attempts to regain legal title to traditional lands, to establish self-government, and to assert control over education, social services, and health delivery services.[204]

These studies present some evidence that Aboriginal populations are more likely to be healthy if they have control not just over health decisions, but also over their communities in general. In contrast, some observers advocate approaching the issue of who ought to oversee Aboriginal public health with caution.

In the Naylor Report,[205] the National Advisory Committee, whose agenda involved conceiving of a new public health agency and program for Canada, was unwilling to take a position on whether the public health of Aboriginal communities ought to be placed within the mandate of a state forum (the new agency), or within the control of Aboriginal communities. The Naylor Report found that Aboriginal health would only be improved through a "wide-angle approach to health determinants and community development", and that this approach must be both guided and supported by the affected Aboriginal communities.

However, the report authors were uncertain that community designed, controlled and delivered public health programming is the answer.[206] This hesitance was based on an observed tension between the goal of Aboriginal peoples to practice greater self-determination within the Canadian federation, "and the uncertain effectiveness and efficiency of reinforcing the extant patterns of separate health systems for First Nations and Inuit communities".[207] In other words, the Naylor Report queried whether the public health needs of Aboriginal Canadians would be better served through multiple smaller communities being responsible for their own programming, or by a more centralized entity that embedded community health programming within a federal or provincial organization. A related question is whether the health of the Aboriginal population will benefit from the existence of a third level of jurisdiction, which must form its own connections with the existing web of federal and provincial departments, laws, policies and practices.

Mental Health of Aboriginal Peoples in Canada (Vancouver: University of British Columbia Press) [forthcoming].

[204] *Ibid.*, at 18.

[205] National Advisory Committee on SARS and Public Health, *Learning from SARS: Renewal of Public Health in Canada* (Ottawa: Health Canada, 2003) (Chair: Dr. D. Naylor) ["Naylor Report"].

[206] *Ibid.*, at 79.

[207] *Ibid.*

Such partnerships can only succeed if there is political will, commitment and co-ordination at all levels of government. Ontario's Aboriginal Healing and Wellness Strategy, which funds and supports community based health and mental health care services in Aboriginal communities, has made great strides in this area.[208] The Strategy employs a consensus model for decision-making that involves ten ministries and eight Aboriginal organizations. This intersectoral governance structure has facilitated effective programming and delivery. First Nations in British Columbia have similarly made considerable progress in forming relationships with provincial departments and agencies. Even within these sorts of formats, however, there remains some fragmentation of health care services.[209]

Given the complexity and political character of health and the relationship between Aboriginal peoples and Canada, it is not surprising that the authors of the Naylor Report chose to refrain from drawing any conclusions. Instead, they felt the issue ought to be grappled with by a policy body which had a longer timeline, and the ability to properly review and consider public health service provision and health promotion for First Nations and Inuit Canadians. To this it is essential to add the need to include the best approach for all Aboriginal peoples, not just those who are currently served by the federal government.

Health Canada has, however, chosen to move forward in creating the new public health agency, and it appears that the agency will address at least some Aboriginal public health issues. The consultation on the structure of this agency, and how it can improve the health of Aboriginal Canadians, has been and continues to be ongoing.[210]

VI. CLOSING COMMENTS

It is evident that Aboriginal peoples fare poorly with regard to all markers of population health. Remedying this situation requires reshaping

---

[208] M. Maar, "Clearing the Path for Community Health Empowerment: Integrating Health Care Services at an Aboriginal Health Access Centre in Rural North Central Ontario" (2004) 1 Journal of Aboriginal Health 54 at 55.

[209] Ibid., at 63.

[210] For example, the Hon. Minister of State (Public Health) Carolyn Bennett hosted a workshop in Ottawa on March 8, 2004 on the proposed agency. The workshop participants were leaders and representatives from five national Aboriginal organizations, including the Assembly of First Nations, Inuit Tapiriit Kanatami, Métis National Council, Congress of Aboriginal Peoples, and the Native Women's Association of Canada. This workshop focused on identifying gaps and priorities for Aboriginal public health, as well as structures to ensure appropriate Aboriginal oversight of the Agency's operations. A second roundtable was held May 3, 2004, to follow up on four issues that had been identified at the March meeting. One of these issues was dealing with jurisdictional barriers to access to health. The author was a participant at this second roundtable.

existing law and policy to better address a broad range of social, economic, political and legal issues. In some cases, great strides can be made through identifying and addressing gaps, such as the jurisdictional void regarding water safety on reserves.

Policy development is more complex in situations where Aboriginal communities claim an Aboriginal right to a standard — such as adequate housing — that is not being met. It is unclear whether such outstanding legal issues must be addressed for Aboriginal peoples to obtain health standing which is comparable to the non-Aboriginal population. In these sorts of situations, Aboriginal communities are unlikely to abandon their legal claims until the situation is abated. Other questions, such as whether Aboriginal peoples possess a right to practice traditional healing, and how or whether that right ought to be regulated, are clearly best answered through community supported conversations and negotiations, not litigation.

There is evidence that the health of Aboriginal populations will benefit from communities taking control over their own affairs. Canada seems committed to promoting some form of Aboriginal self-determination. Although the Health Transfer Policy has been critiqued as only granting administrative powers and not being tied in with transfers of other powers relating to community health, it is a policy that can be implemented fairly quickly. As well, the Policy is, arguably, a small step towards communities practising self-determination.

Through several of the examples detailed in this chapter, Canada requires, or attempts to require, Aboriginal peoples to meet and adjust to the regulatory practices and categories of the state. One can argue that this is the proper policy for producing an accommodation, so as to recognize and enhance indigenous practices, and is essential given that Canada is spending public monies and is engaged in a national project. Alternately, one can take the position that it is a *de facto* form of neo-colonialism, where non-indigenous frames of knowing and validity are imposed upon indigenous ones. Such radical contradictions of perspectives are not easily overcome. Perhaps a key starting point is the recognition that they exist, and that such radical views demand radical new ways of thinking and generating new policy and legislation.

11

PUBLIC HEALTH AND ENVIRONMENTAL PROTECTION IN CANADA

Jamie Benidickson[*]

I.   INTRODUCTION

Relationships between public health and environmental conditions are increasingly of concern to medical specialists and other health care experts researching the origins of particular diseases or their pathways of transmission. More generally, contemporary policy makers have acknowledged the significance of environmental conditions on public health. Indeed, with reference to climate change, the 2007 Speech from the Throne called for action "to ensure our quality of life, particularly for those most vulnerable to health threats from the environment".[1] Measures to enhance environmental quality have clearly become important elements of any comprehensive program to guard against a variety of health risks.

This chapter is intended to provide an introduction to both legal and institutional aspects of environmental protection with reference to the opportunities and challenges that Canada's environmental regime presents from a public health perspective. The chapter begins with a brief review of changing perceptions of the health-environment relationship. This is followed by an overview of the legal framework for environmental protection in Canada. A series of case studies on mercury pollution, pesticide regulation, drinking water contamination and smog is then used to illustrate circumstances in which environmental quality and health

---

[*]   Professor, Faculty of Law, University of Ottawa.

[1]   Canada, Governor General, "Strong Leadership. A Better Canada" (Speech from the Throne, 16 October 2007) at 14, online: Government of Canada <http://www.sft-ddt.gc.ca/grfx/docs/sftddt-e.pdf>.

protection have been closely interrelated. The final section of the chapter analyzes in somewhat greater detail legal and institutional mechanisms available to safeguard public health through environmental protection. These include the common law, regulatory arrangements, procedural opportunities for public participation, initiatives to foster institutional collaboration, and emerging principles of decision-making such as precaution.

II. HEALTH AND ENVIRONMENT

Over at least two centuries, attempts to explain the prevalence of disease generally or to account for more specific incidences of particular illnesses have intermittently identified environmental conditions as either causal or contributory factors. Although some of the suggested explanations — for example, the early 19th-century belief that many prominent maladies originated in noxious vapours, or miasmas — have proven fanciful, and although medical intervention has become focused heavily on individualized treatment and remedial care, environmental influences on public health are again attracting considerable interest from a research and policy perspective.[2]

Contemporary concerns are less likely to involve contemplation of the environment as an independent or autonomous source of disease. Instead, human interference with or disruption of environmental conditions is the more common subject of investigation on the part of those examining the origins of certain adverse impacts on human health. Local water supplies are vulnerable to contamination from municipal, industrial or agricultural sources. Adverse health effects have also been associated with soil contamination attributable to waste disposal or industrial use. Urban atmospheric conditions deteriorate intermittently as a result of emissions from manufacturing processes or transportation with significant impacts on rates of respiratory illness. And, on an even wider scale, people are increasingly vulnerable to various forms of skin cancer because of ozone depletion resulting from the dispersal of certain chemicals into the atmosphere.[3]

---

[2]   See, for example, the work of the Western Ecosystem Health Centre, online: <http://www.med.uwo.ca/ecosystemhealth/aboutus.htm>; the McMaster Institute of Environment & Health, online: <http://www.mcmaster.ca/mieh>; the Department of Public Health Sciences at the University of Alberta, or the R. Samuel McLaughlin Centre for Population Health Risk Assessment at the University of Ottawa, online: <http://www.mclaughlincentre.ca>.

[3]   For a survey of health impacts associated with contamination of air, water and soil, see Health Canada, Health and Environment (Ottawa, 1997).

Greenhouse gas emissions contributing to global climate change represent the most recent example of human interference with environmental conditions in a manner that increases health risks to the general population. It is anticipated that morbidity and mortality related to summer heat will increase as the number of hot days (above 32 degrees Celsius) and days of extremely high temperature (above 36 degrees Celsius) become more common. Toronto's heat-related death rate (currently 19 per year), could increase between ten and 40-fold. The prevalence of water-borne diseases may also increase in areas where more frequent episodes of extreme precipitation occur.[4]

In light of the range of adverse health impacts associated with environmental conditions on both local and global levels, the capacity of the Canadian legal system to prevent or alleviate such threats through environmental protection is of considerable importance.

III. OVERVIEW OF THE CANADIAN ENVIRONMENTAL PROTECTION FRAMEWORK

Traditional common law principles such as nuisance and negligence, (and in Québec analogous provisions in the civil code), continue to anchor civil litigation arising from environmental injuries. We are now more inclined, however, to regard governments as the primary agents of environmental protection.

Responsibility for environmental protection is divided between the federal and provincial governments with each exercising authority derived from areas of jurisdiction allocated under general constitutional arrangements.[5] In the case of the federal government, potential authority for environmental initiatives includes constitutional responsibility for navigation and shipping, seacoast and inland fisheries, and Indians and lands reserved for the Indians as well as more general powers relating to peace, order and good government, or criminal law.[6] For their part, provincial environmental measures may be constitutionally grounded in authority over property and civil rights, the management and sale of

---

[4]   D.F. Charron *et al.*, "Vulnerability of Waterborne Diseases to Climate Change in Canada: A Review" in Steve E. Hrudey, *Drinking Water Safety: A Total Quality Management Approach* (Waterloo: University of Waterloo, Institute for Risk Research, 2003) at 189. For a more comprehensive review, see *Human Health in a Changing Climate: A Canadian Assessment of Vulnerabilities and Adaptive Capacity* (Health Canada, 2008).

[5]   For more extensive discussion, see Jamie Benidickson, *Environmental Law*, 3d ed. (Toronto: Irwin Law, 2008) c. 2.

[6]   *R. v. Crown Zellerbach Canada Ltd.*, [1988] S.C.J. No. 23, [1988] 1 S.C.R. 401 (S.C.C.); *R. v. Hydro Quebec*, [1997] S.C.J. No. 76, [1997] 3 S.C.R. 213 (S.C.C.); *Whitbread v. Walley*, [1990] S.C.J. No. 138, [1990] 3 S.C.R. 1273 (S.C.C.); *Friends of the Oldman River Society v. Canada (Minister of Transport)*, [1992] S.C.J. No. 1, 88 D.L.R. (4th) 1 (S.C.C.).

public lands, municipal institutions, or natural resources, among other powers.

The most significant piece of federal environmental legislation from the perspective of public health is the *Canadian Environmental Protection Act, 1999* ("*CEPA, 1999*").[7] This statute, for whose administration the ministers of environment and of health share responsibility, is more fully described as "an Act respecting pollution prevention and the protection of the environment and human health in order to contribute to sustainable development".[8] *CEPA, 1999*'s various parts and divisions address toxic substances, biotechnology, air and water pollution, as well as hazardous waste and hazardous recyclable materials, among other environmental concerns. Specific provision has also been made for environmental emergencies, including releases of substances that constitute or may constitute a danger to the environment on which human life depends or that constitute or may constitute a danger in Canada to human life or health.[9] Other prominent pieces of federal environmental legislation include the *Canadian Environmental Assessment Act*[10] and the *Fisheries Act*.[11]

The provinces have also adopted environmental legislation designed to protect air, land and water, or ecological resources within their jurisdiction from pollution and other forms of degradation. Provincial statutes ordinarily establish environmental licensing and approval procedures alongside regulatory standards that are enforced by means of monitoring and inspection requirements, administrative supervision and the ultimate threat of prosecution. Considerations of human health may be integrated in a variety of ways. Manitoba legislation, for example, incorporates this concern within the concept of "environmental health" which means "those aspects of human health that are or can be affected by pollutants or changes in the environment".[12] Ontario legislation, on the other hand, seeks to prevent "adverse effects", a concept whose definition encompasses "an adverse effect on the health of any person".[13]

The simultaneous involvement of both federal and provincial governments in environmental protection legislation measures has encouraged the development of coordination mechanisms. These include

---

[7]   S.C. 1999, c. 33.

[8]   *Ibid.*

[9]   *Ibid.*, Part 8; *Environmental Emergency Regulations*, S.O.R./2003-307.

[10]   S.C. 1992, c. 37.

[11]   R.S.C. 1985, c. F-14.

[12]   *Environment Act*, C.C.S.M. c. E125.

[13]   *Environmental Protection Act*, R.S.O. 1990, c. E.19. See also Alberta's *Environmental Protection and Enhancement Act*, R.S.A. 2000, c. E-12, which also included the concept of adverse effects.

statutory provisions expressly intended to avoid potential conflicts and inconsistencies[14] as well as inter-governmental harmonization agreements and institutional forums such as the Canadian Council of Ministers of the Environment ("CCME").[15]

In addition to the efforts of senior governments, municipalities across Canada exercise environmental authority at the local level in relation to issues ranging from water supply and wastewater management through noise controls and the regulation of chemicals in the community.

Some appreciation of the actual operation of the overall environmental protection regime, and of its practical significance for public health may be provided through a brief examination of selected case studies.

IV. ENVIRONMENTAL PROTECTION AND PUBLIC HEALTH: CASE STUDIES

(a) Mercury Pollution

In 1977, Romeo LeBlanc, then federal Fisheries Minister sharply underlined connections between the protection of fisheries and the well-being of the human population: "Our water resists pollution no more than the water in Minimata",[16] LeBlanc remarked, referring to the site of devastating mercury contamination in a Japanese coastal fishing community. "If our laws can protect the water", he continued, "if we give the fish a place to live, we can have a better place for man to live".[17] Pointing to the notorious results of mercury discharges, LeBlanc continued: "We have made of progress a god. But mercury was named for the messenger of the gods, and mercury has warned us clearly that the gods of progress have a darker side".[18] The dark side was by then alarmingly apparent to observers of behavioural consequences attributable to the impact on the functioning of the human brain of mercury accumulated through fish-based diets. Thus Minister LeBlanc had reasoned: to protect human health we should safeguard fish, and to safeguard fish we should protect the aquatic environments they inhabit.

It had been understood for many years that certain constituents of the pulp and paper process could be toxic to fish and other aquatic life, should they be found in "abnormally high concentrations". Yet mid-20th

---

[14]   *Canadian Environmental Protection Act, 1999*, S.C. 1999, c. 33; *Canadian Environmental Assessment Act*, S.C. 1992, c. 37.

[15]   See online: <http://www.ccme.ca>.

[16]   House of Commons Debates, 16 May 1977 at 5667.

[17]   *Ibid.*

[18]   *Ibid.*, 16 May 1977 at 5670.

century opinion still favoured the formulaic response that dilution was sufficient to prevent harmful concentrations from accumulating in the aquatic environment, or that many possible contaminants would settle harmlessly in lake or river beds, or at the ocean bottom. Understanding of toxic pathways was in transition, however. As a *New York Times* editorial explained in the summer of 1970, even though mercury was a known poison, its toxicity had not previously been linked to waterways: "Until recently neither Government officials nor scientists gave much thought to the possible harmful effects of mercury-containing wastes dumped into sewer systems by industrial plants. There was evidently a widespread assumption that mercury was insoluble and would lie forever quietly and inertly at the bottom of any body of water it reached."[19] It would soon be observed however that "one tablespoon of mercury in a body of water covering a football field to a depth of fifteen feet is enough to make fish in that water unsafe to eat".[20]

How often such concentrations might be reached — and more pointedly, where — challenged those responsible for measurement and calculation when the risk came to the attention of the North American public in 1970. Canadian mercury users, including chlor-alkali plants producing pulp and paper, were successful in reducing mercury losses dramatically as soon as the problem had been identified. By that time, however, an uncertain legacy of contamination had accumulated in river sediments and severe damage was underway.

When mercury contamination forced the suspension of commercial fishing in parts of Manitoba, the provincial government distributed approximately $2 million in compensation to roughly 1,600 people who had been adversely affected by the closure. The province first secured the rights of victims to sue those responsible for the damage. Manitoba then applied for an injunction against further discharges and attempted to recover its financial loss from the polluting industries. Among these companies, Dryden Chemicals Limited in northwestern Ontario and Interprovincial Cooperatives Limited in Saskatchewan were discharging industrial mercury on the basis of permits from their respective provincial governments. The recipient rivers, the Wabigoon and the South Saskatchewan, both drained through connecting watercourses into Manitoba, where mercury damage to the fisheries had taken place. Manitoba, as residents of the province have had frequent occasion to note, is "downstream from everywhere".

---

[19]   *New York Times* (25 July 1970), quoted in H.R. Jones, *Mercury Pollution Control* (New Jersey: Noyes Data Corporation, 1971).

[20]   R. Howard, *Poisons in Public: Case Studies of Environmental Pollution in Canada* (Toronto: James Lorimer, 1980) at 19.

Manitoba's claim against the out-of-province companies was founded on a provincial statute of its own — the *Fishermen's Assistance and Polluters' Liability Act*. This legislation sought to impose liability on any person who discharged a contaminant "into waters in the province or into any waters whereby it is carried into waters in the province".[21] The Manitoba statute went further, declaring that a permit to discharge the contaminant provided no lawful excuse for damage to the fishery outside the jurisdiction of the issuing authority. This provision, among other features of the *Fishermen's Assistance and Polluters' Liability Act*, was directly challenged by the two companies in proceedings that eventually reached the Supreme Court of Canada.[22]

In March 1975, a Supreme Court of Canada majority struck down Manitoba's initiative in a complicated ruling.[23] Some members of the court asserted that Manitoba's legislative authority did not extend outside the province's borders. Manitoba legislation, accordingly, could not operate so as to undermine the statutory arrangements of neighbouring jurisdictions, even in an effort to safeguard interests of its own residents, and even in the context of a "truly interprovincial" pollution problem.[24] Another judge, who also rejected the Manitoba legislation, expressed the opinion that if Dryden Chemicals and Interprovincial had valid authorizations from Ontario and Saskatchewan, then "the acts were authorized by licence and therefore justifiable in the places where they were done, [therefore] they were not civil wrongs and [could] form no basis for a damage action".[25]

Only Chief Justice Bora Laskin and two fellow dissenters appreciated the legal situation from Manitoba's downstream perspective. It is "plain enough",[26] Laskin C.J. wrote with characteristic clarity, that a province is entitled to protect its property rights against injury. Equally, provinces are entitled to protect the interests that others might have in such property.[27] Turning his attention to the provision in question, Chief Justice Laskin explained that it did indeed make Manitoba law applicable to the activities of Interprovincial and Dryden Chemicals originating in their respective provinces, but only because these operations had damaged

---

[21]   C.C.S.M. 1970, c. F100, s. 4(1).

[22]   *Interprovincial Co-operatives Ltd. v. Dryden Chemicals Ltd.*, [1975] S.C.J. No. 42, [1976] 1 S.C.R. 477, [1975] 5 W.W.R. 382 (S.C.C.).

[23]   Joost Blom, "The Conflict of Laws and the Constitution — *Interprovincial Co-operatives Ltd. v. The Queen*" (1977) U.B.C. L. Rev. 11 at 144-57.

[24]   *Interprovincial Co-operatives Ltd. v. Dryden Chemicals Ltd.*, [1975] S.C.J. No. 42, [1976] 1 S.C.R. 477, [1975] 5 W.W.R. 382 at 390 (S.C.C.).

[25]   *Ibid.*, at 398 W.W.R.

[26]   *Ibid.*, at 413 W.W.R.

[27]   *Ibid.*, at 413 W.W.R.

a Manitoba fishery by discharging a contaminant into waters flowing into Manitoba.[28]

Hinted at, but not conclusively resolved, was the question of the lawfulness of the mercury discharge within the boundaries of Ontario and Saskatchewan. If residents of the jurisdictions which had licensed — and thereby seemingly approved — the operations that resulted in mercury contamination had suffered injury (either as fishermen or as consumers of contaminated fish) would they be deprived of a claim to compensation on the grounds that mercury had been lawfully released into the waterways? That disturbing possibility was soon faced, at least in Ontario.

The impact of mercury contamination from Dryden Chemical on downstream Aboriginal residents was enormous. The fishery, an important source of both food and income, was lost; signs of illness associated with mercury poisoning were endemic. Moreover, communal existence was severely undermined for members of the Islington and Grassy Narrows Bands, as community institutions and traditions disintegrated around them.[29] In 1977 Aboriginal communities at Islington and Grassy Narrows launched a $25 million lawsuit against corporate owners of the Dryden operation and against the Ontario government. Yet, as apparent as their injuries were, it was far from clear whether these victims of a degraded river system would be any more successful than the Province of Manitoba had been in securing compensation through the courts.

In their search to find a key to the lock of compensation, the bands consulted Robert Sharpe, an experienced litigator and respected academic lawyer. On their behalf, Sharpe surveyed the applicability of such common law doctrines as riparian rights, negligence and nuisance to the known facts of the situation — and to its uncertainties. He explored legal claims not only against the polluting companies but also against the provincial government itself for its role in the devastation. There was doubt about whether any of the legal alternatives would work and also some question about the extent to which compensation could be recovered, even if liability were to be established. Sharpe cautioned that personal injury losses — notably relating to the adverse health impacts of mercury poisoning — would have to be proven in each case. Health effects could not simply be asserted. Other types of loss — purely economic losses and social losses accompanying the devastation of the community — were even more problematic.

---

[28]   *Ibid.*, at 416 W.W.R.

[29]   Anastasia M. Shkilnyk, *A Poison Stronger Than Love: The Destruction of an Ojibwa Community* (New Haven: Yale University Press, 1985).

Almost a decade after the original legal claim, the situation was resolved for around $17 million in exchange for the abolition of all future claims arising from the prolonged ordeal. Complementary federal and provincial legislation confirmed the settlement agreement and established an administrative mechanism, the Grassy Narrows and Islington Bands Mercury Disability Board, to distribute funds to applicants who could demonstrate "exposure to mercury and neurological conditions consistent with mercury poisoning".[30]

(b) Pesticide Regulation

Insecticides and herbicides, among other products intended for pest control, are extensively employed throughout Canada in commercial and domestic applications. Pesticide users may experience direct contact with the substances, while the general public is exposed to pesticides through food residues and to a lesser extent in drinking water. The federal *Food and Drugs Act*[31] provides mechanisms for constant monitoring of pesticide residues in foods, while the *Guidelines for Canadian Drinking Water* outline acceptable residue levels for pesticides that have entered the water supply system either directly through spills, off-target aerial spraying, surface run-off or after filtering through the soil to groundwater. Possible health risks associated with pesticide use have aroused public concern.

The Canadian regulatory framework for pesticides combines federal controls on the registration of chemical ingredients with provincial regimes addressing licensing issues and the supervision of pesticide handling and application procedures. Municipal governments, often demonstrating a particular concern for the vulnerability of children, are increasingly involved in regulating the use of pesticides within their own boundaries.

The federal *Pest Control Products Act* ("*PCPA*") establishes a registration requirement for any product, device, organism, substance or thing sold or used to control, prevent, destroy, mitigate, attract or repel any pest.[32] These so-called control products now also include control products derived from biotechnology. The pesticide registration process, emphasizing health and risk assessments for control products, is carried out under the supervision of the Pest Management Regulatory Agency

---

[30]   "The Grassy Narrows and Islington Bands Mercury Disability Board" in Mario Faieta *et al.*, *Environmental Harm: Civil Actions and Compensation* (Toronto/Vancouver: Butterworths, 1996) at 465-70.

[31]   *Food and Drugs Act*, R.S.C. 1985, c. F-27.

[32]   S.C. 2002, c. 28.

("PMRA").[33] Some 500 active chemical ingredients for pesticides have been registered of which approximately 100 are in regular use.

As described by Justice Cullen of the Federal Court, the *PCPA* was designed to protect the health of the general public from the impact of products that may be dangerous, and imposes significant control mechanisms before a product is registered.[34] In the context of an application for registration, the applicant is required to furnish sufficient information to permit an assessment of the "safety, merit, and value"[35] of the relevant control product and bears the burden of proof in meeting this test. The Minister of Health has authority to refuse registration where the information furnished by the applicant "is insufficient to enable the control product to be assessed or evaluated".[36] Moreover, it must be determined that use of the pesticide will not result in an "unacceptable risk of harm"[37] to public health, plants or the environment.

The risks posed to human health from pesticide use are in some respects distinctive, arising as they do from "the public's routine, involuntary exposure to pesticides contained in virtually all food and drinking water, and their deliberate emission into the environment".[38] The rationale for pesticide regulation thus extends beyond reasons applicable to regulation of therapeutic products where human exposure is voluntary, and beyond reasons underlying the regulation of substances that present risks of purely environmental harm. "Health concerns associated with pesticides tend to centre on long-term effects that are very difficult to attribute to specific products or events. The opposite tends to be true with therapeutic products for people where adverse reactions are generally acute."[39]

---

[33]   For a description of the registration process, see the Report of the House Standing Committee on Environment and Sustainable Development, *Pesticides: Making the Right Choices for the Protection of Health and the Environment* (May 2000) c. 8, online: <http://www2.parl.gc.ca/HousePublications/Publication.aspx?DocId=1031697&Language=E&Mode=1&Parl=36&Ses=2>.

[34]   *Monsanto Canada Inc. v. Canada (Minister of Agriculture)*, [1986] F.C.J. No. 31, 1 F.T.R. 63 (F.C.T.D.).

[35]   *Pest Control Products Regulations*, C.R.C., c. 1253, s. 9(1).

[36]   *Pest Control Products Regulations*, C.R.C., c. 1253, s. 18(*b*).

[37]   *Pest Control Products Regulations*, C.R.C., c. 1253, s. 18(*d*).

[38]   Ivo Krupka, "The Pest Management Regulatory Agency: The Resilience of Science in Pesticide Regulation" in G. Bruce Doern & Ted Reed, eds., *Risky Business: Canada's Changing Science-Based Policy and Regulatory Regime* (Toronto: University of Toronto Press, 2000) at 236.

[39]   *Ibid.*

The manner in which determinations about acceptability are made has aroused controversy; legal challenges are not uncommon.[40] In a report preceding recent statutory revisions to the *PCPA*, the House of Commons Standing Committee on Environment and Sustainable Development canvassed public concerns, many directly associated with health risks. Consideration was given to a recommendation that the PMRA rather than the applicant seeking registration should conduct risk assessments. On the basis of existing procedural controls and general practice in other settings, this proposal was not pursued. There were widespread calls, however, which the committee supported, for a greater degree of certainty, comprehensiveness and transparency in the PMRA's approach to risk assessment. The PMRA's product-by-product approach to determining maximum exposure limits, and in particular to maximum pesticide residue levels ("MRLs") on food, was also questioned. As the committee observed, "many pesticides act in a similar fashion. MRLs, however, continue to be established on a pesticide by pesticide basis, ignoring the cumulative effects of residues from similar pesticides that could also be present on food and in the environment. Assessing pesticides on an individual basis also ignores possible interactions between different pesticides".[41] These circumstances potentially contribute to "a severe underestimation of the risks to which we are being subjected".[42] It is difficult to conclude that the acceptability of risks that have not been fully acknowledged and appreciated, can be effectively established.

At the provincial level, pesticide-management legislation generally provides for a licensing and permit scheme setting out conditions of pesticide sale and use in a range of applications including agriculture, forest management and commercial-extermination services. Notwithstanding prior federal registration of the relevant control product, issues relating to pesticide risk and safety arise in the provincial licensing context. The approach to toxicity and risk taken by British Columbia's Environmental Appeal Board ("EAB") in considering licence applications for pesticide use under the province's *Pesticide Control Act*[43] has been examined by the Court of Appeal.[44] With regard to toxicity, the court supported one trial judge's observations to the effect that it was not a jurisdictional error to assume

---

[40]   *Pulp, Paper & Woodworkers of Canada, Local 8 v. Canada (Minister of Agriculture)*, [1994] F.C.J. No. 1067 (F.C.A.); *Kuczerpa v. Canada*, [1993] F.C.J. No. 217 (F.C.A.).

[41]   Report of the House Standing Committee on Environment and Sustainable Development, *Pesticides: Making the Right Choices for the Protection of Health and the Environment* (May 2000) c. 8, online: <http://www2.parl.gc.ca/HousePublications/Publication.aspx?Doc Id=1031697&Language=E&Mode=1&Parl=36&Ses=2>.

[42]   *Ibid.*, at 8.29.

[43]   See *Integrated Pest Management Act*, S.B.C. 2003, c. 58.

[44]   *Canadian Earthcare Society v. British Columbia (Environmental Appeal Board)*, [1988] B.C.J. No. 3109, 3 C.E.L.R. (N.S.) 55 (B.C.C.A.).

the general safety of a federally — registered pesticide: "Common sense dictates that the fact that a federally registered pesticide that has undergone extensive testing must have some probative value ...".[45] With respect to the relevance of alternative approaches to pest control, the court also agreed with the trial judge's reasons:

> Only by making a comparison of risk and benefit can the Board determine if the anticipated risk is reasonable or unreasonable. . . . If the same benefits could be achieved by an alternative risk-free method then surely the risk method would be considered unreasonable.[46]

In subsequent decisions, British Columbia's EAB demonstrated a greater willingness to impose additional controls over the conditions under which pesticides may be used, to explore alternatives to chemical pest control and to acknowledge the importance of post-registration toxicity data for decision-making.[47]

The desirability of pursuing alternatives and of strengthening controls on the use of pesticides was underlined by a decision of the BC Provincial Court. When, in the course of a storage shed relocation and repair project, several unused bags of a highly toxic restricted pesticide were inexplicably placed with piles of waste material in a gully by a hired hand whose pesticide applicator's licence had long-since expired, the employer presented a due diligence defence. He argued, in other words, that he had taken reasonable care to avoid committing an offence. The claim succeeded. In the court's opinion, no right-minded individual would have imagined that someone with a pesticide applicator's certificate "would have done something so stupid as to dump these chemicals".[48] The facts of this case, suggest that right-minded individuals, including right-minded regulators, might more readily imagine stupid actions and reflect further on measures to reduce their likelihood or avert their consequences.

In response to civic dissatisfaction with existing controls on pesticide use, municipal initiatives restricting pesticide use have proliferated. Municipalities have considered several alternative approaches to pesticide regulation. Some focus on the protection of populations considered to face the most severe risks, children in particular. Others emphasize the elimination of pesticide use by municipalities themselves. By way of example, the Regional Municipality of Halifax prohibits pesticide application on municipally owned property and within a specified distance of properties occupied by such institutions as schools and hospitals. Except in the case

[45]   *Ibid.*, at 59 C.E.L.R.

[46]   *Ibid.*, at 60 C.E.L.R.

[47]   *Wier v. British Columbia (Environmental Appeal Board)*, [2003] B.C.J. No. 2221 (B.C.S.C.).

[48]   *R. v. Rezansoff*, [2003] B.C.J. No. 763, 1 C.E.L.R. (3d) 125 at para. 131 (B.C. Prov. Ct.).

of "permitted pesticides" as designated by the Halifax Regional Council, and in cases where use has been specifically authorized in connection with a danger to human beings over an insect infestation, pesticide applications within the municipality were prohibited as of April 2003.[49] The City of Toronto, exercising general residual authority under the *Municipal Act, 2001*[50] implemented comparable measures, as did a significant number of Québec municipalities.

Municipal implementation of local pesticide controls alongside the existing federal and provincial arrangements provoked challenges from industrial interests. Having been licensed at the provincial level to use federally approved pesticides, a lawn care company challenged a municipal pesticide by-law enacted by the town of Hudson, Québec.[51] The company argued that such a by-law was beyond the powers of the municipality (*ultra vires*) and that it was inconsistent with federal and provincial legislation. The Supreme Court of Canada upheld the by-law as a valid exercise of the general power of the municipality to make by-laws for the general welfare of the municipality. In upholding Hudson's pesticide regime, the Court noted that the by-law regulated but did not prohibit pesticide use, that it was enacted for legitimate purposes, and that courts should exercise caution before holding that elected municipal bodies have exceeded their powers. In connection with the alleged inconsistency between the by-law and the federal and provincial framework for pesticide management, Justice L'Heureux-Dubé concluded that there was no conflict sufficient to nullify the by-law; indeed, Québec's *Pesticide Act* was intended to operate in conjunction with more stringent municipal controls.[52]

(c) Drinking Water Contamination

Drinking water supplies, and hence the health of the human population dependent upon them, are vulnerable to contamination by bacteria and other pathogens, organic chemicals and metals resulting from municipal and industrial pollution, septic arrangements, and agricultural

---

[49]   Regional Municipality of Halifax, By-Law P-800 Respecting the Regulation of Pesticides, Herbicides and Insecticides.

[50]   *Municipal Act, 2001*, S.O. 2001, c. 25, s. 130 authorizes a municipality to "regulate matters not specifically provided for by this Act or any other Act for purposes related to the health, safety and well-being of the inhabitants of the municipality". See *Croplife Canada v. Toronto (City)*, [2005] O.J. No. 1896, 75 O.R. (3d) 357 (Ont. C.A.), leave to appeal to S.C.C. refused [2005] S.C.C.A. No. 329 (S.C.C.).

[51]   *114957 Canada Ltée (Spraytech, Societé d'arrosage) v. Hudson (Town)*, [2001] S.C.J. No. 42, 2001 SCC 40 (S.C.C.).

[52]   R.S.Q. c. P-9.3. The province of Québec subsequently strengthened province-wide controls on pesticide use in the Québec *Pesticides Management Code*, R.Q. c. P-9.3, r.0.0.1.

and other land-use practices. These risks apply to both surface and ground waters. They may result from both "point sources" such as effluent discharges, and from "non-point sources" of contamination such as land use practices in agriculture and forestry, or as a consequence of airborne pollutants.[53]

In Walkerton, Ontario, seven deaths and over 2,300 cases of illness, some involving lasting effects, were attributed to contamination of a municipal well by *E. coli 0157:H7* and *Campylobacter jejuni* in May 2000. Roughly one year later, in April 2001, between 5,800 and 7,100 people in the North Battleford area of Saskatchewan were affected by an outbreak of gastro-intestinal illness caused by the parasite *Cryptosporidium parvum* which entered the community water system. Quite apart from these two dramatic occurrences and the severe personal and community losses they entailed,[54] it has been estimated that the annual costs of water-borne diseases on a national basis in Canada approximate $200 million.[55]

Long-standing arrangements to ensure the quality of drinking water supplies in Canada have involved inter-governmental collaboration in the formulation of drinking water standards, provincial adoption of these either as guidelines or in some instances on the basis of regulation, and municipal implementation, subject to regulatory conditions and approvals, of water supply, treatment and distribution systems. Additional procedures for monitoring and reporting on the quality of municipal supply, as well as for the supervision of responsible personnel have also been employed to maintain water quality standards.

In the Walkerton and North Battleford cases, however, judicial inquiries pointed to a disturbing inclination to take for granted public health advances that are only as effective as the continuing means provided to maintain them on a daily basis. In the North Battleford case, Justice Robert Laing concluded that there were "no villains", although he found "a great deal of indifference to the public health safety aspects of drinking water, on the part of the city who had the responsibility to produce potable water, and on the part of the SERM (Saskatchewan Environment and Resource Management) who had the mandate to regulate it".[56] The Commissioner put the overall deficiency in more

---

[53]   Linda Nash, "Water Quality and Health" in Peter H. Gleick ed., *Water in Crisis* (Health Canada, 1997) at 25-39.

[54]   Not including human suffering and loss of life, the economic impact of the Walkerton contamination was estimated at in excess of $64.5 million (Walkerton Report), Part II at 7.

[55]   Report of the Commission of Inquiry into matters relating to the safety of the public drinking water in the City of North Battleford, Saskatchewan (Hon. Robert D. Laing, Commissioner) (28 March 2002) at 281.

[56]   *Ibid.*, at 8.

diplomatic terms: "there remains a hiatus between knowing the problem and how to solve it on the one hand, and doing anything about it on the other".[57] In a similar vein, following his assessment of the Walkerton experience, Justice Dennis O'Connor gravely warned "that we may have become victims of our own success, taking for granted our drinking water's safety. The keynote in the future should be vigilance. We should never be complacent about drinking water safety".[58]

In assessing the position of drinking water in the regulatory landscape, Justice Laing drew a distinction between health and environmental matters. "Drinking water is a public health category", he insisted, "separate from the regulatory functions that may be performed by other branches of SERM on other aspects of municipal activity that are more related to the traditional environmental mandate".[59] By way of example, Justice Laing expressed the view that while wastewater regulation falls within the environmental mandate, the production of drinking water does not.[60] Despite this drawing of lines, there is increasing reluctance to exclude drinking water supply from the realm of environmental concerns. Thus, in connection with recommendations designed to forestall the likelihood of reoccurrences of the Walkerton or North Battleford experiences, both commissioners endorsed what has come to be known as the multi-barrier approach to drinking water security, sometimes also described as "source to tap" protection. Beginning with source or watershed protection, such an approach endeavours to ensure that supplies are drawn from high quality and reliable sources. Standard-setting and technological systems, including treatment, distribution and monitoring systems, must then be regularly kept up to date in light of technological advances and evolving understanding of risks to water supply arrangements. Effective financial and administrative structures are needed to maintain operational capability and each of these elements must be appropriately supervised on a province-wide basis by an agency or agencies with suitable authority, including emergency response and enforcement capability.[61]

---

[57]   *Ibid.*, at 281.

[58]   Report of the Walkerton Inquiry (Hon. Dennis R. O'Connor, Commissioner) (14 January 2002), Part I at 8.

[59]   Report of the Commission of Inquiry into matters relating to the safety of the public drinking water in the City of North Battleford, Saskatchewan (Hon. Robert D. Laing, Commissioner) (28 March 2002) at 289.

[60]   *Ibid.*

[61]   Report of the Walkerton Inquiry (Hon. Dennis R. O'Connor, Commissioner) (14 January 2002), Part II at 8-15, 72-78.

(d)   Air Quality Standards and Smog

Members of the medical community have been at the forefront of campaigns to highlight linkages between air quality and public health for many years.[62] Smog has been described as representing "a health crisis" which constitutes "a serious threat to the health of many Canadians".[63] Health Canada research has attributed roughly six per cent of hospital admissions for respiratory illnesses to smog. On an annual basis, as many as 5,000 premature deaths and a billion dollars in health-care expenses can be associated with air pollution.[64] Particular concern in Canada is associated with conditions along the heavily-populated Windsor-to-Québec corridor, throughout British Columbia's lower Fraser Valley, including Vancouver, and in parts of the southern Atlantic region, notably along the Bay of Fundy and the Saint John area. Sixty-one per cent of Canadian respondents to a survey in 1999 indicated that they were "very concerned about air quality" while the following year 89 per cent agreed that pollution was affecting the health of children.[65]

The diverse and often distant origins of the factors contributing to smog, create distinctive policy problems. The ingredients of smog — airborne particulate matter in combination with ground level ozone resulting from the interaction of nitrogen oxides and volatile organic compounds — come from a range of sources. Fossil fuel consumption contributes substantially to the gaseous ingredients while particulates are produced by industrial and mining activity, vehicle emissions and thermal power production. Point sources, mobile sources and so-called area sources such as wood-burning homes, forest fire debris and agricultural operations contribute to smog and to the regulatory challenges it poses.

Environment Canada, provincial environment ministries, or in some cases municipal officials monitor air quality. The accumulated data, when converted to a standardized index and combined with information on

---

[62]   World Health Organization, Air Pollution (Geneva, 1961).

[63]   Report of the Commissioner of the Environment and Sustainable Development (May 2000), Chapter 4, "Smog: Our Health at Risk" at paras. 4.30, 4.31, online: Office of the Auditor General of Canada <http://www.oag-bvg.gc.ca/internet/docs/c004ce.pdf>.

[64]   Debora L. VanNijnatten & W. Henry Lambright, "Canadian Smog Policy in a Continental Context: Looking South for Stringency" in Robert Boardman, ed., Canadian Environmental Policy (Oxford: Oxford University Press, 2002) at 256; for discussion of health impacts, see Smog: Our Health at Risk, ibid., at paras 4.31-4.43. See also OECD, Environmental Performance Reviews: Canada (OECD, 2004) at 133-34. The first national assessment of the costs of illness associated with air pollution has recently been completed: No Breathing Room: National Illness Costs of Air Pollution (Canadian Medical Association, August 2008).

[65]   Canada; Earth Summit 2002 Canadian Secretariat, Sustainable Development: A Canadian Perspective, "Health and Environment", c. 5, at 40, online: <http://www.un.org/jsummit/ html/prep_process/national_reports/canadaenglish_908.pdf>.

current and anticipated weather conditions, forms the basis of graduated public warnings in the form of smog watches, smog advisories or smog alerts. These notify the community, and in particular vulnerable members of the population — young children, the elderly, and anyone with a respiratory ailment — to avoid exposure to increased concentrations of contaminants in the air. Even healthy adults are discouraged from outdoor exercise until conditions improve and the combination of ground level ozone and airborne particulates constituting smog has dissipated.

"The most significant obstacle to taking effective action", according to one recent analysis, "is that air pollution is a regional problem that transcends conventional political boundaries and requires co-operation among many levels of government".[66] There are indications that the easiest gains have already been made while population expansion and increases in levels of energy consumption compound the challenge of further progress. "Tackling the smog problem", it has been argued, "will require an approach that addresses all the pollutants and integrates initiatives on other air problems like climate change, air toxics and acid rain".[67]

Canada's control regime is founded on a set of National Air Quality Objectives. These guidelines for ambient levels of exposure to "indicator" pollutants are set on a non-binding basis by the federal government. Individual provinces then formulate control programs intended to bring local conditions into alignment with those objectives, as adopted (sometimes in the form of enforceable standards) or modified. In endeavouring to promote compliance with their declared objectives, provinces have employed measures ranging from voluntary initiatives to detailed prescriptive intervention.

Federal initiatives on the smog front and inter-governmental proposals emerging from the CCME have progressed in the past 15 years as more refined understanding of the health implications of ground level ozone and exposure to particulates has been achieved. A major milestone was the formulation in 1990 of a management plan for nitrogen oxides and volatile organic compounds. The NOx/VOCs Management Plan consisted of 31 initiatives directed towards emission reductions, 27 remedial initiatives for regions already experiencing severe ozone problems and two dozen research initiatives. Subsequent phases of the

---

[66] Debora L. VanNijnatten & W. Henry Lambright, "Canadian Smog Policy in a Continental Context: Looking South for Stringency" in Robert Boardman, ed., *Canadian Environmental Policy* (Oxford: Oxford University Press, 2002) at 253.

[67] Report of the Commissioner of the Environment and Sustainable Development (May 2000), Chapter 4, "Smog: our Health at Risk" at para. 4.94, online: Office of the Auditor General of Canada <http://www.oag-bvg.gc.ca/internet/docs/c004ce.pdf>.

1990 plan were expected to offer opportunities to refine and renew the overall smog response.

The 1990 NOx/VOCs Management Plan, although a major achievement at the time of its origin, was plagued by limitations in implementation. An evaluation by the federal Commissioner for the Environment and Sustainable Development reported that the failure of the federal and provincial governments to sign formal agreements setting out their respective responsibilities for prevention, remediation and research, and specifying the consequences of non-performance compromised the initiative. "In our opinion, when the proposed federal-provincial agreements failed to materialize by November 1991, the 1990 Plan was destined to fail."[68] Aspects of the overall initiative have continued nevertheless, and have included the 2000 Ozone Annex to the 1991 Canada-U.S. Air Quality Agreement. Steps taken pursuant to the Ozone Annex were intended to bring about emission reductions of nitrogen oxides and volatile organic compounds of 39 and 18 per cent, respectively, of 1990 levels by 2007.[69] This latter arrangement is one indication of the international dimension of environmental protection measures with public health implications.

V. ENVIRONMENTAL LAW AND HUMAN HEALTH

Case studies such as the foregoing brief accounts of mercury pollution, pesticides, drinking water protection and smog could be multiplied many times over. These examples, however, are sufficient to illustrate several aspects of the inter-relationship between environmental quality and human health as well as to introduce basic elements of the surrounding environmental protection regime.

In its concern for the protection of species, natural resources, landscapes, ecosystems and other components of the overall environment, law is often most forceful where documented human health impacts of environmental harm strengthen the resolve of advocates, policy-makers and other participants in the legal process to address public concerns. Even in the case of endangered species where forceful arguments support protection on the basis of intrinsic values or ethical considerations, the possibility that cures for diseases faced by humans could be found in some rare ecosystem is often invoked as re-enforcement.

---

[68] *Ibid.*, at para. 4.176.

[69] Canada, Earth Summit 2000 Canadian Secretariat, *Sustainable Development: A Canadian Perspective*, c. 5.1, "Air", online: <http://www.oag-bvg.gc.ca/internet/docs/c20060900ce.pdf>.

The environmental law framework is comprised of an array of legal instruments. Those discussed here include the processes of civil litigation (tort claims, in particular) and the prosecution of statutory offences; regulatory controls and standard-setting programs, administered through approvals, licensing and inspection procedures, or involving environmental assessment.

(a) Civil Litigation

As the northwestern Ontario experience with mercury pollution illustrated, common law claims such as nuisance, negligence or riparian rights involving the health impacts of environmental contamination may face formidable obstacles from the perspective of procedure, burden of proof, and remedies, not to mention costs. The mercury situation involved the use of the common law to secure compensation after the damage had occurred, but the common law has also been employed in attempts to prevent anticipated health impacts by means of injunction proceedings. Equally, if not more formidable litigation challenges arise.

In a prominent and controversial case, *Palmer v. Nova Scotia Forest Industries*, the court considered an injunction claim brought by rural residents who were concerned about risks to their health associated with the use of certain herbicides (2,4-D and 2,4,5-T) on neighbouring forest lands.[70] The trial judge distilled the legal problem before him down to one question: "Have the plaintiffs offered sufficient proof that there is a serious risk of health and that such serious risk of health will occur if the spraying of the substances here is permitted to take place?"[71] As he put the matter elsewhere in the judgment, "The complete burden of proof, of course, rests upon the plaintiffs throughout for all issues asserted by them."[72] Because the plaintiffs could not establish to the satisfaction of the court that the registered and licensed substances being used in forest management operations posed a probability rather than a mere possibility of risk, they failed.

In a stimulating academic commentary on *Palmer*, Bruce Wildsmith observes: "This translates into saying that *if* the plaintiffs must prove the human health dangers of the chemicals, but the scientists themselves have not agreed or settled this issue in scientific terms, then the plaintiffs lose. Scientific uncertainty results in the benefit of the doubt being given to the

---

[70]   *Palmer v. Nova Scotia Forest Industries*, [1983] N.S.J. No. 534, 2 D.L.R. (4th) 397 (N.S.T.D.).

[71]   *Ibid.*, at 496 D.L.R.

[72]   *Ibid.*, at 495 D.L.R.

chemicals. In a court of law chemicals are presumptively innocent."[73] The Nova Scotia decision illustrates some of the challenges surrounding causation[74] that private litigants face where health concerns arise from environmental contamination.[75] The inter-connections between human health and the environment are often extremely complex. Some impacts are indirect; others direct. Some may be immediate and acute; others chronic, or perhaps only observed in subsequent generations.[76] It is still possible, of course, for common law claims arising from environmental risks to health to be advanced under a claim for public nuisance which was recently said by Canada's Supreme Court to encompass "any activity which unreasonably interferes with the public's interest in questions of health, safety, morality, comfort or convenience".[77] However, the burden of proof, the complexities of causation, and litigation costs may deter prospective complainants from pursuing private claims through the courts.

Measures to strengthen, streamline or otherwise facilitate tort litigation offer some potential to increase the utility of common law claims in the context of health risks arising from environmental conditions. Among the more prominent recent developments, legislative elaboration of principles governing class actions in several provinces appears attractive where significant numbers of people who have experienced health risks or adverse effects as a consequence of exposure to environmental contaminants wish to proceed collectively with litigation that might not be pursued on an individual basis.[78] In determining whether certification of a proposed class action is appropriate, courts seek to balance the efficiency and fairness of litigation having regard to such

---

[73] Bruce Wildsmith, "Of Herbicides and Human Kind: Palmer's Common Law Lessons" (1986) 24 Osgoode Hall L.J. 161 at 177.

[74] Multiple exposure situations involving a mix of substances present even more difficulty in terms of causation and remain extremely challenging for researchers. See Robert L. Dixon & Carlton H. Nadolney, "Problems in Demonstrating Disease Causation Following Multiple Exposure to Toxic or Hazardous Substances" in S. Draggan et al., eds., Environmental Impacts on Human Health (New York: Praeger, 1987) at 117-38.

[75] For a discussion of innovative solutions to causation problems in toxic tort litigation, see Brenda H. Powell, "Cause for Concern: An Overview of Approaches to the Causation Problem in Toxic Tort Litigation" (2000) 9 JELP 227.

[76] For a more comprehensive discussion, see Richard T. DiGiulio & William H. Benson, eds., Inter-connections between Human Health and Ecological Integrity (Society of Environmental Toxicology and Chemistry, 2002) at 52-60.

[77] Ryan v. Victoria (City), [1999] S.C.J. No. 7, [1999] 1 S.C.R. 201 at para. 52 (S.C.C.).

[78] Class action legislation has been enacted in British Columbia, Newfoundland, Ontario, Québec and Saskatchewan. Representative actions pursuant to rules of court offer alternative avenues for groups of individuals to pursue common litigation.

underlying considerations as judicial economy, access to justice and behavioural modification.[79]

Health-related claims attributed to environmental damage, where individualized aspects of the litigation may be substantial in comparison with common elements, have had a mixed record of success in securing approval to proceed on a class action basis.[80] In one such case, *Pearson v. Inco Ltd.*, the trial judge on the certification application elaborated on the complexities that might be anticipated from the involvement of some 20,000 class members to contamination:

> [T]o determine exposure, an individual by individual examination is necessary. Coupled with that ... is the need to know the person's health history, their occupation, their habits in terms of the amount of time they spend in their homes as opposed to outside in their gardens as opposed to other places, their travelling habits, their personal habits (e.g. smokers v. non-smokers), their work or school histories and so on.[81]

A smaller group of plaintiffs whose claims were restricted to more manageable issues associated with the loss of property value were eventually granted certification by the Court of Appeal.[82]

From a doctrinal perspective, efforts to clarify and extend the scope of regulatory negligence also offer potential for aggrieved litigants. Legislation intended to safeguard the environment and its inhabitants, including humans, is typically formulated in permissive terms; it is considered to be enabling rather than mandatory. The "matrix of legislation, political realities and discretionary decision-making" has not proven to be fertile ground for those who seek to establish a governmental duty of care toward those who might suffer in consequence of governmental action or inaction.[83] This is in part a consequence of judicial apprehension about establishing indeterminate liability or creating costly public insurance schemes not otherwise intended. It is also in part a reflection of the importance of preserving governmental authority to exercise judgment where multi-dimensional matters affecting political, social and economic considerations may be involved. Nevertheless, negligent implementation or performance of operational activities, in

---

[79]   *Western Canadian Shopping Centres Inc. v. Dutton*, [2000] S.C.J. No. 63, 2001 SCC 46 (S.C.C.); *Hollick v. Toronto (City)*, [2001] S.C.J. No. 67, [2001] 3 S.C.R 158 (S.C.C.); *Rumley v. British Columbia*, [2001] S.C.J. No. 39, 2001 SCC 69 (S.C.C.).

[80]   *Pearson v. Inco Ltd.*, [2004] O.J. No. 317 (Ont. Div. Ct.); *Comité d environnement de la Baie Inc. c. Societé d'électrolyse et de chimie Alcan Ltée*, [1990] J.Q. no 216 (Qué. C.A.).

[81]   [2002] O.J. No. 2764 at para. 120 (Ont. S.C.J.).

[82]   *Pearson v. Inco Ltd.*, [2005] O.J. No. 4918 (Ont. C.A.), leave to appeal to S.C.C. refused [2006] S.C.C.A. No. 1 (S.C.C.).

[83]   Philip H. Osborne, *The Law of Torts*, 2d ed. (Toronto: Irwin Law, 2003).

contrast with what are considered to be policy or planning matters, can entail liability.[84] Government's responsibilities in this regard relate to a duty to warn where risks are identified and adequacy of the disclosure or notice provided to those who might be affected, as well as to the qualifications of personnel involved in responding to problems that have arisen.[85] Litigation arising from cases of the West Nile virus in Ontario failed to establish the existence of a private law duty towards members of the general population affected by the disease. The surveillance and prevention plan adopted by the province was of a policy nature and accordingly did not entail direct operational obligations.[86]

(b) The Prosecution of Environmental Offences

Federal and provincial environmental legislation sets out a range of offence provisions some of which deal with technical compliance matters such as obligations to provide timely information reports while others are explicitly directed toward the prevention of environmental harm. Adverse human health effects will not necessarily figure in environmental prosecutions although there are many possible linkages. Interference with human use or enjoyment of the environment, including interference involving negative health impacts, may constitute the type of "adverse effect" on which prosecutions rest in some jurisdictions.[87] In other settings the offence of "pollution" may be committed with pollutant defined to include the introduction to the environment of something that "is or is likely to be injurious to the health or safety of persons".[88]

Environmental prosecutions most commonly fall within that category of regulatory offences classified as strict liability in contrast with *mens rea* offences or absolute liability offences. The distinguishing characteristic of strict liability offences is the opportunity available to the defence to avoid conviction by demonstrating the exercise of due diligence. As explained by Dickson J. in the seminal decision establishing strict liability offences:

> While the prosecution must prove beyond a reasonable doubt that the defendant committed the prohibited act, the defendant must only establish on the balance of probabilities that he has a defence of reasonable care ... The defence will be available if the accused reasonably

---

[84]   *Cooper v. Hobart*, [2001] S.C.J. No. 76, [2001] 3 S.C.R. 537 (S.C.C.).

[85]   *Jane Doe v. Metropolitan Toronto (Municipality) Commissioners of Police*, [1998] O.J. No. 2681, 39 O.R. (3d) 487 (Ont. Gen. Div.).

[86]   *Eliopoulos Estate v. Ontario (Minister of Health and Long-Term Care)*, [2006] O.J. No. 4400, 2006 CanLII 37121 (Ont. C.A.), leave to appeal to S.C.C. refused [2006] S.C.C.A. No. 514 (S.C.C.).

[87]   *Environmental Protection Act*, R.S.O. 1990, c. E19, s. 1(1).

[88]   *Environment Act*, C.C.S.M. c. E125, s. 1(2).

believed in a mistaken set of facts which, if true, would render the act or omission innocent, or if he took all reasonable steps to avoid the particular event.[89]

It was on this basis, therefore, that the employer whose unlicensed employee had abandoned dangerous pesticides alongside other waste avoided conviction in the British Columbia decision described above.[90] Nonetheless, given the crucial importance of factual determinations peculiar to each assertion of due diligence, controversy persists about the precise relationship between the wrongful act and measures taken to avoid its occurrence.[91]

In the case of conviction for an environmental offence, sentencing typically takes the form of a monetary fine. Yet the determination of a sentence may be affected by the nature or severity of harm or risk, including human health risk, attributed to the wrongful conduct in question, and, in some circumstances, remedial orders issued by the convicting court may address human health concerns. The *Canadian Environmental Protection Act, 1999* permits a sentencing court to order a convicted offender to make a payment to "environmental, health or other groups to assist in their work in the community where the offence was committed".[92] Under some legislative regimes, where water supplies have experienced contamination an obligation may arise to provide alternative supplies.

(c) Administrative Controls: Standards, Permits and Monitoring

(i) Standard Setting

Individualized assessments of a very wide range of threats or risks to health and the environment have been oriented around the task of identifying acceptable levels of exposure for human populations.[93] In addition to pesticide approvals as noted above, such inquiries are constantly underway in relation to toxic and hazardous substances and other chemicals to which the population may be exposed through the environment or related pathways. Workplace health and safety receive

---

[89] *R. v. Sault Ste. Marie*, [1978] S.C.J. No. 59, [1978] 2 S.C.R. 1299 at paras. 1325-26 (S.C.C.).

[90] *Ibid.*

[91] *R. v. Imperial Oil Ltd.*, [2000] B.C.J. No. 2031, 36 C.E.L.R. (N.S.) 109 (B.C.C.A.); *R. v. Petro-Canada*, [2003] O.J. No. 216, 63 O.R. (3d) 219 (Ont. C.A.).

[92] *Canadian Environmental Protection Act, 1999*, S.C. 1999, c. 33, s. 291(*o*).

[93] For a review of approaches to risk assessment, see Cindy G. Jardine *et al.*, "Risk Management Frameworks for Human Health and Environmental Risks" (2003) 6 Journal of Toxicology and Environmental Health 569 at 720.

particular attention in this regard, for occupational exposure not only affects employees directly, but may represent a pathway of exposure for family members.

Limitations of established approaches to risk assessment and management have been the subject of extensive commentary.[94] Substances that are known to be inherently toxic, persistent and subject to bio-accumulation are considered ill-suited to regulation oriented around acceptable levels of exposure. Observers have also noted the uncertainty involved in extrapolating from animal experiments to humans, or the disregard of cumulative effects from multiple exposures to related chemicals, or the distinctive vulnerabilities of sub-groups within the general population. Concern has also been expressed about significant delays or even failures in re-assessing the impacts of exposure to certain substances in light of advances in research. In some cases (ozone and particulate matter are prominent recent examples), researchers have been unable to identify safe levels of exposure. In this instance, therefore, even if existing objectives were to be achieved, this would not protect health.[95]

In the regulatory context, steps have been taken in some specific circumstances to address the needs of vulnerable populations, Aboriginal communities, for example, or children.[96] The House of Commons Standing Committee on Environment and Sustainable Development recommended principles to be applied in relation to pesticide regulation. The committee emphasized that protection of human and environmental health should be an "absolute priority" and public safety should not be traded off against industrial "needs".[97] It argued further that preventive measures should be taken "where there is reason to believe that a pesticide is likely to cause harm" even without conclusive evidence of causation.[98] The Committee's recommendations were not adopted in full when the PCPA was revised.

The primary objective of the new legislation is specifically stated in the preamble to be "to prevent unacceptable risk to people and the environment from the use of pest control products". In this regard, the

---

[94] Theresa McClenaghan et al., "Environmental Standard Setting and Children's Health in Canada: Injecting Precaution into Risk Assessment" (2003) 12 JELP 245 at 249-59.

[95] Report of the Commissioner of the Environment and Sustainable Development (May 2000), Chapter 4, "Smog: Our Health at Risk" at paras. 4.6 and 4.45, online: Office of the Auditor General of Canada <http://www.oag-bvg.gc.ca/internet/docs/c004ce.pdf>.

[96] Theresa McClenaghan et al., "Environmental Standard Setting and Children's Health in Canada: Injecting Precaution into Risk Assessment" (2003) 12 JELP 245 at 258-59.

[97] Report of the House Standing Committee on Environment and Sustainable Development, Pesticides: Making the Right Choices for the Protection of Health and the Environment (May 2000) c. 8, online: <http://www2.parl.gc.ca/HousePublications/Publication.aspx?DocId=103 1697&Language=E&Mode=1&Parl=36&Ses=2>.

[98] Ibid.

legislation offers an important formulation of acceptability: "... the health or environmental risks of a pest control product are acceptable if there is reasonable certainty that no harm to human health, future generations or the environment will result from exposure to or use of the product, taking into account its conditions or proposed conditions of registration".[99]

The manner in which the evaluation of pest-control products is to be carried out is described at some length. The applicant for registration "has the burden of persuading the Minister that the health and environmental risks and the value of the pest control product are acceptable".[100] The Minister is not restricted to considering information provided by the applicant, but where the Minister takes account of additional information, the applicant must be given a reasonable opportunity to comment on it. The legislation explicitly provides that in evaluating health and environmental risks, the Minister shall "apply a scientifically based approach".[101] Still more guidance is set out in relation to evaluating health risks where the Minister is instructed to "apply appropriate margins of safety".[102]

Water quality is another area where the integrity of standards is of exceptional importance. In Canada, these are under continuous review by an inter-governmental panel charged with formulating *Guidelines for Canadian Drinking Water Quality*. Provinces have thereafter tended to adapt the guidelines to their own circumstances occasionally in the form of regulations.[103]

Wherever cause for concern about a particular substance is established, the nature of an appropriate regulatory response arises. The range of alternatives, much debated in each individual instance, might involve a ban or phase-out of the substance in question, or restricted

---

[99]   *Pest Control Products Act*, S.C. 2002, c. 28, s. 2(2).

[100]   *Ibid.*, s. 7(6)(*a*).

[101]   *Ibid.*, s. 7(7) (*a*).

[102]   As described in the statute, *ibid.*, appropriate margins of safety would "take into account, among other relevant factors, the use of animal experimentation data and the different sensitivities to pest control products of major identifiable subgroups, including pregnant women, infants, children, women and seniors, and in the case of a threshold effect, if the product is proposed for use in or around homes or schools, apply a margin of safety that is ten times greater than the margin of safety that would otherwise be applicable in respect of that threshold effect, to take into account potential pre- and post-natal toxicity and completeness of the data with respect to the exposure of, and toxicity to, infants and children unless, on the basis of reliable scientific data, the Minister has determined that a different margin of safety would be appropriate": *Ibid.*, s. 7(7)(*b*)(ii-iii). See also s. 7(7)(*b*)(i).

[103]   See, for example, *Safe Drinking Water Regulation*, B.C. Reg. 230/92; *Potable Water Regulation — Clean Water Act*, N.B. Reg. 93-203; *Drinking Water Quality Standards Regulation*, Man. Reg. 41/2007; *Ontario Drinking-Water Quality Standards*, O. Reg. 169/03.

and controlled uses. Voluntary measures and preventive initiatives are also possible, along with warnings accompanied by information and monitoring programs.

(ii) Permits, Licences, Approvals and Plans

One regulatory mechanism aimed at controlling adverse environmental impacts is the use of individualized permits embodying detailed terms and conditions. These specify the circumstances in which certain activities may be undertaken or substances used and released into the environment. Such measures might also encompass requirements for the training and qualifications of personnel, or concerning the availability of equipment and supplies, including emergency response equipment. Warning and notification requirements may govern the use and transport of certain substances posing health and environmental risks. Specific conditions governing the disposal of waste and contaminants may also be applicable.

Location decisions respecting activities with potential adverse environmental and health consequences are also now subject to closer scrutiny. For this purpose, in relation to water supply, Ontario has moved to establish source protection committees with planning responsibilities.[104]

(iii) Supervision and Monitoring and Administrative Orders

In the absence of actual experience, standard-setting and licensing processes depend heavily upon an understanding of anticipated impacts that may be derived from modelling, other forms of theoretical projection or inferences drawn from comparable situations. From an environmental and health protection perspective it is therefore vital to ensure that reliable information based on experience is made available to inspectors through monitoring or through reporting requirements. Where environmental officials observe that damage is underway, or where a risk has become apparent, authorization for remedial and preventive administrative orders may be available. Where the continued use of an environmental contaminant poses an immediate threat to human life or health, administrative officials may order that the activity be stopped. The officials responsible for the initial authorization ordinarily retain statutory powers to cancel or amend such authorizations on the basis of additional information that emerges following initial approvals, although it may be difficult as a practical matter to review individual situations systematically.

---

[104] *Source Protection Committees*, O. Reg. 288/07.

In British Columbia, pursuant to its authority under the *Health Act*,[105] the local board of health for the Sunshine Coast Regional District issued an order against certain forestry operations in the Chapman Creek Watershed, which is the source of a public drinking water supply. The board, after following up on citizen complaints, concluded that the logging activity constituted a "health hazard" in so far as it was "a condition or thing that ... is likely to endanger the public health".[106] The decision reflects a growing awareness of how operational practices with adverse environmental effects have potential impacts on community health.

VI. ENVIRONMENTAL ASSESSMENT

The accumulation of relevant operational data, including indications of adverse human health impacts that may be attributable to changing environmental conditions, underpins the capacity of regulatory institutions to adapt as circumstances alter. Environmental assessment procedures which are intended to identify and evaluate potential impacts prior to actual development or policy initiatives being undertaken rely heavily on data and research.

Procedures designed to assess anticipated environmental impacts in the context of proposals for industrial and resource development, or other human activities, offer opportunities to consider the implications of such initiatives for human health. Initiatives most likely to entail health effects include mining and processing projects, energy production, manufacturing where chemicals are involved, natural resource projects, transportation, municipal infrastructure and waste management.[107] In cases such as this where environmental assessment procedures apply, those responsible for undertaking the proposed initiative will be expected to provide information for review. This may include information on potential environmental impacts, alternatives to the project, monitoring and contingency plans, and efforts to minimize the production or release of substances that may have adverse effects on the environment. Alberta legislation specifically provides that the terms of reference developed to

---

[105] *Health Act*, R.S.B.C. 1996, c. 179.
[106] *Western Forest Products Inc. v. Sunshine Coast (Regional District)*, [2007] B.C.J. No. 2204, 2007 BCSC 1508 at para. 19 (B.C.S.C.).
[107] Katherine Davies & Barry Sadler, "Environmental Assessment and Human Health: Perspectives, Approaches and Future Directions: A Background Report for the International Study of the Effectiveness of Environmental Assessment" (Health Canada, May 1997) at 25.

guide an environmental assessment may call for "identification of issues related to human health that should be considered".[108]

Where a proposal under review may entail adverse health consequences, environmental assessment procedures typically call for mitigation measures to alleviate those impacts. There are indications however that substantial scope remains for more effective incorporation of health impacts into environmental assessment, for, according to one estimate, more than 90 per cent of EAs either neglect or deal inadequately with health.[109] There are opportunities not only to minimize adverse effects, but possibly for the purpose of enhancing the beneficial implications of development for health.[110]

Improvements from a health protection perspective have been suggested to virtually all aspects of environmental assessment. Of fundamental importance are improvements to the existing knowledge base. These include defined indicators of health; more extensive baseline information on health and environmental conditions; more refined procedures for assessing effects; and more systematic follow-up monitoring to ensure the effectiveness of mitigation measures.[111] Initiatives along these lines are certainly underway. In relation to indicators, for example, information on respiratory effects, the incidence of cancer, and effects on fertility and development, including congenital anomalies, has been identified for its general relevance to assessment processes.[112]

Legal responses to the environment/health interface are also subject to a further set of considerations derived from the broader context that influences all aspects of the operation of legal instruments and policy development.

VII.   FRAMEWORK CONSIDERATIONS AND INSTITUTIONAL CONTEXT

The specific legal procedures described above operate within a context that encompasses intergovernmental, interdepartmental and

---

[108] Alberta, *Environmental Protection and Enhancement Act*, R.S.A. 2000, c. E-12, s. 47.

[109] Katherine Davies & Barry Sadler, "Environmental Assessment and Human Health: Perspectives, Approaches and Future Directions: A Background Report for the International Study of the Effectiveness of Environmental Assessment" (Health Canada, May 1997) at 17.

[110] *Ibid.*, at 14.

[111] *Ibid.*, at 40.

[112] Health Canada; *Canadian Handbook on Health Impact Assessment, Volume 1: The Basics,* ch. 3, Table 3.1 (Ottawa: Health Canada, 2003), online: <http://www.hc-sc.gc.ca/ewh-semt/alt_formats/hecs-sesc/pdf/pubs/eval/handbook-guide/vol_1/hia-Volume_1.pdf>.

international considerations as well as important and evolving procedural norms. The latter relate to public participation, transparency and accountability, and — most recently — to the precautionary principle. These diverse factors may either constrain or enhance the likelihood that environmental procedures will contribute effectively to the protection of public health in Canada.

(a) The Democratic Context

Fundamental commitments to opportunities for participation in decision-making and, more generally, to openness in government contribute to the legitimacy and acceptability of decisions surrounding environmental impacts on health and will often contribute to the knowledge base on which such decisions are founded.

(i)   Participation

Permits, licences and other forms of regulatory approval are almost by definition initiated by the proponents of new projects or by the developers of products that require some form of official authorization as a precondition of lawful use. While these proceedings have traditionally been treated essentially as matters between the applicant and the official decision-maker (with the latter generally understood to be a representative of the public interest), opportunities do arise for wider forms of public participation.

Under principles of administrative law, those whose interests are affected may be entitled to notice of the hearing and to a fair opportunity to present their views to the tribunal responsible for the decision. Legislative arrangements occasionally also provide appeal mechanisms where further opportunities exist for third parties to make relevant representations. The Alberta *Environmental Protection and Enhancement Act*, for example, allows those "directly affected" by a decision to participate, although that language has been construed narrowly to encompass only "persons having a personal rather than a community interest in the matter".[113]

The Ontario *Environmental Bill of Rights* also affords opportunities for public involvement through a public registry process to provide advance notice of certain upcoming decisions and through avenues of appeal respecting statutory permits and other authorizations. Any person resident in Ontario with an interest in the decision on such instruments

---

[113]   *C.U.P.E. Local 30 v. Alberta (Public Health Advisory and Appeal Board)*, [1996] A.J. No. 48, 34 Admin. L.R. (2d) 172 at 178 (Alta. C.A.).

may seek leave to appeal from the relevant appellate body. Although eligibility is broader than under Alberta's "directly affected" requirement, applicants for leave to appeal face a strict two-part test. Leave to appeal should be granted only where, in light of applicable law and policy, there is good reason to believe that the decision was unreasonable and where it appears that significant environmental harm could result from the decision.[114]

In *Residents Against Company Pollution Inc.*, applications were made for leave to appeal air-emissions and sewage-works approvals issued to Petro Canada. Among the arguments put forward to suggest that the approval had been unreasonably granted, it was urged that ambient air quality testing was being ignored in favour of modelling estimates. On other grounds, generally relating to procedural irregularities, the environmental appeal board concluded that the first part of the test was satisfied. In turning to the second test of significant harm to the environment, the board ruled that the possibility of such harm (in this case associated with SO2 concentrations in a nearby apartment building) was sufficient.

(ii)   The Charter and the Environment

Constitutional protection for the right to "life, liberty and security of the person" under s. 7 of the *Canadian Charter of Rights and Freedoms* has ordinarily been understood to apply to governmental action affecting the interests of specific or identifiable individuals rather than of the public at large or of undefined components of the community.[115] Yet some attempts to explore the possible application of s. 7 protection to the creation of environmental public health risks have been made.[116] For example, where licences, permits or other approvals authorize the use of substances entailing environmental or health risks generally and the possibility or even probability of actual injury to some as yet unidentified members of the public, the government action in question may arguably be sufficient to trigger the safeguards required by fundamental justice. As summarized in the most recent survey of the question: "if a government has chosen to legislate for the purpose of protecting public health (including providing for the issuance of permits, licences, approvals or other authorizations), it must do so in a manner that protects the public's right to life, liberty and security of the person, or ensures that those rights

---

[114]   *Environmental Bill of Rights, 1993*, S.O. 1993, c. 28, s. 41.

[115]   *Operation Dismantle Inc. v. Canada*, [1985] S.C.J. No. 22, [1985] 1 S.C.R. 441 (S.C.C.).

[116]   Martha Jackman, "Cabinet and the Constitution — Participatory Rights and Charter Interests: Manicom v. County of Oxford" (1990) 35 McGill L.J. 943.

are only interfered with in accordance with the principles of fundamental justice".[117]

While fundamental justice may involve substantive elements[118] it is most likely to call for procedural preconditions such as notice and disclosure, participation in a fair hearing and other elements of lawful administrative decision-making. Even if the constitutional threshold of "life, liberty and security of the person" is not established in cases of environmental decision-making involving potential health risks, procedural norms are equally vital.[119]

The federal Commissioner for Environment and Sustainable Development reports a petition calling for the explicit introduction of a substantive right to a healthy environment in the *Charter* along the lines of similar provisions in other jurisdictions.[120]

(iii) Access to Information and Disclosure

The availability of information on environmental quality and conditions provides opportunities for those who may be concerned about potential adverse health impacts to consider preventive measures or to direct public attention towards efforts to eliminate the cause of the problems. Some information is available on the basis of disclosure requirements that apply to the operators of water supply systems, or sources of pollutant discharge, for example, while other data, reports and records may be obtained pursuant to freedom of information legislation.[121] Certain environmental decision-making arrangements contain their own disclosure requirements.[122] Environmental registries advise members of the public and of the NGO community about forthcoming decisions so as

---

[117] Andrew Gage, "Public Health Hazards and Section 7 of the Charter" (2004) 13 JELP 1-46 at 26.

[118] *Reference re Motor Vehicle Act (British Columbia) S. 94(2)*, [1985] S.C.J. No. 73, [1985] 2 S.C.R. 486 (S.C.C.).

[119] For discussion of human rights possibly including a right to a healthy environment, see E. Hughes & D. Iyalomhe, "Substantive Environmental Rights in Canada" (1998-1999) 30 Ottawa L. Rev. 229; Erin Eacott, "A Clean and Healthy Environment: The Barriers and Limitations of this Emerging Human Right" (2001) 10 Dal. J. Leg. Stud. 74.

[120] Report Commissioner of the Environment and Sustainable Development to the House of Commons, *The Commissioner's Perspective — 2006* at 10, 34, online: <http://www.oag-bvg.gc.ca/internet/docs/c20060900ce.pdf>.

[121] For a recent survey of the operation of freedom of information regimes in the environmental context, see Lynda M. Collins *et al.*, "Accessing Environmental Information in Ontario: A Legislative Comment on Ontario's Freedom of Information and Protection of Privacy Act" (2004) 13 JELP 267.

[122] *Canadian Environment Assessment Act*, S.C. 1992, c. 37, s. 55.

to facilitate their involvement in the processes of government.[123] Corporate environmental reporting, often provided in conjunction with health and safety data, represents a further source of relevant information.[124]

Air quality is an area where significant advances have been encouraged through systematic data collection and dissemination. The International Joint Commission's long-standing interest in airborne pollutants affecting the Great Lakes region was echoed and magnified under the auspices of the Commission for Environmental Co-operation into a more comprehensive examination of "continental pollutant pathways". The regular release of CEC data on sources and emissions for dozens of distinct substances allows observers to identify problem polluters at the individual and jurisdictional levels, and thereby also to alert communities at risk. Ontario's smog control record did not stand up well in this comparative light. Canada's largest smog producer tended to rely on voluntary measures to reduce emissions that contribute to the production of ground level ozone. In the context of public criticism and international negotiations, however, the province agreed to introduce regulatory controls on the emission of nitrogen oxides by electricity producers and eventually accepted the need for more stringent measures corresponding to U.S. standards established by the Environmental Protection Agency.[125]

As this experience illustrates, information buttresses public participation as a fundamental pre-condition for holding governments accountable for the effectiveness of environmental protection programmes. With reference to planned efforts to deal with Canada's smog situation on the basis of a ten-year program, the federal Commissioner of the Environment and Sustainable Development observed that transparent information is essential, but was not delivered. Environment Canada failed to produce "meaningful, comprehensive and timely information" concerning the results of national efforts to reduce smog. "The lack of transparent information means that the public and Parliament cannot determine whether Canada is addressing its smog problem at a reasonable pace."[126]

---

[123] *Ontario Environmental Bill of Rights, 1993*, S.O. 1993, c. 28; *Canadian Environmental Protection Act, 1999*, S.C. 1999, c. 33, s. 12.

[124] For discussion, see Commission for Environmental Co-operation, Taking Stock: North American Pollutant Releases and Transfers (Montreal: CEC, 1997), c. 9.

[125] Debora L. VanNijnatten & W. Henry Lambright, "Canadian Smog Policy in a Continental Context" in Robert Boardman & Debora L. VanNijnatten, eds., *Canadian Environmental Policy* (Oxford: Oxford University Press, 2002) at 267.

[126] Report of the Commissioner of the Environment and Sustainable Development (May 2000), Chapter 4, "Smog: Our Health at Risk" at para. 4.13, online: Office of the Auditor General of Canada <http://www.oag-bvg.gc.ca/internet/docs/c004ce.pdf>.

(b) The International Context

Domestic and international settings are interconnected in numerous ways. International law may affect national practice; international institutions may influence national actions and priorities, and trade regimes have important implications for domestic environmental protection measures with health-related implications. In addition, international environmental treaty-making often directly addresses health issues associated with environmental deterioration.

In *Baker*, Canada's ratification of international instruments on children's rights, though not legislatively implemented and therefore not directly applicable in Canadian law, was offered as a reflection of values that might serve to "inform the contextual approach to statutory interpretation and judicial review".[127] A comparable assertion was made in a later case to support the domestic applicability of the precautionary principle which is discussed below.[128]

The International Joint Commission ("IJC") and institutions associated with it in carrying out responsibilities established pursuant to the Great Lakes Water Quality Agreement have a lengthy record of drawing attention to the linkages between human health and the environment. In 1990, the IJC underlined the threat posed by contaminants in the Great Lakes watershed: "When available data on fish, birds, reptiles and small mammals are considered along with this human research", the Commission concluded in reference to a study of the consequences for mothers and infants of consuming Lake Michigan fish, "there is a threat to the health of our children emanating from our exposure to persistent toxic substances, even at very low ambient levels".[129] The IJC has consistently pursued the matter of health effects from environmental contamination, asserting forthrightly that "[w]hat we do to the Great Lakes we do to ourselves and to our children".[130] Consisting of five to seven members from Canada and an equivalent number of counterparts from the United States, the Health Professionals Task Force assists and advises the IJC with respect to public health issues in the context of transboundary environmental health. In particular, the

---

[127] *Baker v. Canada (Minister of Citizenship and Immigration)*, [1999] S.C.J. No. 39, [1999] 2 S.C.R. 817 (S.C.C.); *114957 Canada Ltd. (Spraytech, Société d'arrosage) v. Hudson (Town)*, [2001] S.C.J. No. 42, [2001] 2 S.C.R. 241 at para. 70 (S.C.C.).

[128] *Baker v. Canada (Minister of Citizenship and Immigration)*, [1999] S.C.J. No. 39, [1999] 2 S.C.R. 817 (S.C.C.); *114957 Canada Ltd. (Spraytech, Société d'arrosage) v. Hudson (Town)*, [2001] S.C.J. No. 42, [2001] 2 S.C.R. 241 (S.C.C.). In each case, readers are referred to firm expressions of dissent concerning the distorting impact of this position on the established relationship between executive and legislative authority.

[129] International Joint Commission, Fifth Biennial Report on Great Lakes Water Quality at 15.

[130] IJC, Seventh Report at 4.

task force addresses information exchange, health training and education, and emerging clinical and public health issues in relation to transboundary environmental health.

Following more than a decade of further research, both experimental and epidemiological, carried out by the Agency for Toxic Substances and Disease Registry in the U.S. and in Canada by the Great Lakes Health Effects Program, the IJC more forcefully reported that "a convincing body of scientific research clearly links human health exposure to toxic substances in the Great Lakes to serious injury to health".[131] These findings underpin the IJC's continuing efforts within the context of the Canada-U.S. water quality regime to strengthen regulatory, reporting and other measures to alert and protect citizens on both sides of the border about adverse health risks. "Solid studies substantiate harm to both mental and reproductive functions in fetuses and adults ... We strongly urge actions to stop the cycling of contaminants from sediment to people, fish, and wildlife, and to end known injury to ecosystem health."[132] The IJC's authoritative interventions are among the most influential voices pointing to the long-term health consequences of environmental neglect.

International dimensions of the inter-relationship between environmental law and health might also include Canada's active participation in the Stockholm Convention on Persistent Organic Pollutants, an initiative strongly encouraged by evidence of the adverse effects of certain chemicals on the Aboriginal population of northern Canada. Canada has been involved in the development of international treaties dealing with the transportation of hazardous waste and biotechnology where questions of public health have also been addressed.[133]   In addition, domestic measures to achieve national greenhouse gas reduction commitments under the Kyoto Protocol to the United Nations Framework Convention on Climate Change may also offer health-related benefits. As the National Round Table on the Environment and the Economy has observed, "climate change policies focused on improved energy efficiency also will lower air pollutants associated with producing energy, thereby improving local air quality".[134] Revised International Health Regulations adopted in 2005 represent a further

---

[131]   IJC, Eleventh Biennial Report on Great Lakes Water Quality at 14.

[132]   IJC, 11th Biennial Report at vi.

[133]   For an overview of these and related agreements, see David Hunter *et al.*, *International Environmental Law and Policy* (New York, Foundation Press, 2002).

[134]   National Round Table on the Environment and the Economy, *Getting to 2050: Canada's Transition to a Low-emission Future* (Ottawa, 2008), at 35 online: <http://www.nrtee-trnee.ca/eng/publications/getting-to-2050/Getting-to-2050-low-res-eng.pdf>.

example of possible integration between health protection and environmental law.[135]

In an era of increasingly extensive international trade and of economic integration, the trade/environment relationship also figures in the calculation. In a series of closely watched and often controversial decisions, trade panels and supervising appellate bodies have considered the interaction between domestic regulations promulgated in the interests of environmental protection and public health and principles designed to promote the free flow of goods and services across international borders. The dynamic arises because of certain exceptions to provisions generally intended to eliminate impediments to international trade pursuant to the regime governed by the World Trade Organization ("WTO") with reference to principles of the General Agreement on Tariffs and Trade ("GATT"). Of immediate relevance here is the possibility provided for in Article XX (b) of the GATT that a country's "measures ... necessary to protect human, animal or plant life or health" might be successfully defended against assertions by a trading partner that the measures in question operate to restrict trade unlawfully.

The potential for health protection measures to survive trade-based challenges has varied along with the interpretation of "to protect human life or health", "necessary" and other elements of the exception provisions in trade agreements.[136] By way of example, when Canada, an exporter of asbestos or products containing asbestos, challenged a French decree affecting such material, several related issues arose during the course of the trade dispute resolution process. Canada asserted that a French prohibition against asbestos could not be considered "necessary" given that controlled use of asbestos was a "reasonably available" alternative. In the view of the World Trade Organization Appellate Body, however, WTO members enjoyed an undisputed "right to determine the level of protection of health that they consider appropriate in a given situation".[137] This was a conclusion of singular importance. France, having chosen to halt the spread of asbestos-related health risks, "could not reasonably be expected to employ any alternative measure if that measure would involve

---

[135]   The new International Health Regulations, put forward by the World Health Organization and in force as of 15 June 2007, address "public health emergencies of international concern", associated with microbiological, chemical and other risks to human health. Examples of situations encompassed within the intended scope of coverage are events "caused by an environmental contamination that has the potential to spread across international borders" at 45, online: <http://www.who.int/csr/ihr/IRH_2005_en.pdf>.

[136]   Measures provisionally justified as necessary to protect human life or health are subject to further scrutiny related to the possibility that they might nevertheless constitute "arbitrary or unjustifiable discrimination" among other factors.

[137]   *European Communities — Measures Affecting Asbestos and Asbestos-Containing Products*, WT/DS135/AB/R, 12 March 2001.

a continuation of the very risk that the Decree seeks to halt".[138] Canada had, in fact, also challenged France's assertion that the prohibition on asbestos was a measure "to protect human ... life or health". Neither the initial panel nor the appellate tribunal were prepared to accept the Canadian position.

(c)   The Institutional Context

(i)   *Intergovernmental Relations*

With constitutional authority for both environmental protection and health divided between Canada's federal and provincial governments, considerable potential exists for overlap, conflict and uncertainty. As the smog experience reveals, where responsibilities are shared, opportunities to ensure accountability may be blunted or lost.

Some degree of co-ordination is achieved on the basis of harmonization agreements and similar accords developed under the auspices of the CCME.[139] The CCME has identified the linkages between environment and health as a subject for ongoing attention, notably through the work of the federal-provincial-territorial Committee on Health and Environment.

Questions may also be raised within the framework of provincial operations as to whether governments with authority are exercising it appropriately in circumstances where substantial elements of operational responsibility are assigned to municipal governments. This particular issue engaged the attention of Justice Laing during his investigation of contamination of North Battleford's water system. Justice Laing was interested to know whether Saskatchewan could fulfill its constitutional obligations concerning public health and water quality "by devolving onto the municipalities all responsibility to produce safe drinking water, without also providing a regulatory framework which gives some assurance to the public that the municipalities will carry out the devolved responsibility in a manner that will in fact provide safe drinking water".[140] He suggested, in light of available commentary on the question, that "the answer is a very strong 'no'".[141] Municipalities face significant challenges from changes at the operational level, changes in elected officials, changes in technology and in industry. It was thus, "simply too much to expect that

---

[138]   *Ibid.*

[139]   Canada-wide Accord on Environmental Harmonization (January 1998) is one example.

[140]   Report of the Commission of Inquiry into matters relating to the safety of the public drinking water in the City of North Battleford, Saskatchewan (Hon. Robert D. Laing, Commissioner) (28 March 2002) at 282.

[141]   *Ibid.*

every little municipality is going to manage its way through all of these changes without some form of effective supervision from senior government".[142]

(ii) Departmental Responsibilities and Interdepartmental Relations

The aims and objectives specifically assigned to Manitoba's department of the environment include responsibility "to protect the quality of the environment and environmental health of present and future generations of Manitobans ...".[143] What might be involved in exercising a mandate of such scope was outlined in Saskatchewan's North Battleford inquiry where Justice Laing reviewed the essential elements of a drinking water quality regime: a clear mandate, and an effective organization. Elements of the regulatory mandate would include source water protection; standard-setting and regulations for the design, construction and operation of water treatment facilities; a licence or permit system; and a suitable program for compliance and enforcement. On the organizational side, Justice Laing identified requirements for legislative jurisdiction; for technical and policy capability; adequate staffing; and sufficient funding.[144]

At the national level, Health Canada participates actively with Environment Canada on a number of files where environmental quality and health protection intersect. Within Health Canada, environmental matters are addressed in the context of programs and bureaus administered by various branches of the department. Chief amongst these is the Healthy Environment and Consumer Safety Branch ("HECS") with responsibility — along with tobacco, product and workplace safety issues — for such programs as "Safe Environments" and "Sustainable Development". Specific initiatives within the "Safe Environments" program are directed towards radiation exposure and other environmental contaminants. In connection with the latter, Health Canada, in collaboration with Environment Canada and provincial and territorial counterparts, is engaged in assessing human health hazards attributable to airborne pollutants and in assessing risks associated with substances regulated under CEPA, 1999. The Water, Air and Climate Change Bureau, also within HECS, works in collaboration with provincial and territorial officials on such matters as the evaluation of drinking water contaminants

---

[142]   Ibid.

[143]   Manitoba, Environment Act, C.C.S.M. c. E125, s. 2(1). It is also noteworthy that one of the goals of Manitoba's Ministry of Water Stewardship is to ensure that Manitobans have safe drinking water and are protected from water- and fish-related health threats.

[144]   Report of the Commission of Inquiry into matters relating to the safety of the public drinking water in the City of North Battleford, Saskatchewan (Hon. Robert D. Laing, Commissioner) (28 March 2002) at 283.

and the development of *Guidelines for Canadian Drinking Water Quality*. An office of Risk, Impact Assessment is responsible for Health Canada's participation in proceedings under the *Canadian Environmental Assessment Act*. Other branches of Health Canada where environmental considerations figure prominently include the PMRA and the First Nations and Inuit Health Branch.

The need for interdepartmental collaboration inevitably arises, for environmental health protection efforts more typically than not require participation by numerous agencies. At the federal level, the breadth of interdepartmental collaboration is illustrated in the smog file through the involvement alongside Health and Environment of Transport Canada, Agriculture Canada and Natural Resources Canada.

Although interdepartmental co-operation might be considered a basic element of effective governance, and thus hardly remarkable, some statutory schemes have, out of an abundance of caution one might hope, specified such duties. In Alberta, for example, the Minister of Environment "shall, in recognition of the integral relationship between human health and the environment, co-operate with and assist the Minister of Health and Wellness in promoting human health through environmental protection".[145] It would be disheartening indeed to imagine that in the absence of a similar statutory exhortation, there is no expectation of co-operation between health and environment departments. Tensions between departmental agendas are sufficiently common, however, especially when health and environment issues intersect with natural resource development and the economy that an effort to underline common purposes is not entirely unwelcome.

(d) The Scientific Context and Precaution

Among the most significant recent developments in the context within which health-related environmental decisions are made, endorsement of the precautionary principle or approach to decision-making must surely be front-ranked. The concept came to prominence in the aftermath of the 1992 Rio Declaration on Environment and Development where one formulation of precaution appears: "Where there are threats of serious or irreversible damage, lack of full scientific certainty shall not be used as a reason for postponing cost-effective measures to prevent environmental degradation."[146] Although its formulation has since varied, certain essential aspects of the precautionary

---

[145] Alberta *Environmental Protection and Enhancement Act*, R.S.A. 2000, c. E-12, s. 11; see also New Brunswick *Clean Air Act*, S.N.B. 1997, c. C-5.2, s. 8(2)(a).
[146] Declaration of the UN Conference on Environment and Development, Rio de Janiero, 3-14 June 1992, Principle 15.

principle and the principle's relationship to health and environment have been more elaborately described, as the following account from a recent report by the Royal Society of Canada indicates:

> The Precautionary Principle is a rule about handling uncertainty in the assessment and management of risk, and the rule recommends that the uncertainty be handled in favour of certain values — health and environmental safety — over others. Uncertainty in science produces the possibility of error in the prediction of risks and benefits. The Precautionary Principle makes the assumption that if our best predictions turn out to be in error it is better to err on the side of safety. That is to say, all other things being equal, it is better to have forgone important benefits of a technology by wrongly predicting risks of harm to health or the environment than to have experienced those serious harms by wrongly failing to predict them.[147]

Encouraged by some indications of international support for the precautionary principle, the Supreme Court of Canada in *Spraytech v. Hudson* entertained the concept to buttress its conclusions on the validity of measures taken at the local level to regulate the use of pesticides for cosmetic purposes.[148]

The precautionary principle now appears in several pieces of Canadian federal legislation, including *CEPA, 1999*, where it appears in the preamble in this form: "where there are threats of serious or irreversible damage, lack of full scientific certainty shall not be used as a reason for postponing cost-effective measures to prevent environmental degradation". The significance of the precautionary principle's location in the preamble of *CEPA, 1999*, as explained by Marcia Valiante, is that: "if a regulation adopted in conformity with it is challenged, it could assist a tribunal or court in interpreting the specific operative sections of the Act".[149]

Difficulties arise, however, because "there is no guidance in the statute as to how much and what kinds of scientific evidence could justify a shift to a lesser standard" and because of the decision to refer to "cost-effective" measures.[150] These factors contribute to unpredictability, "making it difficult for the government to withstand a legal challenge to a

---

[147] Royal Society of Canada, Elements of Precaution: Recommendations for the Regulation of Food Biotechnology in Canada (Ottawa, January 2001) at 198.

[148] *114957 Canada Ltée (Spraytech, Société d'arrosage) v. Hudson (Town)*, [2001] S.C.J. No. 42, 2001 SCC 40 (S.C.C.).

[149] Marcia Valiante, "Legal Foundations of Canadian Environmental Policy" in Debora L. VanNijnatten and Robert Boardman, eds., *Canadian Environmental Policy: Context and Cases*, 2d ed. (Oxford: Oxford University Press Canada, 2002) at 13.

[150] *Ibid.*

regulation based on this provision".[151] In Valiante's view, "[g]overnments thus far have not regulated when the science was quite uncertain and this provision is unlikely to encourage them to do so".[152]

Precaution now also appears in the revised *PCPA* where it is specifically applicable to re-evaluations of certain pesticides. The Minister is authorized to suspend registration without completing the re-evaluation process where, "in the course of a re-evaluation or special review, the Minister has reasonable grounds to believe that the cancellation or amendment is necessary to deal with a situation that endangers human health or safety or the environment, taking into account the precautionary principle".[153] This provision provides one example of a legislature's resolution of the issue of the appropriate relationship or proportionality between risks to human health and measures that could be taken to prevent or avoid such possible injury.

The question of proportionality is one of several considerations that have been analyzed by federal policy-makers in their ongoing exploration of the implications of implementing precaution.[154] A Privy Council Office paper setting out a framework for the application of precaution in science-based decision-making about risk described aspects of the proportionality principle. The paper suggests that the role of precaution in responding to uncertainty must ultimately be gauged in light of scientific evidence and social acceptance of risk, alongside economic and international considerations.[155] This multi-dimensional view of the application of

[151]   *Ibid.*

[152]   *Ibid.* Where Ministers of Health and Environment are considering toxic substance assessments, they are instructed to apply a "weight of evidence" approach and the precautionary principle: *Canadian Environmental Protection Act, 1999*, S.C. 1999, c. 33, s. 76.1.

[153]   *Pest Control Products Act*, S.C. 2002, c. 28, s. 20(1)(*b*).

[154]   Environment Canada, *A Canadian Perspective on the Precautionary Approach/Principle* (Discussion Document, September 2001), online: <http://www.ec.gc.ca/econom/discussion_e.htm>.

[155]   Canada, Privy Council Office, *A Framework for the Application of Precaution in Science-Based Decision Making About Risk* (2003), online: <http://www.pco-bcp.gc.ca/docs/information/publications/precaution/precaution_e.pdf>. See esp. (at 11): "There is an implicit need to identify, where possible, both the level of society's tolerance for risks and potential risk-mitigating measures. This information should be the basis for deciding whether measures are proportional to the severity of the risk being addressed and whether the measures achieve the level of protection, recognizing that this level of protection may evolve. While judgments should be based on scientific evidence to the fullest extent, decision makers should also consider other factors such as societal values and willingness to accept risk and economic and international considerations. This would allow for a clearer assessment of the proportionality of the measure and ultimately help maintain credibility in the application of precaution. Generally, the assessment of whether measures are considered proportional to the severity of risk should be in relation to the magnitude and nature of potential harm in a particular circumstance, not in comparison with measures taken in other contexts."

precaution is a further indication that participatory and democratic norms should continue to figure prominently in the legal framework for safeguarding the health and environment interests of Canadians.

The multi-faceted complexity of applying the precautionary principle in the context of a particular decision is very effectively explored in a thoughtful paper on Toronto's response to the West Nile Virus. As Dayna Scott observes, "in the case of the WNV, on the surface at least, the precautionary principle seemed to point *two ways*, taking precaution with respect to public health would lead to a widespread aerial spraying campaign using chemical pesticides; taking precaution with respect to the environment would preclude that action".[156]

VIII. CONCLUSION

Although understanding of the relationships between environment and human health has evolved, and new issues continue to arise, environmental conditions are fundamental to human well-being. Environmental disruption such as climate change and the degradation of air quality and water supplies have wide-ranging health impacts which the legal system has had some capacity to influence or mitigate. Arrangements to provide compensation or to penalize those responsible for environmental harms represent one aspect, largely responsive, of legal measures, while environmental assessment and other regulatory techniques, now buttressed perhaps by an emerging endorsement of precaution offer some possibility that environmental harms and consequent injury to human health may be prevented. In Canada, all of these initiatives associated with the health-related implications of environmental quality frequently require both interdepartmental and intergovernmental co-ordination, and are often connected to developments on the international front as well.

---

[156] Dayna N. Scott, "When Precaution Points Two Ways: Confronting West Nile Fever" (2005) 20 C.J.L.S. 27 at 28.

12

FOODBORNE ILLNESS AND PUBLIC HEALTH

Ronald L. Doering[*]

I.   INTRODUCTION

The remarkable success in controlling many foodborne diseases must be considered as one of the great achievements of public health in the 20th century. Due largely to public health laws, food safety regulatory agencies have almost eradicated human disease and deaths from, for example, scarlet fever, bovine tuberculosis, brucellosis and botulism from commercial food products. However, several recent factors such as increases in world food trade, new emerging pathogens, the role of food processing operations, and the aging population have combined to create major new challenges and food safety is once again a significant public health issue in Canada today.

There are more than 250 different types of bacteria, parasites, viruses and toxins that are known to cause foodborne illness (commonly known as food poisoning) and it is now the largest class of emerging infectious diseases in Canada. There is growing evidence that pathogenic Escherichia coli ("E. coli"), especially the 0157:H7 strain, is becoming more common as a source of foodborne illness from a wide range of food products. Multidrug-resistant salmonellae are causing growing concern about reduced treatment options for severe human cases. New foodborne pathogens are emerging at an alarming rate. We are now aware of more than five times the number of foodborne pathogens than were identified 60 years ago. Many of these pathogens can be deadly, especially for people at highest risk — pregnant women, children, the elderly and the

*   Partner, Gowling Lafleur Henderson LLP, Ottawa.

immuno-compromised. The size of the vulnerable population is growing, with aging baby boomers and increased longevity.

This chapter begins with an overview of the incidence of foodborne illness in Canada, which provides stark evidence of the magnitude of this public health problem. Next, the chapter identifies the jurisdictional basis for food safety regulation in Canada and highlights the role of federal, provincial/territorial, and local levels of government. The chapter then addresses the specific topic of food safety investigation and recall and discusses the roles of various actors in those critical functions. The chapter concludes with analysis of several current challenges confronting food safety regulation in Canada: the ability to trace food items from origin to consumption; the problematic reality of fragmented jurisdiction over food safety in Canada; the dilemma of risk perception, analysis and management in the context of food; and international trade issues.

II.   INCIDENCE OF FOODBORNE ILLNESS

Surprisingly, it is not possible to be very precise about the incidence of foodborne illness in Canada. The most common symptoms include stomach cramps, nausea, vomiting, diarrhea and fever, and because these symptoms resemble the stomach flu, most cases of foodborne illness go unreported. Only the serious cases or large outbreaks of illness are investigated.

To be included in Canada's national statistics, a person must be infected, become ill, consult a doctor and be sent for tests. A lab test must identify the illness-causing bacterium, recognize it as foodborne and report it to the local health department, which, in turn, must report it. Any break in the chain will cause the case to be described as estimated rather than confirmed. Estimates among epidemiologists vary widely on the percentage of actual cases that are reported, but there is a clear consensus that foodborne illness is under-reported around the world. Surveys in a few countries indicate that foodborne diseases may be 300 to 350 times more frequent than the reported cases suggest. While the global incidence of foodborne disease is difficult to estimate, the World Health Organization ("WHO") reports "that in 2005 alone 1.8 million people died from diarrhoeal diseases. A great proportion of these cases can be attributed to contamination of food and drinking water".[1]

In industrialized nations, reports suggest that up to 30 per cent of the population may experience foodborne illness each year.[2] In the United

---

[1]   World Health Organization, "Food Safety and Foodborne Illness", Fact Sheet No. 237 (2007), online: <http://www.who.int/mediacentre/factsheets/fs237/en/>.

[2]   Ibid.

States, for example, annual cases are estimated to be more than 75 million, resulting in 325,000 hospitalizations and 5,000 deaths.[3] In the U.S., known foodborne pathogens account for 14 million of the illnesses, 60,000 hospitalizations and 1,800 deaths. In other words, unknown agents account for approximately 81 per cent of foodborne illness and hospitalizations and 64 per cent of deaths. Three pathogens, salmonella, listeria and toxoplasma, kill 1,500 each year, more than 75 per cent of those killed by known pathogens. Campylobacter, salmonella and shigella top the list in known causes of illness. This study also demonstrates that food-related illnesses are on a huge increase overall in the United States, although it could be that improved surveillance and reporting account for much of this increase. Allard has identified several factors that have contributed to the significant increase in foodborne illness and predicts that increases will continue.[4]

According to Health Canada estimates, "there are as many as 13 million cases of foodborne illness each year in Canada. A majority of these cases can be attributed to microbial foodborne illness and traced back to poor food handling practices in the home. Currently, foodborne illness is estimated to cost Canadians up to 3.8 billion dollars each year to the health care system alone".[5] In the United States, annual costs of health care and lost productivity related to foodborne illness are pegged at USD $35 billion.[6]

Although most people recover, foodborne illnesses can result in chronic health problems in some cases. Illnesses such as chronic arthritis and hemolytic uremic syndrome, which can lead to kidney failure, have long-term consequences for the individual affected and for society and the economy. And, of course, certain zoonotic diseases can lead to death, as in the case of bovine spongiform encephalopathy (BSE or "mad cow" disease) being responsible for more than 100 deaths in the United Kingdom so far.

The science of foodborne illness is often remarkably uncertain. Perhaps because it is so under-reported and, in the past, rarely fatal, there are huge knowledge gaps on almost all the foodborne pathogens. Food

---

[3]   P.S. Mead *et al.*, "Food-Related Illness and Death in the United States" (1999) 5(5) Emerging Infectious Diseases 607.

[4]   Denis G. Allard, "The 'Farm to Plate' Approach to Food Safety — Everyone's Business" (2002) 13:3 Canadian Journal of Infectious Diseases 185. Some of the factors Allard identifies include increasing global travel, growing consumption of imported food products, global warming and microbial evolution.

[5]   Canada, News Release, "Government of Canada Supports Launch of *Be Food Safe* Program to Educate Consumers About Safe Food Handling Practices" (3 June 2008), online: <http://www.healthycanadians.ca/media/2008-06-03_e.html>.

[6]   World Health Organization, "Food Safety and Foodborne Illness", Fact Sheet No. 237 (2007), online: <http://www.who.int/mediacentre/factsheets/fs237/en/>.

safety regulators are regularly confronted with managing outbreaks in the face of very uncertain science. Dr. John Frank, scientific director with the Canadian Institutes of Health Research, reportedly observed that most health research is "pretty useless" for solving real health problems.[7] Nowhere is this more evident than in the absence of adequate research on foodborne illness. Useful research on the causes and management of foodborne illness is urgently required.

III. JURISDICTIONAL BASIS FOR FOOD SAFETY REGULATION IN CANADA

Canada's food inspection system operates in a complex jurisdictional context involving federal, provincial/territorial and municipal authorities. Under the provisions of Canada's Constitution, all levels of government have enacted food safety and quality legislation to achieve their respective policy objectives. Fragmentation exists both across and within levels of government. Historically, enforcement of 13 federal statutes and seventy provincial statutes has been divided among agriculture, health, fisheries, environment and natural resource departments.

Federal jurisdiction to enact food inspection legislation is derived primarily from two constitutional provisions. Section 91(2) of the *Constitution Act, 1867*[8] confers on Parliament the power to make laws in relation to the regulation of "trade and commerce", which has come to mean both inter-provincial or international trade and commerce, and "general" trade and commerce. This broad federal power has to be accommodated with s. 92(13), which confers on provincial legislatures the exclusive power over "property and civil rights", which has come to mean intra-provincial trade and commerce.

The other main area of federal jurisdiction comes under s. 91(27), which gives the federal government power over "criminal law". Food, drug and labelling legislation that makes illegal the manufacture or sale of dangerous, adulterated or misbranded products, is within the scope of criminal law and is not restricted to interprovincial or international activity. At the same time, provincial legislatures have enacted health legislation under their authority over matters of a "local or private" nature.[9] This has resulted in provincial food safety legislation focused primarily on local food processing, food retail and food service.

---

[7]   Francine Kopun, "Medical researchers told to get relevant" *National Post* (11 November 2004) A22.

[8]   *Constitution Act, 1867* (U.K.), 30 & 31 Vict., c. 3, reprinted in R.S.C. 1985, App. II, No. 5.

[9]   See *ibid.*, s. 92(16).

Enforcement is sometimes carried out by the provinces but this is increasingly left to be done at the municipal health agency level.

On April 1, 1997, Canada consolidated all federal food inspection and related activities along the food chain into one new agency, the Canadian Food Inspection Agency ("CFIA"). The CFIA carries out inspection, enforcement and compliance activities that were formerly carried out by four federal departments: Health Canada, Agriculture and Agri-Food Canada, Fisheries and Oceans, and Industry Canada. The CFIA enforces 13 federal statutes (and 34 sets of regulations), including the main federal food laws such as the *Food and Drugs Act,*[10] the *Meat Inspection Act,*[11] the *Fish Inspection Act,*[12] and the *Canada Agriculture Products Act.*[13]

Underlying the food inspection system are the agricultural inputs, feeds, seeds and fertilizers, as well as plants and animals that are included in the 13 acts for which the CFIA is responsible. Federal legislative authority for these lies in the agricultural power in s. 95 of the *Constitution Act, 1867.*[14] While under s. 95, parallel legislative authority in relation to agriculture is granted to both the federal and provincial governments, nonetheless provincial legislation is only effective as long as it is not repugnant to any federal legislation. With the 1990 amendment to the *Health of Animals Act*[15] with respect to animal diseases transmissible to humans, that statute has, as a further constitutional basis, the criminal law power for the protection of the public.

Provincial governments have also enacted legislation relating to food safety. For instance, the *Food Safety and Quality Act, 2001*[16] is enabling legislation in Ontario that is designed to implement food safety inspection programs and enhances the provincial government's capacity to maintain high standards of food safety. Under the Act, improved enforcement actions and timely and effective responses to a food safety

---

[10]   R.S.C. 1985, c. F-27.

[11]   R.S.C. 1985, c. 25 (1st Supp.).

[12]   R.S.C. 1985, c. F-12.

[13]   R.S.C. 1985, c. 20 (4th Supp.).

[14]   *Constitution Act, 1867* (U.K.), 30 & 31 Vict., c. 3, reprinted in R.S.C. 1985, App. II, No. 5. Section 95 states:

> In each Province the Legislature may make Laws in relation to Agriculture in the Province ... and it is hereby declared that the Parliament of Canada may from Time to Time make Laws in relation to Agriculture in all or any of the Provinces ... and any Law of the Legislature of a Province relative to Agriculture ... shall have effect in and for the Province as long and as far only as it is not repugnant to any Act of the Parliament of Canada.

[15]   S.C. 1990, c. 21.

[16]   S.O. 2001, c. 20.

crisis — including the ability to trace back to find the source of a contaminated food as well as determine where it has been distributed — have been set forth. Through the implementation of this legislation, the provincial government aims to improve consumer protection from foodborne hazards and to increase the marketability of Ontario food products.

At times, the modernization of food safety legislation can create controversy between government and industry stakeholders. In 2004, the Province of British Columbia enacted a new *Meat Inspection Regulation*[17] under the *Food Safety Act*[18] requiring that by September 2007, all slaughterhouses producing meat for human consumption be provincially or federally licensed. The Regulation aims at improving British Columbia's food safety by creating a consistent province-wide standard for inspecting meat sold to the public. Pursuant to the Regulation, unlicensed facilities in many regions of the province require upgrading to meet the new standards. The implementation of the Regulation has not been embraced by industry workers, as small- and medium-scale producers have struggled to meet the new licensing requirements. In an attempt to mitigate the problem, the provincial government has had to provide financial support to help stakeholders meet the new standards. Nonetheless, these difficulties in compliance have been blamed for reducing the slaughter capacity of the region.

Municipalities derive regulatory authority from provincial legislation and partial funding from provincial ministries. Municipal governments also enact and enforce by-laws that affect food inspection. While the practice varies from province to province, generally speaking, local health units/authorities provide inspection services in food retail and food service establishments as well as institutions such as hospitals, nursing homes, community kitchens and food banks.

Legislative power may not be delegated from one level of government to the other: federal Parliament cannot delegate power to a provincial legislature, and vice versa. Therefore, government officials attempting to work in an area of shared jurisdiction, such as food inspection, are confronted daily with a profound challenge. Even where it might be convenient and desirable to do so, it is not possible to exchange jurisdictional responsibilities. Partnership and collaboration — working together — is the only option.

---

[17]   B.C. Reg. 349/2004.
[18]   S.B.C. 2002, c. 28.

IV. FOOD SAFETY INVESTIGATION AND RECALL

The most visible exercise of public law in food safety is the food safety recall. Hundreds of these are managed every year with the larger ones gaining front-page attention. Both the law and practice in this area is quite complex. While some mostly voluntary recalls are carried out under a variety of statutes and by-laws by provinces and municipalities, most food safety recalls are carried out by the CFIA, with assistance from Health Canada.

The CFIA has wide powers under its various Acts to investigate, search, seize and detain food products that violate legislative requirements. For example, under the *Meat Inspection Act*, an inspector has full authority to enter any place or stop and enter any vehicle and may open any package that contains a meat product that the inspector believes does not comply with the statute or the regulations. The inspector may take samples and require full production of all administrative material. It is a criminal offence to obstruct inspectors in their work, including making false statements. Similarly, inspectors may seize and detain any product they believe, on reasonable grounds, may contravene any regulation and, in certain circumstances, detained products can be forfeited.[19] The CFIA has equally broad powers in relation to imported meat products. For example, an inspector may seize an imported product and require the importer to remove it from Canada.[20] Similar wording exists in many of the other 13 statutes and 34 sets of regulations for which the CFIA has responsibility, including the *Food and Drugs Act*, the *Fish Inspection Act* and the *Canada Agricultural Products Act*.

Since its creation in 1997, the CFIA has exercised its investigative and enforcement powers in the management of several thousand investigations that ultimately culminated in 1,509 public recalls in its first five years.[21] All but three of these were voluntary; while the CFIA may have exercised various investigative powers, once a product recall was considered necessary, the company involved voluntarily removed the product from sale and either the company, the CFIA, or both, issued public notice of the recall.

While recalls are typically voluntary, the CFIA has broad authority in s. 19 of the *Canadian Food Inspection Agency Act*[22] ("*CFIA Act*") to order mandatory recalls. Under this provision, the CFIA Minister has the power to order recall of food products where he or she is of the view that

---

[19] *Meat Inspection Act*, R.S.C. 1985, c. 25 (1st Supp.), ss. 13-17.

[20] *Ibid.*, s. 18.

[21] Ronald L. Doering, "Ready for a Recall" (2002) 62:9 Food in Canada: The Voice of the Canadian Food & Beverage Industry.

[22] S.C. 1997, c. 6.

the product poses a risk to public, animal or plant health.[23] Non-compliance is punishable by fine or imprisonment. Coupled with the authority in s. 18 to apply for an interim injunction to prevent contravention of the *CFIA Act*, the CFIA has very broad powers to order recalls and to ensure control over unsafe products. This mandatory power is rarely exercised, and in the very few cases in which it was necessary to resort to s. 19, one case involved a manufacturer that could not be located and, in others, the manufacturer refused to recall the product voluntarily. Despite its uncommon use, mandatory recall power adds to the Agency's capacity to work with industry prior to any outbreak and to achieve voluntary recalls of unsafe food products.[24]

With the creation of the CFIA, Health Canada gave up all activities relating to carrying out food safety recalls but it still plays an important role as it retains responsibility for establishing health, safety and nutritional standards for food and for assessing the CFIA's food safety activities. Health Canada's Food Directorate conducts and co-ordinates research activities and provides health risk assessments associated with physical, biological and chemical hazards to the CFIA.

The Public Health Agency of Canada, established in 2004, also has a role to play as it takes on functions previously carried out by the Population and Public Health Branch ("PPHB") of Health Canada. PPHB was responsible for the co-ordination of investigations into human illness outbreaks occurring in multiple provinces and territories. PPHB also maintained links with the CFIA during the course of investigations and advised CFIA upon confirmation of the epidemiological risk of an outbreak with a food product.

The Bureau of Veterinary Drugs at Health Canada has also played a significant role in carrying out risk analysis when the food safety problem has related to the presence of an unapproved veterinary drug residue. A key example is the extensive recall of honey imported from China in spring 2002 because of contamination with chloramphenical, a veterinary antibiotic. Chloramphenical was a popular drug in Canada for many years until it was determined that a very small number of people have a remote chance of experiencing a serious allergic response from the drug's residue in food products. This discovery led to a Canadian ban on using the drug in food-producing animals. The presence of chloramphenical in Chinese honey was detected through CFIA investigations and following a Health Canada risk assessment, the CFIA issued a recall of products on the

---

[23]   This contrasts with the situation in the United States where there is no mandatory recall power.

[24]   Ronald L. Doering, "Ready for a Recall" (2002) 62:9 Food in Canada: The Voice of the Canadian Food & Beverage Industry.

market and detained all incoming shipments of honey from China for further testing.

With the wide differences in veterinary drug approvals around the world, the Canadian standard of zero tolerance and the increasingly sophisticated technology for testing, this is likely to be a fruitful area for recalls in the future, especially as "zero" keeps getting smaller. In the chloramphenical case, no contamination was detected when the technology could only identify parts per billion ("ppb"), but when the technology was improved to detect at the level of .3 ppb, then there was a violation. No one really knows what the health hazards of such trace amounts are, but so long as the standard is zero, recalls will be required.

The risk analysis, risk management and risk communication functions must be closely co-ordinated and often involve a difficult iterative process. Health Canada does a preliminary health risk assessment and provides a determination of the level of recall, classified according to the relative degree of health risk presented by the product being recalled. Recall classification follows the following numeric designation that outlines the consequences of exposure. "Class I" involves a situation where there is a reasonable probability that the use of, or exposure to, a product will cause serious adverse health consequences or death. "Class II" situations exist where temporary adverse health consequences may occur or where the probability of serious adverse health consequences is remote. "Class III" denotes a situation in which no adverse health consequences are likely to occur.[25]

The CFIA receives the Health Canada risk analysis and then reviews risk management options and takes the lead in dealing with industry on both risk management and risk communication. However, the process is considerably more complicated than this framework suggests. In carrying out the risk management function, the CFIA will encounter feasibility problems or discover that new information will require additional assistance or analysis. New scientific opinions are provided, new risk management options reviewed, and difficult choices often have to be made. The science is critical but is rarely determinative, particularly when it is incomplete. The actual decisions on the nature and scope of the recall arise from a complex interplay among many actors both within Health Canada and the CFIA. For example, if Health Canada has already made a clear health risk assessment determination that the presence of E. coli 0157:H7 requires a full Class I recall, then the CFIA will proceed to deal

---

[25]   For further discussion of these recall classification categories, see Ronald L. Doering, "Ready for a Recall" (2002) 62:9 Food in Canada: The Voice of the Canadian Food & Beverage Industry.

with an affected company without requiring another health risk assessment.

It is remarkable how many companies are ill prepared when they are confronted with a product recall. There is really no excuse for this. The CFIA publishes detailed recall manuals and procedures that can be readily downloaded from its website.[26] Public warning "generic" templates are available for allergens, E. coli contamination, listeria, salmonella and C. botulism. The CFIA will assist a company at every stage of the recall including the provision of translation service for national public warnings.

Detailed protocols have been developed with consumers and industry associations to deal with often difficult cases of alleged tampering. Although general provisions of the *Criminal Code*[27] may have application, the Code does not contain specific provisions that relate directly to product tampering. Bill C-80, the *Canada Food Safety and Inspection Bill*, was introduced in 1999 to address this legislative gap by specifically prohibiting tampering or threats of tampering of food products but, unfortunately, a lack of political support caused the bill to die after First Reading. Bill C-80 represented a major consolidation and modernization of Canadian food law, but a similarly ambitious legislative reform effort has not materialized. In November 2004, the federal government introduced the *Canadian Inspection Agency Enforcement Act*, which was aimed at modernizing and enhancing the CFIA's inspection and enforcement powers[28] but the bill was not passed and passage is now not likely.

In December 2007, Prime Minister Stephen Harper announced Canada's Food and Consumer Safety Action Plan. The Action Plan aims at modernizing and strengthening Canada's safety for food, health and consumer products by better supporting the collective responsibilities of government, industry and consumers for product safety. The Action Plan involves legislative amendments to the *Food and Drugs Act*, as well as expanded program measures to improve Canada's food safety system. The federal government intends to prevent future food safety problems by broadening the coverage of potentially unsafe food imports and enhancing authority to require industry to implement food safety controls to prevent potential problems. In its Action Plan, the government also provides for the strengthening of its authority to verify the safety of food at all points

---

[26]   The CFIA has developed recall guides for distributors, manufacturers, importers and retailers. These are available from the CFIA website: <http://www.inspection.gc.ca/english/fssa/recarapp/recarappe.shtml#rp>.

[27]   R.S.C. 1985, c. C-46.

[28]   Bill C-27, First Session, 38th Parl., 53 Elizabeth II, 2004. See also Canadian Food Inspection Agency, News Release, "Government Introduces New Food Inspection and Enforcement Bill in the House of Commons" (26 November 2004).

in the food continuum, including prior to importation into Canada. Finally, the Action Plan sets out support measures to improve rapid responses to a food safety crisis by providing new authority to require adequate records be kept by those who handle food; strengthening access to the information that is needed to respond effectively to identified problems; and modernizing and streamlining inspection systems.[29]

V. CURRENT ISSUES IN FOOD SAFETY REGULATION

(a) Traceability

While the concept of food origin tracing is not new, for a variety of reasons the issue of traceability has achieved renewed prominence in the last decade. Increased globalization of supply chain sourcing and distribution, more rapid spread of contamination and disease, several major recent foodborne illness outbreaks, the increased public health risks of zoonotic diseases, and the growing threat of international terrorism, have all combined to thrust traceability to the forefront as a food safety issue in Canada and around the world.[30]

"Traceability is the ability to trace the history, application or location of an entity by means of recorded information."[31] In the context of food safety, traceability is the ability to track a food item (of animal or plant origin, finished product or ingredient) forwards or backwards through the food continuum or supply chain.

Improved traceability systems can contribute to food safety in a number of critical ways. Most directly, it is a critical tool in emergency response situations. The timeliness, scope, cost and effectiveness of a recall are often determined by the capability for traceability. Increasingly, all along the food chain, producers, processors and retailers need the ability to trace a food safety problem both backwards and forward in order to get the product off the shelf as quickly as possible. Only more sophisticated traceability systems can achieve this.

Improved traceability systems are also necessary to support health and safety label claims and to support marketing claims for specialized

---

[29]   Health Canada, *Strengthening and Modernizing Canada's Safety for Food, Health and Consumer Products: A Discussion Paper on Canada's Food and Safety Action Plan* (10 January 2008), online: <http://www.healthycanadians.gc.ca/alt_formats/pdf/Cons_ActionPlan_Paper_eng_06.pdf>.

[30]   Ronald L. Doering, "Prove It" (2003) 63(1) Food in Canada: The Voice of the Canadian Food & Beverage Industry.

[31]   *Ibid.*

products such as organic produce or "Omega 3" eggs.[32] Manufacturers, processors and retailers are increasingly demanding segregation process documentation and identity preservation systems all along the food chain to support the truth and integrity of claims and to meet a range of audit-based inspection and verification systems, all of which are designed to improve the quality and safety of food products.

Government-industry collaboration has already created some excellent national systems that are in operation, such as our Canadian Cattle ID Program which was critical to managing both the threat of foot and mouth disease and the recent cases of BSE in cattle.[33] Demonstrating the ability to trace back the origin of the diseased cattle and the credibility of the regulatory system significantly contributed to the fact that beef sales actually went up during the recent BSE crisis.

The most ambitious project is the government-funded, industry-managed voluntary whole-chain tracking and tracing initiative called Can-Trace. Launched in July 2003, with the lead by the Canadian Council of Grocery Distributors, the Food and Consumer Products Manufacturers of Canada, the Canadian Federation of Independent Grocers, and the Electronic Commerce Council of Canada, Can-Trace now has participation from 20 national trade associations, several provincial governments, and the federal government. Can-Trace was funded by Agriculture and Agri-Food Canada to develop industry standards for traceability and to pilot test the standards for beef, pork, fruits and vegetables. With federal government funding from Can-Trace ending in 2007, its future is uncertain.

The marketplace was the initial driver for the Can-Trace initiative as large food retailers have begun to demand that suppliers certify particular attributes of their product, such as being free of certain ingredients (for example, products of genetic engineering) or complying with specific quality requirements (such as having been produced under certain food safety systems or by good manufacturing practices). As these warranties are required by retailers, food processors will drive the requirement for traceability back up the food chain to the producer. The implications of this for small farmers may be quite problematic in that compliance requirements may be too onerous for small scale producers and they may also face difficulties obtaining liability insurance.

---

[32]   "Omega 3" eggs are produced by hens that are fed a diet supplemented with ground flax seeds, which are rich in omega-3 fatty acids.

[33]   The Canadian Cattle Identification Program was established under the *Health of Animals Regulations*, C.R.C., c. 296. For a program description, see Canadian Food Inspection Agency, *Canadian Cattle Identification Program — Enforcement Provisions*, online: <http://www.inspection.gc.ca/english/anima/trac/catbetide.shtml>.

While the market, not federal regulation, has pushed for improved traceability systems in Canada, recent regulatory initiatives have given the concept some urgency. First, the U.S. *Bioterrorism Act*[34] now requires trace back documentation for many food products being imported to the United States. Second, the European Union has passed legislation that stipulates that "the traceability of food, feed, food producing animals, and any other substance intended to be, or expected to be, incorporated into a food or feed shall be established at all stages of production, processing and distribution".[35] This means that in order to export food products to our largest markets, the U.S. and Europe, Canada will have to have greatly improved traceability systems. In addition, the Province of Québec has introduced regulations that will require enhanced traceability for products produced in that province.

The requirement for improved traceability capacity has prompted the development of a number of new technologies. For example, bar coding on a tag affixed to an animal or a product that can be read electronically is already being used and some companies are beginning to use radio frequency identification (known as "RFID") where the data is attached to an ear tag, injected under the skin of an animal, or attached to product labels, so that data can be collected by a proximity reader and does not require direct contact with the tag.

The most active area of current research and development in food and feed traceability is DNA analysis that allows a product to have a genetic bar code that would allow very detailed tracing all along the food chain from production to consumption. Maple Leaf Foods is already using this technology to trace pork sold to Japan from the maternal sows with all of their offspring and all meat and meat products derived from them. DNA sampling has great potential for food derived from plant products; it could, for example, be used to detect or confirm absence of genetically engineered traits.[36] From a public health point of view, DNA tracing will make a significant contribution to epidemiological investigations because it will be possible to trace from stool samples back through the food chain to the retailer or even the producer.

Obviously, these traceability technologies and systems will have a huge impact on food safety in the coming years. However, the legal implications are not so clear. While large retailers will be able to demand traceability warranties to enhance the safety of the foods they sell, it is not

---

[34] *Public Health Security and Bioterrorism Preparedness and Response Act of 2002*, 42 U.S.C. 201 (2002).

[35] Ronald L. Doering, "Prove It" (2003) 63(1) Food in Canada: The Voice of the Canadian Food & Beverage Industry.

[36] Canada, Agriculture and Agri-Food Canada, *Agriculture and Agri-Food Canada Scan of Current & Emerging Traceability Technologies — Final Report* (10 September 2004).

so clear how processors and producers will be able to respond to the demands or how they will be able to cope with legal liabilities that they may never have anticipated and for which they are not insured.

(b) Fragmented Jurisdiction

Food safety is necessarily a shared responsibility all along the food chain from the producer to the consumer and across all levels of government. In federal systems of government, there can be a high degree of fragmentation of responsibility between the central and regional governments. Even in unitary systems there is usually at least a division of responsibility between agriculture and fishery officials on one hand and health officials on the other. Indeed, the most pervasive issue in food safety regulation internationally is the debate about whether food safety is essentially a matter of public health (with health departments having primacy) or of food production (with agriculture and fishery departments having the lead responsibility). Of course, in reality, it is increasingly obvious that both departments must be involved. Food safety must be the primary goal and this can only be achieved by a close collaboration among all relevant departments at all levels of government.[37]

Happily, even though Canada is a federal system, our situation is remarkably more integrated than is the case in many countries. While there are still many challenges and an ongoing need to strengthen collaboration, two developments in the last ten years have served to significantly strengthen intergovernmental co-operation on food safety in Canada.

First, Canada led the world in 1997 by placing the enforcement of all regulations all along the food chain — seeds, feeds, fertilizer, plants, animals, all commodities, including fish — within one agency. The creation of the CFIA has proven to be a real asset to enhance accountability by bringing a co-ordinated and focused approach to food safety at the federal level.[38] Many countries are studying the Canadian experience. A single food agency has been recommended almost yearly since early in the last century by some entity in the United States. However, a major structural reform that would centralize U.S. Department of Agriculture food safety activities with the Food and Drug Administration appears to be unlikely at this time.

---

[37] Ronald L. Doering, "Reforming Canada's Food Inspection System: The Case of the Canadian Food Inspection Agency (CFIA)" (1998) 62 Journal of the Association of Food and Drug Officials 3.

[38] Michael J. Prince, "Banishing Bureaucracy or Hatching a Hybrid? The Canadian Food Inspection Agency and the Politics of Reinventing Government" (2000) 13(2) Governance: An International Journal of Policy and Administration 215.

The other major development in Canada has been a little publicized but remarkable process carried out by the Canadian Food Inspection System Implementation Group ("CFISIG"). Recognizing the need to have a more comprehensive and systematic process to promote food law harmonization, provincial health, agriculture and environment officials, municipal level public health officials, and federal health, agriculture and fishery officials held several meetings in the early 1990s to promote a more co-operative and integrated inspection approach and system delivery with more uniform procedures and practices. Their work culminated in a Blueprint for the Canadian Food Inspection System ("CFIS"),[39] which was adopted by federal and provincial/territorial Ministers of Agriculture in 1994 and by Health Ministers the following year.

The CFIS Blueprint outlines a structure and process for developing an integrated food inspection system where "[i]ndustry has primary responsibility for the safety and quality of product..." and "[c]onsumers have a right to be informed and the responsibility to handle food properly".[40] The responsibilities of governments include establishing and enforcing health and safety standards, monitoring adequacy of product information released by industry, providing consumer information, and representing consumer and producer interests at the international level.

To oversee the implementation of the Blueprint, Ministers created the CFISIG. The principal focus of this group has been to develop consensus-based national harmonized standards. In a historic development, CFISIG formally approved a National Dairy Code, which, when adopted by the respective governments, will create for the first time a national standard for fluid milk products (both production and processing) replacing the ten standards that exist now.[41]

Working groups are also developing national regulations and voluntary codes for the meat, fruit and retail service sectors. In all cases, there is a desire to not only have harmonized standards but to have more streamlined, outcome-based regulations that are supported by non-regulatory codes that describe best practices in more detail. While the importance of public health and federal-provincial co-operation are factors encouraging co-operation, it is interesting to note that the main driver for harmonization stems from the implications of free trade agreements. CFIS members recognize that the rights and obligations that result from the World Trade Organization ("WTO") and the North American Free Trade

---

[39] A copy of the Blueprint is available online: <http://www.cfis.agr.ca/english/blupr/blueprinte.shtml>.
[40] *Ibid.*
[41] Report of the Meat Regulatory and Inspection Review, *Farm to Fork — A Strategy for Meat Safety in Ontario* (Ontario, 2004) (Chair: The Honourable Roland J. Haines).

Agreement ("NAFTA") provide strong reasons for developing harmonized standards consistent with international standards (such as Codex Alimentarius, the international standard setting body for food established under the WHO and the Food and Agriculture Organization) in particular as they relate to "national treatment" provisions and to establishing equivalency with trading partners.[42]

CFISIG is also engaged in developing model legislation. The goal of this process is to provide a basis for consistency in Canada's food laws — the over 77 federal, provincial and territorial statutes that regulate food. The model legislation outlines a set of common standards and requirements against which existing federal, provincial and territorial legislation can be compared and harmonized. Jurisdictions are developing a report card to identify variances between existing legislation and the model. This will help to ensure equivalence of all food legislation in the country.[43]

Work in this area is necessarily slow because, at the multilateral level, all decisions require full consensus and this work will never be complete; Canadian federation has more to do with process than product. Food inspection harmonization over the coming years will present a real test of Canada's ability to manage interdependence in this area of jurisdictional complexity.[44] Regulatory harmonization and co-operation among levels of government and between health and agriculture departments is one of the most significant issues for food safety in all countries of the world.

(c) Risk Analysis

Managing public health risks is an increasingly complex task. As in other areas of public health, food safety regulators are constantly faced with having to make regulatory decisions that can have profound implications for their citizens, often without clear safety standards and with serious lack of scientific certainty. For almost any decision that becomes controversial, critics will emerge, who often have the benefit of hindsight and who disguise their economic interests as public health

---

[42]   Under the WTO, national governments agree not to require higher standards of exporting countries than they require of their industry and countries are urged to negotiate equivalency of standard agreements in order to facilitate trade.

[43]   For additional information on efforts to develop a common legislative framework for Canadian food law, including model food safety and inspection legislation, see Canadian Food Inspection System, online: <http://www.cfis.agr.ca/english/regcode/clb/clb_flic_e.shtml>.

[44]   Ronald L. Doering, "Reforming Canada's Food Inspection System: The Case of the Canadian Food Inspection Agency (CFIA)" (1998) 62 Journal of the Association of Food and Drug Officials 3.

concerns, arguing that the regulator under-reacted or over-reacted. Scientifically illiterate consumers may be at a loss to understand the situation when both sides purport to defend their position as science-based and can point to risk assessments that support their position.

The dilemma is complicated by the fact that the classical risk model is simply not robust enough to adequately describe the deep complexity of risk analysis. In the classical model, risk assessments are carried out by scientists to determine the likelihood of an event (usually expressed in mathematical terms of probability) and the consequences if that should occur. Risk management is carried out by others who take the risk assessment and weigh it against the political, economic, ethical and social considerations, make a policy decision and then explain the decision to the public by way of a risk communication strategy.

Unfortunately, the world is much more complicated than that. In the real world, one cannot separate science from policy. As Covello and Merkhofer emphasize: "In practice, assumptions that have potential policy implications enter into risk assessment at virtually every stage of the process. The idea of a risk assessment that is free, or nearly free, of policy considerations is beyond the realm of possibility."[45] Risk assessments are far more subjective than most scientists want to admit and both risk management and risk communication are more of an art than a science.[46]

Another complicating factor is that for most public health threats — and food safety is no exception — there is always both the science risk and the perception risk. They are quite different and yet they are commonly interchanged. Governments are often forced to introduce measures to deal with the one risk that actually complicates the other.

It is not that science is not important; indeed, it is absolutely essential. But science is not sufficient, especially when we so frequently deal not just with mere risk, but ambiguity and deep uncertainty. Science-based quantitative expert risk assessments often disguise the underlying subjective framework of assumptions and understate the high degree of uncertainty. The classical model of risk analysis falls short both in describing what regulators actually do and in providing much useful guidance on how they should practice their regulatory craft.

Perhaps we need to develop a whole new model and language for describing public health regulation in a field like food safety. While a new approach cannot be described yet with any precision, it would seem that

---

[45]   V.T. Covello & M.W. Merkhofer, *Risk Assessment Method: Approaches for Assessing Health and Environment Risks* (New York: Plenum Press, 1993).

[46]   Ronald L. Doering, "Risky Business" (2004) 64(5) Food in Canada: The Voice of the Canadian Food & Beverage Industry.

we must begin to recognize that the language of risk is not really helpful when one is dealing primarily with uncertainty. Food safety risk assessors do not do double blind laboratory studies over a long period; they generally just review the conclusions of other scientists. In fact, in spite of their name, they typically do not even assess cases of risk (as calculations of probability are usually impossible to determine especially in the context of an urgent food safety problem). "Risk assessors" actually assess situations of uncertainty and then engage in a complex iterative process with decision-makers to try to find ways to manage an immediate issue fraught with multiple perspectives where the science, however uncertain, is important but rarely determinative. It is issue or crisis management, not risk management.

A new model would borrow heavily from the emerging literature on adaptive management: in the face of such uncertainty, making policy choices and implementing regulatory decisions should be recognized as necessarily experimental; decisions are made that expect the unexpected; policies and regulatory responses are adapted as lessons continue to be learned.[47]

The new approach would also have to more fully recognize that while food safety must always be paramount, trade-offs are always a necessary part of the process and there is no current model that adequately describes how risks and benefits are to be weighed when there cannot be zero risk. For example, the only way to ensure food safety for sufferers of peanut allergies would be to make the sale of peanuts illegal. But peanuts will be sold and this creates health uncertainty for a sizeable group of Canadians. Managing the associated allergy issues becomes a policy decision, not a science decision.

A new model would also have to grapple with the complex issue of how to communicate this uncertainty to a generally scientifically illiterate consumer who simply expects retailers to only sell safe food, and expects the regulatory system to guarantee such safety. Fortunately, in Canada, consumers continue to have a high degree of confidence in the safety of their food and in the integrity of their regulatory systems. Not all countries enjoy such support. Perhaps this is because our food safety system does generally work in practice, even if it does not yet work in theory.

(d) International Trade Issues

The growth in the international trade of food (and the law regulating its movement) is perhaps the single biggest factor affecting food safety

---

[47]   Kai N. Lee, *Compass and Gyroscope: Integrating Science and Politics for the Environment* (Washington, D.C.: Island Press, 1993).

regulation today. Canada annually exports more than $24 billion of agricultural products and fish and fish products are valued at $3.8 billion.[48] Canada imports food and agricultural products from half the countries in the world with food imports alone valued at over $20 billion annually.[49] Canada, then, has much to gain from trade liberalization. At the same time — and this is at the heart of the current globalization debate — countries like Canada strive to obtain the benefits of trade liberalization without sacrificing certain national sovereignty rights such as the maintenance of national public health standards for safe food.

The WTO recognizes the sovereign right of countries to afford appropriate levels of health and safety protection for their people, animals and plants through a subsidiary agreement called the Agreement on the Application of Sanitary and Phytosanitary Measures ("SPS Agreement"). While enshrining the right of protection, the agreement sets up a regime to prevent these measures from being protectionist; that is, to prevent countries from using domestic standards as disguised barriers to trade. The SPS Agreement places a number of restrictions on how these measures are developed and enforced, particularly requiring that the standards be science-based. Countries that adopt certain international standards are deemed to be trade compliant without the need to establish any other scientific basis. The Agreement specifically references three existing international standard-setting bodies: the Codex Alimentarius for food safety standards; the *Office International des Epizooties* for animal health; and the International Plant Protection Convention for plant health.

These organizations have been fundamentally transformed by the WTO reference. While established to allow technical-level bureaucrats to design voluntary technical standards by consensus, they are now at the heart of the protection-protectionism debate because decisions they make have huge implications for a country. Their standards can be used to justify preventing products from being exported from competitor countries.

There have already been several cases where food safety has been used as a disguised barrier to trade. North American beef still cannot be exported to the European Union because of allegations that American and Canadian use of certain growth hormones in cattle cause a food safety risk. The Codex Committee concluded that the hormone was safe but the E.U. chose to accept trade sanctions rather than allow this perceived threat to its food supply. Similarly, the E.U. has justified its ban on the imports

---

[48] Statistics Canada, 2003, data compiled by Agriculture and Agri-Food Canada, Food Value Chain Bureau.
[49] *Ibid.*

of food containing genetically modified ingredients disguising their protectionist position by citing science that supports a food safety risk.

It is not well-recognized that food safety regulators around the world regularly find themselves thrust into the midst of complex international trade issues in which the science is relevant but rarely determinative.

Of course, Canada's largest trading partner is the United States. Because our economies are so integrated, there is always discussion about the need to harmonize food regulations. Actual regulatory harmonization, however, has not occurred and is not likely to in the foreseeable future as our systems are very different and there is little political will to really tackle the problem.[50]

VI. CONCLUSION

While Canada's food has never been safer and is among the safest in the world, food safety continues to grow as a public health concern. Increased globalization of food trade, new emerging pathogens, high profile food recalls and the central role of food safety in several major trade disputes have all served to once again put food safety among the front ranks of public health issues in this country.

Food safety will undoubtedly be a growing and increasingly complex area of public health law in the years ahead. Even with much more practical research, the field will continue to be characterized by considerable scientific uncertainty. Practitioners will be frustrated by the apparent inability of our sluggish regulatory system to keep up with the pace of technological change. Regulators will continue to struggle with protecting the public in an area where zero risk is impossible and where a multitude of forces combine to present a complex public policy environment. Both practitioners and food safety regulators will have to have a high degree of tolerance for turbulence in the coming years.

---

[50]   Ronald L. Doering, "Canada's Food Laws; Harmonization with U.S. Not in Sight" (January/February 2008) Update 37 (published by the Food and Drug Law Institute).

13

CRIMINAL JUSTICE AND PUBLIC HEALTH

Wayne N. Renke[*]

The relationship between criminal justice and public health is complex — at once tangled and distant, convergent and divergent, hostile and co-operative. The precise relationship of criminal justice and public health can only be discerned in connection with particular circumstances; I can at best only gesture here at some general topographical features where the two great functionalities of criminal justice and public health grind against one another. I shall begin by (I) comparing and contrasting conceptual elements of the public health system and the criminal justice system, then consider (II) criminal justice incursions into the public health system in pursuit of evidence; (III) the incorporation of preventative, public health-style approaches in criminal justice procedures; and (IV) the criminal justice system as a source of public health risks.

I. THE PUBLIC HEALTH SYSTEM AND THE CRIMINAL JUSTICE SYSTEM: CONCEPTUAL COMPARISON AND CONTRAST

The public health system and the criminal justice system might seem to be purely contrasting institutions. The two systems do differ fundamentally. Even so, their conceptual relations are more nuanced than might be immediately apparent. After providing brief accounts of (a) the "public health system" and (b) the "criminal justice system", I shall discuss (c) the systems' conceptual similarities or points of convergence,

[*] Professor, Faculty of Law, University of Alberta. Thank you to Lydia Lau, Colin Ouellette and Gergely Hegedus for their research assistance.

(d) their conceptual differences or points of divergence, and (e) some implications of their similarities and differences.

(a) The Public Health System

Public health as an academic discipline should be contrasted with public health as a system. As a discipline — or set of disciplines — public health studies are contrasted with the study of medicine. Public health studies include epidemiology, economics, sociology, political science, and psychology; the study of medicine, in contrast, includes such disciplines as physiology, anatomy, and histology.[1] As a system, public health links disciplinary experts with health care professionals and facilities, but brings these health system elements into a broader context. The health system *per se* focuses on individual patients, their treatment, and their rehabilitation.[2] The public health system encompasses individual health, but it concentrates on the health of populations. Its tactics and strategies are based on information gathered from surveillance of populations. It supplements treatment and rehabilitation with the design and execution of programs and policies of prevention and management of population health risk factors; and with the design and execution of programs and policies of health promotion, which encourage populations to engage in healthy lifestyles. The public health system also has a reactive aspect, triggered when health emergencies beset populations.

The public health system is an open system of systems. Its component systems include hospitals with front-line staff in emergency rooms, clinics, long-term care facilities, research laboratories, research ethics boards, regional health boards, governmental departments, intergovernmental working groups and professional associations. These systems are supported by government funding (in contrast to privately-funded health care). These systems are epistemologically organized around paradigms of Western medicine and science (in contrast to some alternative modes of health care).

---

[1]   D. Prothrow-Stith, "Strengthening the Collaboration between Public Health and Criminal Justice to Prevent Violence" (2004) 32:1 J.L. Med. & Ethics 82 at 82-83.

[2]   *Ibid.*; Canadian Institutes of Health Research, *The Future of Public Health in Canada: Developing a Public Health System for the 21st Century — Executive Summary* (Ottawa: Institute of Population and Public Health, June 2003), online: <http://www.cihr-irsc. gc.ca/e/19573.html>; Canadian Medical Association, "Answering the Wake-up Call: CMA's Public Health Action Plan" (25 June 2003), online: <http://www.cma.ca/ multimedia/staticContent/HTML/N0/l2/working_on/OfficePublicHealth/pdf/wake-up.pdf>; Canadian Medical Association, "Health Protection and a Canadian Public Health Strategy: A Comprehensive Approach to Public Health" (April 2004), online: <http://www.cma.ca/ multimedia/staticContent/HTML/N0/l2/where_we_stand/political/2004/Health-Protection_e.pdf>.

(b) The Criminal Justice System

The criminal justice system is just one of many subsystems within the law. Its constitutive rules differ from those of (*e.g.*) the civil justice system, corporate-commercial law, intellectual property law, bankruptcy and insolvency law, or labour law. The criminal justice system — like the public health system — is an open system of systems. Criminal justice systems are all clustered around the enforcement, application, administration, and development of the criminal law. At the heart of the criminal law are offences — rules that serve criminal law purposes and that establish prohibitions enforced through penalties.[3] Offence rules are surrounded by intricate sets of rules governing the legal status of criminal justice system personnel, investigative techniques, evidence and proof, procedures before and during trial, sentencing options, and the nature of custodial dispositions. Criminal justice systems include the police, the legal profession (which supplies Crown prosecutors, defence counsel and judges), the judiciary and the courts, probation authorities, custodial facilities and associated professionals, and parole authorities; as well as governmental departments and intergovernmental working groups, professional associations, and non-governmental or volunteer organizations. The criminal justice system too is supported by government funding. Unlike the public health system, the criminal justice system is epistemologically organized around lay common sense and the adversary system.

(c) Convergence

On an abstract level, the public health system and the criminal justice system share some features.

Both are modern public institutions (or better, sets of institutions). They rely on a distinction between credentialed professional service providers and consumer-client-patients who receive those services, a distinction between those with knowledge and those who lack knowledge.[4] If citizens were or perceived themselves as being competent to look after their own health or disputes, neither institution would be

---

[3]   "For a law to be classified as a criminal law, it must possess three prerequisites: a valid criminal law purpose backed by a prohibition and a penalty": *R. v. Malmo-Levine*, [2003] S.C.J. No. 79, [2003] 3 S.C.R. 571 at para. 74 (S.C.C.), *per* Gonthier and Binnie JJ.; *Reference re: Firearms Act (Can.)*, [2000] S.C.J. No. 31, [2000] 1 S.C.R. 783 at para. 27 (S.C.C.). Offences created under federal legislation other than the *Criminal Code* may be classifiable as "criminal law". Offences prosecuted in the manner of criminal offences may not be, technically, criminal law, but law sustained under other legislative authority (*e.g.*, provincial traffic offences).

[4]   I. Illich, "Disabling Professions" in *Disabling Professions* (London: Marion Boyers, 1977) at 11; I. Illich, *Tools for Conviviality* (New York: Harper Colophon, 1980) at 56; see generally D. Cayley, *Ivan Illich in Conversation* (Concord, Ont.: Anansi, 1992).

necessary, at least on their present scale. The status of the service providers is underwritten by the state, which confers on them more-or-less porous official monopolies for providing health and justice services. These service providers are at the core of each institution. They do not belong to a single profession, but to complementary sets of professions — e.g., in the public health system, physicians and surgeons, nurses, pharmacists, physiotherapists, and researchers; in the criminal justice system, judges, prosecutors, defence counsel, police officers and correctional officers. The core professionals are supported by an array of support and administrative staff. What unifies the core professionals is their commitment to and training in a "paradigm" — a group of doctrines, methods, techniques and ethical principles. Certification of possession of the requisite degree of knowledge of the paradigm is (generally) established by the professions themselves. The professions — as befits those with knowledge not shared with ordinary citizens — are allowed significant self-governance. The state, however, provides substantial funding for the systems. Money comes with strings attached. Governmental regulation, management and intervention accompany funding.

Like the public health system, the criminal justice system seeks to maximize Canadians' health. One of the traditionally recognized objectives of true criminal law is the promotion of public health: "Public peace, order, security, health, morality: these are the ordinary though not exclusive ends served by [criminal] law."[5] Because of this convergence of objectives, the public health system and the criminal justice system deal with some of the same social issues — e.g., alcohol and drug abuse, domestic violence, or the transmission of communicable disease.

Like the public health system, the criminal justice system is concerned with the "body politic", with "the population", understood as a structure distinct from individuals. Population is not only a source of information but a target of interventions. It is a new subject and a new object: "population comes to appear above all else as the ultimate end of government".[6] The criminal justice system manifests its population orientation through its assignment of prosecutions to state employees. This differentiates criminal litigation from civil litigation, which leaves plaintiffs to pursue their actions personally. Prosecutors conduct prosecutions on behalf of the state, as indicated by the style of cause of

---

[5]   Reference re: Dairy Industry Act (Canada) S. 5(a), [1948] S.C.J. No. 42, [1949] S.C.R. 1, at 50 (S.C.C.), per Rand J., aff'd [1950] J.C.J. No. 1, [1950] 4 D.L.R. 689 (P.C.); Reference re: Firearms Act (Can.), [2001] S.C.J. No. 31 at para. 31 (S.C.C.); R. v. Malmo-Levine, [2003] S.C.J. No. 79 at para. 74 (S.C.C.).

[6]   M. Foucault, "Governmentality" in G. Burchell et al., eds., The Foucault Effect: Studies in Governmentality (Chicago: University of Chicago Press, 1991) 87 at 100 [translated by C. Gordon].

prosecutions, which pit "Regina", the Queen (or the State, the People, or the Commonwealth), against the accused. Part of the defining myth or rhetoric of criminal justice is that the involvement of the state is justified because criminal offences affect not merely particular victims, but society as a whole. Crimes have a public aspect that private wrongs lack. Furthermore, criminal justice seeks to manipulate the body politic through sentencing. One of the purposes of sentencing is general deterrence — *i.e.*, to stop others from doing what the offender has already done.[7] Sentencing steers the body politic. Thus, offences harm "the population", and are prosecuted on behalf of "the population," for the purpose of managing "the population". Criminal justice is thoroughly interested in the body politic.

Like the public health system, the criminal justice system pursues prevention initiatives. Prevention is a goal of court-based judicial processes. Section 718 of the *Criminal Code* provides that "[t]he fundamental purpose of sentencing is to contribute, *along with crime prevention initiatives*, to respect for the law and the maintenance of a just, peaceful and safe society . . ." (emphasis added). Prevention techniques administered by judges target individuals, seeking to prevent those individuals from offending in the future. Prevention techniques include "peace bonds" (criminal restraining orders)[8] and the more recent prohibition order provisions respecting anticipated terrorism or criminal organization offences, sexual offences, or serious personal injury offences.[9] Prevention may be achieved by denying a suspect judicial interim release on the "secondary ground", when detention is necessary for the protection or safety of the public.[10] The dangerous offender provisions of the *Criminal Code*, which permit detention for what an offender has not done (yet), are an example of the preventative jurisdiction of the criminal law.[11] The "not criminally responsible on account of mental disorder" provisions of the *Criminal Code* are also supported by the preventative jurisdiction of the criminal law.[12]

The police have always had prevention and "safe lifestyle" promotion mandates. The sheer presence or probability of presence of police officers has a preventative function. Community policing programs, such as "broken windows" initiatives, involve work with communities to

---

[7] *Criminal Code*, R.S.C. 1985, c. C-46, s. 718(*b*).

[8] *Ibid.*, s. 810.

[9] *Ibid.*, ss. 810.01, 810.1 and 810.2, respectively.

[10] *Ibid.*, s. 515(10)(*b*).

[11] Part XXIV of the *Criminal Code, ibid.*; see *R. v. Lyons*, [1987] S.C.J. No. 62, [1987] 2 S.C.R. 309 at 329 (S.C.C.), *per* La Forest J.

[12] Part XX.1 of the *Criminal Code, ibid.*; see *R. v. Swain*, [1991] S.C.J. No. 32, [1991] 1 S.C.R. 933 at 1000-1001 (S.C.C.), *per* Lamer C.J.C.

reduce factors that lead to crime or to serious types of crime.[13] The police may engage in educational campaigns to ensure individuals' safety and security or to promote healthy, offence-free lifestyles (*e.g.*, anti-drug abuse programs in schools).

Governments are now embracing prevention as a pillar of justice administration. Prevention's allure is based on a simple cost benefit hypothesis ("an ounce of prevention is worth a pound of cure"): in the mid- to long-run, the costs of preventing, reducing and managing risks of criminal conduct are less than the costs (particularly the social and individual non-pecuniary damage) incurred by relying too extensively on reactions to criminal conduct after it happens. The emphasis on prevention in criminal matters is not altogether new. It has been recommended by United Nations agencies[14] and has been championed in Canada by Irvin Waller[15] and the Institute for the Prevention of Crime at the University of Ottawa.[16] Several provinces, including British Columbia,[17] Nova Scotia[18] and Alberta, have recently embarked on crime prevention programs. In 2007, Premier Stelmach and Alberta Justice sponsored a Crime Reduction Task Force which, following cross-province consultations, made a variety of recommendations, all based on a crime prevention perspective.[19] The province responded positively, and has

---

[13]   U.S., Department of Justice, *"Broken Windows" and Police Discretion* by G.L. Kelling (Washington, D.C.: National Institute of Justice Research Report, October 1999); J.Q. Wilson & G.L. Kelling, "Broken Windows" *The Atlantic Monthly* (March 1982) 29; J.Q. Wilson & G.L. Kelling, "Making Neighborhoods Safe" *The Atlantic Monthly* (February 1989).

[14]   United Nations Economic and Social Council, Commission on Crime Prevention and Criminal Justice, "Guidelines for the Prevention of Crime", online: United Nations Human Settlements Program <http://ww2.unhabitat.org/programmes/safercities/documents/declarations/ny.pdf>; and E. Krug, L. Dahlberg, J. Mercy, A. Zwi, R. Lozano, eds., *World Report on Violence and Health*, online: World Health Organization <http://whqlibdoc.who.int/hq/2002/9241545615.pdf>.

[15]   I. Waller, *Less Law, More Order: The Truth about Reducing Crime* (Westport, CT: Praeger, 2006).

[16]   Institute for the Prevention of Crime, online: University of Ottawa, Faculty of Social Sciences <http://www.sciencessociales.uottawa.ca/ipc/eng/>.

[17]   In 2007, British Columbia established a Criminal Justice Reform Secretariat: Criminal Justice Reform, online: Attorney General of British Columbia <http://www.ag.gov.bc.ca/justice-reform-initiatives/criminal/index.htm>.

[18]   Nova Scotia struck a Justice Minister's "Task Force on Safer Streets and Communities in 2006", online: Nova Scotia Department of Justice <http://www.gov.ns.ca/just/Public_Safety/safer_communities.asp>.

[19]   "Keeping Communities Safe: Report and Recommendations of Alberta's Crime Reduction and Safe Communities Task Force" (6 November 2007), online: Alberta Justice <http://www.justice.gov.ab.ca/publications/default.aspx?id=5328>.

created a Safe Communities Secretariat (housed in Alberta Justice) which will facilitate and support crime prevention initiatives in Alberta.[20]

Finally, like the public health system, the criminal justice system is concerned with treatment. Yet another objective of sentencing is to assist in "rehabilitating" offenders.[21] Rehabilitation may involve treatment. Treatment may be made available to individuals who are diverted from standard criminal law processes, to offenders bound by probation orders, or to offenders either within custodial settings or as part of conditional release. As an example, an express sentencing option in impaired driving or driving with excessive blood/alcohol cases is the "curative discharge", which allows the offender to be sentenced to a type of conditional discharge; the terms of probation include a condition requiring the offender to attend for alcohol or drug curative treatment.[22]

Treatment and rehabilitation figure prominently in government-sponsored crime prevention initiatives. Some of these initiatives will be discussed below. An important feature of these initiatives is their interdisciplinary, inter-Ministerial, broadly based nature. Interventions may be supported for expectant mothers, families with young children, children in primary and secondary schools, persons with addictions, and persons with mental health issues. These non-traditional crime reduction strategies are linked to treatment initiatives connected with criminal justice processes.

(d) Divergence

Despite their points of convergence, the public health system and the criminal justice system are, of course, very different systems. This difference lies not only in the general lack of overlap between the systems' physical plant, personnel, and education and training programs.

While the criminal justice system is concerned with social effects, its primary tactical focus is on individuals: it seeks social effects through manipulating individuals. Outside of the prevention context, the criminal justice system attends to whether this particular individual committed a particular offence in the particular circumstances; and, if a penal disposition is warranted, to the particular disposition appropriate to that individual in those circumstances.

A critical point of difference between the public health system and the criminal justice system is that the criminal justice system seeks to

---

[20]   Alberta's Safe Communities Secretariat, online: Alberta Justice <http://www.justice. gov.ab.ca/safe/default.aspx>.

[21]   *Criminal Code*, R.S.C. 1985, c. C-46, s. 718(*d*).

[22]   *Ibid.*, s. 255(5); although this provision is not yet in force in all provinces.

assess the fault or blame of rule-breakers, and paradigmatically, to punish those who deserve punishment.[23] The public health system is not concerned with fault or punishment, but with identifying factors that heighten risks of illness, with reducing risks of illness, and with treating those who contract illness (the public health system may concern itself with intentional acts that cause or cause risks of injury or illness).

Even when the criminal justice system engages in treatment, another important distinction must be recognized. Criminal justice system treatment is, directly or indirectly, compulsory. It takes place in the shadow of the state's monopoly on legitimate violence. This is most plain in drug treatment court contexts, where judges supervise treatment, and require periodic in-court reporting by offenders — on pain of punishment in the ordinary fashion, should offenders fail to abide by judge-imposed conditions of treatment. In contrast, public health system interventions are generally non-compulsory; they rely on informed consent or choice. In emergency situations, however, public health tactics may be compulsory, as when quarantine or isolation are imposed on individuals.

The epistemologies of the public health system and the criminal justice system differ as well. The criminal law system, like science and medicine, does search after truth, and does seek truly effective interventions promoting justice and safety. The criminal justice system is open to medical and scientific research, whether in investigations (*e.g.*, DNA analysis), in trials (*e.g.*, expert evidence generally), or in sentencing (*e.g.*, in designing terms of probation); but, at root, it could not be said to follow a medico-scientific paradigm. Instead, it relies primarily on lay investigators and witnesses (*e.g.*, police officers or "eye witnesses") to supply data for analysis. Analysis, the determination of the facts, occurs through the adversary system of trials (the judge or jury as passive arbiter; counsel for either side as active proponents of their respective positions). Even in cases that do not go to trial, lawyers and judges negotiate the facts. Factual conclusions are drawn through "common sense inferences" from the evidence, and sentencing dispositions are arrived at through precedent and speculation (*e.g.*, virtually all judicial reasoning concerning "deterrence").

There is an exception to this epistemological divergence: efforts are being made to ensure that crime-prevention initiatives are evidence-based — in contrast to the traditional intuitivist approach of criminal justice

---

[23]   A principle of fundamental justice is that "punishment must be proportionate to the moral blameworthiness of the offender . . . the fundamental principle of a morally based system of law [is] that those causing harm intentionally be punished more severely than those causing harm unintentionally": *R. v. Martineau*, [1990] S.C.J. No. 84, [1990] 2 S.C.R. 633 at 645 S.C.R. (S.C.C.), *per* Lamer C.J.C.

policy. Crime prevention initiatives are regularly assessed and evaluated. To the extent possible, large-scale social experimentation is employed (finding like communities, determining relevant baseline rates, introducing initiatives in some communities but not others, attempting to control for other variables, and assessing the impact of initiatives). Crime prevention should be informed by research and should incorporate scientific method.

(e) Implications

The points of convergence between the public health system and the criminal justice system establish the possibility of inter-institutional co-operation, collaboration and complementarity. Both systems seek to maximize health, to manage the body politic, to use tools of prevention and promotion, and to support treatment. At the same time, convergence creates the possibility of conflict or inconsistency, if the two systems approach shared issues without shared strategies. One system's tactics may undermine the other's. Each side, operating within its own paradigm, is likely to consider its own tactics to be the best remedies. To bridge the interdisciplinary gap and to facilitate co-operation, recourse must be had to a "meta-authority" — i.e., the state, which may ultimately exert control through its funding powers.

Before turning to collaborative developments, I shall discuss some contexts in which the two systems may come into conflict, beginning with some instances in which criminal justice investigations are pursued within the public health system.

II. CRIMINAL JUSTICE INCURSIONS: COLLECTING EVIDENCE

In the course of treating patients, particularly in emergency wards, public health personnel may gather information about whether individuals were victims of crime, perpetrators of offences, or witnesses to crimes. Caregivers may not only obtain information, but may come into custody of physical evidence, ranging from bodily samples to instrumentalities of crime. While public health workers, like other citizens, may have a natural inclination to co-operate with the authorities in the investigation of offences, the basic rule is that public health workers and facilities must keep information and bodily samples gathered during treatment confidential unless the patient provides informed consent, or the law otherwise permits or requires disclosure.[24] Disclosure issues arise in five main contexts: (a) when the law permits or requires disclosure, regardless of any request for disclosure; (b) when the police request disclosure, but without a warrant; (c) when the police request disclosure under the authority of a warrant or other court process; (d) when disclosure to the defence is required by court order; and (e) when disclosure is required in court through testimony. In the following, I will use the term "caregiver" to describe a public health worker who is in possession of confidential information or bodily samples.

(a)   Permission or Requirement to Disclose, Without Prior Request

(i)   Discretionary Disclosure

In some circumstances, statute or common law permits a caregiver to disclose information without the consent of the subject of the information, even though no "official" request has been made for the information. Alberta's *Health Information Act*, for example, provides that a custodian has the discretion to disclose health information without consent "to any person if the custodian believes, on reasonable grounds, that the disclosure will avert or minimize an imminent danger to the health or safety of any person".[25] In *Smith v. Jones*, the Supreme Court recognized a similar common law "public safety exception" to solicitor/client privilege: a solicitor is entitled to disclose confidential information if there is a "clear risk to an identifiable person or group of persons"; if this is a "risk of serious bodily harm or death"; and the risk is "imminent".[26] This case concerned disclosure by a psychiatrist, but the information was considered to be covered by an aspect of solicitor/client privilege. Because solicitor/client privilege is the "highest privilege recognized by the courts", the common law public safety exception "applies to all classifications of privileges and duties of confidentiality".[27]

---

[24]   Public health workers' obligations of confidentiality are confirmed by professional ethical rules, the common law, Québec's *Civil Code*, statute (particularly statutes such as Alberta's *Health Information Act*, R.S.A. 2000, c. H-5), and the *Canadian Charter of Rights and Freedoms* jurisprudence.

[25]   *Ibid.*, s. 35(1)(m).

[26]   *Smith v. Jones*, [1999] S.C.J. No. 15, [1999] 1 S.C.R. 455 at para. 77 (S.C.C.), *per* Cory J.; see W.N. Renke, "Secrets and Lives: The Public Safety Exception to Solicitor-Client Privilege — *Smith v. Jones*" (1999) 37 Alta. L. Rev. 1045.

[27]   *Smith v. Jones, ibid.*, at para. 44. The Supreme Court decision did not resolve the issue of whether disclosure was mandatory or discretionary. The British Columbia Court of Appeal had held that disclosure was discretionary only. The Supreme Court affirmed the Court of Appeal decision, with some variation, but did not comment on the discretionary nature of

Additional common law authority may support a discretion to disclose information to avoid a "miscarriage of justice". For example, an accused may be at risk of conviction on the basis of the testimony of a witness who is known to the caregiver. The caregiver may have information that the witness is unreliable, for medical or psychiatric reasons, but neither the prosecution nor the defence have this information. The caregiver, then, may be entitled to disclose the information to the Crown or defence or both, "to follow the matter up and clear the air".[28]

The *Health Information Act* was amended in 2006 to provide additional broader discretion to disclose. Section 37.3 provides as follows:

(1) A custodian may disclose individually identifying health information referred to in subsection (2) without the consent of the individual who is the subject of the information to a police service or the Minister of Justice and Attorney General where the custodian reasonably believes

    (a)   that the information relates to the possible commission of an offence under a statute or regulation of Alberta or Canada, and

    (b)   that the disclosure will protect the health and safety of Albertans.

(2) A custodian may disclose the following information under subsection (1):

    (a)   the name of an individual;

    (b)   the date of birth of an individual;

    (c)   the nature of any injury or illness of an individual;

    (d)   the date on which a health service was sought or received by an individual;

    (e)   the location where an individual sought or received a health service;

    (f)   whether any samples of bodily substances were taken from an individual.

(3) If a custodian discloses individually identifying health information about an individual under subsection (1), the custodian may also disclose health services provider information about a health services provider from whom that individual sought or received health services if that information is related to the information that was disclosed under subsection (1).

(4) Health services provider information may be disclosed under subsection (3) without the consent of the health services provider who is the subject of the information.

Bailey and Penney have observed that the legislation provides no concrete guidance respecting the determinations of whether there are grounds to believe that an offence has occurred, whether disclosure will "protect the health and safety of Albertans", or how much information to

---

disclosure. Hence, arguably, the Supreme Court approved of and implicitly confirmed the Court of Appeal's view.

[28] *R. v. Ross*, [1993] N.S.J. No. 18, 79 C.C.C. (3d) 253 at 255 (N.S.C.A.), *per* Chipman J.A.

disclose. They are also concerned that the legislation is not valid, since it arguably infringes s. 8 of the *Charter* and is legislation outside of provincial legislative competence respecting health.[29]

(ii) Mandatory Disclosure

Caregivers may be obligated by statute to disclose information concerning offence-related matters to public authorities. For example, under s. 4(1) of Alberta's *Child, Youth and Family Enhancement Act*, "[a]ny person who has reasonable and probable grounds to believe that a child is in need of intervention shall forthwith report the matter to a director [designated under the Act]". This legislation requires caregivers to report (*inter alia*) child abuse, including physical injury, sexual abuse, and emotional abuse.[30] Disclosure is required, "notwithstanding that the information on which the belief is founded is confidential and its disclosure is prohibited under any other Act".[31] Similarly, under Alberta's *Protection for Persons in Care Act*, "[e]very individual or service provider who has reasonable and probable grounds to believe and believes that there is or has been abuse against a client shall report that abuse to the Minister or a police service or a committee, body or person authorized under another enactment to investigate such an abuse".[32] Again, disclosure is required, despite the confidentiality of the information or prohibitions on disclosure under other statutes.[33] Public health legislation, such as Alberta's *Public Health Act*,[34] may require the reporting of prescribed communicable diseases:

> Where a health practitioner, a teacher or a person in charge of an institution knows or has reason to believe that a person under the care, custody, supervision or control of the health practitioner, teacher or person in charge of an institution is infected with a communicable disease prescribed in the regulations . . . [he or she] shall notify the medical officer of health of the regional health authority . . . .[35]

---

[29] T.M. Bailey & S. Penney, "Healing, not Squealing: Recent Amendments to Alberta's Health Information Act" (2007) 15:2 Health Law Rev. 3, at paras. 12 and 13, 17 and 22.

[30] *Child, Youth and Family Enhancement Act*, R.S.A. 2000, c. C-12 (which reflects the amendments made by S.A. 2003, c. 16). For a more detailed discussion, see W.N. Renke, "Mandatory Reporting of Child Abuse Under the Child Welfare Act" (1999) 7 Health L.J. 91.

[31] *Child, Youth and Family Enhancement Act, ibid.*, s. 4(2). Lawyers alone receive an exemption — "This section does not apply to information that is privileged as a result of a solicitor-client relationship": *ibid.*, s. 4(3).

[32] R.S.A. 2000, c. P-29, s. 2(1).

[33] *Ibid.*, s. 2(2).

[34] R.S.A. 2000, c. P-37.

[35] *Ibid.*, s. 22(1).

Alberta's *Fatality Inquiries Act* requires the medical examiner or an investigator to be notified of deaths that occur under specified circumstances or in specified places.[36]

Ontario recently enacted legislation requiring medical facilities (through prescribed persons) to disclose information respecting gunshot wounds.[37] Saskatchewan broadened the disclosure requirement to include information respecting stabbings.[38] In a parallel Alberta development, the Select Special Health Information Act Review Committee recommended in its October 2004 Report that legislation be enacted in Alberta to require the reporting of gunshot wounds, stabbings and serious beatings.[39] To date, no Alberta legislation has taken up this specific recommendation.[40]

Three observations respecting mandatory reporting obligations are warranted.

First, mandatory reporting obligations established by provinces are province-specific — the obligations attach only in the province that has legislated the obligation. Hence, caregivers in provinces other than Ontario and Saskatchewan are not (yet) obligated to report information respecting gunshot wounds, stabbings, serious beatings of non-institutionalized adults or drug overdoses. This may come as a surprise. Legislation in 48 states requires gunshot wound reporting. While caregivers might gain the impression that they are required to report gunshot wounds from the popular media, American colleagues, or practice in the United States, this is not the law in every Canadian province.

Second, the obligations are engaged only in specific circumstances, in relation to specific types of conduct or specific types of infection. Reporting is mandatory if the defined circumstances obtain, but not otherwise. More extensive mandatory reporting obligations may be on the horizon; but for now, mandatory reporting is required only in limited circumstances.

Third, the specification of the recipient of the information is important. Reports of child abuse are made to the child welfare

---

[36]   R.S.A. 2000, c. F-9, ss. 10-13.

[37]   *Mandatory Gunshot Wounds Reporting Act, 2005*, S.O. 2005, c. 9, s. 2.

[38]   *The Gunshot and Stab Wounds Mandatory Reporting Act*, S.S. 2007, c. G-9.1.

[39]   Alberta, Select Special Health Information Act Review Committee, *Final Report* (October 2004) (Chair: Broyce Jacobs), online: <http://www.assembly.ab.ca/HIAReview/hiawebreport.pdf>.

[40]   This mandatory reporting legislation could be challenged as unjustifiably violating *Charter*-based privacy protections, or on division of powers grounds as an unauthorized venture by provinces into the realm of federal criminal law and procedure. On this latter point, the provinces might reply that the legislation is sustained under provincial authority respecting the administration of justice in the province. See W.N. Renke, "The Constitutionality of Mandatory Reporting of Gunshot Wounds Legislation" (2005) 14:1 Health Law Rev. 3.

authorities. Reports of communicable disease are made to public health authorities. Abuse of persons in care may be reported to institutional or Ministerial authorities — but also to the police. In the child abuse and communicable disease cases, and in some abuse of persons in care cases, the information is not or is at least not directly provided to the police.

(b)   Disclosure in Response to a Request, Without a Warrant

The police may attend at a public health facility seeking information about a patient, without a warrant. While the fundamental stance of caregivers should be to refuse the request, in some instances, disclosure may be permissible.

(i)   No-Request Discretionary and Mandatory Disclosure Provisions

Section 37.3 of Alberta's *Health Information Act*, along with the disclosure provisions described in the previous section, may permit disclosure to the police upon request, if the police are specified as authorized recipients of the information.

(ii)   Fatalities

Under s. 9 of Alberta's *Fatality Inquiries Act*, police officers (including members of the R.C.M.P. and municipal police services) are medical examiners' investigators. Under s. 21(1),

> A medical examiner or an investigator acting under the medical examiner's authorization may, in performing the medical examiner's or investigator's duties under this Act,
>
> > (a)   without a warrant, enter any place where the medical examiner or investigator believes, on reasonable and probable grounds, a body that is the subject of an investigation is located or has been located;
> >
> > (b)   without a warrant, take possession of anything that may be directly related to the death and may place anything seized into the custody of a peace officer . . . .

Under s. 21(3),

> Notwithstanding any other Act, regulation or other law, a medical examiner is entitled to inspect and make copies of any diagnosis, record or information relating to
>
> > (*a*)   a person receiving diagnostic and treatment services in a diagnostic and treatment centre under the *Mental Health Act*, or
> >
> > (*b*)   a patient under the *Hospitals Act*.

Officials acting under this authority are entitled to information and to seize things. Obstruction of an investigator is an offence under the Act[41] and could amount to obstruction of justice under the *Criminal Code*.[42]

(iii) Warrantless Search and Seizure Incident to Arrest

In some limited circumstances, the police are entitled to search for and seize evidence, without a warrant. The main type of legitimate warrantless search likely to confront caregivers is the right of the police to search a person, without a warrant, as an incident of arrest. The law permits a search of the person, and, in some cases, the person's immediate surroundings, to guarantee the safety of the police and the suspect, to prevent the suspect's escape and to gather and preserve evidence.[43] This warrantless search power, however, should not entitle the police to search for or seize a patient's chart or other health information.

The police are entitled to request assistance in effecting an arrest, and a failure to assist may be an offence: "Every one who . . . omits, without reasonable excuse, to assist a . . . peace officer in the execution of his duty in arresting a person . . . after having reasonable notice that he is required to do so . . . is guilty of [an offence] . . . ."[44] A distinction may be drawn between assisting in an arrest and assisting in a search incident to an arrest. If a caregiver were to decline to assist respecting the latter, it is at least possible that he or she would avoid liability, although this argument has not been considered in the cases. If a caregiver were to assist a peace officer, so long as the caregiver acted on reasonable grounds, he or she would be "justified in doing what he is required or

---

[41]   *Fatality Inquiries Act*, R.S.A. 2000, c. F-9, s. 24.

[42]   *Criminal Code*, R.S.C. 1985, c. C-46, s. 139.

[43]   *Cloutier v. Langlois*, [1990] S.C.J. No. 10, [1990] 1 S.C.R. 158 (S.C.C.); *R. v. Caslake*, [1998] S.C.J. No. 3, [1998] 1 S.C.R. 51 (S.C.C.); *R. v. Golden*, [2001] S.C.J. No. 81, [2001] 3 S.C.R. 679 (S.C.C.). Warrantless search may also be an incident of "investigative detention", as explained by Iacobucci J. in the *Mann* case: "[P]olice officers may detain an individual for investigative purposes if there are reasonable grounds to suspect in all the circumstances that the individual is connected to a particular crime and that such a detention is necessary. In addition, where a police officer has reasonable grounds to believe that his or her safety or that of others is at risk, the officer may engage in a protective pat-down search of the detained individual. Both the detention and the pat-down search must be conducted in a reasonable manner. In this connection, I note that the investigative detention should be brief in duration and does not impose an obligation on the detained individual to answer questions posed by the police. The investigative detention and protective search power are to be distinguished from an arrest and the incidental power to search on arrest . . .": *R. v. Mann*, [2004] S.C.J. No. 49, 2004 SCC 52 at para. 45 (S.C.C.). This warrantless search authority would not attract the involvement of caregivers.

[44]   *Criminal Code*, R.S.C. 1985, c. C-46, s. 129(*b*).

authorized to do and in using as much force as is necessary for that purpose"[45] — thereby avoiding criminal or civil liability.

(iv)   Body Cavity Searches

A particularly unpleasant species of warrantless search is the body cavity search. The police may urge caregivers to assist with body cavity searches incident to arrest. It is not clear whether a warrantless body cavity search is permissible at all under s. 8 of the *Charter*, particularly because it involves serious interference with bodily integrity. In the pre-*Charter* era, body cavity searches were countenanced as a form of warrantless search incident to arrest.[46] In *Stillman*, however, the Supreme Court held that the seizure of bodily samples for DNA analysis — involving only minor physical intrusion — fell outside the legitimate scope of warrantless search incident to arrest.[47] *Stillman* might be taken to have decided that warrantless body cavity searches incident to arrest are constitutionally impermissible, at least outside special contexts such as border crossings.[48] Nonetheless, in the later *Golden* case, the Supreme Court appeared to open the constitutional possibility of this sort of warrantless search, although the Court did indicate that a high level of justification would be required and the search would have to be conducted in a very sensitive manner — possibly in a medical facility.[49] The dangers of participating in this fortunately rare type of search are illustrated in the *Nagy* case, in which a passenger who arrived at the Edmonton International Airport was strip-searched, arrested and subjected to invasive bodily searches — all without warrant and all, as it was found, without reasonable grounds. A police officer was found civilly liable for the unlawful search and false imprisonment, while the physician who

---

[45] *Ibid.*, s. 25(1).

[46] *Reynen v. Antonenko*, [1975] A.J. No. 428, 20 C.C.C. (2d) 342 (Alta. T.D.).

[47] *R. v. Stillman*, [1997] S.C.J. No. 34, [1997] 1 S.C.R. 607 at paras. 42-43 (S.C.C.), *per* Cory J.

[48] The Supreme Court has not ruled out the permissibility of body cavity searches in the border crossing context, although it has not yet specified the standards that must be met for such searches to be legal: "it is obvious that the greater the intrusion, the greater must be the justification and the greater the degree of constitutional protection": *R. v. Simmons*, [1988] S.C.J. No. 86, [1988] 2 S.C.R. 495 at para. 28 (S.C.C.), *per* Dickson C.J.C.; see *R. v. Monney*, [1999] S.C.J. No. 18, [1999] 1 S.C.R. 652 at para. 38 (S.C.C.), *per* Iacobucci J. Another context in which warrantless bodily cavity searches are permissible is in association with entry to federal penitentiaries, at least if visitors are notified that they are subject to drug searches: *R. v. Vandenbosch*, [2007] M.J. No. 346, 2007 MBCA 113 (Man. C.A.), leave to appeal to S.C.C. refused [2007] S.C.C.A. No. 554 (S.C.C.), Bulletin of Proceedings (15 February 2008), no. 32356, online: Lexum (University of Montreal) <http://scc.lexum. umontreal.ca/en/bulletin/2008/08-02-15.bul/08-02-15.bul.html>.

[49] *R. v. Golden*, [2001] S.C.J. No. 81 at paras. 87, 101 (S.C.C.), *per* Iacobucci and Arbour JJ.

conducted the bodily searches was found civilly liable for assault and battery.[50]

Since the legitimacy of this type of search is not clear, neither is it clear whether a failure to assist an officer with such a search would constitute obstruction under s. 129(*b*) of the *Criminal Code*; or whether, if assistance were provided, s. 25 of the *Criminal Code* would protect from criminal and civil liability.

(v)   Blood Sample Upon Demand

Under s. 254(3) of the *Criminal Code*,

> Where a peace officer believes on reasonable and probable grounds that a person is committing, or at any time within the preceding three hours has committed, as a result of the consumption of alcohol, an offence under s. 253,[51] the peace officer may, by demand made to that person forthwith or as soon as practicable, require that person to provide then or as soon thereafter as is practicable . . .
>
> (*b*) where the peace officer has reasonable and probable grounds to believe that, by reason of the physical condition of the person,
>
>> (i) the person may be incapable of providing a sample of his breath, or
>>
>> (ii) it would be impracticable to obtain a sample of his breath,
>>
>> such samples of the person's blood . . . as in the opinion of the qualified medical practitioner or qualified technician taking the samples
>
> are necessary to enable proper analysis to be made in order to determine the concentration, if any, of alcohol in the person's blood, and to accompany the peace officer for the purpose of enabling such samples to be taken.

The term "qualified medical practitioner" is defined by s. 254(1) to mean "a person duly qualified by provincial law to practise medicine". Pursuant to s. 254(3), a qualified caregiver could be requested by a police officer to take a suspect's blood for testing in relation to an intoxicated driving offence. In this type of case, the suspect does not object to the testing, but the suspect does not (strictly speaking) "consent", since

---

[50]   *Nagy v. Canada*, [2005] A.J. No. 36, 2005 ABQB 26 (Alta. Q.B.), *per* Ouellette J., aff'd [2006] A.J. No. 1020, 2006 ABCA 227 (Alta. C.A.), *per* Ritter J.A.

[51]   Generally, operation of a vehicle while impaired by alcohol or a drug, or with an alcohol/blood concentration exceeding 80 milligrams of alcohol in 100 millilitres of blood.

refusing to comply is an offence and compliance is therefore not voluntary or free from coercion.[52]

A "qualified medical practitioner" is not guilty of an offence only because he or she refuses to take a sample of blood under s. 254 — that is, a caregiver may refuse to take the sample, without being guilty of obstruction.[53] If the caregiver uses reasonable care and skill in taking blood, he or she is protected from criminal and civil liability.[54]

(c)   Disclosure in Response to a Warrant

If the police have a warrant,[55] the simple rule is that caregivers should co-operate with the police and deliver up the required information or things. Under s. 35(1)(i) of Alberta's *Health Information Act*, a custodian may disclose health information without consent "for the purpose of complying with a subpoena, warrant or order issued or made by a court, person or body having jurisdiction in Alberta to compel the production of information or with a rule of court binding in Alberta that relates to the production of information".[56] Of course, a caregiver (or supervisor on site) should read the warrant, and confirm that the document is indeed a warrant, that it has not expired, that it authorizes search and seizure at the relevant location, and that it authorizes the search for and seizure of the type of things or information claimed by the police.

---

[52] *Criminal Code*, R.S.C. 1985, c. C-46, s. 254(5).

[53] *Ibid.*, s. 257(1).

[54] *Ibid.*, s. 257(2).

[55] A warrant is an official court document issued by a "justice" — a justice of the peace or provincial court judge. A warrant is applied for by a peace officer, on the basis of (usually) a written and sworn "information". Under s. 487(1) of the *Criminal Code, ibid.*, the informant must provide evidence that there are reasonable grounds to believe that (*inter alia*) there is in a building, receptacle or place "(*a*) anything on or in respect of which any offence against [the *Criminal Code*] or any other Act of Parliament has been or is suspected to have been committed, [or] (*b*) anything that there are reasonable grounds to believe will afford evidence with respect to the commission of an offence . . .". If the justice is satisfied that reasonable grounds have been established, the justice may, in his or her discretion, issue the warrant, authorizing a named person or peace officer to search the building, receptacle or place for the thing and to seize it, within a specified time, subject to any appropriate conditions. Subsection 29(1) of the *Criminal Code, ibid.*, provides that "[i]t is the duty of every one who executes a . . . warrant to have it with him, where it is feasible to do so, and to produce it when requested to do so".

[56] The *Health Information Act*, R.S.A. 2000, c. H-5 "does not affect the power of any court or tribunal in Canada to compel a witness to testify or to compel the production of documents": s. 3(b).

(i)   Search Warrants

Compliance with a warrant issued under s. 487 of the *Criminal Code* may require the delivery up of physical objects or the disclosure of records. Warrants do not, however, require persons to provide information orally or to provide pre-trial testimony, sworn or unsworn.[57] A caregiver may be otherwise required to testify in a preliminary inquiry or at trial. This possibility will be considered below.

A warrant issued under s. 487 of the *Criminal Code* cannot authorize an intrusive or invasive bodily search. The human body is not a "building, receptacle or place", which alone may be searched pursuant to a s. 487 search warrant.[58] Bodily searches may, however, be authorized by warrant under other *Criminal Code* provisions, and caregivers may be requested to assist with these searches.

(ii)   Driving While Intoxicated Offences: Warrant for Blood Sample

Under s. 256(1) of the *Criminal Code*, if an informant satisfies a justice that a person has, within the preceding four hours, committed an offence under s. 253 and the person was in an accident resulting in the death of another or in bodily harm to himself or herself or another; and if a qualified medical practitioner has provided the opinion that the person is unable to consent to the taking of a blood sample and taking a sample would not endanger the person's life or health (thus rendering s. 254(3) unavailable), the justice may issue a warrant

> authorizing a peace officer to require a qualified medical practitioner to take, or to cause to be taken by a qualified technician under the direction of the qualified medical practitioner, the samples of the blood of the person that in the opinion of the person taking the samples are necessary to enable a proper analysis to be made in order to determine the concentration, if any, of alcohol or drugs in the person's blood.

Again, a caregiver's mere refusal to take a blood sample is not an offence.[59] And again, so long as the caregiver uses reasonable care and

---

[57] The only procedure in our criminal law that compelled testimony outside of trial or preliminary hearings was the former "investigative hearing" procedure, which applied respecting terrorism offences: *Criminal Code*, R.S.C. 1985, c. C-46, s. 83.28 (this provision expired in 2007, pursuant to s. 83.32).

[58] *Re Laporte and the Queen*, [1972] Q.J. No. 35, 29 D.L.R. (3d) 651 at 661-62 (Qué. Q.B.), *per* Hugessen J.; *R. v. S.A.B.*, [2003] S.C.J. No. 61, [2003] 2 S.C.R. 678 at paras. 41-42 (S.C.C.), *per* Arbour J.

[59] *Ibid.*, s. 257(1).

skill in taking a blood sample, he or she is protected from criminal and civil liability.[60]

(iii) Forensic DNA Analysis Warrant

The *Criminal Code* permits a warrant to be issued for the purpose of taking bodily samples for DNA analysis.[61] The results are used to determine whether a suspect was the perpetrator of a designated offence. Essentially, the warrant is to be used to collect bodily samples from a suspect so that, through analysis, the suspect's bodily samples may be compared with bodily samples found on the victim or at the crime scene (*i.e.*, a "match" is some evidence that the suspect was connected to the offence; the absence of a match excludes the suspect as the source of the bodily sample on the victim or at the crime scene). The *Criminal Code* establishes an interlocking scheme of definitions and ancillary provisions. Section 487.05 authorizes a provincial court judge, if satisfied that there are reasonable grounds to believe that certain criteria have been met, to issue a warrant for the taking of bodily substances by means of investigative procedures set out in s. 487.06(1):

> (*a*) the plucking of individual hairs from the person, including the root sheath;
>
> (*b*) the taking of buccal swabs by swabbing the lips, tongue and inside cheeks of the mouth to collect epithelial cells; or
>
> (*c*) the taking of blood by pricking the skin surface with a sterile lancet.

A caregiver could be requested to assist with these procedures. If he or she acts with reasonable care and skill, he or she is protected from criminal and civil liability.[62]

(iv) DNA Data Bank Orders and Authorizations

The *DNA Identification Act* came into force on June 30, 2000.[63] It establishes "a national DNA data bank to help law enforcement agencies identify persons alleged to have committed designated offences . . . ".[64] The data bank consists of a "crime scene index" and a "convicted

---

[60] *Ibid.*, s. 257(2).

[61] The forensic DNA provisions of the *Criminal Code, ibid.*, have been upheld as constitutional by the Supreme Court: *R. v. S.A.B.*, [2003] S.C.J. No. 61 (S.C.C.).

[62] *Criminal Code*, R.S.C. 1985, c. C-46, s. 487.058.

[63] S.C. 1998, c. 37; see *R. v. Briggs*, [2001] O.J. No. 3339, 157 C.C.C. (3d) 38 (Ont. C.A.), leave to appeal to S.C.C. refused [2002] S.C.C.A. No. 31 (S.C.C.); and *R. v. Ku*, [2002] B.C.J. No. 2316, 169 C.C.C. (3d) 535 (B.C.C.A.), leave to appeal refused [2002] S.C.C.A. No. 541 (S.C.C.), which upheld the constitutionality of the DNA order provisions.

[64] *DNA Identification Act, ibid.*, s. 3.

offenders index".[65] Generally, the crime scene index contains DNA profiles derived from bodily substances found at crime scenes or on victims;[66] the convicted offender index contains DNA profiles derived from bodily substances from convicted offenders.[67] The Commissioner of the R.C.M.P. is responsible for maintaining the data bank.[68] Only law enforcement agencies may submit profiles to and request information from the DNA data bank.[69] A comparison of the DNA profile of a perpetrator's bodily sample left at a crime scene with the crime scene index could show that one perpetrator is linked to multiple offences. A comparison of the DNA profile of a perpetrator's bodily sample with the convicted offender index could identify the suspect as a convicted offender. A comparison of the DNA profile of a convicted offender with the crime scene index could show that the offender is linked to other crimes. Under s. 6(1) of the *DNA Identification Act*, only the following types of information may be communicated to a requesting agency:

(*a*) if the DNA profile is not already contained in the data bank, the fact that it is not;

(*b*) if the DNA profile is already contained in the data bank, the information contained in the data bank in relation to that DNA profile;

(*c*) if the DNA profile is, in the opinion of the Commissioner, similar to one that is already contained in the data bank, the similar DNA profile; and

(*d*) if a law enforcement agency or laboratory advises the Commissioner that their comparison of a DNA profile communicated under paragraph (*c*) with one that is connected to the commission of a criminal offence has not excluded the former as a possible match, the information contained in the data bank in relation to that profile.

In the last type of comparison mentioned, the police would seek a forensic DNA warrant respecting the offender on the strength of the match to compare his or her profile with the crime scene index profile and thereby to establish that he or she was the perpetrator.

Caregivers could be requested to perform investigative procedures to gather DNA from convicted persons for analysis and ultimate submission to the DNA data bank convicted offender index. The specific statutory authority for the judicial order or authorization for testing (not, in these cases, a "warrant") depends on the nature of the offence for which the

---

[65]   *Ibid.*, s. 5(1).

[66]   *Ibid.*, s. 5(3).

[67]   *Ibid.*, s. 5(4).

[68]   *Ibid.*, s. 2, definition of "Commissioner".

[69]   *Ibid.*, s. 6.

offender was convicted,[70] and depends on some timing issues: whether the offender committed the offence or was sentenced or continues to serve his or her sentence before or after the *DNA Identification Act* came into force. Again, so long as the caregiver uses reasonable care and skill in taking bodily samples, he or she is protected from criminal and civil liability.[71]

(d) Disclosure to the Defence[72]

A caregiver may be contacted by defence counsel seeking information respecting a client (a suspect or an accused) or a third party (a complainant or witness). If the request concerns counsel's client, then counsel should have the client provide a consent for the disclosure of the information to the caregiver, following (any) standard procedures for the release of information to patients' own lawyers. If the request concerns information respecting a third party, the stance of caregivers should be the same as that respecting requests from the police: caregivers should refuse to provide the information, unless there is a legal requirement to provide the information.[73] While the defence (as a rule) cannot cause search warrants to be issued, the defence may apply for court orders compelling records custodians (such as caregivers and public health facilities) to disclose information concerning third parties. If the defence does obtain a court order compelling disclosure, caregivers should comply. For example, s. 35(1)(i) of Alberta's *Health Information Act* provides that a custodian may disclose health information without consent "for the purpose of complying with a subpoena, warrant or order issued or made by a court". Again, while compliance with the court order may entail the disclosure of records, the court order will not require caregivers to give information orally or to provide pre-trial testimony, sworn or unsworn.

Orders compelling caregivers or their facilities to disclose records relating to third parties are available to the defence in two main contexts — sexual offence cases and other cases. In both types of cases, caregivers or their facilities will be entitled to participate in the proceedings that determine whether an order will be granted.

---

[70]   See *Criminal Code*, R.S.C. 1985, c. C-46, s. 487.051 (offence committed after coming into force); *ibid.*, s. 487.052 (offence committed before coming into force, but accused convicted after coming into force); *ibid.*, s. 487.055 (accused convicted before coming into force, but continuing to serve sentence for certain offences).

[71]   *Ibid.*, s. 487.058.

[72]   See W.N. Renke, "Applications for Third-Party Records: The Relationship of the *O'Connor* Procedure to Other Application Procedures" (2002) 40 Alta. L. Rev. 593.

[73]   For a discussion of the issues and dangers surrounding physician interviews by defence counsel in civil (personal injury) cases, see *N.M. v Drew (Estate of)*, [2003] A.J. No. 962, 2003 ABCA 231 (Alta. C.A.), *per* Côté J.A.

(i)   Sexual Offence Cases[74]

Sections 278.1-278.91 of the *Criminal Code* establish a special procedure governing the production of records by custodians to accuseds (the "*Mills* procedure").[75] These rules apply to "records" relating to complainants or witnesses in proceedings respecting listed sexual offences.[76] Section 278.1 defines "record" as follows:

> For the purposes of section 278.2 to 278.9, "record" means any form of record[77] that contains personal information for which there is a reasonable expectation of privacy and includes, without limiting the generality of the foregoing, medical, psychiatric, therapeutic, counselling, education, employment, child welfare, adoption and social services records, personal journals and diaries, and records containing personal information the production or disclosure of which is protected by any other Act of Parliament or a provincial legislature, but does not include records made by persons responsible for the investigation or prosecution of the offence.

This definition captures health information records (as "medical, psychiatric, therapeutic, or counselling" records that contain "personal information"). Patients would have reasonable expectations of privacy respecting the information contained in the records. The disclosure of these records is statutorily protected — *e.g.*, by the *Health Information Act*.

An accused must bring the application for production before the trial judge.[78] The application must be in writing, and must set out

(*a*) particulars identifying the record that the accused seeks to have produced and the name of the person who has possession or control of the record; and

---

[74]   For more extensive discussions, see J. Koshan, "Disclosure and Production in Sexual Violence Cases: Situating *Stinchcombe*" (2002) 40 Alta. L. Rev. 655; S. Coughlan, "Complainants' Records After *Mills*: Same As It Ever Was" (2000) 33 C.R. (5th) 300; and W.N. Renke, "Unbalanced Balancing: Bill C-46, 'Likely Relevance,' and Stage-One Balancing" (2000) 11:3 Const. Forum Const. 85.

[75]   This procedure was held to be constitutional in *R. v. Mills*, [1999] S.C.J. No. 68, [1999] 3 S.C.R. 668 (S.C.C.).

[76]   Paragraphs 278.2(1)(*a*)-(*c*) of the *Criminal Code*, R.S.C. 1985, c. C-46, provide the list, which includes sexual assault (s. 271), sexual assault causing bodily harm or with a weapon (s. 272), and aggravated sexual assault (s. 273); also included are any proceedings in respect of two or more offences that include an offence referred to in any of the paragraphs (*a*) to (*c*).

[77]   Including, for example, records in written, audio-visual tape, cassette audio tape, photograph, DVD, CD-ROM, or computer memory form.

[78]   *Criminal Code*, R.S.C. 1985, c. C-46, s. 278.3(1), (2).

(*b*) the grounds on which the accused relies to establish that the record is likely relevant to an issue at trial or to the competence of a witness to testify.[79]

The application must be served on the Crown, the record custodian, the complainant, and any other person to whom the record relates. At the time of serving the application, the accused must also serve a subpoena in Form 16.1 on the record custodian.[80] The application has two stages.

At the first stage, the judge determines in an *in camera* hearing whether to order the record custodian to produce the record to the court for review. The record custodian, the complainant, and any other person to whom the record relates have standing in the hearing, but are neither compellable nor subject to an order for costs.[81] The judge may order production for review if the application was formally correct, if the accused has established that "the record is likely relevant to an issue at trial or to the competence of a witness to testify",[82] and if "the production of the record is necessary in the interests of justice".[83]

If the judge does not order production to the court for review, the application is at an end. If the judge does order production to the court, the application moves to the second stage. In an *in camera* hearing, the judge reviews the record in question and determines whether all or part of it should be produced to the accused.[84] The stage one tests — "likely relevance" and "necessary to the interests of justice" — apply at stage two, and the factors considered at stage one are considered at stage two, but now in light of the actual record before the court.[85]

If the judge orders production of the record to the accused, the judge may impose conditions to protect the interests of justice and the privacy and equality of the complainant.[86] The judge must provide reasons for ordering or refusing to order production to the court, and for ordering or refusing to order production to the accused.[87] For the purposes of an

---

[79] *Ibid.*, s. 278.3(3).

[80] *Ibid.*, s. 278.3(5), (6).

[81] *Ibid.*, s. 278.4(1), (2), (3).

[82] Subsection 278.3(4) of the *Criminal Code, ibid.*, sets out "mere assertions" which, either alone or together, do not establish "likely relevance". The point of these provisions is to bar production on the basis of mere speculation, when there is no evidence that records contain relevant information.

[83] *Ibid.*, s. 278.5(1). Subsection 278.5(2) sets out a list of factors to be considered in determining whether to order production to the court.

[84] *Ibid.*, s. 278.6(1), (2), (3).

[85] *Ibid.*, s. 287.7(1), (2).

[86] *Ibid.*, s. 287.7(3). The judge shall also direct that a copy of the record be provided to the Crown, "unless the judge determines that it is not in the interests of justice to do so": *ibid.*, s. 278.7(4).

[87] *Ibid.*, s. 278.8.

appeal by the Crown or accused, the judge's rulings are questions of law and would be appealed to the court of appeal along with other trial issues.[88] Custodians should be entitled to seek leave to appeal directly to the Supreme Court of Canada, under s. 40(1) of the *Supreme Court Act*.[89]

(ii) Cases Involving Non-sexual Offences

In *R. v. O'Connor*,[90] the Supreme Court of Canada established a procedure for accuseds to apply for the production of records held by record custodians. When this case was decided, no settled common law or statutory procedures permitted defence counsel to obtain pre-trial production of records from custodians. The *Mills* procedure was established after *O'Connor*. The *Mills* procedure leaves the *O'Connor* procedure available for proceedings respecting offences other than the listed sexual offences (*e.g.*, murder, manslaughter, aggravated assault, or assault with a weapon) — so long as the subject of the records has a reasonable expectation of privacy respecting the information contained in those records, and no other production procedure governs.[91]

An *O'Connor* production application should be made to the trial judge.[92] Ordinarily, the accused initiates the application by serving a *subpoena duces tecum* on the record custodian and an application for production on the Crown, the record custodian, and on all persons having privacy interests in the records, supported by an affidavit setting out the grounds for production.[93] *O'Connor* did not specify the notice period.[94] Should justice and the circumstances so dictate, the judge may waive the written application requirement.[95]

[88]   *Ibid.*, s. 278.91.
[89]   R.S.C. 1985, c. S-26; *L.L.A. v. A.B.*, [1995] S.C.J. No. 102, [1995] 4 S.C.R. 536 (S.C.C.).
[90]   [1995] S.C.J. No. 98, [1995] 4 S.C.R. 411, 103 C.C.C. (3d) 1 (S.C.C.) ["*O'Connor*" cited to C.C.C.]. On the production issue, Lamer C.J.C. and Sopinka J. (in a joint decision) wrote for the majority, Cory, Iacobucci and Major JJ. concurring. For further discussion, see W.N. Renke, "Applications for Third-Party Records: The Relationship of the *O'Connor* Procedure to Other Application Procedures" (2002) 40 Alta. L. Rev. 593.
[91]   *R. v. Hunter*, [2000] A.J. No. 656 at para. 20 (Alta. Prov. Ct. (Crim. Div.)), *per* Allen Prov. Ct. J.; *R. v. Zhang*, [2001] A.J. No. 824 (Alta. Prov. Ct. (Crim. Div.)), *per* Lefever Prov. Ct. J.; *R. v. Szczerba*, [2002] A.J. No. 915 at para. 4 (Alta. Q.B.), *per* Rooke J.; *R. v. B.M.*, [1998] O.J. No. 4359, 42 O.R. (3d) 1 (Ont. C.A.), *per* Rosenberg J.A.
[92]   And not to a motions judge or a preliminary inquiry justice: *R. v. O'Connor*, [1995] S.C.J. No. 98, 103 C.C.C. (3d) 1 at 19, 72, 75 (S.C.C.). The application should be made before the empanelling of the jury, along with other pre-trial motions: *ibid.*, at 19.
[93]   *Ibid.*, at 19 (103 C.C.C.).
[94]   The general civil rule (*e.g.*, two clear days' notice) could serve as a guideline: *Alberta Rules of Court*, Reg. 390/68, r. 386.
[95]   *R. v. O'Connor*, [1995] S.C.J. No. 98, 103 C.C.C. (3d) 1 at 18 (S.C.C.).

A *voir dire* is not always necessary. In appropriate cases, the application may be decided on the basis of counsels' submissions. If a *voir dire* is held, *viva voce* evidence may be tendered. The *O'Connor* majority did not decide whether a complainant, record custodian, or other witness is compellable in the application.[96] Even if they are compellable, none could be examined on the contents of the records, since whether those records are to be produced to the accused is the subject of the production application. The examination may only concern general matters, such as the existence or the timing of creation of the records.[97]

As in the *Mills* procedure, the application has two stages. The accused bears the burden of proof at each stage.[98] At the first stage, the accused must satisfy the judge that the records sought are likely to contain information relevant to the "issues in the case" or the competence of witnesses.[99] What the accused must establish is a "reasonable possibility", based on evidence, that the records contain relevant (but not necessarily technically admissible) information.[100] If an accused fails to establish likely relevance, the application is at an end. If the accused succeeds, the judge compels production of the records to the court, to determine whether production to the accused is warranted.

At the second stage, the judge has the records but the records are not provided to the accused or Crown.[101] The judge is to examine the records. In light of the records and the parties' submissions, the judge must balance the salutary and deleterious effects of production, consider whether denying the production "would constitute a reasonable limit on the ability of the accused to make full answer and defence",[102] and

---

[96]   For the court to compel a potential witness to testify, the party proposing to call the witness must establish that the potential witness is likely to be able to testify to material evidence: *R. v. Trang*, [2002] A.J. No. 1008, 2002 ABQB 744 at paras. 379-81 (Alta. Q.B.), *per* Binder J., rev'd on other grounds, [2007] A.J. No. 907, 2007 ABCA 263 (*sub nom. Trang v. Alberta (Edmonton Remand Centre)*) (Alta. C.A.), leave to appeal refused [2007] S.C.C.A. No. 525 (S.C.C.), Bulletin of Proceedings (22 February 2008), no. 32310, online: Lexum (University of Montreal) <http://scc.lexum.umontreal.ca/en/bulletin/2008/08-02-25.bul/08-02-25.bul.pdf>.

[97]   Respecting permissible questioning of a complainant or witness in a preliminary inquiry, see *R. v. B. (E.)*, [2002] O.J. No. 75 at paras. 40, 61 (Ont. C.A.), *per* Cronk J.A., leave to appeal to S.C.C. refused [2002] S.C.C.A. No. 94 (S.C.C.).

[98]   *R. v. O'Connor*, [1995] S.C.J. No. 98, 103 C.C.C. (3d) 1 at 18 (S.C.C.).

[99]   *Ibid.*, at 19. The accused's burden on the "likely relevance" issue should not be understood as "onerous". The reason for imposing this burden is to prevent the accused from engaging in "speculative, fanciful, disruptive, unmeritorious, obstructive and time-consuming requests for production": *ibid.*, at 20.

[100] *Ibid.*, at 19. "Relevance" means "logical relevance" to a fact-in-issue in the litigation: and entails that the information is more than merely "useful" to the accused: *ibid.*

[101] To facilitate argument, the judge might provide a judicial summary of the records to the parties: *ibid.*, at 23.

[102] *Ibid.*

determine whether and to what extent the records should be produced.[103] The *O'Connor* majority ruled that the judge should consider the following factors in the balancing:

(a)   the extent to which the record is necessary for the accused to make full answer and defence;

(b)   the probative value of the record;

(c)   the nature and extent of the reasonable expectation of privacy vested in the record;

(d)   whether the production of the record would be premised on any discriminatory belief or bias; and

(e)   the potential prejudice to the complainant's dignity, privacy or security of the person that would be occasioned by the production to the accused.[104]

Appeals from *O'Connor* procedure decisions take the following routes: A party to the proceedings must await the end of the trial to appeal to the court of appeal, and thereafter to the Supreme Court. Third parties, such as complainants or record custodians have different options. If the trial judge was a provincial court judge, his or her decision is reviewable through *certiorari* in the superior court (in Alberta, the Court of Queen's Bench). If the trial judge was a superior court judge, third parties may seek leave to appeal directly to the Supreme Court, under s. 40(1) of the *Supreme Court Act*.

(e) Caregivers as Witnesses

Caregivers may be called as witnesses in a preliminary inquiry or criminal trial and may be asked to testify respecting patients' health information or other personal information. They may attend voluntarily, upon request by either side, or they may be compelled to attend and provide evidence on being served with a *subpoena*.[105] The information

---

[103]   *Ibid.*

[104]   *Ibid.*, at 23-24, 69. The dissent urged three further considerations: the extent to which production would frustrate society's interest in encouraging the reporting of sexual offences; the extent to which production would frustrate society's interest in encouraging the acquisition of treatment by victims; and the effect of producing or failing to produce the record on the integrity of the trial process: *ibid.*, at 69. In the majority's opinion, the first two considerations could be addressed through the imposition of conditions on production: *ibid.*, at 24. For example, the court might impose a ban on the publication of the record, restrict the persons to whom the record may be disclosed, or restrict the making of copies: *ibid.* The "integrity of the trial process", in the majority's estimation, is a matter to be considered in relation to admissibility at trial, not production.

[105]   See *Criminal Code*, R.S.C. 1985, c. C-46, ss. 697-700.1.

held by the caregiver may have been gathered in medical settings or in the course of research.[106] Caregivers may contend that this information is confidential, and they should not be compelled to disclose this information. This raises the issue of testimonial "privilege".

Testimonial privileges are of two types — "class privileges" and "case-by-case" privileges. Class privileges are recognized for a very limited number of specific relationships. The main class privilege is "solicitor-client" privilege. Once the criteria for a class privilege are established[107] (on a balance of probabilities)[108] the court must recognize the privilege. A judge cannot compel a witness to disclose information falling within the scope of the privilege, unless an exception applies — and exceptions are interpreted strictly. Class privileges cannot be abridged through judicial discretion, or through any procedure involving a balancing of interests (as in the *O'Connor* and *Mills* procedures).[109] It may come as a surprise that public health professionals are not covered by class privilege in criminal cases.

If a caregiver has any privilege to rely on at all, it is "case-by-case" privilege. This type of privilege applies to an open-ended list of relationships, typically officially sanctioned professional "service-provider"-client relationships. Whether or not communications made within these relationships will be compelled to be disclosed depends on the judicial assessment of factors on a case-by-case basis. The person seeking to rely on the privilege bears the burden of establishing that the criteria are satisfied in the particular case.[110] The over-arching test judges employ to determine whether privilege should be recognized is known as the "Wigmore test",[111] which requires the following four criteria to be satisfied:

---

[106] See *Ogden v. Simon Fraser University*, [1998] B.C.J. No. 2288 (B.C. Prov. Ct. (Sm. Cl. Div.)), respecting a euthanasia researcher subpoenaed to appear at a coroner's inquest. This case generated significant controversy at Simon Fraser University. See T. Palys, "Russel Ogden v. SFU" [unpublished], online: Ted Palys, web page <http://www.sfu.ca/~palys/OgdenPge.htm>. See also T. Palys & J. Lowman, "Ethical and Legal Strategies for Protecting Confidential Research Information" (2000) 15 C.J.L.S. 39.

[107] For example, solicitor-client privilege applies to (i) communications, (ii) between solicitor and client, (iii) exchanged in any consultation for legal advice, (iv) if the communications were intended to be kept confidential: see *R. v. Campbell and Shirose*, [1999] S.C.J. No. 16, [1999] 1 S.C.R. 565 at para. 49 (S.C.C.), *per* Binnie J.

[108] *R. v. Trang*, [2002] A.J. No. 1008, at paras. 362-63 (Alta. Q.B.).

[109] *R. v. Leipert*, [1997] S.C.J. No. 14, [1997] 1 S.C.R. 281 at paras. 9-14 (S.C.C.), *per* McLachlin J. (as she then was).

[110] *R. v. Zhang*, [2002] A.J. No. 331 at para. 34 (Alta. Prov. Ct. (Crim. Div.)), *per* Lefever Prov. Ct. J., var'd [2002] A.J. No. 530 (Alta. Prov. Ct. (Crim. Div.)).

[111] See *A.M. v. Ryan*, [1997] S.C.J. No. 13, [1997] 1 S.C.R. 157 (S.C.C.), in which psychiatric records respecting a plaintiff in a civil case were ordered disclosed.

(a)   the communications must have originated in a confidence that they would not be disclosed;

(b)   confidentiality must be essential to the full and satisfactory relationship between the parties;

(c)   the relationship must be one which in the opinion of the community should be fostered and promoted; and

(d)   the injury that would be caused to the relationship by disclosure of the communications would exceed the benefit gained for the litigation by the disclosure of the information.

In health care or research contexts, the first three criteria would typically be relatively easy to satisfy. The last criterion causes difficulties. Its application involves a cost-benefit analysis and a balancing of interests — a weighing of the personal and social consequences of disclosure against the interests of the justice system in arriving at an accurate assessment of the facts. The factors considered are similar to those considered in *O'Connor* and the *Mills* procedures. Since in any particular case the interests in disclosure may be found to outweigh the interests in non-disclosure, no caregiver can ever guarantee that privilege will be recognized and confidentiality will be protected. If a judge does require a caregiver to disclose a communication, the caregiver could nonetheless refuse to disclose — and suffer the consequences of being held in contempt of court.

III. PUBLIC HEALTH APPROACHES IN CRIMINAL JUSTICE PROCESSES

The previous section left open the issue of the types of (alleged) offences that caregivers are likely to encounter, putting them in possession of information sought by the criminal justice system. Because the criminal law has the promotion of health as one of its proper objects, it is inevitable that caregivers would encounter some conduct with adverse public health impacts that is subject to criminal prohibitions. Many offences that are the grist for day-to-day criminal justice processing have public health aspects. These include impaired driving and driving with excessive blood/alcohol content offences, some drug offences, and offences concerning family violence. Not without controversy, individuals have been charged with violence offences (*e.g.*, assault, aggravated assault or sexual assault) in circumstances involving the transmission of communicable diseases.[112]

---

[112]   In *Cuerrier*, the Supreme Court held that non-disclosure of HIV-positive status may be a type of "fraud" that vitiates consent to unprotected sexual intercourse, transforming an ostensibly consensual act into an assault offence (the non-disclosure must have exposed the

But despite the interest of the criminal law in public health, a reasonable observer might be forgiven for the observation that the everyday processing of public health related offences seems to have little to do with public health. Public health objectives, public health impacts, or public health strategies or tactics are seldom mentioned in busy docket or trial courts. One might respond that the criminal justice system is dealing with public health issues in its own way, using its tools of arrest, charging, trials, fines, imprisonment, and not-always-so-creative probation orders. Yet the reasonable observer might reply that in dealing with public health issues in its own way, the criminal justice system may be making things worse, or at least may be hampering efforts to reduce health risks.[113] The problem is not that standard criminal justice approaches should be abandoned; the problem is that, in some contexts, exclusive reliance on these approaches may create social costs that outweigh any benefits achieved.

Awareness of difficulties of the sort raised by the reasonable observer has been growing. The last several decades have witnessed an evolutionary (if not revolutionary) branching in the criminal justice system. The standard criminal justice responses to issues remain. The standard procedures, however, have become linked to other forms of intervention. These recent developments have six interlocking general features — reconceptualization, interdisciplinarity and collaboration, rehabilitative focus, contextualization, specialization, and meta-organization.

First, issues that (from a justice system perspective) had traditionally been conceptualized as issues of individual wrong doing, of anti-social

---

complainant to a risk of bodily harm, and it must be established that the complainant would have refused to have engaged in unprotected sexual intercourse if he or she had known of the accused's HIV-positive status): *R. v. Cuerrier*, [1998] S.C.J. No. 64, [1998] 2 S.C.R. 371 (S.C.C.); *R. v. Williams*, [2003] S.C.J. No. 41, [2003] 2 S.C.R. 134 (S.C.C.). For a detailed discussion, see Chapter 6, "HIV/AIDS and Public Health Law" in this volume. See also W.N. Renke, "Communicable Disease Exposure and Privacy Limitations: Issues Paper" (Paper presented to the Uniform Law Conference of Canada, Civil Division, 10-14 August 2003) Schedule A, online: Uniform Law Conference of Canada <http://www. chlc.ca/en/poam2/Communicable_Disease_Issues_En.pdf>.

[113]   This type of claim has been made in connection with the criminalization of the non-disclosure of HIV-positive status to sexual partners. Criminal prosecutions have been argued to be counterproductive; prosecution exacerbates disease transmission by undermining education, prevention, and care programs: *Handbook for Legislators on HIV/AIDS, Law and Human Rights*, UNAIDS/99.48E (Geneva, Switzerland: Joint United Nations Programme on HIV/AIDS (UNAIDS), November 1999) at 18, online: <http:// www.ipu.org/PDF/publications/aids_en.pdf>. See also Chapter 6, "HIV/AIDS and Public Health Law". Instead of prosecution, education, counselling and support for infected persons are argued to be preferable tactics: R. Elliott, "Criminal Law and HIV/AIDS: Strategic Considerations" (2000) 5:4 Can. HIV/AIDS Pol'y & L. Rev. 66 at 69.

behaviour warranting punishment, have been explicitly re-conceptualized as having social, health-related aspects.

Second, new forms of intervention are interdisciplinary and collaborative. They are based on the recognition by justice system participants — policy-makers, police, judges, prosecutors, defence counsel, probation officials, and correctional officials — that certain issues cannot be addressed adequately by standard approaches, that is, on the recognition that "one size does not fit all". Issues that come before the courts have come to be recognized as having causes and effects that fall outside the zone of legal relevance in litigation. They are recognized as demanding responses that lie outside the usual repertoire of punitive techniques.

This recognition of disciplinary limitation is linked to a recognition that better responses to the issues can only be achieved through interdisciplinary means — through the co-operation, co-ordination, and mutual reinforcement of justice system institutions and personnel, and external institutions and personnel. The importance and novelty of co-operation should not be underappreciated. Justice system stakeholders have tended to work in isolation from one another and from external agencies, in part as an institutional expression of our adversary system, in part to ensure fair treatment through independence (which forestalls some species of bias, partiality, and conflict of interest),[114] and in part as an aspect of the exclusiveness and territoriality of all disciplines and professions (particularly those in competition for public funds). Working in isolation has been a tendency not only of justice system stakeholders — relevant governmental Ministries and agencies (e.g., health, education, children's services, addictions) and non-governmental organizations have operated in silos of their own.

A further aspect of the shift in attention towards interdisciplinarity is the enhanced status granted to victims, to persons affected by antisocial behaviour. If a problem has multiple effects and linkages, and those effects and linkages involve individuals other than the state as prosecutor and the perpetrator as accused, and if the criminal justice system should be concerned with solving social problems, then those other individuals should be granted some standing or consideration in criminal justice system processes.

Third, in conjunction with their external partners, criminal justice participants incorporate treatment and prevention techniques into criminal justice processes. As indicated above, criminal justice as administered by

---

[114] M.M. Clarke, "Best Practices Review, 2nd Draft" (July 2003), prepared as part of the HomeFront evaluation conducted by Synergy Research Group [unpublished] at 73.

the courts has long had a "preventative" jurisdiction. This, though, has tended to be "negative" prevention, designed to stop individuals from doing prohibited acts. Negative prevention is now being supplemented by "positive" prevention, whereby individuals are assisted with transforming themselves and their circumstances, so that motivations for anti-social acts are (it is hoped) attenuated. In particular, again as indicated above, governments are now sponsoring a variety of crime prevention initiatives. These initiatives may operate entirely outside the formal justice system, as with family interventions, school programs, or social marketing campaigns against alcohol or drug abuse or participation in gangs; or even in the formal justice system.

Fourth, trials become explicitly contextualized, as one phase (and not always a necessary phase) in the co-operative co-ordinated response to issues. First contact between social issues and criminal justice occurs with the intervention of the police. Responses to the issues, then, begin with the police. Diversion of potential accuseds out of the system and into programs has become increasingly emphasized. Diversion may be established formally under the *Criminal Code*.[115] Less formally and in addition to this *Criminal Code* authority, peace officers have a discretion,

---

[115]   R.S.C. 1985, c. C-46. Subsection 717(1) creates diversion authority, described as "alternative measures".

Alternative measures may be used to deal with a person alleged to have committed an offence only if it is not inconsistent with the protection of society and the following conditions are met:

   (a)   the measures are part of a program of alternative measures authorized by the Attorney General [of the province] or the Attorney General's delegate or authorized by a person, or a person within a class of persons, designated by the lieutenant governor in council of a province;

   (b)   the person who is considering whether to use the measures is satisfied that they would be appropriate, having regard to the needs of the person alleged to have committed the offence and the interests of society and the victim;

   (c)   the person, having been informed of the alternative measures, fully and freely consents to participate therein;

   (d)   the person has, before consenting to participate in the alternative measures, been advised of the right to be represented by counsel;

   (e)   the person accepts responsibility for the act or omission that forms the basis of the offence that the person is alleged to have committed;

   (f)   there is, in the opinion of the Attorney General or the Attorney General's agent, sufficient evidence to proceed with the prosecution of the offence; and

   (g)   the prosecution is not in any way barred at law.

recognized at common law, not to charge individuals with offences.[116] The police may divert individuals to external agencies. With the assistance of Victims Services Units associated with police services, the police may also direct individuals affected by criminal acts to external agencies for help.

Even if an individual has not been diverted and is brought under the authority of the courts, the courts may offer programs (whether or not premised on a guilty plea) as alternatives to trial. External agencies may deliver the programs. The courts take on supervisory roles; judges become process managers.

Fifth, criminal justice institutions create specialized units. Again, the novelty and importance of specialization should not be underappreciated. The justice system as a whole and criminal justice more particularly have tended to have a generalist orientation. One of the hallmarks of our superior courts, for example, has been their generalist nature — a judge might hear applications in civil litigation matters one day, family law applications the next, and a criminal trial on the day following. In contrast, our provincial courts have tended to be organized into more specialized divisions — concerning, for example, civil litigation (with a maximum damages cap), criminal litigation, and youth and family litigation. Lawyers have become more specialized (although some law societies may not permit "specialist" designations). At least in large communities, most private lawyers who practise criminal law seriously will confine their practices to that area. Of course, prosecutors prosecute criminal offences. But all of this is still fairly unspecialized specialization — there are many different offences, involving many different types of accuseds and victims, arising out of many different types of social situations. Newer forms of institutional and professional specialization have become more focused.

Sixth, for the inter-institutional components of new initiatives to work, governance structures must exist that are distinct from the individual institutions. These structures are not necessarily "above" any of the institutional components; neither do these structures require command and control powers. In fact, what is more typical is that these structures have no formal authority over institutional components; they are organizations formed by representatives of stakeholder groups. What

---

[116] U.S. Department of Justice, *"Broken Windows" and Police Discretion* by G.L. Kelling (Washington, D.C.: National Institute of Justice Research Report, October 1999) at 22; A. Grant, *The Policy — A Policy Paper* (Ottawa: Law Reform Commission of Canada, 1980) at 5; P.C. Stenning, *Legal Status of Police* (Ottawa: Law Reform Commission of Canada, 1982) at 101, 131; Nova Scotia, Royal Commission on the Donald Marshall, Jr., Prosecution, *Volume I: Findings and Recommendations* (Halifax: Nova Scotia, 1989) at 231-32.

these structures must do is facilitate, co-ordinate, and encourage co-operation. These structures exist at local, provincial and federal levels. For example, the City of Grande Prairie, Alberta has established a Community Action on Crime Prevention organization, with participation from (among others) the R.C.M.P. detachment, local and provincial government agencies, the Chamber of Commerce, Native Counselling and the Western Cree Tribal Council, and the Crown Prosecutor's office.[117] As indicated above, Alberta has recently established the Safe Communities Secretariat, which involves the participation of nine government Ministries: Justice and Attorney General, Solicitor General and Public Security, Health and Wellness, Education, Children and Youth Services, Municipal Affairs, Aboriginal Relations, Housing and Urban Affairs, and Culture and Community Spirit.[118] The National Anti-Drug Strategy involves the co-operation of 11 federal Ministries and organizations: Justice, Health, Public Safety, Public Prosecutions, the R.C.M.P., the Border Services Agency, Correctional Service, Foreign Affairs and International Trade, Public Health, Public Works and Government Services, and Canada Revenue.[119]

It would be inaccurate to characterize these recent developments in the criminal justice system as "public health initiatives". These developments do, however, echo some public health themes and strategies: the understanding of issues as having social sources and social effects; the recognition of disciplinary limitation; the fundamental interdisciplinarity of responses to issues; and the focus on treatment and prevention, which often does incorporate health-related intervention.

These recent developments can be observed in cases involving family violence, mental illness and drug offences. One might immediately protest that this classification is arbitrary. Family, mental health and addictions issues are overlapping and inter-related. This is true. But the personal crises that bring individuals before the justice system tend to have a focus, and institutional responses must start somewhere. The classification should be regarded as a typology of institutional entry-points into broad-based personal, family and social problems. The description of the initiatives that follows is illustrative only — it is not and could not be exhaustive. There are simply too many relevant and innovative recent developments to recount here.

---

[117]   See City of Grande Prairie, Crime Prevention, online <http://www.cityofgp.com/citygov/initiatives/crime/default.htm>.

[118]   Alberta Justice, Alberta's Safe Communities Secretariat, online: <http://www.justice.gov.ab.ca/safe/default.aspx>.

[119]   See Government of Canada, National Anti-Drug Strategy, Partners, online: <http://www.nationalantidrugstrategy.gc.ca/part.html>.

(a) Family Violence

A standard criminal justice response to some types of family violence is appropriate. Individuals who attack their spouses or children may be guilty of assault, assault causing bodily harm or assault with a weapon, or aggravated assault; they may be guilty of manslaughter or murder — and they should be punished accordingly. Parents who fail to provide necessaries for their children[120] or who kill or injure their children through negligence[121] may also deserve punishment.

Family violence, though, is also an appropriate target of public health conceptualization and strategies. Certainly violence threatens the physical health of victims. It also has emotional and psychological effects.[122] It is therefore a concern for health professionals. Family violence does occur (regrettably) relatively frequently.[123] Risk factors can be identified that aggravate the probabilities of violence. In the United States, public health approaches to violence have been promoted by — among other agencies — the Centers for Disease Control and Prevention and the Surgeon General's office.[124]

---

[120] *Criminal Code*, R.S.C. 1985, c. C-46, s. 215. A recent and shocking case is *R. v. C.M.R.*, [2004] O.J. No. 3356 (Ont. C.J.), *per* Halikowski J., var'd [2004] O.J. No. 4490 (Ont. C.A.).

[121] *Criminal Code*, *ibid.*, ss. 219, 220, 221. "About 235,315 investigations for child maltreatment were done in Canada in 2003. This adds up to a rate of almost 38 investigations per 1000 children between the ages of 0 and 15. Almost half (49 percent) of the investigations were found to be valid. Six percent of these investigations involved alleged sexual abuse. Of these, 24 percent were found to be valid (Canadian Incidence Study of Reported Child Abuse and Neglect - 2003)": Department of Justice (Canada), "About Family Violence in Canada", online: <http://www.justice.gc.ca/eng/pi/fv-vf/about-aprop.html>.

[122] "Family violence harms others besides the primary victim. Children living in close to half a million households in Canada saw or heard one parent being assaulted by the other in the five-year period covered by the 1999 General Social Survey. . . ." Department of Justice (Canada), "About Family Violence in Canada", *ibid.* The text refers to M. Dauvergne & H. Johnson, "Children Witnessing Family Violence" 21:6 Juristat, (Ottawa: Canadian Centre for Justice Statistics, Statistics Canada, Cat. No. 85-002-XPE, 2001).

[123] "In 2003, there were 5,921 spousal abuse incidents reported to police in Alberta. During the same period, 3,666 charges related to spousal abuse were laid and six deaths were attributed to spousal abuse": Alberta Roundtable on Family Violence and Bullying, *Finding Solutions Together: Report Presented to Government* (Fall 2004) at 6, online: Government of Alberta <http://www.familyviolenceroundtable.gov.ab.ca/pdf/fstr_low.pdf>. "Based on responses from around 24,000 people, about 7 percent of adults in Canada (that is, about equal to 653,000 women and 546,000 men) experienced some form of violence in their marriage or common-law relationship in the five years prior to the 2004 General Social Survey (GSS). The overall violence rates for spouses have remained about the same since the 1999 GSS": Department of Justice (Canada), "About Family Violence in Canada", *ibid.*

[124] D. Prothrow-Stith, "Strengthening the Collaboration between Public Health and Criminal Justice to Prevent Violence" (2004) 32:1 J.L. Med. & Ethics 82.

Since the 1990s, criminal justice system responses to family violence have become highly collaborative and co-operative. The membership of various coalitions stretches from federal and provincial government Departments, municipal governments, policing services, Crown prosecutors' offices, duty counsel offices, and community corrections offices, to community groups at the grassroots level. Within the levels of government itself, an *ad hoc* working group has been established to review spousal abuse policies and legislation, involving federal, provincial, and territorial governmental participants.[125] The federal government has developed the Family Violence Initiative, which involves several governmental departments, provincial governments, women's organizations, and community organizations:

> The [Family Violence Initiative] promotes public awareness of the risk factors of family violence and the need for public involvement in responding to it; strengthens the criminal justice, housing, and health systems to respond; and supports data collection, research and evaluation efforts to identify effective interventions.[126]

In 2004, Alberta held a comprehensive province-wide roundtable process on family violence and bullying, involving victims, experts, community organizations, Aboriginal peoples, and others.[127] An important conclusion was that "[n]o single entity — whether that's an individual, family, community, or the provincial government — can solve this problem alone".[128]

Calgary has been the site of highly collaborative efforts respecting domestic violence. Justice Canada contributed nearly $1 million in funding from the *National Strategy on Community Safety and Crime Prevention* Investment Fund for a four-year pilot project. Project partners include Alberta Justice, the City of Calgary, community organizations, and Status of Women Canada. The partnership now operates under the name "HomeFront".[129]

---

[125] Alberta Justice, *2002-2003 Annual Report*, at 43 (Goal 1, Strategy 1.4), online: <http://www.justice.gov.ab.ca/publications/downloads/annual_report/2003/alberta_justice_annual_report_2003.pdf>.

[126] Public Health Agency of Canada, "The Family Violence Initiative (FVI)[:] Reducing Family Violence - A Comprehensive Federal Approach", online: <http://www.phac-aspc.gc.ca/ncfv-cnivf/familyviolence/initiative_e.html>.

[127] Alberta Roundtable on Family Violence and Bullying, *Finding Solutions Together: Report Presented to Government* (Fall 2004) at 3, online: Government of Alberta <http://www.familyviolenceroundtable.gov.ab.ca/pdf/fstr_low.pdf>.

[128] *Ibid.*, at 8.

[129] HomeFront Calgary, online: <http://www.homefrontcalgary.com/printer/baknov05pf.htm>; Canada, National Crime Prevention Strategy, *Home Front Project: Interim Project Findings*, online: Public Safety and Emergency Preparedness Canada <http://ww4.ps.sp.gc.ca/en/library/publications/research/summaries/homefront.html>.

Through the resources and expertise of collaborators, a variety of interventions respecting domestic violence can be deployed. These include public education, making health services available to victims — including mental health services for children[130] — and making counselling and therapeutic programs available to batterers.

For all this, some might observe that a significant element of the response to domestic violence has not been new techniques, but more law.[131] For example, child-welfare legislation has been amended to characterize violence against a spouse in the presence of a child as a form of child abuse, which could allow child welfare authorities to intervene.[132] In Alberta, the *Protection Against Family Violence Act* was enacted to permit family members to obtain emergency protection orders from provincial court judges or justices of the peace, or protection orders from Court of Queen's Bench justices, in circumstances of family violence.[133] Provisions in these orders may (among other things) grant exclusive possession of the family home to applicants and may restrain respondents from contacting the applicants. Conduct which may not have easily fit under other offence provisions is criminalized through new legislation — *e.g.*, in 1993, "criminal harassment" (*i.e.*, "stalking") was made an offence in Canada.[134] On the "more

---

[130]   See D. Whitcomb, "Prosecutors, Kids, and Domestic Violence Cases" (2002) 248 Nat'l Inst. Just. J. 2 at 6.

[131]   *Ibid.*

[132]   See ss. 1(2)(f) and 1(3)(a)(ii)(C) of Alberta's *Child, Youth and Family Enhancement Act*, R.S.A. 2000, c. C-12.

[133]   R.S.A. 2000, c. P-27, ss. 2, 4. Other provinces, including Saskatchewan and Prince Edward Island, have similar legislation (the Saskatchewan and P.E.I. legislation pre-dates Alberta's).

[134]   More recent federal legislative amendments were made through Bill C-2, S.C. 2005, c. 32, Parliament of Canada, online: <http://www2.parl.gc.ca/HousePublications/Publication.aspx?DocId=2334051&Language=e&Mode=1&File=19>. The Bill's Summary provides as follows: This Act amends the *Criminal Code* to

    (a)   amend the child pornography provisions with respect to the type of written and audio material that constitutes child pornography, and with respect to the child pornography offences, defences and penalties;

    (b)   add a new category to the offence of sexual exploitation of young persons and make additional amendments to further protect children from sexual exploitation;

    (c)   increase the maximum penalty for child sexual offences, for failing to provide the necessaries of life and for abandoning a child;

    (d)   make child abuse an aggravating factor for the purpose of sentencing and direct the courts to give primary consideration to the objectives of denunciation and deterrence in sentencing for offences involving abuse of a child;

    (e)   amend and clarify the applicable test and criteria that need to be met for the use of testimonial aids, for excluding the public, for imposing a publication ban, for using video-recorded evidence or for appointing counsel for self-represented accused to conduct a cross-examination of certain witnesses; and

    (f)   create an offence of voyeurism and the distribution of voyeuristic material.

The Act also amends the *Canada Evidence Act* to abolish the requirement for a competency hearing for children under 14 years of age.

legislation" front, the response to domestic violence differs from the responses to mentally ill offenders and drug offenders. The reason for the difference is that there has been no lack of laws criminalizing the conduct of the mentally ill and drug addicts; the problem is not that we lack law, but that there may be too much of it. In the case of family violence, the starting point was not over-regulation but under-regulation. Family violence takes place within the sphere of the "private" and has not been a preoccupation of legislators. With the growing official awareness of family violence, in all its complexity, the legislative deficit is being addressed.

Police services have developed specialized domestic violence units, with specially selected and specially trained members.[135] These units do not merely charge batterers, but (in association with Victim Services Units) provide assistance to family members, and contribute to educational campaigns aimed at the public and other police officers.[136] They assist family members with safety planning, and follow up with family members after incidents have occurred.[137] They notify family members of "high risk releases" of batterers, whether on bail, conditional release, or at the conclusion of sentences.[138]

Domestic violence courts have been developed across Canada, based on a variety of models.[139] A domestic violence court was established in the Provincial Court in Calgary in 2000 as a component of the HomeFront project. It began as an "intake" court only, dealing with first appearances and guilty pleas, but expanded to hearing domestic violence trials in 2005.[140] The court relies on specialized participants — Crown prosecutors, community corrections staff, Legal Aid duty counsel, and Domestic Court

---

[135]   For example, the Calgary Police Service's Domestic Conflict Unit: see "Domestic Conflict Unit", online: <http://www.calgarypolice.ca/sections/major/domestic.html>; Alberta Justice, *2002-2003 Annual Report*, at 43 (Goal 1, Strategy 1.4), online: <http://www.justice.gov.ab.ca/publications/downloads/annual_report/2003/alberta_ justice_annual_report_2003.pdf>; and the Ottawa Police Service's Partner Assault Unit, online: <http://www.ottawapolice.ca/en/serving_ottawa/support_units/partner_assault.cfm>.

[136]   "Alberta Justice and Alberta Solicitor General, in co-operation with Alberta Children's Services and police services, are involved in a major initiative to provide training to staff involved in the criminal justice system including, but not limited to, police, Crown prosecutors, court personnel, corrections and victim service workers": Alberta Roundtable on Family Violence and Bullying, *Finding Solutions Together, Report Presented to Government* (Fall 2004) at 21, online: Government of Alberta <http://www.familyviolenceroundtable.gov.ab.ca/pdf/fstr_low.pdf>.

[137]   Calgary Police Service, "What does the Domestic Conflict Unit do?", online: <http://www.calgarypolice.ca/sections/major/domestic.html#7>.

[138]   *Ibid.*

[139]   E.J. Ursel, "The Family Violence Court of Winnipeg" (1992) 21 Man. L.J. 100; M.M. Clarke, "Best Practices Review, 2nd Draft" (July 2003), prepared as part of the HomeFront evaluation conducted by Synergy Research Group [unpublished] at 73.

[140]   H. Johnson, "Measuring Violence Against Women: Statistical Trends 2006", Institutional and community-based responses, at 48; Statistics Canada, Catalogue no. 85-570-XIE, online: <http://www.statcan.ca/english/research/85-570-XIE/85-570-XIE2006001.pdf>.

Case Workers (formerly known as Victim Services workers). Initially the court had specialized judges, but because of judicial interest in the project and concerns respecting judicial independence and impartiality, judges are now rotated into the court. Information exchange and early case resolution are promoted. Sentences focusing on treatment are strongly considered by judges. Through community corrections, batterer treatment is facilitated for offenders. HomeFront and the Alberta Mental Health Board deliver treatment. Community corrections supervises treatment completion.[141]

A second domestic violence court was established in the Provincial Court in Edmonton in 2002. It is a docket and trial court, dedicated to domestic violence cases. It relies on a team of three prosecutors, who prosecute domestic violence cases exclusively. Unlike the Calgary court, this court does not enjoy an extensive collaborative infrastructure.[142] Domestic violence courts have also been introduced in the Provincial Courts in Lethbridge, Medicine Hat, Red Deer, Fort McMurray and Airdrie (the first provincial circuit court with a specialized family violence sitting).[143]

Domestic violence courts have also been established in Winnipeg (the earliest domestic violence court in Canada, established in 1990); North Battleford, Saskatoon and Regina (in development); Whitehorse and Watson Lake, Yukon; and at least 49 court sites in Ontario. New Brunswick is developing a domestic violence court.[144]

(b) Mentally Disordered Offenders

The criminal justice system accommodates mentally disordered offenders. Their circumstances do engage special rules, but those rules are integrated into the basic criminal law. These special rules concern fitness

[141] M.M. Clarke; Alberta Justice, *2002-2003 Annual Report*, at 43 (Goal 1, Strategy 1.4), 53 (Goal 4); online: <http://www.justice.gov.ab.ca/publications/downloads/annual_report/ 2003/ alberta_justice_annual_report_2003.pdf>; Alberta Justice, *2001-2002 Annual Report* (September 2002) at 36 (Strategic Objective 3), online: <http://www.justice.gov.ab.ca/ publications/default.aspx?id=2223>.

[142] *Alberta Justice 2002-2003 Annual Report, ibid.*, at 53 (Goal 4); C. Christopher, "Domestic Violence Courts" *Law Now* (February/March 2002) 5 at 6; Alberta Roundtable on Family Violence and Bullying, *Finding Solutions Together: Report Presented to Government* (Fall 2004) at 22, online: Government of Alberta <http://www.familyviolenceroundtable.gov. ab.ca/pdf/fstr_low.pdf>.

[143] H. Johnson, "Measuring Violence Against Women: Statistical Trends 2006", Institutional and community-based responses, at 48; Statistics Canada, Catalogue no. 85-570 XIE, online: <http://www.statcan.ca/english/research/85-570-XIE/85-570-XIE2006001.pdf>.

[144] H. Johnson, "Measuring Violence Against Women: Statistical Trends 2006", Institutional and community-based responses, *ibid.*, at 47-48; Ursel claims that the Family Violence Court in Winnipeg, which was founded in 1990, was "the first of its kind in North America": E.J. Ursel, "The Family Violence Court of Winnipeg," (1992) 21 Man. L.J. 100.

to stand trial and the verdict of "not criminally responsible on account of mental disorder".

Individuals accused of offences may be unfit to stand trial because of mental disorder, in that they are unable to conduct a defence or instruct counsel to do so.[145] The *Criminal Code* sets out procedures to deal with accuseds who are unfit to stand trial. These provisions were recently amended, in response to a Supreme Court determination that earlier provisions were overbroad.[146] The earlier procedures failed to deal fairly with permanently unfit accuseds who were not significant threats to public safety. The basic procedures are as follows: If the issue of fitness is raised, the court may order the issue of fitness to be tried.[147] The court may make an assessment order, requiring the filing of an assessment report with the court within a prescribed time.[148] If the accused is found to be unfit to stand trial, the court may make a disposition,[149] or if it does not, a provincial Review Board makes the disposition.[150] A court may order a stay of proceedings against a permanently unfit accused if the accused poses no threat to public safety.[151]

An accused who is fit to stand trial, but whose mental disorder rendered him or her "incapable of appreciating the nature and quality of the act or omission or of knowing that it was wrong" cannot be convicted for committing a prohibited act, since the accused could not have formed the *mens rea* or have had the fault requisite for attracting criminal liability.[152] The appropriate verdict is not one of guilt, but of "not criminally responsible on account of mental disorder".[153] Following this verdict, the court may make a disposition, or, if it does not, the Review Board makes the disposition.[154]

The *Criminal Code* establishes procedures for disposition hearings[155] and sets out possible dispositions — absolute discharge (for "not criminally responsible" accuseds only), conditional discharges, or

---

[145] See the definition of "unfit to stand trial" in s. 2 of the *Criminal Code*, R.S.C. 1985, c. C-46.

[146] S.C. 2005, c. 22.

[147] *Criminal Code*, R.S.C. 1985, c. C-46, s. 672.23.

[148] *Ibid.*, ss. 672.12, 672.2.

[149] *Ibid.*, s. 672.45.

[150] *Ibid.*, s. 672.46.

[151] *Ibid.*, ss. 672.851 and 672.852.

[152] *Ibid.*, s. 16; *R. v. Chaulk*, [1990] S.C.J. No. 139, [1990] 3 S.C.R. 1303 (S.C.C.).

[153] This verdict is established in s. 672.34 of the *Criminal Code, ibid.*

[154] *Ibid.*, ss. 672.45, 672.47. For an overview of the post-verdict process and Review Boards' "inquisitional" duties, see *Winko v. British Columbia (Forensic Psychiatric Institute)*, [1999] S.C.J. No. 31, [1999] 2 S.C.R. 625 (S.C.C.) and *R. v. LePage*, [2006] O.J. No. 4486, 214 C.C.C. (3d) 105 (Ont. C.A.).

[155] *Ibid.*, s. 672.5.

detention on appropriate conditions.[156] Review Boards must review dispositions other than absolute discharges annually.[157]

Mental disorder, however, has a public health aspect that has not been adequately addressed by the criminal justice system; or, put another way, the criminal justice system has contributed to a public mental health crisis:[158]

Consider the American experience:

> The prevalence of mental disorders among persons with criminal justice system involvement is staggering. Each year about 700,000 adults with serious mental illness come into contact with the criminal justice system. Justice Department statistics indicate that sixteen percent of jail and prison inmates have a serious mental illness, but these estimates rise to 35% when they include less serious disorders. About 70% of those admitted to correctional facilities have active symptoms of serious mental illness, making the Los Angeles, Cook County (Chicago and surrounding suburbs) and Rikers Island (New York City) jails the largest mental hospitals in the country . . . . Serious mental illness is not just prevalent among those who have been convicted, however. A recent large-scale study of pre-trial arrestees in Brooklyn, New York found that 18.5% had a serious mental disorder (schizophrenia, bipolar disorder, or major depression) and that 3% had a moderately serious mental disorder (post traumatic stress disorder, depression, or generalized anxiety disorder) . . . .[159]

The Canadian experience is similar:

> Portions of our jails are now the "new asylums" but without many of the psychiatric resources available to mental health hospitals. A 1999 Alberta study found that a full 34% of male inmates in provincial jails suffer a serious form of mental disorder like schizophrenia or bipolar disorder and

[156] *Ibid.*, s. 672.54. On Review Boards' authority to make conditions, see *Mazzei v. British Columbia (Director of Adult Forensic Psychiatric Services)*, [2006] S.C.J. No. 7, [2006] 1 S.C.R. 326 (S.C.C.).

[157] *Ibid.*, s. 672.81.

[158] For remarks respecting the social impact of mental illness, see Sunil Patel, "Toward a National Strategy on Mental Illness and Mental Health", Canadian Medical Association Presentation to the Senate Standing Committee on Social Affairs, Science and Technology (31 March 2004), online: Canadian Medical Association <http://www.cma.ca/index.cfm/ci_id/33248/la_id/1.htm>.

[159] R.E. Redding, "Why it is Essential to Teach About Mental Health Issues in Criminal Law (And a Primer on How To Do It)" (2004) 14 J.L. & Pol'y 407 at 408-10 [footnotes omitted].

22% have attempted suicide. Suicide is now the number one cause of death for Canadians in Correctional facilities.[160]

In 1997, seven percent of male offenders coming into the federal correctional system were diagnosed as having a mental health problem. By 2007, the proportion had jumped to one in eight — a 71 percent increase. A similar rate of increase has been seen for women offenders, at least 25 percent of whom are now diagnosed as having mental health problems at the time they're admitted to federal institutions.[161]

In response, "[s]ome jurisdictions are trying to improve how they handle mentally ill people by developing innovative 'prebooking' diversion programs that give police alternatives to arrest and enable police to directly refer mentally ill people to community-based treatment programs. Prebooking diversion programs often involve novel police training practices and collaboration with local consumer and family groups".[162]

In 1997, Ontario addressed the issue of mentally disordered offenders through a joint effort of the Ministries of Health, Attorney General, Solicitor General, Community and Social Services, and the Provincial Court. A "mental health" court pilot project was established in Toronto: "The overall aim of the project [was] to put the mentally disordered accused back into the hands of the mental health system where he or she belongs and to reduce, as much as possible, their criminalization."[163] The project applied only to accuseds required to appear in two Toronto courthouses. The process was designed to deal with accuseds for whom fitness to stand trial was in issue, and accuseds whose criminal responsibility was in issue — so long as trials were not

---

[160] Canadian Mental Health Association, Alberta Division, "Promoting the 'diversion' of mentally ill people from the criminal justice system" in *Advocacy: Current Issues*, online: <http://www.cmha.ab.ca/bins/print_page.asp?cid=284-285-1247&lang=1>.

[161] "CSC Launches a Comprehensive Mental Health Strategy" (2007) 32:1 *Let's Talk*, online: Correctional Service of Canada <http://www.csc-scc.gc.ca/text/pblct/lt-en/2007/32-1/2-eng.shtml>; see also "Mental Health Strategy: Quick Facts", online: Correctional Service of Canada <http://www.csc-scc.gc.ca/text/pblct/qf/11-eng.pdf>.

[162] "At-A-Glance: Recent Research Findings", respecting H.J. Steadman *et al.*, "Police Response to Emotionally Disturbed Persons: Analyzing New Models of Police Interactions with the Mental Health System" (2002) 248 Nat'l Inst. Just. J. 33. See the Ontario police manual: Centre for Addiction and Mental Health, "Not Just Another Call . . . Police Response to Persons with Mental Illnesses in Ontario" (2004), online: Ontario Association of Chiefs of Police <http://www.oacp.on.ca/content/news/article.html?ID=60>.

[163] The Hon. R.D. Schneider, "Mental Disorder in the Courts" (December 1998) 19:4 *Criminal Lawyers Association Newsletter*. See also The Hon. R.D. Schneider, H. Bloom & M. Heerema, *Mental Health Courts: Decriminalizing the Mentally Ill* (Toronto: Irwin Law, 2006). The Toronto Mental Health Court was an inspiration for the three-season CBC courtroom comedy-drama, "This is Wonderland".

required.[164] The Ontario Review Board shared the courtroom with the Provincial Court. Forensic psychiatrists were on site. The process involved specially trained duty counsel and selected Crown prosecutors and judges, with experience in mental disorder cases. Mental Health Court workers were also employed — social workers with, again, training and experience in mental disorder matters. One objective of the project was to divert appropriate accuseds out of the criminal justice system. The Mental Health Court workers were to assist individuals in connecting with appropriate services, to ensure that they attended at appointments, and to "assist with maintaining a higher than usual level of compliance".[165] Referrals to external agencies could also be made conditions of judicial interim release ("bail"). If individuals were not diverted, issues of fitness could be dealt with expeditiously. If no trial was required, the court could consider whether the accused was not criminally responsible. The presence of the Review Board on site ensured that its hearings could be conducted quickly. If trials were required, standard procedures before trial courts were followed. The project — with variations — has now expanded to other Toronto provincial courts.[166] Other provinces have established or are establishing mental health courts, including New Brunswick[167] and Nova Scotia.[168] A mental health court for Alberta's Provincial Court is currently under discussion.[169]

(c) Drug Offences

Some drug offences demand a standard and intense criminal justice response: traffickers may belong to criminal organizations, of varying

---

[164] Schneider, "Mental Disorder in the Courts", *ibid.*

[165] *Ibid.*

[166] See Canadian Mental Health Association (Toronto), "Mental Health Court Support and Diversion Program", online: CMHA Toronto Branch <http://www.toronto.cmha.ca/ct_services_we_offer/mh_court_support.asp>; "Mental Health Court Support Services", in *Programs Services*, online: CMHA Hamilton Branch <http://www.inform.hamilton.ca/details.asp?UseCICVw=47&RSN=28670>; "Mental Health Court Support", online: CMHA – York Branch <http://www.cmha-yr.on.ca/prog-mentalhealthcourt.asp>.

[167] Mental Health Court — St. John, online: <http://www.mentalhealthcourt-sj.com>.

[168] See Bill No. 21 (2007), "An Act Respecting a Mental Health Court Program in the Provincial Court of Nova Scotia", online: Nova Scotia Legislature <http://www.gov.ns.ca/legislature/legc/bills/60th_2nd/1st_read/b021.htm>. See generally D. Moulton, "Mental health courts gain popularity across Canada" (2007) 28:23 *The Lawyers Weekly*, online: <http://www.lawyersweekly.ca/index.php?section=article&articlid=484>.

[169] In Alberta, a "multi-department/community committee" is currently developing a "Diversion Framework" for consideration by the Ministries of Health and Justice: Canadian Mental Health Association, Alberta Division, "Promoting the 'Diversion' of Mentally Ill People from the Criminal Justice System" in *Advocacy: Current Issues*, online: Canadian Mental Health Association <http://www.cmha.ab.ca/bins/print_page.asp?cid=284-285-1247&lang=1>.

degrees of sophistication, who use violence and intimidation, who seek to corrupt legitimate government, and who are willing to victimize children or anyone else to maximize their profits. These offenders should be investigated, prosecuted, and punished. Some drug use offences, though, have a public health aspect: drug addiction is a form of illness; injection drug users are exposed to high risks of HIV and hepatitis C infection — and if users are infected, they may infect others. Substance abuse has become understood as a "multi-faceted problem", which affects the health and welfare of individual abusers, their families, and third parties with whom they come into legal and illegal contact.[170]

This multi-faceted problem requires a multi-faceted response involving all levels of government, health care professionals, social workers, non-governmental organizations, and the criminal justice system.[171] Through the efforts of a variety of federal governmental departments, Canada's *National Anti-Drug Strategy* has been developed.[172] The Strategy

> . . . provides a focused approach involving three action plans to deliver on priorities aimed at reducing the supply of and demand for illicit drugs, as well as addressing the crime associated with illegal drugs. The new approach will lead to safer and healthier communities by taking action in three priority areas:
>
> • Preventing illicit drug use;
>
> • Treating illicit drug dependency; and
>
> • Combating the production and distribution of illicit drugs.[173]

The Strategy's "Prevention Action Plan" will

- refocus existing community-based prevention strategies, programs and services on youth;
- develop resources and tools for preventing drug use — such as tool kits for parents, educators, and health professionals, and materials for school-based awareness and prevention strategies for both elementary and secondary school students;
- launch a new awareness campaign to discourage young people from using drugs; and
- provide assistance to communities affected by drug-related crime.[174]

---

[170]   Public Safety and Emergency Preparedness Canada, "Drug Strategy: Substance Abuse Affects Canadians", online: <http://ww2.ps-sp.gc.ca/policing/drug_strategy_e.asp>.

[171]   *Ibid.*

[172]   *National Anti-Drug Strategy*, online: Government of Canada <http://www.national antidrug strategy.gc.ca/nads-sna.html>.

[173]   *Ibid.*

[174]   *Ibid.*

The Strategy's "Treatment Action Plan" will "promote collaboration with provinces and territories to support drug treatment services where needed (*e.g.*, services for youth, Vancouver's Downtown Eastside)", including

- improvements to the treatment system through investment in foundation pieces such as developing national benchmarks for evaluation, and data collection;

- enhanced treatment and support for First Nations and Inuit;

- provide diversion and treatment programs that are outside the justice system for youth offenders with drug-related problems at the various stages of the criminal justice system; and

- develop new tools for the R.C.M.P. to refer youth at risk to treatment programming.[175]

The Strategy's "Enforcement Action Plan" enhances traditional law enforcement approaches to drug crime.

Treatment and prevention have been incorporated into the criminal justice process. Since 1995, "HEP" — "Health and Enforcement in Partnership"[176] — has encouraged such projects as "drug awareness videos, programs for street youth, pre-charge diversion options for young offenders and referral programs".[177] Through community-based policing programs which now exist in many cities, police officers work collaboratively with community agencies, work with needle-exchange projects, shelters and detoxification centres, and emphasize diversion and referral.

Canada currently has six drug treatment courts financed through the federal Drug Treatment Court Funding Program — Toronto (established in 1998), Vancouver (2001), Edmonton (2005), Winnipeg (2006), Ottawa

---

[175]   *Ibid.*; Government of Canada, Department of Justice, News Release, "Government of Canada Announces Funding for Innovative New Drug Treatment Program for Youth" (11 August 2008); Government of Canada, Department of Justice, News Release, "Government of Canada Invests in Addiction Support Programs for Youth in Prince Edward Island" (12 August 2008).

[176]   This involves the Canadian Centre on Substance Abuse, Health Canada, the Alberta Alcohol and Drug Abuse Commission, the National Advisory Commission on AIDS, Correctional Services Canada, the Canadian Association of Chiefs of Police, the R.C.M.P., Department of the Solicitor General, and Justice Canada.

[177]   Public Safety Canada, "About HEP" in *Collaborate! Health and Enforcement in Partnership — How to Build Partnership 8 for Alcohol and other Drug Projects* (Ottawa: August 1997), online: <http://ww2.ps-sp.gc.ca/publications/policing/199708b_e.asp>.

(2006) and Regina (2006).[178] The objectives of the Funding Program are as follows:

- To promote and strengthen the use of alternatives to incarceration with a particular focus on youth, Aboriginal men and women and street prostitutes;

- To build knowledge and awareness among criminal justice, health and social service practitioners, and the general public about drug treatment courts; and

- To collect information and data on the effectiveness of [drug treatment courts] in order to promote best practices and the continuing refinement of approaches.[179]

Drug treatment courts establish processes that are alternatives to trials and custodial punishments, including court-monitored drug treatment programs.[180] Drug treatment court processes are made available to offenders who meet defined criteria. For example, eligible offenders may include non-violent offenders whose offences were motivated by drug (not alcohol) addictions and who have been charged with low-level possession, trafficking or prostitution offences. Generally, Crown prosecutors select eligible offenders, in consultation with defence counsel.[181] The offender must plead guilty and agree to be bound by the terms of the Drug Treatment court program. Participants then follow a program to reduce their drug dependency, which may involve individual and group counselling, medical treatment, and random testing. Regular court appearances to monitor progress may also be required. Programs may take about a year to complete. If a program is completed successfully, the offender will receive no disposition or only a non-custodial disposition. If the program is not completed successfully, the offender will be sentenced in the ordinary way. Very clearly, drug

---

[178] National Anti-Drug Strategy, "Drug Treatment Courts", online: Government of Canada <http://www.nationalanti drugstrategy.gc.ca/comm-coll/dtc-ttt.html>.

[179] National Anti-Drug Strategy, "Backgrounder — Drug Treatment Court Funding Program", online: Government of Canada <http://www.nationalantidrugstrategy.gc.ca/back-fich/doc2008_02_21.html>.

[180] For details concerning the Edmonton Drug Treatment and Community Restoration Court, see its website, online: <http://www.edtcrc.ca/pages/home>. Information is available respecting its legal foundation, vision and mission, program and key principles (which incorporate community justice and restorative justice concepts with the drug treatment court model), two processing tracks (pre-plea stream ("Track One") and post-plea stream ("Track Two")), the Court Team (including, among others, the presiding Provincial Court Judge, Crown Counsel, duty counsel, defence counsel, Case Manager/Treatment, and Case Manager/Probation), process, eligibility, rewards and sanctions. See also B. Gelinas, "Drug court helps addicts kick habit and get a life" *Edmonton Journal* (17 March 2006) B3.

[181] Department of Justice, "Backgrounder", online: <http://www.justice.gc.ca/eng/news-nouv/nr-cp/2003/doc_30916.html>.

treatment courts require substantial inter-agency co-operation to be effective.[182]

In some very limited circumstances, a far more thoroughgoing readjustment of the relationship between standard criminal justice processes and public health techniques has occurred, to the point that public health techniques have displaced criminal justice. This approach might be called "radical non-intervention". It is distinguished from "de-criminalization." If de-criminalization occurs, conduct is no longer an offence.[183] In the non-intervention situation, the conduct generally remains an offence, remains contrary to the law, and remains punishable by serious fines and imprisonment. The authorities, however, through an express exemption, decline to investigate or prosecute the conduct, so long as it occurs within prescribed areas and meets prescribed conditions. In the case of drug offences, the federal Minister of Health is entitled to create an exemption, under s. 56 of the *Controlled Drugs and Substances Act*,[184] which provides as follows:

> The Minister may, on such terms and conditions as the Minister deems necessary, exempt any person or class of persons or any controlled substance or precursor or any class thereof from the application of all or any of the provisions of this Act or the regulations if, in the opinion of the Minister, the exemption is necessary for a medical or scientific purpose or is otherwise in the public interest.

Like the integrative approaches considered above, non-intervention requires institutional coalitions. The police agree not to intervene, but other institutions must step in to manage the prosecution-insulated area.

The prime example of the non-intervention approach to drug use is Vancouver's "safe injection site" program (known as "Insite") which commenced in September 2003.[185] It was a three-year pilot project to determine whether allowing injection drug users to inject drugs in a safe, clean and supervised environment would reduce overdoses and HIV and

---

[182] Public Safety Canada "Toronto Drug Treatment Court Project", online: <http://www.publicsafety.gc.ca/prg/cp/bldngevd/2007-es-09-eng.aspx>.

[183] The conduct may no longer be an offence of any sort at all. Alternatively, the conduct may no longer be prohibited as a criminal offence by the *Criminal Code*, R.S.C. 1985, c. C-46 or *Controlled Drugs and Substances Act*, S.C. 1996, c. 19, but may remain a "contravention", penalized by fines, in the manner of minor traffic offences.

[184] S.C. 1996, c. 19.

[185] "Vancouver crack users want 'safe smoking' site" *Canadian Press* (5 August 2004), online: CTV.ca <http://www.ctv.ca/servlet/ArticleNews/story/CTVNews/20040804/crack_ smoking_ 040804/20040804/>. See "Insite — Supervised Injection Site", online: Vancouver Coastal Health <http://www.vch.ca/sis/>. Other similar projects include needle-exchange programs in Ottawa and Toronto and crack-pipe parts exchange programs in Ottawa, Toronto and Vancouver Island (free, clean, rubber-tipped glass pipes are provided, in order to reduce the spread of hepatitis and HIV through pipe-sharing).

hepatitis C infections.[186] The program was funded by Health Canada ($1.5 million) and the Province of British Columbia ($3.2 million).[187] The police agreed not to arrest users within a ten-block radius around the site.[188] To make the project work, "Vancouver Coastal Health expanded health services, including addiction treatment services and harm reduction services."[189] The program has been evaluated, and has been found to have positive health impacts.[190]

The Ministerial exemption for Insite was set to expire on June 30, 2008, and renewal was not contemplated. PHS Community Services Society, the Vancouver Area Network of Drug Users and some others therefore commenced actions in the British Columbia Supreme Court seeking relief that would obviate the need for Ministerial exemption. Justice Ian Pitfield found that ss. 4(1) (possession) and 5(1) (trafficking) of the *Controlled Drugs and Substances Act* unjustifiably limited rights under s. 7 of the *Charter* (life, liberty and security of the person).[191] Justice Pitfield suspended the declaration of constitutional invalidity until June 30, 2009. In the meantime, he declared a constitutional exemption permitting Insite to continue operations. The critical passage in Justice Pitfield's reasons is as follows:

In my opinion, s. 4(1) of the *CDSA*, which applies to possession for every purpose without discrimination or differentiation in its effect, is arbitrary. In particular it prohibits the management of addiction and its associated risks at Insite. It treats all consumption of controlled substances, whether addictive or not, and whether by an addict or not, in the same manner. Instead of being rationally connected to a reasonable apprehension of harm,

[186] Four Pillars Coalition (City of Vancouver), "A Dialogue on the Prevention of Problematic Drug Use" in *A Summary of the Proceedings from the Symposium "Visioning a Future for Prevention: A Local Perspective" (20 and 21 November, 2003)* (February 2004) at 5, online: City of Vancouver <http://www.city.vancouver.bc.ca/fourpillars/pdf/4Pillars_Report_Final.pdf>.
[187] "B.C. safe-injection site worries UN" *Canadian Press* (3 March 2004), online: *The Globe and Mail* <http://www.theglobeandmail.com/servlet/story/RTGAM.20040303.wnarcotics0303_/BNStory/National/>.
[188] Crack users are now seeking a safe smoking site: *ibid.*
[189] Four Pillars Coalition (City of Vancouver), "A Dialogue on the Prevention of Problematic Drug Use" in *A Summary of the Proceedings from the Symposium "Visioning a Future for Prevention: A Local Perspective" (20 and 21 November, 2003)* (February 2004) at 4, online: City of Vancouver <http://www.city.vancouver.bc.ca/fourpillars/pdf/4Pillars_Report_Final.pdf>.
[190] "Research Results", online: Vancouver Coastal Health <http://www.vch.ca/sis/research.htm>; Expert Advisory Committee, Final Report, "Vancouver's INSITE service and other Supervised injection sites: What has been learned from research?", online: Health Canada <http://www.hc-sc.gc.ca/ahc-asc/pubs/_sites-lieux/insite/index-eng.php>.
[191] *PHS Community Services Society v. Canada (Attorney General)*, [2008] B.C.J. No. 951, 2008 BCSC 661 (B.C.S.C.).

the blanket prohibition contributes to the very harm it seeks to prevent. It is inconsistent with the state's interest in fostering individual and community health, and preventing death and disease. That is enough to compel the conclusion that s. 4(1), as it applies to Insite, is arbitrary and not in accord with the principles of fundamental justice. If not arbitrary, then by the same analysis, s. 4(1) is grossly disproportionate or overbroad in its application.

The conclusion I have reached in relation to s. 4(1) applies equally to s. 5(1) of the *CDSA*. It is possible that staff at Insite who handle used equipment contaminated by controlled substances, or staff who take possession of any controlled substance for delivery to police, could be alleged to be engaged in "trafficking", which is broadly defined by the *CDSA* to the administration or transfer of a controlled substance. Failure to protect the staff against such an allegation would negative the utility of any determination that s. 4(1) is contrary to s. 7.[192]

The federal government plans to appeal.[193]

The Insite program and related Canadian programs have been criticized by the International Narcotics Control Board, a United Nations agency, on the grounds that these programs violate Canada's obligations under international drug control treaties. The Board has called on Canada to eliminate these programs.[194]

IV. THE CRIMINAL LAW AS A SOURCE OF PUBLIC HEALTH RISKS

One should also recall that the movement for reforming the prisons, for controlling their functioning is not a recent phenomenon. It does not even seem to have originated in a recognition of failure. Prison "reform" is virtually contemporary with the prison itself: it constitutes, as it were, its programme.[195]

---

[192] *Ibid.*, at paras. 152-153.

[193] Canwest News Service, "Ottawa to appeal BC ruling allowing injection site to stay open" *Edmonton Journal* (30 May 2008) A5; and see "Remarks for the Honourable Tony Clement, Minister of Health and Minister Responsible for the Federal Economic Development Initiative for Northern Ontario, Before the House of Commons Standing Committee on Health" (29 May 2008), online: Health Canada <http://www.hc-sc.gc.ca/ahc-asc/minist/speeches-discours/2008_05_29-eng.php>; and A. Picard, "Supporting Insite unethical, Clement tells doctors" *The Globe and Mail* (19 August 2008) 1, 5.

[194] International Narcotics Control Board, *Annual Report, 2007*, Chapter 3, para. 369, online: <http://www.incb.org/pdf/annual-report/2007/en/chapter-03.pdf>. "B.C. safe-injection site worries UN" *Canadian Press* (3 March 2004), online: *The Globe and Mail* <http://www.theglobeandmail.com/servlet/story/RTGAM.20040303.wnarcotics0303_/BNStory/National/>.

[195] M. Foucault, *Discipline and Punish: The Birth of the Prison*, trans. by A. Sheridan (New York: Vintage Books, 1979) at 234.

The public health system may create sites for the commission of crimes; it may create collection points for evidence respecting offences. But the criminal justice system, conversely, may create public health risks, through its species of compulsory confinement. Legal compulsory confinement has two broad types — imprisonment as punishment for an offence, and pre-trial confinement (*i.e.*, when "bail" is denied or revoked, or an accused cannot meet the terms of bail).[196]

(a) Imprisonment and Public Health

If a sentence of imprisonment is for a period greater than two years, it is served in a federally-regulated and administered penitentiary. If a sentence of imprisonment is for a period of less than two years, it is served in a provincially-regulated and administered prison. Most of the Canadian literature concerns offenders serving "federal time".

Imprisonment creates two main sorts of health risks.[197]

First, imprisonment exposes inmates to elevated risks of contracting disease.[198] Drug abuse and criminality are linked; since injection drug use attracts risks of infection, the population entering prisons is likely to have relatively high rates of infection.[199] Penitentiaries, then, have a sort of concentrating effect. This effect is exacerbated by inmates being lodged in confined spaces with relatively high population densities. High-risk

---

[196] Arrest or detention are also forms of confinement, but they are or should be fleeting, and they should not pose health risks — although that may be a function of police discipline and detainee conduct.

[197] The aging of Canada's inmates is also emerging as a health challenge within institutions: Canada, Strategic Planning and Integrated Justice Directorate, "Offender Health" in *Corrections in the 21st Century* (March 2000), online: Public Safety Canada <http://ww2.ps-sp.gc.ca/publications /crim_jus/corrections_21 _e.asp>.

[198] Corrections staff, of course, are also at risk.

[199] "The war on drugs took the group that was at greatest risk for H.I.V. infection and made sure that they would be locked up, without ever considering what to do when they got out": R.E. Fullilove, quoted in L. Clemetson, "Links Between Prison and AIDS Affecting Blacks Inside and Out" *The New York Times* (6 August 2004). In tests done in 1998, over 97 per cent of the total number of offenders with positive tuberculin skin tests results were identified upon entry to penitentiaries: Correctional Service Canada, *Tuberculosis Prevention and Control in Canadian Federal Prisons 1998* (2000) at 1, 11, online: <http://www.csc-scc.gc.ca/text/pblct/antituberculeuse/tuberculosis.pdf>.

behaviours such as injection drug use, the sharing of needles, and unprotected sexual acts do occur in custodial environments.[200] In 2001,

(a)   the prevalence of reported HIV infection in federal facilities was over 10 times greater than in the general population;[201]

(b)   the prevalence of hepatitis C infection was about 20 times greater than in the general population;[202]

(c)   the rate of acute hepatitis B infection was 320 per 100,000 population, in comparison to a rate of about 2.3 per 100,000 in the general population;[203] and

(d)   the rates for sexually transmitted diseases or infections were higher than in the general population.[204]

---

[200]   "In the present study, over a 6-year period, 50% of [injection drug user] participants reported being incarcerated and 15% of those incarcerated reported injecting in prisons. Furthermore, syringe lending, syringe borrowing and inconsistent condom use with casual sexual partners were all independently associated with incarceration .... Regardless of the exact nature of this association, however, our findings nevertheless have serious public health implications, particularly considering the high rate of syringe borrowing and lending in correctional institutions that study participants reported. A recent study suggested that the number of known HIV cases in Canadian prisons has risen by 35% in the last 5 years, while studies have reported HIV rates several times that of the national average among prisoners in the United States": D. Werb, T. Kerr, W. Small, K. Li, J. Montaner & E. Wood, "HIV Risks Associated with Incarceration Among Injection Drug Users: Implications for Prison-Based Public Health Strategies" (2008) 30:2 Public Health 126 at 129 (footnotes omitted).

[201]   See "HIV/AIDS and HCV in Prisons: A Select Annotated Bibliography", online: Health Canada <http://www.hc-sc.gc.ca/ahc-asc/pubs/int-aids-sida/hiv-vih-aids-sida-prison-carceral-eng.php>; Correctional Service Canada, *Infectious Diseases Prevention and Control in Canadian Federal Penitentiaries 2000-01* (2003) at 6, online: <http://www.csc-scc.gc.ca/text/pblct/infectiousdiseases/en.pdf>; P. De, "Infectious Diseases in Canadian Federal Penitentiaries, 2000-2001" in *Forum on Corrections Research* (May 2002) Vol. 14, No. 2 at 24; Canada, Strategic Planning and Integrated Justice Directorate; "The Spread of Diseases in Correctional Institutions" in *Corrections in the 21st Century* (March 2000), online: Public Safety Canada <http://ww2.ps-sp.gc.ca/publications/crim_jus/corrections_21_e.asp>. In the United States in 2001, the rate of HIV infection in State and Federal prisons was more than three times higher than in the general population: U.S., Bureau of Justice Statistics (Dept. of Justice), "HIV in Prisons, 2001" in *Bureau of Justice Statistics Bulletin* (January 2004) (by L.M. Maruschak) at 5.

[202]   De, *ibid.*, at 25; *Infectious Diseases Prevention and Control, ibid.*, at 14.

[203]   Correctional Service Canada, *Focus on Infectious Diseases* (Spring 2002) at 3.

[204]   *Ibid.*; P. De, "Infectious Diseases in Canadian Federal Penitentiaries, 2000-2001" in *Forum on Corrections Research* (May 2002) Vol. 14, No. 2 at 26.

Inmates are also at risk of contracting tuberculosis.[205] Sexual transmission and injection drug use are the most common causes of HIV and hepatitis C infection.[206]

Second, individuals who leave penitentiaries (who had elevated risks of contracting disease while imprisoned) may transmit disease to individuals with whom they come into contact, and thereby to the public at large:[207]

> The diseases that incubate behind bars don't just stay there. They come rushing back to the general population — and to the overburdened health system — with the nearly 12 million inmates who are released [in the United States] each year.[208]

The *Corrections and Conditional Release Act* requires the Correctional Service of Canada ("CSC") to provide every inmate with essential health care conforming to professionally accepted standards.[209] The CSC has adopted standards for health care service,[210] and, more precisely, has adopted public health measures to address the risks of disease transmission associated with imprisonment. It pursues health promotion and "harm reduction" strategies through inmate and staff

---

[205] *Ibid.*, at 24; B. Staples, "Treat the Epidemic Behind Bars Before it Hits the Streets" *The New York Times* (22 June 2004). However "[r]elatively few offenders had documented conversion of their TST status within federal correctional facilities in 1998": Correctional Service Canada, *Tuberculosis Prevention and Control in Canadian Federal Prisons 1998* (2000) at 11, online: <http://www.csc-scc.gc.ca/text/pblct/antituberculeuse /tuberculosis.pdf>.

[206] Correctional Service Canada, *Infectious Diseases Prevention and Control in Canadian Federal Penitentiaries 2000-01* (2003) at 6, 14, online: <http://www.csc-scc.gc.ca/text/pblct/ infectiousdiseases/en.pdf>; P. De, "Infectious Diseases in Canadian Federal Penitentiaries, 2000-2001" in *Forum on Corrections Research* (May 2002) Vol. 14, No. 2 at 26; M.B. Pongrac, "HIV, Hepatitis C virus (HCV) in Women Offenders — Why Are the Rates So High?" in *Focus on Infectious Diseases* Vol. 1, No. 2 (Fall 2002) at 5; "The Spread of Disease in Correctional Institutions" and see fn. 50 in *Corrections in the 21st Century* (March 2000), online: Public Safety Canada <http://ww2.ps-sp.gc.ca/publications/crim_jus/corrections_21_ e.asp>. Tattooing, which involves needles or other skin piercing equipment, involves risks of transmission: *Infectious Diseases Prevention and Control, ibid.*, at 6.

[207] De, *ibid.*, at 24; see also L. Clemetson, "Links between prison and AIDS affecting blacks inside and out" *The New York Times* (6 August 2004), quoting Dr. David Wohl: "Many inmates who have been locked up for a while want two things when they come out . . . . One of them is a Big Mac. The other is sex. If you're going to get to them with condoms or health messages, you have to be quick."

[208] B. Staples, "Treat the epidemic behind bars before it hits the streets" *The New York Times* (22 June 2004).

[209] *Corrections and Conditional Release Act*, S.C. 1992, c. 20, s. 86. For materials respecting the U.S. experience, see the website of the National Commission on Correctional Health Care, online: <http://www.ncchc.org>.

[210] Correctional Service Canada, "Preface" (2002), online: <http://www.csc-scc.gc.ca/text/ prgrm/fsw/hlthstds/toc-eng.shtml>.

education;[211] makes available condoms, dental dams, water-based lubricants, and bleach; promotes immunization for hepatitis A and B;[212] and provides methadone maintenance programs to assist drug addicts.[213] It has developed testing and screening programs[214] and counselling and treatment programs.[215] It has no plans, however, to implement a needle exchange program.[216] The CSC's steps may seem obviously appropriate. Some U.S. prisons, apparently, for budgetary or politico-moral reasons, have not pursued such strategies, with the result that prisoners' infection rates have grown alarmingly.[217]

The CSC has also initiated a "health surveillance" program — the CSC Infectious Diseases Surveillance System: "[h]ealth surveillance is the continuous, systematic use of routinely collected health data to guide health action".[218] Data collected are used "for various purposes, including measuring performance for health service provision and creating new initiatives for infectious disease prevention and control".[219] In 2004, the CSC and the Centre for Infectious Disease Prevention and Control of Health Canada signed a Memorandum of Understanding respecting the control and management of infectious disease in penitentiaries.[220] Health Canada provides expertise concerning educational strategies and

---

[211] For example, the CSC began publishing *Focus on Infectious Diseases*, a quarterly newsletter, in 2002; *Infectious Diseases Prevention and Control in Canadian Federal Penitentiaries 2000-01* (2003) at 3, online: CSC <http://www.csc-scc.gc.ca/text/pblct/infectiousdiseases/en.pdf>.

[212] *Ibid.*, at 21.

[213] P. De, "Infectious Diseases in Canadian Federal Penitentiaries, 2000-2001" in *Forum on Corrections Research* (May 2002) Vol. 14, No. 2 at 26; *Infectious Diseases Prevention and Control, ibid.*, at 4. See Correctional Service Canada, *Correctional Service of Canada: Specific Guidelines for Methadone Maintenance Treatment* (November 2003), online: <http://www.csc-scc.gc.ca/text/pblct/methadone/english/meth_guidelines_e.pdf>.

[214] M.B. Pongrac, "STI Prevention and Treatment" in *Focus on Infectious Diseases*, Vol. 2, No. 1 (Fall 2003) at 3.

[215] Correctional Service Canada, *Infectious Diseases Prevention and Control in Canadian Federal Penitentiaries 2000-01* (2003) at 3, online: <http://www.csc-scc.gc.ca/text/pblct/infectiousdiseases/en.pdf>.

[216] M. Munro, "Prisons helping spread AIDS: study" *Edmonton Journal* (7 August 2008) A7.

[217] B. Staples, "Treat the epidemic behind bars before it hits the streets" *The New York Times* (22 June 2004). But for information concerning services that are provided, see U.S., Bureau of Justice Statistics (Dept. of Justice), "Hepatitis Testing and Treatment in State Prisons" in *Bureau of Justice Statistics: Special Report* (April 2004) (by A.J. Beck & M.M. Maruschak).

[218] Correctional Service Canada, *Focus on Infectious Diseases*, Vol. 1, No. 1 (Spring 2002) at 2; Correctional Service Canada, *Infectious Diseases Prevention and Control in Canadian Federal Penitentiaries 2000-01* (2003) at 4, online: <http://www.csc-scc.gc.ca/text/pblct/infectiousdiseases/en.pdf>.

[219] Correctional Service Canada, *Focus on Infectious Diseases*, Vol. 1, No. 1 (Spring 2002) at 2.

[220] Correctional Service Canada, *Focus on Infectious Diseases*, Vol. 2, No. 2 (Winter 2004) at 1.

educational programs, and support for the infectious disease surveillance system.

Bridges are required between the federally regulated penitentiary system and provincial public health systems.[221] For example, the CSC has a partner notification program.[222] Information respecting sexually transmitted infections should be transmitted to public health authorities, in accordance with public health legislation (the issue of whether provincial mandatory reporting requirements apply respecting information gathered by federal workers in the course of their duties shall not be pursued here). Bridges must be built not only between institutions, but to individuals in the community who are at heightened risk of transmitting infection or becoming infected. In the United States, "[r]esearchers trying to prevent the spread of H.I.V. are urging strategies that connect education and treatment among three groups of people: inmates, those recently released, and those in the social networks through which they move".[223] The need for such strategies has been recognized in Canada: "strategies may have to be developed to deal with this population upon release . . . . It may become incumbent on the Ministry to develop effective strategies to facilitate the effective reintegration of this particular population of individuals".[224]

(b)   Pre-Trial Confinement and Public Health

Often individuals charged with offences remain free until trial. Depending on the nature of the offence or offences with which the individual has been charged, on whether the individual is a flight risk, and on whether confinement is necessary to establish the individual's identity, to preserve evidence, or to prevent the commission of offences, the individual may be released by the police and be required to attend court on the basis of an appearance notice, summons, promise to appear, or recognizance. If not released by the police, the individual is entitled to a "bail hearing" before a justice (justice of the peace or Provincial Court

---

[221]   See U.S., National Commission on Correctional Health Care, *The Health Status of Soon-to-be-released Inmates: A Report to Congress*, online: <http://www.ncchc.org/pubs/pubs_stbr.html>.

[222]   P. De, "Partner Notification and STI Case Management" in *Focus on Infectious Diseases*, Vol. 2, No. 1 (Fall 2003) at 4; Correctional Service Canada, *Infectious Diseases Prevention and Control in Canadian Federal Penitentiaries 2000-01* (2003) at 26, online: <http://www.csc-scc.gc.ca/text/pblct/infectiousdiseases/en.pdf>.

[223]   L. Clemetson, "Links between prison and AIDS affecting blacks inside and out" *The New York Times* (6 August 2004).

[224]   "The Spread of Disease in Correctional Institutions" in *Corrections in the 21st Century* (March 2000), online: Public Safety Canada <http://ww2.ps-sp.gc.ca/publications/crim_jus/corrections_21_e.asp>.

judge).[225] Very generally, the individual is entitled to be released upon an undertaking or recognizance, unless the prosecutor shows cause for the detention of the individual, on the grounds that the detention is necessary to ensure his or her attendance in court, to ensure the protection of the public, or on "any other just cause being shown".[226] Under s. 11(e) of the *Charter*, persons charged with an offence have the right "not to be denied reasonable bail without just cause".

Nevertheless, in a significant number of cases individuals are confined until trial. They are housed in jails or "remand centres". In 2002, the total number of admissions to remand was 130,021 — while the total number of custodial sentencing admissions was (only) 88,129.[227] Although confinement in these facilities would replicate some of the structural features of confinement in prison (*e.g.*, living in close quarters with relatively large numbers of individuals; engaging in high-risk activities), the population is more transient, and the periods of confinement in such facilities are (or should be) shorter than periods of confinement in federal penitentiaries. These factors could mitigate the health risks associated with confinement in these facilities.

A difficulty with remand facilities, however, is their funding. Because of lack of funding, the living conditions in these facilities may be below the standards of federal penitentiaries — *e.g.*, respecting overcrowding (particularly because of "double-bunking" or higher multiple-bunking), the quality of living quarters, the cleanliness of living quarters, the availability of showers and hot water, the quality and quantity of food, temperature controls, clothing, time for exercise and exercise facilities, and the availability of medical treatment.[228] The

---

[225]   Unless the offence is an offence listed in s. 469 of the *Criminal Code*, R.S.C. 1985, c. C-46 (very serious offences, such as murder), in which case the bail hearing is held by a superior court judge.

[226]   *Ibid.*, s. 515(10)(c).

[227]   Statistics Canada, "Adult Correctional Services, Admissions to Provincial, Territorial and Federal Programs", online: <http://www.statcan.ca/english/Pgdb/legal30a.htm>.

[228]   These sorts of concerns were raised in a *habeas corpus* application brought by former inmates against the Edmonton Remand Centre. An application for interim relief was dismissed, on the basis (generally) that the evidence did not establish the "likelihood of irreparable harm": *Trang v. Alberta (Director of the Edmonton Remand Centre)*, [2001] A.J. No. 1124, 2001 ABQB 659 (Alta. Q.B.). Nonetheless, Marceau J. made the following observation respecting the main application: "The public has an interest in seeing that the citizens of this country are not imprisoned in a manner which offends the *Charter*. The humane treatment of its prisoners is surely one of the hallmarks of a free and democratic society. The issue is clearly one of great importance": *Trang v. Alberta (Edmonton Remand Centre)*, [2002] A.J. No. 1469, 2002 ABQB 1042 at para. 32 (Alta. Q.B.), *Trang v. Alberta (Edmonton Remand Centre)*, [2004] A.J. No. 796, 2004 ABQB 497 (Alta. Q.B.), Marceau J., aff'd [2005] A.J. No. 157, 2005 ABCA 66 (Alta. C.A.), leave to appeal to S.C.C. refused [2005] S.C.C.A. No. 161 (S.C.C.). After the commencement of the proceedings, changes

Supreme Court of Canada has recognized the harsh nature of pre-trial custody.[229] In *Wust*, Arbour J. relied on a passage from Trotter's *The Law of Bail in Canada*: "[d]ue to overcrowding, inmate turnover and the problems of effectively implementing programs and recreation activities, serving time in such institutions can be quite onerous".[230] Spending time in jail is not good for one's health. And if going to jail makes an individual sick, it may also make his or her friends and family sick, through contact. And so illness spreads, again, into the community.

If human rights concerns are not sufficient to warrant decent treatment of people in jail, public health concerns may be.

V. CONCLUSION

This chapter has, I hope, fulfilled its promise of demonstrating the intricacies of the relationships between the criminal justice system and the public health system. At least at our present level of civilization, we cannot do without both systems. Our challenges are to preserve each in its proper role, to foster collaborations for the public benefit, and to minimize inevitable clashes, confrontations, and misunderstandings. This chapter is offered as a small contribution toward meeting those challenges.

---

occurred at the Remand Centre: "a long term remand unit has been developed for detainees expected to be held for more than six months, the food menu now has greater caloric content, [and] a methadone treatment program has been established . . .": [2004] A.J. No. 796, 2004 ABQB 497 at para. 69 (Alta. Q.B.).

[229] *R. v. Wust*, [2000] S.C.J. No. 19, [2000] 1 S.C.R. 455 at para. 28 (S.C.C.), *per* Arbour J.

[230] *Ibid.*, at para. 41, quoting G. Trotter, *The Law of Bail in Canada*, 2d ed. (Scarborough, Ont.: Carswell, 1999) at 37.

14

GENETICS AND PUBLIC HEALTH: LEGAL, ETHICAL AND POLICY CHALLENGES

Timothy Caulfield[*]

I. INTRODUCTION

Few areas of science have received as much attention and have moved forward as quickly as human genetics. The Human Genome Project (the massive, international effort to map the human genome that took off in the early 1990s[1]) was the initiative that shifted our focus to genetics. But since the completion of Human Genome Project in 2003,[2] many other advances and developments have kept the field in the public eye, such as completion and release of the first individual genome,[3] the emergence of new areas like nutrigenomics,[4] and the increased interest in direct-to-consumer genetic testing.[5]

[*] Canada Research Chair in Health Law and Policy; Professor, Faculty of Law and Faculty of Medicine & Dentistry, Research Director, Health Law Institute, University of Alberta.

[1] Robert Cook-Deegan, *The Gene Wars: Science, Politics and the Human Genome* (New York: W.W. Norton & Co., 1994).

[2] National Human Genome Research Institute, National Institutes of Health, "International Consortium Completes Human Genome Project" (14 April 2003), online: <http://www.genome.gov/11006929>.

[3] S. Levy *et al.*, "The diploid genome sequence of an individual human" (2007): 10 PLoS Biology e254; Carolyn Abraham, "This human's life, decoded," *The Globe and Mail* (3 September 2007), online: <http://www.theglobeandmail.com/servlet/story/RTGAM.20070903.wgenemap0903/BNStory/Science/home>.

[4] Nola Ries & Timothy Caulfield, "First Pharmacogenomics, Next Nutrigenomics: Genohype or Genohealthy?" (2006) 46 Jurimetrics 281-8.

[5] Carolyn Abraham, "Click here to unlock your DNA code" *The Globe and Mail* (23 January 2008) A1; American College of Medical Genetics, ACMG Statement on Direct-to-

While the benefits and limits of the emerging genetics to health care continue to stir debate,[6] there is no doubt that biomedical researchers are gaining an unprecedented amount of knowledge about the role of genes in disease development. This has led to speculation about the potential role of emerging genetic technologies and services in the area of public health. In this chapter, I outline both the promise and perils associated with the application of genetics in the context of public health. We will see that while there are, indeed, reasons to be optimistic about potential public health applications, such as the development of more precise preventive strategies, there are also many profound social, ethical and legal challenges.

This chapter is not meant to be a comprehensive analysis of all relevant social concerns. Rather, I seek to provide the reader with a sense of the primary legal and policy issues. It begins with an overview of the science and the possible public health applications. This is followed by a discussion of the principal ethical tension relevant to the area (*i.e.*, the conflict between respecting individual rights and seeking to advance the public good) and the health policy obstacles that may stall implementation of genetic strategies. Next, I consider relevant research ethics issues, with an emphasis on consent and confidentiality. The chapter ends with a discussion of the broadest and most controversial social concerns, the long shadow of past eugenic justifications for the use of genetics in the area of public health.

II.   THE PROMISE OF PUBLIC HEALTH GENETICS

While there are already a number of public health initiatives that involve genetic analysis, most notably newborn screening programs,[7] the

---

Consumer Genetic Testing (2008), online: <http://www.acmg.net/StaticContent/StaticPages/DTC_Statement.pdf>.

[6]   See, for example, Wylie Burke & B.M. Psaty, "Personalized Medicine in the Era of Genomics" (2007) 298 JAMA 1682. See also, James P. Evans, Cécile Skrzynia & Wylie Burke, "The Complexities of Predictive Genetic Testing" (2001) 322 BMJ 1052 at 1055: "The utility of testing varies widely, however, depending on the magnitude of risk, the accuracy of risk prediction, options available to reduce risk, an individual's previous experience, and the needs and experience of family members. In addition, the utility of a given predictive genetic test is likely to change over time as knowledge grows, new strategies for prevention are developed, and costs change."

[7]   These programs, which exist in most developed nations, usually screen newborns for treatable, serious, congenital diseases, such as phenylketonuria ("PKU") and congenital hypothyroidism. In recent years, largely as a result of technological advances, there has been a push for an expansion of newborn screening programs. See, for example, Jeffrey R. Botkin, Ellen Wright Clayton, Norman C. Fost, Wylie Burke *et al.*, "Newborn Screening Technology: Proceed with Caution" (2006) 117 Pediatrics1793; U.S. Department of Health and Human Services, Maternal and Child Health Bureau, "Newborn screening: toward a

rapid advances that have occurred in human genetics may soon result in a much broader application of genetics technologies — including the possibility of the introduction of whole or partial genome sequencing as a routine part of clinical care.[8] Indeed, as we learn more about the role of genetics in complex diseases, there is potential for genetics to provide insight for a wide variety of preventative public health strategies. Some commentators have gone so far as to suggest that "the sequencing of the human genome and the subsequent demonstration of variation in numerous genes in health and disease will surely stimulate a golden age for the public health sciences".[9]

For example, emerging genetic analysis may, one day, provide greater information about the relationship between genetic characteristics, environmental factors and the distribution of disease within the general population.[10] In addition to increasing our basic understanding of human disease, this knowledge may help in the development of preventative health care strategies. We may, for instance, be able to identify particularly carcinogenic environments and individuals or populations that are especially susceptible to the adverse health effects associated with those environments.

The science of genetics may also allow for what has been called "individualized medicine", including the development of targeted drug therapies that maximize individual therapeutic benefit while reducing adverse reactions.[11] If successful, such a trend could have important implications for health care costs and policy development.[12] For instance,

---

uniform screening panel and system — report for public comment", online: <http://www.mchb.hrsa.gov/screening>. In Canada, all provinces provide newborn screening, but there is a degree of variation. W.B. Hanley, "Newborn screening in Canada — are we out of step?" (2005) 10:4 Paediatric & Child Health 203.

[8]   A.L. McGuire, M.K. Cho, S.E. McGuire & T. Caulfield, "The Future of Personal Genomics" (2007) 317 Science 1687.

[9]   Gilbert Omenn, "Public Health Genetics: An Emerging Interdisciplinary Field for the Post-Genomic Era" (2000) 21 Annu. Rev. Public Health 1 at 1.

[10]   Melissa Austin et al., "The Interface of Genetics and Public Health: Research and Educational Challenges" (2000) 21 Annu. Rev. Public Health 81 at 82-83. See also, Muin Khoury and the Genetics Working Group, "From Genes to Public Health: The Application of Genetic Technology in Disease Prevention" (1996) 86 American Journal of Public Health 1717 at 1718-19: "The study of gene-environment interaction can provide an important basis for refining the predictive value of traditional epidemiological risk factors and for targeting intervention and prevention activities for individuals in high-risk groups."

[11]   This area of research is often referred to as "pharmacogenetics". See, for example, Jai Shah, "Economic and Regulatory Considerations in Pharmacogenomics for Drug and Licensing and Healthcare" (2003) 21 Nature Biotechnology 747.

[12]   As noted by Shah, ibid., at 747, the potential for the more efficient use of drug therapies creates a number of interesting market dilemmas. Because pharmacogenetics could lead to the more targeted use of pharmaceuticals (that is, the identification of individuals who would benefit from a particular drug therapy and the elimination of those for whom the

by maximizing the impact of useful pharmaceuticals, individualized medicine may help reduce the burden of disease and, concomitantly, the cost to the health care system. As noted by geneticist, Jim Evans:

> With increases in the ability to parse individual risk, screening programs for everything from heart disease to cancer can be more efficiently tailored, resulting in possible savings of time and money and reduced morbidity.[13]

It has also been suggested that genetic information may lead to the identification of individuals who are at particular risk for infectious diseases[14] and will provide new insight into well established areas of public health, including the health impact of nutrition and physical activity.[15] In short, the science of genetics could, one day, create myriad opportunities for public health researchers, practitioners and policy makers. However, as we will see below, there are also profound scientific and social challenges associated with the use of genetics in the context of public health.

III. ETHICAL AND LEGAL TENSIONS

One of the underlying challenges associated with the use of genetic technologies in public health relates to the conflict between the ethical principles that have traditionally informed public health and clinical genetics. Public health policy is dedicated to the health of populations. There is a focus on the greater good which may, in some circumstances, require a de-emphasis of individual rights (*e.g.*, mandatory vaccination and screening programs). In genetics, the emphasis has been on informed

---

drug is no benefit), it may actually reduce the market for a drug. "Pharmacogenomics creates a dilemma between a move toward a broad spectrum of highly stratified personalized medicines (with corresponding high efficacy), and the reduced revenue that results from market segmentation."

[13] Jim Evans, "Health Care in the Age of Genetic Medicine" (2007) 298 JAMA 2670 at 2670. See also Karen Steinberg *et al.*, "The Role of Genomics in Public Health and Disease Prevention" (2001) 286 JAMA 1635 at 1635.

[14] See generally, Jean-Laurent Casanova & Laurent Abel, "Human Genetics of Infectious Diseases: A Unified Theory" (2007) 26 The EMBO Journal 915.

[15] See Gilbert Omenn, "Public Health Genetics: An Emerging Interdisciplinary Field for the Post-Genomic Era" (2000) 21 Annu. Rev. Public Health 1 at 4. Omenn suggests that genetics could play a greater role in understanding unhealthy behaviour. For example, he notes (at 9) that genes likely play a role in the "initiation, maintenance, cessation, and recurrence" of addictive behaviour like smoking and alcoholism. However, it should also be noted that the area of "behavioural genetics" is surrounded by a good deal of social controversy. While there is little doubt that genes play a role in human behaviour, the cause of these traits is invariably complex involving, *inter alia*, a mix of genes and environment. See generally, Nuffield Council on Bioethics, *Genetics and Human Behaviour: The Ethical Context* (London: Nuffield Council on Bioethics, 2002).

individual decision-making. As summarized by Gerard, Hayes and Rothstein:

> Almost by definition, however, public health and genetics are incompatible. Public health is based on utilitarianism and paternalism. The benefit to society as a whole, justifies coercive measures that outweigh individual rights. Consequently, a whole range of interventions — from immunization to isolation — may be justified. Genetics, on the other hand, has a completely different philosophical grounding. The intensely personal, inter-generational, and reproductive aspects of genetics have given rise to a professional ethos of non-directive counselling, autonomous decision-making, and individual rights — the very opposite of the approach of public health.[16]

As we will see below, this conflict may make it difficult, rightly or not, to do population-based public health genetics research and to implement public health genetic programs. With few exceptions, Canadian health law jurisprudence has long viewed individual autonomy as the dominant ethical consideration, as highlighted in our informed consent laws and autonomy-centred research ethics policies.[17] There are, of course, exceptions to the dominance of individual autonomous decision-making, such as public health and child welfare laws. But the exceptions that do exist are usually legislated and are viewed as a necessary deviation from the dominant norm of individual consent. To date, there are no legislative regimes designed specifically for public health genetics.[18] For instance, there are no legislative provisions that would allow for the collection of genetic information — at least without specific, informed, consent — for the sole purpose of public health surveillance.[19] As one commentator notes: "There is no population-based

---

[16]   Susan Gerard et al., "On the Edge of Tomorrow: Fitting Genomics into Public Health Policy" (2002) 30 J.L. Med. & Ethics 173 at 175.

[17]   See Bernard Dickens, "Informed Consent" in Jocelyn Downie et al., eds., Canadian Health Law and Policy, 2d ed. (Markham, Ont.: Butterworths Canada, 2002).

[18]   Julian Little, Beth Potter, Judith Allanson et al., "Canada: Public Health Genomics" (2008) Public Health Genomics [forthcoming].   Even in the context of newborn screening programs, only two provinces, Saskatchewan and Québec, have relevant law.

[19]   There are legislative regimes that mandate the collection of health information that would, no doubt, be relevant to this area, most notably provincial cancer registries. See generally, Barbara von Tigerstrom et al., "Legal Regulation of Cancer Surveillance: Canadian and International Perspectives" (2000) 8 Health L.J. 1. Likewise, population genetic information could be collected as part of a research project. However, "[t]he distinction between surveillance and research is important" because the latter is governed by ethics policies designed to protect human research subjects: Ellen Wright Clayton, "Genetics, Public Health and the Law" in Muin Khoury et al., eds., Genetics and Public Health in the 21st Century (New York: Oxford University Press, 2000) at 494.

counterpart to the principle of autonomy and the practice of informed consent by individuals in medical ethics."[20]

This tension between individual rights and the public good is hardly unique to public health genetics — indeed, it is a principal theme in all areas of public health ethics. However, the tension appears to be particularly acute in the context of genetics. In part, this is due to the fact that individuals seem especially concerned about keeping genetic information private and controlling access to it.[21] There is some evidence that Canadians believe that genetic information is special. For example, a 2001 survey that found that 90 per cent either strongly agree (61 per cent) or agree (29 per cent) that genetic information is different and rules governing access should be stricter than for other forms of personal information.[22] Another survey found that the number of Canadians "very willing" to contribute genetic information to research has decreased substantially, from 56 per cent in 2003 to only 37 per cent in 2004. Similarly, more Canadians feel that privacy (39 per cent) should be given a greater focus than research (26 per cent).[23] In a 2003 survey, Canadians were asked directly "whether access to genetic information should be more strictly regulated than other health information" and 58 per cent said it should be.[24] In follow up focus groups, it was found that, for many, "genetic information is more personal and more fundamental to identity".[25] People said they would be more upset "if their personal genetic

---

[20]   Gilbert Omenn, "Public Health Genetics: An Emerging Interdisciplinary Field for the Post-Genomic Era" (2000) 21 Annu. Rev. Public Health 1 at 10.

[21]   For a review of relevant empirical data, see generally Timothy Caulfield & Nola M. Ries, "Consent, Privacy and Confidentiality in Longitudinal, Population Health Research: The Canadian Legal Context" (2004) Health L.J. (Supp.) 1.

[22]   Pollara & Earnscliffe, Public Opinion Research into Biotechnology Issues, Third Wave (December 2001) at 51. This finding is consistent with other research. See generally Lidewij Henneman et al., "Public Experiences, Knowledge and Expectations about Medical Genetics and the Use of Genetic Information" (2004) 7 Community Genetics 33. See also Mairi Levitt & Sue Weldon, "A Well Placed Trust?: Public Perceptions of the Governance of DNA Databases" (2005) 15 Critical Public Health 311 at 314: "[a]s the discussion moved from personal information in general to medical information and then to genetic information so the participants became more concerned".

[23]   Jeff Walker, Decima Research, Public Opinion Research on Biotechnology (Prepared for the Biotechnology Assistant Deputy Minister Coordinating Committee, Government of Canada, March 2004), online: Government of Canada <http://www.bioportal.gc.ca/english/View.asp?x=588&mp=524>.

[24]   Pollara Research and Earnscliffe Research and Communications, Public Opinion Research Into Genetic Privacy Issues (Prepared for the Biotechnology Assistant Deputy Minister Coordinating Committee, Government of Canada, March 2003) online: <http://biotech.gc.ca/epic/site/cbs-scb.nsf/vwapj/Wave_1_GPI_ExSum.pdf/$FILE/Wave_1_GPI_ExSum.pdf>.

[25]   Ibid.

information was inadvertently made public than if their health records had been".[26]

This "essentialist" view of genetics — that is, that genetic information is unique — has been adopted in policies relevant to genetic research and public health initiatives. The best known example is in Article 4 of UNESCO's *International Declaration on Human Genetic Data* which states that human genetic data has special status because:

> ... they can be predictive of genetic predispositions concerning individuals and that the power of predictability can be stronger than assessed at the time of deriving the data; they may have a significant impact on the family, including offspring, extending over generations, and in some instances on the whole group to which the person concerned belongs; they may contain information the significance of which is not necessarily known at the time of the collection of the biological samples; they may have cultural significance for persons or groups.[27]

As a result of this unique status, UNESCO suggests that "an appropriate level of protection for these data and biological samples should be established special protection should be afforded to human genetic data and to the biological samples".[28]

However, not all agree that genetic data is significantly different from other forms of sensitive health information. For example, the U.K.'s Nuffield Council on Bioethics has suggested that many of the allegedly unique features of genetic information, such as its predictive nature, apply to other sensitive health information (*e.g.*, HIV status and cholesterol testing).[29] The Nuffield Council suggests that given the "similarities between genetic and other forms of personal information, it would be a mistake to assume that genetic information is qualitatively different in some way".[30] Others have noted that we should be careful not to cast genetics as special as we risk legitimizing inappropriate and scientifically inaccurate views of genetics that may, paradoxically, heighten the chance that genetic data will be used to stigmatize and discriminate.[31]

---

[26] *Ibid.*
[27] UNESCO's *International Declaration on Human Genetic Data* (October 2003).
[28] *Ibid.*
[29] Nuffield Council on Bioethics, *Pharmacogenetics: Ethical Issues* (London: Nuffield Council on Bioethics, 2003) at 6.
[30] *Ibid.*
[31] See Scott Burris *et al.*, "Public Health Surveillance of Genetic Information: Ethical and Legal Responses to Social Risk" in Muin Khoury *et al.*, eds, *Genetics and Public Health in the 21st Century* (New York: Oxford University Press, 2000) at 538: "Treating genetics as distinct from the rest of medicine may enhance the stigma of genetics testing, even as legislators attempt to remove its stigmatizing effects. This can create public fears and

Regardless of whether one accepts the essentialist view of genetics information, the public increasingly views genetic information as special.[32] This will likely have an impact on policy development (as exemplified by the genetic discrimination policies emerging throughout the world)[33] and will ensure that the tension between individual rights and the public good will remain especially sharp in the area of genetics. The Nuffield Council notes: "If there is widespread belief that genetic data are special, then proper account must be taken of this fact. A belief does not need to be true to have real effects."[34] And, to be fair, given some of the horrendous historical uses of genetics in the context of public health, to be discussed more fully below, it is understandable that there is a continuing hesitancy both to combine public health policies with genetics and to move away from an autonomy driven ethos.[35]

IV. HEALTH CARE POLICY CONSIDERATIONS

Public health genetics also faces a number of significant health care policy challenges,[36] the most obvious being the need for more evidence regarding the role of genetics to inform the development of appropriate

---

misapprehensions about genetics that could discourage individuals from seeking testing and treatment, and thwart future scientific progress."

[32] It is worth considering the source of this essentialist view of genetics. I have argued elsewhere that the scientific enthusiasm needed to attract public and private funds, and the media coverage of that message, may be at least partially responsible. See Timothy Caulfield, "Perceptions of Risk and Human Genetic Databases: Consent and Confidentiality Policies" in G. Arnason *et al.*, eds., *Blood and Data: Ethical, Legal and Social Aspects of Human Genetics Databases* (Reykjavik: University of Iceland Press and Centre for Ethics, 2004) at 283-89. See also, Muin Khoury *et al.*, "Challenges in Communicating Genetics: A Public Health Approach" in Lawrence O. Gostin, ed., *Public Health Law and Ethics: A Reader* (Berkeley: University of California Press, 2002) at 476: "Popular representations of genetics are often deterministic, reinforcing a view of humans as a product of their genes, to the exclusion of nongenetic factors."

[33] Amy Harmon, "Congress Passes Bill to Bar Bias Based on Genes" *The New York Times* (2 May 2008). Indeed, though there is a great deal of public concern about genetics discrimination, there is, in fact, little evidence that it is a widespread problem. See, for example, Hank Greely, "Banning Genetic Discrimination" (2005) 357 New Eng. J. Med. 865 at 865: ". . . studies have shown that although there is widespread concern about genetic discrimination, there are few examples of it — and no evidence that it is common".

[34] Nuffield Council on Bioethics, *Pharmacogenetics: Ethical Issues* (London: Nuffield Council on Bioethics, 2003) at 7.

[35] Scott Burris *et al.*, "Public Health Surveillance of Genetic Information: Ethical and Legal Responses to Social Risk" in Muin Khoury *et al.*, eds, *Genetics and Public Health in the 21st Century* (Oxford University Press, 2000) at 530: "The concern that progress in genetics could create social risk is founded on historical experience with other health conditions."

[36] Brenda Wilson, "The Challenge of Developing Evidence-Based Genetics Health Care in Practice" (2006) 5 Familial Cancer 55-59.

public health strategies.[37] Few would dispute that genes often play a significant role in the development of disease, even many complex diseases with a strong environmental component. However, the role of genetics in most human diseases is tremendously complicated and, to date, remains largely unclear. For some diseases, such as Huntington's and Tay Sachs, there is a direct relationship between genetics and the presence of the disease. If you have the gene you will have the disease. But these purely genetic diseases — also called "monogenetic" — are relatively rare.[38] Most common diseases, such as heart disease and cancer, "result from a more complex interaction between single or multiple mutations and factors in the social and physical environment".[39] These more common conditions are generally the focus of public health initiatives. While the study and treatment of monogenetic diseases remains important, the rarity of these conditions means that their identification and treatment will have only a marginal impact on the broader public health goal of reducing overall morbidity and mortality.

As a result of the complexity created by gene/environment interaction, the near future significance of genetics to practical public health initiatives is far from clear. Indeed, the clinical value of available genetic testing, particularly in the context of macro health care policy, is still a topic of great debate.[40] This is because there are few tests that provide concrete, clinically useful, information. As noted in a 2008 article by Janssens *et al.*: "Although genomic profiling may have potential to enhance the effectiveness and efficiency of preventive interventions, to

---

[37]   It has also been noted that there is a need to invest resources in clinical research and practice. See, for example, A. Silversides, "The Wide Gap Between Genetic Research and Clinical Needs" (2007) 176 C.M.A.J. 315.

[38]   See, for example, Neil Pearce *et al.*, "Genetics, Race, Ethnicity and Health" (2004) 328 British Medical Journal 1070 at 1070: "The constant interaction between genes and the environment means that few diseases are purely hereditary (even if they are genetic). Purely hereditary diseases are very rare (1/2300 births for cystic fibroses, 1/3000 for Duschenne's muscular dystrophy, and 1/10,000 for Huntington's disease) and account for a small proportion of overall disease." See also, Marieke Dekker & Cornelia Duijn, "Prospects of Genetic Epidemiology in the 21st Century" (2003) 18 European Journal of Epidemiology 607.

[39]   Scott Burris *et al.*, "Public Health Surveillance of Genetic Information: Ethical and Legal Responses to Social Risk" in Muin Khoury *et al.*, eds. *Genetics and Public Health in the 21st Century* (New York: Oxford University Press, 2000) at 529.

[40]   See, for example, Gilbert Omenn, "The Crucial Role of the Public Health Sciences in the Postgenomic Era" (2002) 4 Genetics in Medicine 21S-26S at 21S; and Gilbert Omenn, "Public Health Genetics: An Emerging Interdisciplinary Field for the Post-Genomic Era" (2000) 21 Annu. Rev. Public Health 1 at 1: "It is far too simplistic, especially for common diseases, to associate individual genes and individual variants or single nucleotide polymorphisms of genes with disease risk." See also H. Welch & W. Burke, "Uncertainties in Genetic Testing for Chronic Disease" (1998) 280 JAMA 1525; L.B. Andrews, "Past as Prologue: Sobering Thoughts on Genetic Enthusiasm" (1997) 27 Seton Hall L. Rev. 893.

date the scientific evidence for most associations between genetic variants and disease risk is insufficient to support useful applications."[41]

There have, however, been a few recent examples of genetic testing services being integrated into healthcare systems. In September 2008, for instance, the U.S. government explored the possibility of Medicare coverage of a pharmacogenetic test to identify differences in patient response to warfarin, a commonly prescribed anticoagulant. In this context, genetic testing could help prevent serious and potentially fatal adverse events, including strokes.[42] In the U.K., the National Institute for Health and Clinical Excellence released a guidance document in August 2008 that recommends genetic testing in certain circumstances to identify individuals, including children, who are at high risk of familial hypercholesterolemia ("FH").[43] But despite these developments and a handful of tests for relatively high penetrance genes,[44] genetic services have yet to have a broad impact on the treatment of individual patients.

The uncertainty regarding the role of genetic services becomes even greater when viewed from the level of common diseases and public health policy.[45] Another layer of ambiguity is created by the fact that there are few preventative strategies available for individuals with a known genetic predisposition. In other words, at the current time, there is not much we can do, clinically, with information about genetic predisposition. In addition, we still are not sure how people will react to genetic predisposition information. It has been suggested by some, for example, that the emerging area of nutrigenomics, a field that brings together genetics and nutrition, will lead to new preventative public health strategies. Afman and Müller claim that, "[u]ltimately, nutrigenomics research will lead to development of evidence-based healthful food and

---

[41]   A.C. Janssens *et al.*, "A Critical Appraisal of the Scientific Basis of Commercial Genomic Profiles Used to Assess Health Risks and Personalize Health Interventions" (2008) 82 American Journal of Human Genetics 593 at 598.

[42]   See U.S. Department of Health and Human Services, Centers for Medicare and Medicaid Services, "National Coverage Analysis Tracking Sheet for Pharmacogenetic Testing for Warfarin Response", online: <http://www.cms.hhs.gov/mcd/viewtrackingsheet.asp?id=224>.

[43]   See U.K. National Health Service, National Institute for Health and Clinical Excellence, "Identification and Management of Familial Hypercholesterolaemia" (28 August 2008), online: <http://www.nice.org.uk/nicemedia/pdf/CG071NICEGuideline.pdf>. FH is a genetic disorder that leads to extremely high levels of cholesterol and, if untreated, can result in heart disease and premature death.

[44]   "Penetrance" refers to the relationship between the presence of the gene or mutation and the manifestation of the disease.

[45]   See Kathleen Ries Merikanges & Neil Risch, "Genomic Priorities and Public Health" (2004) 302 Science 599 at 601: "there is a growing consensus that widespread genomic profiling will not be useful until the full potential of genomics and its intersection with public health has been more fully exploited."

lifestyle advice and dietary interventions for contemporary humans".[46] Such benefits, while exciting, depend on individual behavioral changes.[47] In other words, people would need to use the genetic information to motivate healthier eating habits. But it remains unclear how people will respond to such risk information. Public health experts, such as Carlsten and Burke, have suggested that, in fact, "genetic risk information may be ineffectual in motivating behavior change or potentially may even be harmful by inducing fatalism, feelings of impotency, or loss of willpower".[48]

Given this uncertainty, it is not surprising that genetic testing and surveillance strategies have yet to play a significant role in Canadian public health policy.[49] There is, however, great potential, as noted above. But more research is required to provide a sharper picture of the role of genetics in disease development, a fact that was noted over ten years ago by a well known group of public health experts: "If the public health applications of the Human Genome Project are to be widespread, the impact of genes in the population at large has to be carefully evaluated

[46] Lydia Afman & Michael Müller, "Nutrigenomics: From Molecular Nutrition to Prevention of Disease" (2006) 106 Journal of the American Dietetic Association 569 at 572. See also Kaput et al., who contend, "[d]iagnostics, preventive lifestyle guidelines, more efficacious dietary recommendations, health-promoting food supplements, and drugs are some of the anticipated end-products of nutrigenomics research": Jim Kaput, Janelle Noble & Betul Hatipoglu, "Application of Nutrigenomic Concepts to Type 2 Diabetes Mellitus" (2007) 17 Nutrition, Metabolism & Cardiovascular Diseases 89 at 98.

[47] For a more indepth discussion of this challenge, see Theresa M. Marteau & Caryn Lerman, "Genetic Risk and Behavioural Change" (2001) 322 British Medical Journal 1056 and Susanne B. Haga, Muin J. Khoury & Wylie Burke, "Genomic Profiling to Promote a Healthy Lifestyle: Not Ready for Prime Time" (2003) 34 Nature Genetics 347.

[48] Chris Carlsten & Wylie Burke, "Potential for Genetics to Promote Public Health: Genetics Research on Smoking Suggests Caution about Expectations" (2006) 296 JAMA 2480 at 2480-481. See also Hans-Georg Joost, Michael J. Gibney, Kevin D. Cashman et al., (2007) "Personalised Nutrition: Status and Perspectives" (2007) 98 British Journal of Nutrition 26 at 30, who observe, "[t]he possibility cannot be excluded that, in some individuals, knowledge of a genetic predisposition might lead to a fatalistic attitude and a reduced compliance with any intervention". See also J. Heshka, C. Palleschi, H. Howley, B. Wilson & P. Wells, "A Systematic Review of Perceived Risks, Psychological and Behavioral Impacts of Genetic Testing" (2008) 10 Genetics in Medicine 19-32 at abstract where they come to a rather startling conclusion about the influence of predisposition testing: "Overall, predispositional genetic testing has no significant impact on psychological outcomes, little effect on behavior, and did not change perceived risk."

[49] To date, there is no nationally co-ordinated strategy for the integration of genetics into the Canadian healthcare system. See, for example, Julian Little, Beth Potter, Judith Allanson et al., "Canada: Public Health Genomics" (2008) Public Health Genomics [forthcoming]. However, the Public Health Agency of Canada has established an Office of Biotechnology, Genomics and Population Health to facilitate co-ordination of relevant activities. See Public Health Agency of Canada, Report on Plans and Priorities, 2006-2007 (Ottawa: Treasury Board of Canada, 2006), online: Treasury Board of Canada Secretariat <http://www.tbs-sct.gc.ca/rpp/0607/phac-aspc/phac-aspc02_e.asp>.

through epidemiological studies. Such studies quantify the impact of susceptibility alleles on disease incidence and prevalence."[50]

If and when we move closer to the development of genetic services that can play a useful role in public health policy and clinical care, there will also be a need for evidence that can appropriately inform the technology assessment process.[51] Public health care systems will need to make tough decisions about which genetic technologies they ought to implement and fund. For example, a genetic screening program would create "immediate service costs (*e.g.*, clinical, counselling and laboratory services, laboratory and counselling costs) but also the costs of actions taken on the basis of the information that the tests provide (*e.g.*, detection, prevention, or intervention into disease processes)".[52] In fact, the economic impact of implementing genetics testing services could increase, rather

---

[50]   Muin Khoury and the Genetics Working Group, "From Genes to Public Health: The Application of Genetic Technology in Disease Prevention" (1996) 86 American Journal of Public Health 1717 at 1718. In fact, to maximize the impact on broader health care policy, it has been suggested that future research priorities should be framed through the lens of public health policy. This is because such an approach will ensure that genetic research will benefit the greatest portion of the population and, as a result, have the most dramatic impact on health care systems. Kathleen Ries Merikangas & Neil Risch, "Genomic Priorities and Public Health" (2004) 302 Science 599 at 601: "When making choices in research, the potential for advancing our understanding of human biology, insight into disease pathogenesis, and the impact of those findings on the individuals and families affected by rare, severe diseases must always be balanced with the public health impact of ameliorating more common diseases with lower mortality but high levels of disability."

[51]   In 2001, an international, interdisciplinary group of researchers and policy makers met to consider what evidence would be required and what processes should be in place to implement effective and ethical genetic screening programs. The group looked at the classic criteria used to make determinations about public health screening programs and applied them to an analysis of genetic tests. The conclusions are instructive for policy makers considering the role of genetics in public health and the development of research priorities.

Among the issues to be examined with this test are the criteria for selecting the target population; the natural course and burden of disease; the interventions that could be offered to those who are screened, particularly in young people; the psychological and social effects of being tested; and the balance of economic, psychological, and social effects. System issues are paramount: screening programmes should be efficient, accessible, of high quality, ensure consumer choice, and respect the fundamental principles of human rights.

Vivek Goel, for the Crossroads 99 Group, "Appraising Organised Screening Programmes for Testing for Genetic Susceptibility to Cancer" (2001) 322 British Medical Journal 1174 at 1177. See also Francis Collins & Alan Guttmacher, "Genetics Moves into the Medical Mainstream" (2001) 286 JAMA 2322 at 2322: "before moving such diagnostic tests into mainstream medicine, it is critical to collect data about their clinical validity and utility. Premature introduction of predictive tests, before the value of the information have been established, actually could be quite harmful."

[52]   Mita Giacomini *et al.*, "Economic Considerations for Health Insurance Coverage of Emerging Genetic Tests" (2003) 6 Community Genetics 61 at 61.

than decrease, costs to the system.[53] As such, this decision-making process ought to be informed by the best available information, including an understanding of the short- and long-term economic implications of implementing and funding a genetic program.[54]

V. POPULATION GENETIC RESEARCH: ETHICAL AND LEGAL CHALLENGES

The need for more research in this area is largely agreed upon.[55] As a result, there is growing interest in the development of large, population-based, longitudinal research projects that include the collection, storage and long-term analysis of identifiable genetic samples. Because these large databanks provide an unprecedented ability to tease out the complex interaction between genes and environment in the disease process, they are emerging as an important methodological tool for exploring the research questions raised by public health genetics.

In general, population genetic studies involve the recruitment of thousands of research participants and the collection of identifiable genetic samples. These samples are stored in a manner that will allow ongoing linkage to other sets of data relevant to disease development, including health records, demographic data and, even, lifestyle information. This ability to link and cross-reference data is one of the reasons that genetic databanks — or "biobanks", as they are commonly called[56] — have so much scientific value. For example, Francis Collins, the individual who led the efforts by the U.S. National Institutes of Health

---

[53] Steve Morgan & Jeremiah Hurley (August 2002) *Influences on the "Health Care Technology Cost-Driver"*, online: Commission on the Future of Health Care in Canada <http://dsp-psd.pwgsc.gc.ca/Collection/CP32-79-14-2002E.pdf >.

[54] See M. Giacomini & F. Miller, "Confronting the 'Gray Zones' of Technology Assessment: Evaluating Genetic Testing Services for Public Insurance Coverage in Canada" (2003) 19 International J. of Tech. Assess. in Health Care 301. I. Blancquaert, "Availability of Genetic Services: Implementation and Policy Issues" (2000) 3 Community Genetics 179; and Timothy Caulfield *et al.*, "Providing Genetic Testing Through the Private Sector: A View From Canada" (2001) 2 ISUMA: Canadian Journal of Policy Research 72.

[55] See, for example, David Melzer, Stuart Hogarth, Kathy Liddel *et al.*, *Evidence and Evaluation: Building Public Trust in Genetic Tests for Common Diseases* (February 2008), online: PHG Foundation <http://www.phgfoundation.org> at 5: "There was therefore near universal support for improving the generation of good clinical evidence on tests and for this evidence to be made easily available to doctors, patients and consumers."

[56] It should be noted that not all "biobanks" are the same. They range from a small collection of biological samples to large scale, initiatives. Here, we are primarily concerned with the latter. For a discussion of the challenges associated with the definition of "biobanks" see: Jane Kaye, "Do We Need a Uniform Regulatory System for Biobanks Across Europe?" (2006) 14 European Journal of Human Genetics 245.

to map the human genome,[57] has argued that biobanks are "vital for defining the genetic and environmental factors that contribute to health and disease".[58]

The research potential of these large population-based studies has led many countries throughout the world to get involved in genetic data banking projects.[59] A major banking initiative in Iceland, which involves almost the entire country's population, has been up and running for years.[60] In the United Kingdom, the government has developed a research project, known as U.K. Biobank, that involves the collection of samples from 500,000 individuals. Recruitment of research participants for this major initiative started in March 2007.[61] They plan to follow the research participants for approximately 30 years, linking the analysis of genetics to

---

[57]   On the Human Genome Project, see <http://www.ornl.gov/sci/techresources/Human_Genome/home.shtml>.

[58]   Francis Collins, "The Case for a US Prospective Cohort Study of Genes and Environment" (2004) 429(6990) Nature 475 at 475. For Omenn, this type of research is essential to achieving the goals of public health genetics. See Gilbert Omenn, "The Crucial Role of the Public Health Sciences in the Postgenomic Era" (2002) 4 Genetics in Medicine 21S-26S at 21S: "In order to achieve this goal genetic information must be linked with information about nutrition and metabolism, lifestyle behaviours, diseases and medications, and microbial, chemical, and physical exposure." See also William Lowrance, Editorial, "The Promise of Human Genetic Databases" (2001) 322 British Medical Journal 1009 at 1009: "Genetic databases are now helping elucidate gene function, estimate the prevalence of genes in populations, differentiate among subtypes of diseases, trace how genes may predispose to or protect prevent against illnesses, and improve medical intervention. They achieve this by bringing together several streams of data about individuals: molecular genetic data; high quality standardized clinical data; data on health, lifestyle, and environment; and in some cases, genealogical data." Finally, for a relevant policy report, see: Academy of Medical Sciences, *Personal Data for Public Good: Using Health Information in Medical Research* (January 2006) at 4, online: <http://www.acmedsci.ac.uk/images/project/Personal.pdf>.

[59]   See generally Melissa Austin *et al.*, "Genebank: A Comparison of Eight Proposed Genetic Databases" (2003) 6 Community Genetics 37; Anne Cambon-Thomsen, "The Social and Ethical Issues of Post-Genomic Human Biobanks" (2004) 5 Nature Reviews Genetics 866; and Timothy Caulfield & Nola M. Ries, "Consent, Privacy and Confidentiality in Longitudinal, Population Health Research: The Canadian Legal Context" (2004) Health L.J. (Supp.) 1. A new organization, P3G, is a consortium of many of the large population genetic projects. For more information, see P3G (Public Population Project in Genomics) online: <http://www.p3gconsortium.org>.

[60]   For a discussion of the social challenges associated with the Icelandic project, see: Vilhjámur Árnason, "Coding and Consent: Moral Challenges of the Database Project in Iceland" (2004) 18 Bioethics 27.

[61]   See Press Release, "Manchester First For UK Biobank" (21 March 2007), online: <http://www.ukbiobank.ac.uk/docs/Manchesterinvites.pdf>. The U.K. Biobank website indicates that as of September 2008, over 175,000 individuals have been recruited, see <http://www.ukbiobank.ac.uk/>.

health data and other personal information. In Canada, a number of similar initiatives are in planning phases.[62]

Though the research potential of large genetic databanks is tremendous,[63] the databanks have also created a number of challenging legal and ethical issues, most notably around the process of consent.[64] Bernice Elger and Arthur Caplan have suggested that they are forcing us to "question fundamental ethical milestones".[65] Why is this so? The law imposes tight restrictions on the use of identifiable tissue and health information for research purposes. In general, the research participants must give fully informed consent,[66] so researchers must provide participants with information about the exact nature of, and risks associated with, a given research project. However, most of the large databank projects are designed to be long-term research platforms. The scope of all the studies that will be involved is impossible to know at the beginning of the research initiative, when the genetic material is likely to be collected. As such, it will often be impossible to obtain truly informed consent at that stage of the project.

Regardless, many commentators have suggested that if the genetic sample remains linkable to identifiable information, a fresh consent would be needed for each new research project.[67] In other words, a one time "blanket consent" (also known as "broad consent") would not be sufficient. In a recent report by the World Health Organization it was

---

[62]   See, for example, CartaGene <http://www.cartagene.qc.ca>. This Québec project is in the process of recruiting 20,400 individuals aged 40-69 years to be randomly selected from the index of the Régie de l'assurance maladie du Québec.

[63]   This said, there are those who question the value of these large, and expensive, research initiatives. See, for example, P. Ghosh, "Will Biobank pay off?" BBC News (23 September 2003), online: <http://news.bbc.co.uk/1/hi/health/3134622.stm>. See also, Hilary Rose, "From Hype to Mothballs in Four Years: Troubles in the Development of Large-Scale DNA Biobanks in Europe" (2006) 9 Community Genetics 184.

[64]   There are a variety of legal issues associated with biobanks, including issues associated with commercialization, "look back" liability, benefit sharing, community consent and patenting. In this chapter, I focus only on the issue of consent. See generally Timothy Caulfield, "Biobanks and Blanket Consent: The Proper Place of the Public Perception and Public Good Rationales" (2007) 18 King's L.J. 209. See also Report of the Secretary's Advisory Committee on Genetics, Health, and Society, *Policy Issues Associated with Undertaking a New Large U.S. Population Cohort Study of Genes, Environment and Disease* (March 2007), online: Department of Health and Human Services <http://www4.od.nih.gov/oba/sacghs/reports/sacghs_lps_report.pdf>.

[65]   Bernice Elger & Arthur L. Caplan, "Consent and Anonymization in Research Involving Biobanks: Differing Terms and Norms Present Serious Barriers to an International Framework" (2006) 7(7) EMBO Reports 661 at 661.

[66]   Timothy Caulfield *et al.*, "DNA Databanks and Consent: A Suggested Policy Option Involving An Authorization Model" (2003) 4 BMC Medical Ethics 1.

[67]   See, generally, Timothy Caulfield, "Biobanks and Blanket Consent: The Proper Place of the Public Perception and Public Good Rationales" (2007) 18 King's L.J. 209.

suggested that: "Blanket consent for future research [on DNA samples] is only permissible in circumstances where anonymity of future data can be guaranteed."[68] But, as noted by the UN's ethics committee (UNESCO), "[a] system which required fresh consent would be extremely cumbersome and could seriously inhibit research".[69] Imagine, for example, the need to obtain new consent from thousands of people for the hundreds of research projects that may be associated with any given population genetic research project. On the one hand, satisfying this legal requirement could create an insurmountable barrier to valuable population genetic research. On the other hand, moving away from the need for individual consent could be viewed as a dangerous erosion of autonomy. The World Health Organization Report noted this as a classic tension between individual rights and the public good:

> We have, then, a fundamental tension between the possibility of considerable public good on the one hand, and the potential for significant individual and familial harm on the other. The basic interests that lie in the balance are those between human dignity and human rights as against public health, scientific progress and commercial interests in a free market.[70]

The countries that already have biobanking projects have attempted to resolve this issue using a variety of policy strategies. In Iceland, for instance, specific legislation, the *Health Sector Database Act*, was passed to allow for the collection, storage and linkage of genetic data. The

---

[68]   Graeme Laurie, "Genetic Databases: Assessing the Benefits and the Impact on Human and Patient Rights — A World Health Organisation Report" (2004) 11 European Journal of Health Law 79.

[69]   UNESCO's *Human Genetic Data: Preliminary Study by the IBC Draft Report on its Collection, Processing Treatment, Storage and Use of Genetic Data* 2002. The U.K. Human Genetics Commission ("HGC") has noted that getting consent for all future research uses of information collected through Biobank could be a tremendous challenge. The HGC concluded that "the difficulties involved in tracing and securing re-consent for different forms of medical research may make obtaining fresh consent impractical and would seriously limit the usefulness of large-scale population databases". See Human Genetics Commission, *Inside Information: Balancing Interests in the Use of Personal Genetic Data* (London: Human Genetics Commission, May 2002), online: <http://www.hgc.gov.uk/UploadDocs/Contents/Documents/iiintroduction.pdf>.

[70]   Graeme Laurie, "Genetic Databases: Assessing the Benefits and the Impact on Human and Patient Rights — A World Health Organisation Report" (2004) 11 European Journal of Health Law 79. It is worth noting that most research ethics norms do not allow the goals of science, no matter how laudable, to override individual rights. See, for example, the Helsinki Declaration where it is emphasized that "[i]n medical research on human subjects, considerations related to the well-being of the human subject should take precedence over the interests of science and society". World Medical Association, *The Revised Declaration of Helsinki: Interpreting and Implementing Ethical Principles in Biomedical Research* (Edinburgh: 52nd WMA General Assembly, 2000).

Icelandic approach is based on a model of presumed consent.[71] Individuals are considered to be participants unless they explicitly decline.[72] In the U.K., BioBank uses a form of "blanket consent" coupled with a robust governance structure that will carefully monitor the use of databank information.[73]

It is worth noting, however, that there have been protests and formal objections in virtually every jurisdiction that has established a large public biobanking project.[74] For example, in a recent case in Iceland, *Guomundsdottir v. Iceland*,[75] a woman challenged the constitutionality of the legal framework used to create the genetic databank. In the case, it was argued that the automatic inclusion of health information violated privacy rights in the Icelandic Constitution (in this situation, it was the health information of the plaintiff's deceased father). The Icelandic Supreme Court noted that the database contains highly private information and ruled "the legislature must ensure, *inter alia*, that legislation does not result in any actual risk of information ... involving the private affairs of identified persons falling into the hands of parties who do not have any legitimate right of access to such information ...".[76] The court concluded that the presumed consent approach to participation in the national health sector database was not necessarily unconstitutional, but the legislation must be amended to ensure a higher level of privacy protection.

---

[71] See Jon F. Merz *et al.*, "'Iceland Inc.'? On the Ethics of Commercial Population Genomics" (2004) 58 Social Science & Medicine 1201.

[72] However, see Anne Cambon-Thomsen, "The Social and Ethical Issues of Post-Genomic Human Biobanks" (2004) 5 Nature Reviews Genetics 866 at 868, where it is noted that over 20,000 Icelandic individuals have chosen to opt out.

[73] This is an approach that is being used in other projects. See, for example, Blair Smith *et al.*, "Generation Scotland: The Scottish Family Health Study; A New Resource for Researching Genes and Heritability" (2006) 7:74 BMC Medical Genetics 1. For a discussion of governance issues see Susan M.C. Gibbons *et al.*, "Governing Genetic Databases: Challenges Facing Research Regulation and Practice" (2007) 34 J.L. & Soc'y 163.

[74] See, for example, Melissa Austin *et al.*, "Genebank: A Comparison of Eight Proposed Genetic Databases" (2003) 6 Community Genetics 37. In Tonga, poor handling of consent issues was at least partially responsible for the termination of the population study. There has also been a degree of organized protest in Iceland and the United Kingdom. For example, Dr. Helen Wallace, the president of GeneWatch UK, has suggested that "Biobank would tear up [consent] rules and say: 'Give your sample to us and we'll decide how it's going to be used.'" P. Ghosh, "Will BioBank Pay Off?" *BBC News* (24 September 2003), online: <http://news.bbc.co.uk/go/pr/fr/-/2/hi/health/3134622.stm>.

[75] November 2003, Icelandic Supreme Court. A summary of the court decision, as well as an English translation of the ruling, is available at the website of the Association of Icelanders for Ethics in Science and Medicine, online: <http://www.mannvernd.is/english/lawsuits/Mannvernd_PressRelease_SupremeCourt.html>.

[76] *Ibid.*

In Canada, there is a complicated patchwork of provincial and federal privacy legislation and judge-made consent law that needs to be considered.[77] As such, it is difficult to predict how the existing Canadian legal environment might accommodate the consent issues created by large biobanking projects. At a minimum, it is safe to conclude that profound challenges remain. As noted above, the existing common law has long put an emphasis on individual autonomy and informed consent, though emerging health information legislation is altering some of the existing consent laws relevant to health information.[78] In addition, Canadians feel strongly about privacy issues and the protection of health information, especially genetic information. As such, there are reasons to believe that Canadian population genetic research projects have the potential to create legal controversies similar to those seen in other jurisdictions.

VI. EUGENICS, "RACE" AND PUBLIC HEALTH GENETICS

The misapplication of the science of genetics to justify state sponsored eugenic programs has, understandably, caused a degree of caution to be associated with any future use of genetic information in the context of public health. In the first half of the 20th century, numerous North American "state-mandated" eugenic programs led to the sterilization of thousands and the "wholesale stigmatization of numerous groups, resulting in, among other things, extremely restrictive immigration laws".[79]

In Alberta, for example, the *Sexual Sterilization Act* was passed in 1928, revised in 1937 and again in 1942.[80] This law was in force until 1972. During that time, nearly three thousand individuals, many of them children and adolescents, were sterilized.[81] There is little doubt that this law was motivated by the emerging science of genetics and a eugenic philosophy — that is, the hope that genetic information could be used to

---

[77]   See generally, Timothy Caulfield & Nola M. Ries, "Consent, Privacy and Confidentiality in Longitudinal, Population Health Research: The Canadian Legal Context" (2004) Health L. J. (Supp.) 1.

[78]   *Ibid.*

[79]   Ellen Wright Clayton, "Genetics, Public Health and the Law" in Muin Khoury *et al.*, eds., *Genetics and Public Health in the 21st Century* (New York: Oxford University Press, 2000) at 497-98.

[80]   See Timothy Caulfield & Gerald Robertson, "Eugenic Policies in Alberta: From the Systematic to the Systemic?" (1996) 35 Alta. L. Rev. 59; Alberta Institute of Law Research and Reform, *Sterilization Decisions: Minors and Mentally Incompetent Adults*, Report for Discussion No. 6 (Edmonton: Institute of Law Research and Reform, 1988); and Bernard Dickens, "Eugenic Recognition in Canadian Law" (1975) 13 Osgoode Hall L.J. 547.

[81]   Caulfield & Robertson, *ibid.*

improve the health of populations by stopping the birth of individuals who were potentially "genetically unfit".[82] Indeed, well-known individuals such as Emily Murphy and Louise McKinney supported both eugenics generally and the Alberta law specifically. Likewise, health care professions viewed the laws as a wise application of emerging scientific information. In 1934, the president of the University of Alberta, Dr. R.C. Wallace, gave an address in support of eugenics to the annual meeting of the Canadian Medical Association.[83]

Similar laws were passed throughout the United States. As demonstrated by the famous decision of the United States Supreme Court in *Buck v. Bell*,[84] eugenics was the dominant philosophy at play. In this case, the U.S. Supreme Court upheld the constitutional validity of the sterilization laws of Virginia, explicitly comparing sterilization with another public health initiative, compulsory vaccination. As Justice Holmes stated:[85]

> It is better for all the world, if instead of waiting to execute degenerate offspring for crime, or to let them starve for their imbecility, society can prevent those who are manifestly unfit from continuing their kind. The principle that sustains compulsory vaccination is broad enough to cover cutting the Fallopian tubes ... Three generations of imbeciles are enough.

Of course, the Nazi's use of eugenics to justify genocide has had the greatest impact on the development state mandated public health initiatives. The Nuremberg Code and the Declaration of Helsinki,[86] both of which emphasize the importance of individual autonomy in the area of health, were a direct result of the Nazi atrocities. Some commentators have noted that the gross misapplication of genetics in the World War II era has led contemporary health care providers to recoil from "the public health model that dominated the eugenic movement" to "adopted an almost absolute commitment to 'nondirectiveness' in their relations with

---

[82] Eugenics as a "science" was described by its founder, Sir Francis Galton, as: "The study of agenciesegis under social control that may improve or impair the racial qualities of future generations either physically or mentally." See F. Ledley, "Distinguishing Genetics and Eugenics on the Basis of Fairness" (1994) 20 Journal of Medical Ethics 157 at 158.

[83] R.C. Wallace, "The Quality of the Human Stock" (1934) 31 C.M.A.J. 427.

[84] 274 U.S. 200 (1927).

[85] *Ibid.*, at 207.

[86] See, the Nuremberg Code, from Trials of War Criminals before the Nuremberg Military Tribunals under Control Council Law No. 10. Nuremberg, October 1946–April 1949. Washington, D.C.: U.S. G.P.O, 1949–1953, online: <http://www.ushmm.org/research/doctors/Nuremberg_Code.htm>, article 1: "The voluntary consent of the human subject is absolutely essential." See also, World Medical Association, *The Revised Declaration of Helsinki: Interpreting and Implementing Ethical Principles in Biomedical Research* (Edinburgh: 52nd WMA General Assembly, 2000).

those seeking genetic services".[87] This means that decisions about whether to use a particular genetic testing service will be left to the informed individual patient and, in all likelihood, will rarely be "mandated" by the government.[88]

However, there remains concern that the application of genetics in public health will reinforce inappropriate notions of race and "genetic essentialism". Because public health genetics is more focused on populations than on individuals, there is concern that this approach will lead to a re-emphasis on superficial differences among identifiable populations.[89] As noted above, "race" has been used, typically disastrously,[90] as a blunt proxy for categorizing groups for the purposes of public health, such as in the case of sickle cell screening.[91] However, it is now recognized that relying on race is problematic on a number of levels. First, it seems to confuse the concepts of genetics and race.[92] Race is largely a social construct that often does not correspond with true genetic variation.[93] While there is no doubt that genes play a central role in superficial characteristics, such as skin and eye colour, there is much more

---

[87]   Allen Buchanan et al., "Two Models for Genetic Intervention" in Lawrence O. Gostin, ed., Public Health Law and Ethics: A Reader (Berkeley: University of California Press, 2002) at 482. The authors later note that most clinical geneticists "publicly endorse the view that genetic tests and interventions are simply services offered to individuals — goods for private consumption — to be accepted or refused as individuals see fit". Ibid.

[88]   This is not to say that screening programs, such as existing newborn screening programs, will not be implemented. However, it seems unlikely, at least in the short term, that governments will compel individuals to, for example, get a particular genetic test for the purpose of satisfying a public health goal.

[89]   See, for example, Ellen Wright Clayton, "Genetics, Public Health and the Law" in Muin Khoury et al., eds., Genetics and Public Health in the 21st Century (New York: Oxford University Press, 2000) at 497: "Some relatively well-defined ethnic groups, such as American Indians and Ashkenazi Jews, have also expressed concern that genetic research and testing will cause them to be perceived to be unusually unhealthy and, therefore, burdens onto society."

[90]   It must be noted that defining "race" is tremendously difficult. The term will mean different things to different people — and its meaning will change with perspective. For the purposes of this paper, I am largely referring to the broad, crude, social categories that have the most traction in the Western world: such as black, white and Asian. For a discussion of the challenges associated with defining race, see D. Fullwiley, "Race and Genetics: Attempts to Define the Relationship" (2007) 2 BioSocieties 221.

[91]   Troy Duster, Backdoor to Eugenics (New York: Routledge, 1990).

[92]   Neil Pearce et al., "Genetics, Race, Ethnicity and Health" (2004) 328 British Medical Journal 1070.

[93]   See, for example, K. Owens & M.C. King, "Genomic Views of Human History" (1999) 286 Science 451 at 453, who note that existing racial categories are not "consistent with genetic evidence".

genetic variation within socially defined "racial" groups than between them.[94]

Data from the Human Genome Project has often been used to buttress the idea that there is little genetic biological basis to the concept of race.[95] In short, genetic differences do not necessarily correspond to traditionally "racial" groups.[96]

Second, and most significantly, relying on race has the potential to reinforce existing social stereotypes. As we seek to use emerging genetic technologies to explore relationships between genetic variation and the health of populations we must guard against simplistic views of genetic variation. There is no doubt that certain sub-populations express a genetic similarity that may have relevance to population health policies.[97] And often, these sub-populations may fall within a broader socially constructed race category. For example, individuals of Chinese ancestry may have a gene that causes them to metabolize a drug differently from individuals with a particular European background. This does not mean, however, that all "Asians" and all "Caucasians" will respond the same way. Likewise, "categorical population identities (such as African or European) imply single origins and mutually exclusive distributions for genetic variants" that likely do not exist.[98] In other words, the use of existing categories of race usually confuse and inappropriately simplify a very complex biological situation.[99]

---

[94] See, for example, S.S-J. Lee, J. Mountain & B.A. Koenig, "The Meanings of 'Race' in the New Genomics: Implications for Health Disparities Research" (2001) 1 Yale J. Health Policy, L. & Ethics 1: 33 at 39 who declare that the "widely accepted consensus among evolutionary biologists and genetic anthropologists is that biologically identifiable human races do not exist". Neil Pearce et al., "Genetics, Race, Ethnicity and Health" (2004) 328 British Medical Journal 1070.

[95] Margaret Winker, "Measuring Race and Ethnicity: Why and How?" (2004) 292 JAMA 1612. M. Rothstein & P.G. Epps, "Pharmacogenomics and the (ir)relevance of race" (2001) 1 The Pharmacogenomics Journal 104 at 106.

[96] See Morris Foster & Richard Sharp, "Beyond Race: Towards a Whole-Genome Perspective on Human Populations and Genetic Variation" (2004) 5 Nature Reviews Genetics 790 at 790: "when used to define populations for genetic research, race has the potential to confuse by mistakenly implying biological explanations for socially and historically constructed health disparities".

[97] Valentine Burroughs, "The Importance of Individualizing Prescribing Among Genetically and Culturally Diverse Groups" (March 2003) Group Practice Journal 1.

[98] Morris Foster & Richard Sharp, "Beyond Race: Towards a Whole-Genome Perspective on Human Populations and Genetic Variation" (2004) 5 Nature Reviews Genetics 790 at 790.

[99] See ibid., at 795: "Human genetic variation and human social identity and ancestry are complex, multifaceted phenomena that promise great rewards when investigated in their entirety, but that have distinctive risks when one or both are reduced to less sophisticated typologies." See also Margaret Winker, "Measuring Race and Ethnicity: Why and How?" (2004) 292 JAMA 1612 at 1613: "Genetic similarity cannot be inferred simply based on

The concerns associated with the issues of race were recently highlighted by controversial statements made by James Watson, co-discover of the double-helix and Nobel laureate. Watson suggested that individuals of African descent are genetically predisposed to have inferior intelligence. The statements led to an immediate international reaction from the scientific community and, eventually, a retraction by Watson.[100]

In the end, we need to recognize that population genetic research is going to reveal subtle differences between groups that may be of importance to areas such as drug selection and susceptibility to certain diseases.[101] But the crude category of race is an increasingly archaic notion that is likely of marginal biological use or clinical value. Moreover, nnecessary and possibly inaccurate reference to socially constructed notions of race have the potential to re-enforce existing prejudices. In a recent study, Celeste Condit and colleagues found that "some messages linking race, genes, and health produce increases in racist attitudes in some audiences".[102] The authors provide the following caution:

> If these results are replicated, and if medical research eventually indicates that there are clinically useful differences in frequencies of conditions that have components that are strongly linked to particular genetic variations, the benefits of utilizing these tools will need to be weighed against the social harm of discussing them.[103]

Recognizing both the value of population research and the dangers inherent in the simplistic categorizing of human populations, a number of policy recommendations have emerged.[104] The recommendations highlight

racial categories ... socioeconomic status, not race, is likely the greater determinant of health and health-related qualities."

[100] M. Kahn, "Scientist Watson returns to U.S. over race row" Reuters (19 October 2007), online: <http://www.reuters.com/article/newsOne/idUSN1844930820071019?sp=true>. The marketing of the first "race based" drug, known as BiDil, serves as another example of the potential challenges associated with the use of race in this context. See, for example, P. Sankar & J. Kahn, "BiDil Race Medicine or Race Marketing" (2005) Health Affairs, Web Exclusive, W5-455. See also, Timothy Caulfield & Simrat Harry, "Popular Representations of Race: The News Coverage of BiDil" (2008) J.L. Med. & Ethics [accepted for publication].

[101] Timothy Caulfield, "Nutrigenomics, Popular Representations and the Reification of 'Race'" (2008) 16:3 Health Law Review 50.

[102] See, for example, Celeste Condit et al., "Exploration of the Impact of Messages about Genes and Race on Lay Attitudes" (2004) 66 Clinical Genetics 402, where the authors report on a study that shows the potential for public health statements that associated race with disease predisposition to reinforce notions of racism. They conclude that: "The presentation of such messages to the public is not recommended until additional research clarifies this finding and perhaps describes mitigating vocabularies or approaches." Ibid., at 402 [abstract].

[103] Ibid., at 407.

[104] See, for example, Timothy Caulfield, Stephanie M. Fullerton, Sarah E. Ali-Khan et al., "Race and Ancestry in Biomedical Research: Exploring the Challenges" (2008) Genome Medicine [forthcoming]; Race, Ethnicity and Genetics Working Group, "The Use of Racial,

the need to use the term race carefully, to justify its use and, when necessary, to use the term in a consistent and scientifically appropriate manner.

VII.   CONCLUSION

There are many other legal, ethical and policy challenges associated with the use of genetics in the context of public health that have not been covered in this chapter.[105] For example, it will be necessary to educate health care providers, particularly primary care physicians, with the basic knowledge necessary to provide the public with information about the role of genetics in health. Public education will also be needed. Indeed, some commentators have gone so far as to suggest that the "most important factor for determining whether genetics will enhance or impede public health goals is the extent to which the public is adequately informed about genetics".[106] Perhaps more vital, however, is to develop systems that allow for the ongoing and meaningful engagement of the public on the policy issues associated with public health genetics. Such an exercise would help inform policy development and build and maintain public trust, an essential element for any public health initiative.

This chapter has provided a brief overview of some of the central issues associated with public health genetics. Many of these issues are the result of the classic public health ethics conflict between individual rights and a desire to advance the public good. However, for a number of reasons, this tension may be especially problematic in the context of genetics, including the emerging essentialist view of genetics and the history of past misuses of genetic information.

Ethnic, and Ancestral Categories in Human Genetics Research (2005) 77 Am. J. Hum. Genet. 519; and F.P. Rivara & L. Finberg, "Use of the Terms Race and Ethnicity" (2001) 155 Arch. Pediatr. Adolesc. Med. 119.

[105] For instance, the potential role of genetics in improving global health was not addressed here, but for discussion, see e.g., Peter A. Singer & Abdallah S. Daar, "Harnessing Genomics and Biotechnology to Address Global Health Equity" (2001) 291 Science 87.

[106] Toby Citrin & Stephen Modell, "Genomics and Public Health: Ethical, Legal and Social Issues", Chapter 8, online: <http://www.cdc.gov/genomics/activities/ogdp/2003.htm> at 55.

INDEX